For over a decade *Pears Med... ...* guide to health and ailments i... ...unrivalled authority, and ser... ...admirable work for laymen.

The original work was compiled by Dr James Alexander Campbell Brown, M.B., B.Chir. (1911–1964), who, after studying medicine at Edinburgh and in several European countries, became a specialist in social psychiatry and psychology and was the author of several books, including *The Distressed Mind* (1946), *The Evolution of Society* (1947), *The Social Psychology of Industry* (1954), *Freud and the Post-Freudians* (1961) and *Techniques of Persuasion* (1963). Since it was first published in 1962 by Pelham Books, *Pears Medical Encyclopaedia* has been revised and updated several times to take account of new methods and techniques. The present edition has been thoroughly revised and largely rewritten by Dr Michael Hastin Bennett, M.A., M.B., B.Chir., F.R.C.S., a specialist in neuro-surgery as well as a family doctor and general surgeon.

In the course of the revision of the present edition, many entries have been expanded and a number of entirely new entries have been introduced, such as Cardiac Massage, Cell, Chromosomes, Defibrillation, Incisions, Ionizing Radiation, Kwashiorkor, L.S.D., Myelogram, Pacemaker, Plastic Surgery, Poisonous Plants, Thermography, Trachoma, Ultrasonics, Weights and Measures.

In this new edition *Pears Medical Encyclopaedia* is truly international, covering many tropical diseases and conditions, and providing advice for the world traveller. To allow for this internationalization a few words will be found cross-referred from their usual British spelling to an alternative and internationally accepted form: for example, Oedema and Oesophagus will be found under Edema, Esophagus; Haemophilia and Haemorrhage will be found under Hemophilia and Hemorrhage; Paediatrics under Pediatrics; and so on. Despite these changes in appearance, the aim of *Pears Medical Encyclopaedia* remains the same as that of the original edition: to encourage co-operation between doctor and patient, to present sensible articles about many controversial and taboo topics and to provide the individual or family with a valuable home reference to good health.

Pears Medical Encyclopaedia

J. A. C. BROWN, M.B., B.Chir.
Revised by A. M. HASTIN BENNETT,
M.A., F.R.C.S.

SPHERE BOOKS LIMITED

SPHERE BOOKS LTD

Published by the Penguin Group
27 Wrights Lane, London W8 5TZ, England
Viking Penguin Inc., 40 West 23rd Street, New York, New York 10010, USA
Penguin Books Australia Ltd, Ringwood, Victoria, Australia
Penguin Books Canada Ltd, 2801 John Street, Markham, Ontario, Canada L3R 1B4
Penguin Books (NZ) Ltd, 182–190 Wairau Road, Auckland 10, New Zealand

Penguin Books Ltd, Registered Offices: Harmondsworth, Middlesex, England

First published in Great Britain by Pelham Books Ltd in association with
Rainbow Reference Books 1971
Published by Sphere Books 1977
Reprinted 1977, 1979, 1981, 1983, 1986, 1988

The modern translation of the Hippocratic Oath is reproduced from
The Doctor's Oath by W. H. S. Jones, with the permission of
Cambridge University Press

Printed and bound in Great Britain by
Cox & Wyman Ltd, Reading
Set in Monotype Baskerville

Introduction

This book is designed for the layman, assuming no medical knowledge on his part, but since its aim is to be scientific, and, within the limits imposed by space, reasonably detailed, it may also prove useful to nurses and others who wish to refresh their memories or refer to something outside their own immediate field. It has been written in the belief that so far as possible all knowledge should be available to anyone who seeks it and that in the particular case of medical information those who feel that it can be harmful are wrong because the choice is no longer between some knowledge or none at all but between correct and incorrect information. With an increasingly educated population learning daily about medical matters from newspapers, radio and television, it is impossible to keep people in the dark. Every family doctor knows that rumour and old wives' tales flourish where the truth is withheld.

The *Encyclopaedia* cannot take the place of a doctor's opinion and care. The experienced physician never seeks to heal himself. How much less should a layman, relying not on a lifetime's skill and knowledge but on the pages of a small book, try to diagnose and treat his own illness. No book can be a substitute for the doctor, for diagnosis and treatment are not mechanical matters but depend in part upon the doctor's estimate of his patient's total condition, including his character and personality.

It follows that the patient must always be frank with the doctor, answering all his questions carefully although they may not at first seem to be relevant. There must be no false modesty about any sort of examination that may be required. Conversely, the doctor must be worthy of his patient's trust, and answer his questions truthfully. If the patient wants a second opinion he should ask his family doctor to arrange the consultation. It is not wise for a patient to go directly to a specialist, because symptoms are often misleading and it is easy to choose the wrong specialist. If a patient does not trust his family doctor he must change to another.

A layman should never believe what he hears from non-medical sources, and he should never give medical advice to others. Nevertheless, there is every reason why we should all try to understand something of what goes on inside our bodies. It is the aim of this *Encyclopaedia* to help the layman to co-operate with his family doctor in dealing with the every-day problems of health and disease by providing him with an accurate source of general medical information.

A

Abdomen: that part of the trunk between the thorax (chest) and the pelvis. It is separated from the thorax by a muscular partition called the diaphragm, but is continuous below with the cavity of the pelvis. It is well protected behind by the bone of the vertebral column and the lower ribs, but is vulnerable in front and at the sides where the abdominal contents are covered only by muscular layers – the transverse, internal and external oblique muscles at the sides, and the vertical rectus abdominis muscle in the mid-line. The structures which make up the abdominal wall are skin, fat of varying thickness, muscle, another layer of fat, and the thin slippery membrane called the peritoneum which lines the abdominal cavity. The peritoneum, which is rather like wet cellophane, covers all the internal organs in the abdominal cavity. The principal contents of the abdominal cavity are the organs of the digestive system: the stomach, small and large intestine with the appendix and caecum, and the liver and pancreas. The end of the intestine, the rectum, lies in the pelvis. The kidneys lie at the back of the abdomen up under the lower ribs at each side of the spinal column. Tubes called ureters run down the back wall of the abdomen from the kidneys to the bladder, which is in the pelvis. On the left side, under the diaphragm, lies the spleen, corresponding roughly in position to the liver on the right. The liver is much larger than the spleen, which is pushed back and up by the stomach. At the back, running down along the spinal column, are the abdominal aorta and vena cava, the biggest artery and vein in the body, and on each side of the spinal vertebrae runs the abdominal autonomic nervous system with its chain of ganglia. The prostate gland in the male and the uterus, ovaries and Fallopian tubes in the female are in the pelvis below the abdominal cavity. Diseases of the abdomen and pelvis are dealt with under the various systems affected or under their commonly known names.

Abdominal Injuries: although the front of the abdomen is relatively unprotected (*see* above) serious abdominal injuries affecting the internal organs are fairly uncommon in civilian life. They occur most often in car accidents, crushing accidents and falls from a height, when the liver or spleen may be ruptured. If a large blood vessel is torn the bleeding may be so severe that the patient dies before operation is possible. Leakage from the stomach or intestines is most likely to follow a penetrating wound of the abdomen, and in these cases antibiotics and operation are urgently needed to avoid the spread of peritonitis. The kidneys are sometimes injured by a blow in the back, and in these cases the urine is stained with blood. If the condition does not improve, or is very severe, operation on the kidney may be needed. In the interval between the injury and the arrival of skilled help, the patient should be kept still and should be moved as little as possible.

Abortion: the death and expulsion of the foetus before the 28th week of pregnancy. It may be accidental (natural) or procured, and procured abortions may be lawful or criminal. By the Abortion Act of 1967 in Great Britain abortion may be procured legally under the following circumstances:
1. Two registered medical practitioners must be of the opinion, formed in good faith, (a) that the risk of the continuation of the pregnancy to the life of the mother, or the risk of injury to the mental and physical health of the mother or any existing children of the family, is greater than the risk of terminating the pregnancy, (b) that there is a substantial risk that if the child were born it would suffer from such mental or physical abnormalities as to be seriously handicapped.
2. In forming the opinion on the risk of injury to health account may be taken of the woman's actual or foreseeable environment.
3. Treatment for the termination of pregnancy must be carried out in a National Health Service Hospital or in a place approved for the purpose by the Minister of Health.
A woman who endeavours to procure an abortion on herself does not commit any offence, but if she allows anyone else to try to procure an abortion on her she is guilty of an offence. If death results from criminal abortion the offence is manslaughter if the operator was skilled, but the charge is murder if the abortionist was unskilled.

In the U.S.A., since laws concerning abortion differ from state to state, it is advisable to consult one's own doctor or the County Medical Society for accurate information.

Abrasion: an abrasion is an area from which the surface layer of the skin has been rubbed, for example by contact with a rough surface, as when a boy falls off his bicycle and his knee hits the road. When a very large area is affected it is obviously best to consult a doctor, but a minor abrasion may be dealt with by careful washing with soap and water to clear away any foreign matter. The abrasion will heal most quickly if it is left open to the air without a dressing, but a dressing will keep it from being rubbed by clothes. A piece of porous adhesive tape with antiseptic gauze dressing attached is convenient; if it becomes dirty it should be changed, but the less interference the better. If the abrasion is badly contaminated with soil it is wise to go to the doctor immediately for an injection against tetanus (q.v.).

Abreaction: a technique in psychiatry. The doctor brings to the patient's conscious attention details of an incident partially or completely suppressed in the memory. This process can often be made easier by the use of a very light anaesthetic; just enough pentothal or ether is used to produce drowsiness. During abreaction the patient may become very excited, for he feels again the strong emotion which caused him to suppress the memory in the first place.

Abscess: an abscess forms in the tissues as the result of irritation, usually because of bacterial infection. Increased blood flow leads to effusion of fluid into the tissue spaces and the collection of a great number of white blood corpuscles. The area of infection becomes cut off from the healthy tissue; and in time the dead white blood cells, bacteria, and exuded fluid form pus. The earliest outward sign of abscess formation on the surface of the body is an area of redness which is hard and painful to the touch. As the abscess becomes localized and pus forms so the area of redness becomes sharply defined, and its centre starts to soften. Usually the pus tracks towards the area of least resistance, which in the case of a surface abscess or boil is the surface of the body, and points.

9

Eventually the abscess will burst and discharge, but much pain and illness can often be avoided if it is lanced or incised as soon as it has localized and pus has formed. It is worse than useless to stick a knife into an abscess, or a needle into a pimple, before the pus has formed and the inflammation has become localized, since this spreads the infection. Two courses of action are possible – to diminish the infection by the use of antibiotics, and to help increase the local flow of blood by keeping the part warm and at rest. Poultices are often used to apply local heat but their effect only lasts for a short while, and they are likely to make the area soggy. It is sensible to ask for skilled advice on the treatment of all but the smallest abscesses. When the abscess discharges it will heal quickly, providing the drainage is free and the part is prevented from becoming soggy. Use plain dry dressings to cover the discharging abscess, and change the dressing often. Abscesses on the skin are caused by infection entering through a small cut or abrasion, or through the small lubricating glands of the skin and the hair follicles (see Skin). Internal abscesses can be caused by the entry of a foreign body, as in the case of knife or bullet wounds, or, in the lungs, by accidental inhalation of food or a tooth. Other internal abscesses are caused by the spread of local infections, as in a burst appendix which causes a pelvic abscess, or the spread of infection from the middle ear into the brain. Abscesses of the liver in amoebic dysentery and the 'cold' abscesses of tuberculosis are different in nature and are described under the diseases producing them. See Inflammation.

Acarus: a genus of very small creatures called mites which often live as parasites on the external surface of larger animals. They cause various skin diseases such as itch and mange. See Mites.

Accidents: the number of people killed on the roads of Great Britain during 1968 was 6,810, and there were 88,563 serious injuries. The corresponding figures for the U.S.A. during 1969 were 56,400 killed and 2,000,000 injured. In Great Britain the number of people killed in accidents in and about their homes was 7,561, and 120,000 were seriously injured, and in the U.S.A. 27,000 were killed by domestic accidents and 4,100,000 seriously injured – remarkable figures which show that in Great Britain more people were killed by domestic accidents than by accidents on the roads. Analysis of the British figures by the Royal Society for the Prevention of Accidents reveals that 68% of the victims of home accidents were aged 65 or over, and that a further 13% were under 5 years of age. The common causes of death in the home are falls, poisoning, burns and scalds, suffocation and choking.

The Royal Society for the Prevention of Accidents lists these causes of road accidents as the most common:

1. Speed too fast for the conditions.
2. Overtaking improperly.
3. Turning without due care.
4. Misjudging speed, distance or intended direction of movement.
5. Loss of control (for example, skidding).
6. Vehicle defects such as faulty tyres or brakes.
7. Vehicles crossing carelessly at junctions.
8. Alcohol or drugs.
9. Lack of experience.
10. Jay-walking by pedestrians, or thoughtless misuse of the roads.

Although none of us believe that we commit these faults in our driving, it is quite clear that it is sensible to wear seat belts designed to stop the body coming into contact with hard pieces of machinery in an accident. A simple strap across the lap is not satisfactory, for the body can jack-knife in an impact; moreover it has been found that restraint applied over the abdomen can in a severe impact result in rupture of the liver or spleen, or damage to other internal organs. It is therefore important that the harness should keep the upper part of the body as well as the hips from coming forwards. A great deal of thought is going into the design of motor cars to try to lessen the effects of accidents, but it is obvious that once a man ventures outside his natural 'envelope of performance' or his natural environment he is running a risk; if he hits something at a speed greater than he can run, if he falls from a height greater than he can jump, if he tries to venture into reduced or increased atmospheric pressure, indeed if he stays under water longer than he can hold his breath, sooner or later he is going to have an accident.

Accommodation: the lens of the eye is made of elastic tissue so that its shape can be altered by the contraction of the ciliary muscle which surrounds it. When the ring of muscle contracts or relaxes, the lens alters shape, becoming more or less convex. The result is like focusing the lens of a camera or a telescope – images of things at varying distances are made sharp. The process is called accommodation. As we get older, so the lens loses its elasticity and accommodation becomes less easy. *See* Eye.

Acetic Acid: the essential principle of vinegar, which is produced from the fermentation of wine or malt. Commercial acetic acid is derived from the distillation of wood with subsequent separation from tar. In its pure form it is solid and is called glacial acetic acid. It is used in medicine for destroying warts. Ordinary vinegar was once used as a cooling toilet preparation and in the proportion of two or three tablespoons to a quart of water it may be used to sponge patients suffering from the sweats of fever, from which it gives pleasant if temporary relief. Headaches may be helped by a cold vinegar compress applied to the forehead. A dilute preparation of vinegar and water may be used for cleansing vaginal douches.

Acetone: a substance found in the urine primarily in severe cases of diabetes, sometimes in chronic wasting diseases such as cancer, and after prolonged vomiting. It has a distinctive smell which can often be detected in the breath of those in diabetic coma. *See* Diabetes.

Acetylcholine: a substance normally found in many parts of the body. It is used in the transmission of nervous impulses between nerve fibres and the muscles and in the workings of the parasympathetic nervous system (*see* Nervous System). Normally it is broken down in the body by the substance cholinesterase. If the amount of cholinesterase in the blood is lowered, for example by exposure to phosphorus insecticides, the effect is to increase the amount of circulating acetylcholine and therefore to produce too much stimulation of the parasympathetic nervous sytem. The action of the heart is slowed down, the muscles become weak, and the patient suffers from nausea, giddiness, headache, and disturbance of sight (the pupils of the eyes become small).

If the condition is not relieved by the injection of atropine, which counteracts the excess of acetylcholine, the patient develops colic and more severe symptoms which eventually end in convulsions and coma.

Acetylsalicylic Acid: *see* Aspirin.

Achalasia: the term means 'no relaxation' and is applied to a condition of the oesophagus in which the mechanism of swallowing is disturbed. Food normally stimulates the muscle of the wall of the gullet to begin a series of contractions which pass food towards the stomach in waves. Where achalasia is present this does not happen, nor does the muscle surrounding the opening to the stomach relax to allow food to pass from the oesophagus to the stomach. The muscle only opens when the column of food which builds up in the oesophagus is heavy enough to force its way through, which occurs when the column is about 20 cm high. The patient is troubled by discomfort rather than pain, and complains of food sticking in his throat. Young people of both sexes are affected, and treatment is surgical.

Achilles Tendon: according to Greek myth, Achilles' mother dipped her son into the river Styx to make him invulnerable. She held him by the back of the ankle – and the heel was the only part of the hero which remained dry. Not until he was struck in the heel could he be wounded: it was his only weak point. The tendon, which runs from the great muscles of the calf to the calcaneum, the bone which forms the heel, draws the foot downwards about the hinge of the ankle. It is the tendon we use to stand on tip-toe. The Achilles tendon becomes the weak point of some athletes as they get older, and if it is suddenly put under great strain it is liable to rupture.

Achlorhydria: this means an absence of the normal hydrochloric acid in the gastric juice. It is found in 4–5% of normal people, in whom it leads to no ill effects, but it is the rule in cancer of the stomach, pernicious anaemia, and often in chronic gastritis.

Achondroplasia: this is a form of dwarfism which is inherited, of unknown cause, and unalterable. The trunk is of normal size while the arms and legs are abnormally short and the head relatively large. Most of the dwarfs seen in circuses are of this type; the less frequently seen dwarf of the 'Tom Thumb' type who has perfectly proportioned limbs and body is suffering from a defect of the pituitary gland (q.v.) resulting in a deficiency of the growth hormone.

Acidity and Acidosis: two much misused terms, the former when employed in a general sense meaning nothing at all, the latter referring to a condition which occurs in such serious illnesses that it cannot be what people ordinarily mean when they make use of the word. In fact, the blood is always alkaline, so that even in the proper use of the word acidosis, all that is meant is that the blood is less alkaline than it should be. Examples of acidosis are found in diabetic coma or starvation where the metabolism is grossly disordered, or in failure of the kidneys or the process of respiration. In these conditions the appearance of acidosis is of grave significance. 'Acidity' is used sometimes to signify excess of acid thought to be the cause of pain in the stomach, which can be relieved by taking mildly alkaline medicines or drinking milk, but as a diagnosis it leaves a lot to be desired.

Acne: a chronic skin disease affecting the sebaceous (i.e. fat or grease) glands on the face, shoulders, back and chest. It occurs most often in people between the ages of 14 and 20, and the typical 'blackheads' and pimples cause a good deal of embarrassment at an age when people tend to be particularly sensitive about personal appearance. A plug forms in the canal through which the sebaceous gland normally discharges its secretion to the surface of the skin, and the top of the plug becomes black and hard. Sometimes the gland goes on secreting although the canal is blocked, and a cyst forms containing the glandular secretion. The sebaceous plug contains vast numbers of acne bacilli, but sometimes the blocked gland becomes infected with other bacilli and pus is formed. The medical name for a blackhead is 'comedo'; comedones are found not only in the acne of puberty but also as a result of exposure to oil and grease. They may also form when susceptible patients are given

14

bromides or iodides by mouth, and when workers in industry are exposed to some compounds containing chlorine.

TREATMENT: in the first place this must be aimed at dealing with the fundamental state, which is the greasy condition of the skin and scalp; the hair should be shampooed at least twice a week, preferably with a non-soapy medicated hair-wash, and the face washed frequently with soap and water. The blackheads may be squeezed out either with clean hands or with a special comedo expressor obtainable at chemist's shops, but when they are inflamed, large or have no 'head' they are best left alone since squeezing will only worsen the condition and tend to spread the infection. Lotions can be used providing they are not greasy; the best contain sulphur. Further treatment is possible in obstinate cases, but this is a matter for a skin specialist. Diet is not regarded as being as important as once it was, but it is probably best to cut down on carbohydrates such as sweets or cakes. The acne of puberty normally disappears spontaneously.

Acne Rosacea: more often known as rosacea, and formerly described as 'grog-blossom', this condition of the skin of the face is primarily dependent upon changes in the small blood vessels of the skin. These become enlarged and the result is a red, greasy and coarsened area shaped like a butterfly spreading across the nose and extending out over both cheeks. Associated with this may be chronic dyspepsia or gastritis, and in some cases a meal, hot drink or alcohol will make the butterfly area flush. The name 'grog-blossom' arose from the belief that rosacea was invariably associated with chronic indulgence in alcohol; but this is less than kind to the commonest type of sufferer who is a middle-aged lady of blameless habits except, perhaps, for addiction to frequent cups of strong tea. It is true that in former times such people as coachmen who were exposed both to the elements and to the temptation of frequent noggins of hot rum tended to develop red noses and cheeks, but the alcoholic of today is no more likely to bear such stigmata than is the teetotaller, for it is associated with anything that leads to frequent flushing of the blood vessels of the face – prolonged exposure to harsh weather, the change of life in women, hot foods such as curries, and hot and irritant drinks which produce gastritis when carried to excess, such as strong and stewed tea.

Treatment obviously includes the cure of the underlying gastritis and in women the correction of any glandular irregularity. Much can be done to improve the appearance by the use of cosmetic preparations which mask the discoloration.

Acoustic Nerve Tumour: the acoustic nerve is one of the cranial nerves (q.v.); it connects the brain with the ear. Upon it there may rarely form a fibrous tissue tumour which as it grows presses upon the brain stem and on the other cranial nerves which originate there, for on one side of the tumour is the hard temporal bone which contains the inner ear and upon the other side the relatively soft brain tissue. Giddiness, double vision, deafness, weakness of one side of the face, and various other signs point to the presence of an acoustic nerve tumour. The only treatment is removal; the operation is for the specialist, and bearing in mind the situation of the tumour, the results are satisfactory.

Acriflavine: a powerful yellow antiseptic derived from aniline and used either in liquid solution (1 in 1,000 of water), in liquid paraffin, or as a cream for dressing wounds. Like iodine and other old antiseptics, it is being replaced by more modern preparations which do not stain the skin and are less irritating to healing tissues.

Acrocyanosis: a condition found especially in young women in which there is coldness and blue discoloration of the skin of the hands and feet, spreading sometimes to the nose and ears. The underlying cause is an undue sensitivity to cold on the part of the small blood vessels of the affected parts, and treatment other than physical exercise and wearing protective clothes is not likely to be effective. *See* Raynaud's Disease.

Acromegaly: a state produced by overactivity of the front part of the pituitary gland (q.v.) at the base of the brain. When this begins in early life before the bones have stopped growing increased height or gigantism results, and the patient develops a prominent forehead and cheek-bones, a large lower jaw, long arms with big hands, big feet, and a tendency to stoop. When the disease begins later in life, an enlargement of the face bones, hands and feet, a bent back and general coarsening of the expression without gigantism result, with a hollow deep voice. Other symptoms such as disorders of vision or sexual impotence may be present. Although the appearance of the acromegalic patient suggests great strength, the reverse may well be true, especially as the disease progresses.

TREATMENT: acromegaly always calls for skilled treatment, which in severe cases may necessitate an operation on the pituitary gland. Diabetes insipidus (*see* Diabetes) is sometimes associated with acromegaly. *See* Gigantism.

Acromion: the point of the shoulder, formed by the outermost part of the spine of the scapula or shoulder-blade.

A.C.T.H.: the abbreviation for adrenocorticotrophic hormone, or corticotrophin, a secretion of the pituitary gland which has the function of stimulating the adrenal gland cortex, causing among other things the production of more cortisone. A.C.T.H. was first isolated in 1933, but was not used to any extent in medicine until 1949. It appeared to be useful in rheumatoid arthritis, but its promise was not fulfilled, and it is now rarely used. *See* Corticosteroids, Pituitary Gland.

Actinomycosis: a chronic disease caused by the 'ray fungus', Actinomyces israeli in man, and Actinomyces bovis in cattle. Infection ordinarily takes place through the mouth, and there is often a history of injury, removal of a tooth, or operation for tonsillitis. The face and neck are commonly affected. A swelling appears at the angle of the jaw, which ultimately discharges pus both into the mouth and outwardly. The infection may spread into the chest, the intestine or the liver.

Diagnosis depends on expert bacteriological investigation; the outlook has changed since the introduction of penicillin, which is used in massive doses for some weeks. Occasionally the fungus is found to be resistant to penicillin, but it is sensitive to other antibiotics, notably tetracycline. The disease in humans is caused by a different organism from

17

that which produces 'lumpy jaw' or 'wooden tongue' in cattle.

Acupuncture: a method of treatment with no known scientific basis, used for the relief of various pains and diseases according to the credulity of the operator. It consists of inserting needles 2–3 in long either into the parts affected, or the parts which, rightly or wrongly, are supposed to influence them. Acupuncture is still practised in the West, where it is sometimes thought that the principle of counter-irritation furnishes some explanation for its survival, but it originated in China centuries ago where it was believed that by such an operation the harmful vapours which allegedly gave rise to certain disorders could be released from the body.

Acute: in medicine, any process which has a sudden onset and runs a relatively severe and short course is called acute. The opposite is 'chronic'.

Acute Abdomen: the patient who is suffering from acute abdominal (or pelvic) pain of sudden onset is said to have 'an acute abdomen'. Such cases include appendicitis, per-forated ulcers, and acute inflammation of the gall-bladder. There is an old rule which says that an acute abdomen which does not get better in 6 hours is a surgical case; and it is a good rule to call a doctor about any abdominal pain which does not improve in a few hours. In the more severe cases, it becomes obvious that professional help is needed immedi-ately. Until medical help arrives, the patient should be kept as still as possible, and given only enough water to keep his mouth moist. Laxatives should not be given in cases of abdominal pain.

Adaptation: the process by which the eye is able to adjust to varying intensities of light. If we come into a shaded room from the bright sunshine, at first everything seems dark, but after a few minutes the light is perfectly adequate. Similarly, the photographer waits to develop his film in the dark room until his eyes have adapted to the dark and he can see some-thing of what he is doing. The same photographer has probably found out by experience what an enormous range of adaptation the human eye enjoys; he knows that he has to use an exposure meter to set his camera because film has nothing like the flexibility of the eye, which is in consequence a bad judge of light. Adaptation has to do with the amount of visual purple (*see* Rhodopsin) in the retina; in dark adaptation, there is an increase, whereas exposure to bright light decreases the amount of visual purple. The formation of visual purple depends on adequate supplies of Vitamin A, and lack of this vitamin in the diet leads to night blindness.

Addison's Disease: a disease first described by Dr Thomas Addison in 1849 (the year in which he also described pernicious anaemia). Born in England near Newcastle upon Tyne and educated at Edinburgh University, Addison became a famous physician at Guy's Hospital in London. His account of the disease which he correctly attributed to destruction of the suprarenal glands (q.v.) is still valid: 'Anaemia, general languor or debility, remarkable feebleness of the heart's action, irritability of the stomach, and a peculiar change of colour in the skin.' The discoloration begins first on exposed areas – the face and hands – and ranges from yellow to dark brown or even black as it spreads over the rest of the body. Extreme weakness on slight exertion, fainting attacks or giddiness and noises in the ears due to low blood pressure, palpitations, nausea with or without actual vomiting, and sometimes diarrhoea, complete the picture.

CAUSE: destruction of the suprarenal glands may be due to tuberculous infection, growths, or haemorrhage and leads to loss of their hormones which are necessary to life, for among other things they maintain the blood pressure and the contractility of the muscles. Addison's disease is rare in childhood or old age, being most common during the twenties and thirties.

TREATMENT: until the introduction of cortisone the only treatment was large doses of common salt which delayed its ultimate fatal conclusion. Today, however, the administration of the missing hormones by mouth or by injection enables most patients to lead a normal and healthy life. Since this is a form of substitution therapy, like the use of insulin in diabetes, it has to be continued permanently.

Adenitis: inflammation of a gland. Usually applied to inflammation of the lymphatic glands. *See* Glands.

Adenofibroma: a tumour composed of connective tissue with glandular elements. *See* Breast Diseases (benign tumours).

Adenoids: swellings formed by the overgrowth of lymphatic glandular tissue at the back of the nose in children, which obstruct the free passage of air through the nose and lead to mouth breathing. In severe cases the adenoids may cover the openings of the Eustachian tubes, and the child suffers from impairment of hearing and an increased liability to infection of the middle ear, as well as recurrent colds, chronic tonsillitis and bronchitis. Treatment may have to be surgical, but removal of the tonsils and adenoids is not advised as often as it used to be.

Adenoma: a tumour, usually benign, composed of glandular tissue, for example a pituitary adenoma or thyroid adenoma. A benign tumour in contrast to a malignant one does not spread throughout the body but remains confined to its place of origin. It is not a cancer.

Adhesions: many structures in the body are normally separated by tissues which are free to move over each other: the lung is separated from the chest wall by the pleural membrane; the inside of the joints is covered by a slippery synovial membrane; and the abdominal organs move over each other easily because they are covered by the peritoneal membrane. Sometimes these membranes become inflamed, often because of disease in the organs they cover, and in the course of inflammation and recovery, fibrous tissue sticks the formerly slippery membranes together and adhesions are the result. Adhesions in the joints lead to limitation of movement and are treated by physiotherapy, but adhesions in the abdomen can lead to obstruction of the gut or twisting of the bowel. If the condition is severe enough surgical operation may be unavoidable, although this in its turn is liable to lead to further adhesions. *See* Obstruction.

Adipometer: an instrument for measuring the thickness of a fold of skin, so that some indication can be gained of the progress of a reducing, or, on occasion, a fattening diet.

Adiposis: an abnormal accumulation of fatty tissue in the body. A form of adiposis found in women is adiposis dolorosa, a disease in which painful fatty swellings form in association with defects in the nervous system.

Adolescence: the period of life beginning with the first development of the secondary sexual characteristics and ending with the cessation of bodily growth. It is the time during which a child matures into an adult. Rapid physiological changes may produce difficulties in psychological development, making for turbulence.

Adrenal Glands: over the upper part of each kidney lies an adrenal gland, weighing about 5 g and coloured yellow. It has a cortex and a medulla, the medulla being derived during development from nervous tissue and the cortex from mesoderm, like the gonads. The gland has a capsule separate from that of the kidney and takes its blood supply from the aorta, renal artery and the arteries running to the diaphragm. The functions of the medulla and cortex are quite separate. The *medulla* secretes the hormones adrenaline and noradrenaline, which are together referred to as the catecholamines; their action was in 1916 described by Cannon as preparation for 'fright, flight or fight'. The modern physiologist tends to say that hormones are released in 'stress situations'. *See* Adrenaline.
The *cortex* of the gland, derived from the same type of tissue as the sex glands, secretes the corticosteroid hormones, and the secretion of these hormones is also strongly influenced by stress situations. *See* Corticosteroids.

Adrenaline: a hormone secreted by the medulla, or central part, of the adrenal glands. Its function in nature is to prepare the body for emergency action, and its effect is to speed up the pulse, divert the blood from the guts and skin to the muscles, and transform glycogen in the liver into glucose, an immediate source of energy. It also dilates the pupils of the eyes, and the bronchi or breathing-tubes in the lungs. Adrenaline was first prepared by Takamine in 1901 from the adrenal glands of animals, but it is now produced synthetically. It is given for asthmatic attacks, as a heart stimulant, or to diabetics suffering from an overdose of insulin; it is combined with local anaesthetic, especially in dentistry, to control bleeding. Adrenaline cream is sometimes used as a treatment for fibrositis, but whether it has any effect in this condition is very much a matter of opinion.

Aerophagy: the neurotic habit of swallowing air, usually unconsciously, which is the cause of gastric flatulence and 'wind'. It may be cured by carrying a cork between the teeth.

Aerosol: a suspension of very finely divided liquid or solid particles in a gas. In medicine aerosols are generally used (a) for destroying insects such as fleas and mosquitoes which carry disease, (b) for 'purifying' the air, (c) for combating disease caused by droplet infection in public places, and (d) for inhalation by patients with diseases of the lungs.

The method of delivery may be a hand-operated spray or nebulizer, a specially designed inhaler, or the common pressurized container. Aerosols are very effective against insects, but those sold to purify the air of a room should be regarded with reserve, for stale air can only be made fresh by ventilation. Antiseptics delivered into the air by a spray are certainly capable of killing germs in a bottle, but whether they remain suspended in the air long enough to be effective in preventing droplet infection from people coughing and spluttering at close range is quite another matter. In a crowded place spraying in order to be effective would have to be carried out so frequently that many would prefer the risk of infection. Aerosols used to relieve spasm of the air passages in the lungs, which are constricted in asthma, contain adrenaline, atropine methonitrite, isoprenaline, or orciprenoline. The introduction of these aerosols has transformed the lives of many patients with asthma, but it is important for the patient to follow instructions with great care; these are powerful drugs and it is easy to take an overdose.

Afterbirth: placenta and membranes expelled in the third stage of labour. *See* Placenta, Labour.

Agar: sometimes known as 'agar-agar', this is a vegetable jelly made from seaweed, used to make soups and jellies, particularly in the East, although its commercial applications have also been thoroughly exploited in the West. Before World War 2, most agar came from Japan, but it is now made in the U.S.A. and in the Commonwealth. In medicine, agar is used by bacteriologists to make bacterial culture media of broth or blood more solid. It can be given as a medicine, either by itself or in combination with other ingredients. Its most common use is in constipation because it absorbs water in the bowel and makes the bowel movement more fluid.

Age: *see* Geriatrics.

Agglutination: the clumping together of small bodies in a fluid suspension. This happens to blood corpuscles when they are brought into contact with the serum of an incompatible blood group, or bacteria exposed to the serum of a person or animal which has developed an immunity against them. The former reaction is important in testing the compatibility of blood groups (q.v.) prior to blood transfusion, and the latter is used in bacteriology, for example in the Widal reaction for typhoid fever, when the addition of a patient's serum to typhoid germs in solution produces agglutination if the disease is typhoid, but fails to do so if it is not.

Agoraphobia: an uncontrollable sensation of fear at the thought of being alone in a large open space. It may lead to panic at the thought of crossing the street. *See* Claustrophobia, Agromania.

Agranulocytosis: a serious but not very common blood disease in which ulceration of the throat and mouth is accompanied by a diminution in the number of granulocytes (one type of white blood cell), initially in the bone marrow where they are produced and subsequently in the bloodstream.

The commonest cause of agranulocytosis is hypersensitivity to drugs, such as the tranquillizer chlorpromazine (Thorazine), the antibiotic chloramphenicol, certain sulphonamides, or thiouracil, a drug used in the treatment of thyroid disease. Such drugs must be used with considerable caution, although it is not sensible to give them up entirely as they are valuable in many cases and can usually be used with perfect safety. One drug that used to cause agranulocytosis is amidopyrine, which was used in place of, or combined with aspirin; the use of this drug has been almost entirely abandoned. Agranulocytosis may occur in a variety of different diseases, such as glandular fever, severe septicaemia, acute leukaemia, chronic suppurative conditions, malaria and kala-azar. It may also occur after over-exposure to radiation.

Agromania: the opposite condition to agoraphobia – an abnormal desire to be alone, to wander about in open fields.

Ague: a vague and now outdated term for malaria or other fevers confused with malaria.

Ainhum: this condition is found mainly in Negroes in tropical countries. A constriction appears in the skin of a toe, commonly the little toe, running round the affected part so that as the contraction gets worse the blood supply is progressively diminished. The toe eventually falls off.

Air Encephalography: *see* Encephalography.

Airsickness: *see* Motion Sickness.

Air Travel: if anyone has any doubt about his fitness to travel by air he must ask for a doctor's advice. The number of people who should not fly as airline passengers is very small; active tuberculosis is a bar to flying, and so is a recent history of coronary thrombosis, or the presence of severe anaemia.

Patients should not fly in the first two weeks after an abdominal operation, nor after a recent operation on the eyeball, nor, obviously, if they are suffering from infective or contagious disease. Epileptics and diabetics will take care that their condition is well controlled and those with severe colds or hay fever are advised to take some decongestant preparation with them, for the mild variation of air pressure inseparable from flying may result in a painful blockage of the ear or sinus.

Airway: in medical use, airway means the path by which the air enters and leaves the lungs – the mouth, throat, trachea or windpipe, and the air passages of the lungs themselves. In anaesthetics, the term is transferred to mean a device for ensuring the free and unobstructed passage of air in and out of the lungs. It is as important in an accident case to make sure that the airway is clear, and is kept clear, as it is to stop bleeding. The easiest way of doing this is to turn the patient over on to his side or on to his face with his head to one side; he cannot then swallow his tongue, and the secretions or vomit will run out of his mouth and not down into his lungs.

Albinism: a condition in which the individual, called an albino, shows an inherited lack of pigment in the skin, hair and eyes. In complete albinism, the skin of the whole body is pale pink, the hair white, and the iris of the eye colourless. The eyes look pink, because the colour of the blood in the vessels of the back of the eye shows through the transparent retina and iris. Too much light is able to enter the eyes of albinos, and they have to wear dark glasses in order to protect them. Albinism may be complete or partial, and in partial albinism there are irregularly shaped white patches in the hair and skin. Curiously, albinism is commonest among Negroes. It occurs in plants and animals as well as in man – white rabbits with pink eyes are albinos – but some animals living in countries which are likely to be covered with snow for part of the year show periodic albinism, the white colour of their fur serving as protective coloration during the winter months; the stoat is a familiar example. Albinism is inherited as a Mendelian recessive characteristic. *See* Heredity.

Albumin: albumins are proteins which enter into the composition of all living organisms. They vary according to their source of origin; but they all contain carbon, hydrogen, nitrogen, oxygen and sulphur. The main ones found in food are egg albumin in the white of egg, fibrinogen and haemoglobin in blood, myosin in meat, caseinogen in milk, casein in cheese, and gluten in flour. Albumins show the following characteristics: they are colloidal and do not pass, as salts do, through parchment membranes or the membranes of normal living cells; they are coagulated by heat, following which they become insoluble in water until treated with caustic alkalies or mineral acids; they are precipitated by various chemicals such as alcohol, tannin, nitric acid, and mercury perchloride.

Albuminuria: albumin (*see* above) is not normally found in the urine, for it does not pass through the kidney cells unless they are damaged by, for example, nephritis or inflammation of the kidneys. However, its presence in the urine does not necessarily mean that the kidneys themselves are damaged, for albumin can be found in any inflammation of the lower part of the urinary tract where pus or blood is produced, for example, in pyelitis, cystitis and urethritis (q.v.). Heart disease, many fevers, severe anaemia, and the administration of drugs and poisons may be accompanied by albuminuria, the significance of which is as serious as the disease causing it. Despite what has been said above, albumin is sometimes found in the urine of a small proportion of perfectly normal people, usually in youth. This condition is described as cyclic, postural or orthostatic albuminuria, and it disappears when the individual lies down, only to reappear when he stands upright. It has no pathological significance. During pregnancy the urine must be tested regularly for albumin, for albuminuria may indicate the presence of complications which can be arrested if they are discovered in time.

Alcohol: the name given to a large class of organic compounds, the only ones relevant to medicine being methyl, or wood alcohol, and ethyl alcohol which is the compound found in alcoholic drinks. Methyl alcohol, known as methanol, is poisonous to drink; methylated spirits is alcohol to which has been added 10% of wood spirit, a little paraffin oil, and an aniline dye. The idea is to make it undrinkable, as it is with denatured or surgical alcohol, where methanol or acetone are the additives; these alcohols are intended for industrial use, and being theoretically undrinkable carry no excise duty. Unfortunately, this fact makes them very cheap, and there are people who drink methylated spirits neat or mixed with cheap wine. This is a dangerous habit which leads to blindness, neuritis and death. Ethyl alcohol when completely free from water and other impurities is called 'absolute alcohol', and its chemical formula is C_2H_5OH. In medicine and science, alcohol is used as a solvent as it is capable of dissolving many substances not soluble in water, particularly fats, oils and resins; in the form of 'rectified spirit', containing 90% alcohol by volume, it is used in the making of tinctures, essences and weaker spirits of 10–20% strength. The alcohol of the United States Pharmacopeia contains not less than 94.9% ethyl alcohol by volume. Outside the laboratory, the medical uses of alcohol are few. It is used externally to remove grease from the skin and sterilize it before giving injections, and to harden the skin particularly in those confined to bed for long periods, where its use lessens the risk of bedsores. 'Rubbing alcohol' is popularly used to massage the body after a bath or exercise in many countries; it is a preparation containing acetone, methyl isobutyl ketone and ethyl alcohol. Internally, there are virtually no indications for the use of alcohol as far as medicine is concerned; that is to say, there are no conditions for which it need be prescribed. But to those accustomed to its use, a drink before a meal, wine during a meal, or the nightcap of whisky, no doubt play their part in aiding digestion by quelling nervous tension or inducing sleep. So-called tonic wines, in which a burgundy or claret type wine is medicated with such substances as glycerophosphates, meat extract, or some protein material which is supposed to build up the nerves, are entirely useless, and in their effect no different from the unmedicated product – except that they taste nastier. Spirits should never be given to those who are in a fainting or collapsed state; they are more likely to choke than revive them. The only good reason for taking alcohol is liking it.

Alcoholism: addiction to alcohol. This is a condition in which there is chronic or periodic drinking of a compulsive nature. It is often both a cause and a reflection of emotional and social difficulties. Abuse of alcohol leads to a great deal of misery, marital unhappiness and broken homes, a certain amount of crime, and produces physical and mental disease both directly and indirectly. Directly, by the physical effect of alcohol on the body, and indirectly by the fact that those in a drunken state are more likely to contract venereal disease, succumb to ordinary illnesses such as pneumonia if they are chronic addicts and, of course, to endanger the lives of themselves and others by causing motor and other accidents. On the other hand, there can be no doubt that some people can drink very considerable quantities of alcohol throughout a long life without showing any apparent ill-effects whatever, and that in most cases alcoholism is a symptom rather than a disease in itself. Thus, although alcohol may be the immediate cause of a broken home, it is extremely likely that adjustment problems of long standing have antedated the obvious problem of alcoholism and perhaps contributed to it. Similarly, it could well be argued that, if the evil effects of alcohol are constantly discussed, its good effects in oiling the wheels of social intercourse and reducing tension have usually been ignored and it might be said with more than a grain of truth that moderate amounts of alcohol have kept some people going who would otherwise have found it difficult to carry on reasonably good relationships with their families or friends. Painstaking statistical study carried out in the United States has demonstrated that, if heavy drinking considerably lowers the average expectation of life, the moderate drinker has a higher than average expectation.

The general (although by no means universally accepted) belief today, among those who have studied the problem scientifically, is that the physical diseases brought about by the excessive' consumption of alcohol are the result of its indirect effect in producing malnutrition rather than any direct toxic one. The repeated consumption of strong spirits, especially on an empty stomach, leads to a chronic gastritis of the stomach and probably inflammation of the intestines which interferes with the absorption of food substances and notably vitamins of the B group; this, in turn, damages the nerve cells causing alcoholic neuritis, injury to the brain cells causing certain forms of insanity, and in some cases cirrhosis of the liver. The alcoholic is not necessarily the sort of person who becomes obviously drunk on frequent occasions; he or she may be the man or woman who drinks steadily throughout the day, often without any immediate effect being apparent to others. Later, however, symptoms which are partly due to physical effects, partly to the underlying neurosis which is at the root of the trouble in most cases, and partly social, begin to show themselves. The person eats less and drinks more, often begins the day with vomiting or nausea which necessitates taking the first drink before he can show himself in public, his appearance tends to become bloated and the eyes are often red and congested, his work suffers, he forgets to keep his appointments and becomes indifferent to his social responsibilities, his craving for drink becomes insatiable and, when he is unable to get it, he becomes shaky, irritable and tense. As he is ashamed of his condition, he tries to hide it and often, instead of drinking openly, conceals bottles throughout the house. His emotions are poorly controlled and he gets angry or tearful readily, tells facile lies, and a minor illness or cessation of drinking may lead to an attack of delirium tremens (D.T.s). In another type, there may be no craving for alcohol for quite long periods, until a sudden impulse makes it seem absolutely necessary to have a drink and the sufferer in a few hours becomes dead drunk and quite uncontrollable; this form is rather less frequent than the other and is known as dipsomania. In severe cases the alcoholic may die from cirrhosis of the liver – although this is not so common a result of drinking as it used to be – or an attack of pneumonia or some other infection not ordinarily fatal to healthy people may be so to him; in other cases there may be a gradual mental deterioration with loss of memory (Korsakow's Psychosis). Nearly all cases of chronic alcoholism should be referred to a psychiatrist who may recommend treatment in an institution or nursing home because it is necessary to have complete control over the situation for several months, and the patient cannot be relied upon to abstain without supervision. The main principles of treatment are: complete abstention, psychotherapy to treat the psychological causes of the condition, and the general building up of impaired physical health. Concentrated injections of vitamins may be given, and in some cases drug treatments designed to create revulsion from alcohol are employed. Among these are apomorphine treatment in which the patient is allowed to drink as much as he likes but given injections to cause severe vomiting with the idea that drink and vomiting will form unpleasant associations. Another method is the Danish drug Antabuse which, when taken regularly, causes the patient to feel so ill after drinking that it may turn him against the habit. Unfortunately, when left to themselves, some patients are more likely to neglect taking Antabuse than alcohol.

Aldomet: proprietary name for methyldopa, a drug recently introduced for the treatment of high blood pressure.

Aldosterone: a steroid secreted by the adrenal cortex, which has the function of regulating the balance of salts in the body. Some rare tumours of the adrenal cortex lead to excessive secretion of aldosterone, and this leads to high blood pressure, muscular weakness, thirst, increased secretion of urine, tetany and changes of sensation in the arms and legs. *See* Corticosteroids.

Alkalies: substances, usually oxides, hydroxides, or carbonates and bicarbonates of metals, which neutralize acids to produce salts. Weak solutions of household alkalies – ammonia or washing soda – are useful to alleviate the discomfort of insect bites or stings, but strong ammonia, caustic soda or potash, and washing soda are caustic poisons. The main use of alkalies in medicine is to neutralize acid in the stomach. The chief agents used are: sodium bicarbonate, calcium carbonate (common chalk), magnesium carbonate, magnesium trisilicate and aluminium hydroxide. They may be used alone or in mixtures. Although there is no harm in using sodium bicarbonate (baking soda) from time to time when nothing else is available, its regular use is unwise because it produces gas in the stomach, and is so strongly alkaline that it has a tendency to upset the acid-alkali balance of the body. Magnesium trisilicate and aluminium hydroxide are the safest in this respect, although it is important to emphasize that prolonged dyspepsia should be medically investigated and not self-treated. *See* Stomach Diseases.

Alkaloids: a large group of alkaline substances found in plants. They are extremely potent and widely used in medicine. They are insoluble to a greater or less extent in water but soluble in alcohol (hence those given by mouth are usually in the form of tablets or tinctures, i.e. alcoholic solution). Most of them have a bitter taste, and are extremely poisonous if taken beyond the correct dosage. Common alkaloids are atropine from the belladonna plant, cocaine from coca leaves, caffeine from tea and coffee, morphine, codeine and other drugs from the opium in poppy-juice, nicotine from tobacco, quinine and quinidine from Peruvian bark, strychnine from nux vomica seeds. It will be noticed that alkaloids have names ending in -ine; certain drugs with similar properties but no alkaline reaction have names ending in -in, for example aloin, digitalin.

Allantotoxicon: a poison formerly supposed to be found in sausages. Fortunately there is no evidence that it exists.

Allergy: every adult reacts to the presence of foreign tissue in his body by bringing into action a process designed to neutralize, kill and expel the invader. The bacteria which cause infectious disease provoke the production in the blood-stream of antibodies, which help to kill the bacteria and to make the task of the white blood cells, which dispose of the dead and dying bacteria, much easier. More than this, the body remembers the antigen that produced the antibody, and future introduction of the same antigen provokes a much quicker response to a smaller amount of antigen than was necessary the first time. This reaction can become changed – the word allergy means an altered capacity to react – so that a foreign protein substance produces in a susceptible individual an allergic reaction. An allergic reaction is the same whatever the nature of the protein which causes it, and bears no relation to the effect produced by the offending protein when given to a normal individual. The reason for this is thought to be that a process similar to the antibody-antigen reaction is set off not in the bloodstream but on the surface of the body cells. This allergen-antibody reaction damages the cell walls and liberates a substance known as histamine which, with other substances, is the cause of the actual allergic response. Histamine produces two main effects: (a) it increases the permeability of the small blood vessels, causing the fluid part of the blood or serum to leak into the tissues; (b) it brings about spasm of

31

certain groups of muscles, notably in the bronchial tubes. The former effect leads to swelling (oedema), blisters, and irritation of the skin, nose and eyes, the latter to the asthmatic attacks in allergic subjects.

It is not known with any degree of certainty what makes a person allergic. In some cases heredity may play a part, and there can be little doubt that in others the psychological element is an important factor. It has been shown that allergic-type symptoms can arise from purely psychological causes, as in the well-known instance of a person allergic to roses developing an asthmatic attack in the presence of artificial flowers mistakenly thought to be real, and nettle-rash (hives) or blisters often arise when there is a history of psychological shock but none of exposure to allergens. Blisters can be produced under hypnosis. Treatment of allergic diseases depends on the individual case, but includes: (1) removal of or from the source of trouble, as when feather-stuffed pillows, animals in the house, flower or grass pollen, or dusts at work are responsible; (2) a course of desensitization by giving increasing doses of the allergen over a long period – which is more likely to be successful in hay-fever than in other allergies; (3) psychotherapy in a very few selected cases; (4) the use of drugs which, by antagonizing the effects of histamine, relieve or even remove the symptoms without permanently curing the condition. There are a considerable number of these drugs and it may be necessary to try out more than one before finding the most suitable. Asthma of allergic origin is by far the most difficult of these conditions to treat, perhaps because of its larger psychological element.

Allopathy: this word is used to describe treatment given by doctors who are not homeopaths.

Alopecia Areata: a form of baldness brought about by factors which are not understood. As the hair grows back again in 99% of cases with or without treatment, there can be little doubt that most of the letters written to makers of 'hair-restorer' by grateful customers are written by those suffering from this condition. *See* Baldness.

Aluminium: the compounds of aluminium are used in

medicine for two main reasons: some are astringent, and some are alkaline. Aluminium acetate, for example, is used as ear-drops to dry up discharges from an infected outer ear, and aluminium hydroxide is used to neutralize gastric acid.

Alveolus: *see* Lung, Bronchus, Gum.

Amaurosis: blindness, in particular the type of blindness that is caused by disease of the optic nerve, the brain or the retina, so that the blind eye looks outwardly normal.

Amazon: a female without breasts (now usually the result of a developmental abnormality).

Ambylopia: dimness of vision without apparent abnormality in the eye.

Amenorrhoea: absence or stoppage of the menstrual flow. The commonest cause of amenorrhoea is pregnancy.

Aminophylline: a combination of theophylline and ethylene diamine which produces an increased flow of urine, dilates the breathing-tubes, and improves the blood supply to the heart. It may therefore be used in the form of injections, suppositories, tablets and capsules (sometimes in combination with a sedative) in the treatment of asthma, angina pectoris, or in order to reduce the amount of fluid in the body as in the oedema of heart disease.

Ammonia: a gas with the chemical formula NH_3. It is soluble in water, and is used in solution for domestic purposes. It is very irritating to the lungs, and if it is inhaled can cause distressing symptoms. Inhalation of the vapour arising from ammonia water is uncomfortable but not dangerous. Inhalation of the gas can lead to oedema of the lungs and to bronchitis, but this is rarely serious. Ammonia can also cause burns.

Amnesia: partial or complete loss of memory, although the latter is almost inconceivable since without memory no intellectual functions would be possible. The commonest form is verbal amnesia where words or names are forgotten,

33

but varying types and degrees of amnesia are found in old
age and other organic conditions in which the brain cells are
impaired by disease directly affecting them or, indirectly,
through a poor blood supply, due, for example, to arteriosclerosis. However, many cases of poor memory or loss of
memory are largely psychological in origin, the poor
memory of anxiety neurosis being caused by lack of attention
in one obsessed with his own troubles, the genuine amnesia
of hysteria being a mechanism of retreat from some intolerable situation. *See* Neurosis, Arterial Disease, Memory.

Amodiaquine: (Camoquin). One of the most powerful
drugs used for suppressing and treating malaria. The drug
acts on the malaria parasite in the red blood cell but has no
action on the parasite in the tissues. Unfortunately, some
strains of malaria have become resistant to Amodiaquine,
especially in regions where it has been used to guard the
population against falciparum, or malignant malaria, so
that although it is simple and in most cases effective as a
suppressant – it only has to be taken once a week – it is not
entirely safe to rely on it.

Amoeba: single-celled microscopic animal belonging to
the group of protozoa. The common amoeba is found in
pond water and is just visible to the naked eye; it is harmless.
Other harmless amoebae are found in the human intestine;
certain amoebae are, however, capable of causing disease,
especially Entamoeba histolytica which is the cause of
amoebic dysentery (*see* Dysentery).

Amphetamine: (Benzedrine, Dexedrine). The amphetamines are drugs which imitate the action of the sympathetic
nervous system (*see* Nervous System); they cause a rise in
blood pressure, quickening of the heartbeat, and constriction of the arteries. They also have an action on the
brain, and produce feelings of excitement, elation and
alertness. Doses which are too high make the patient anxious,
restless, tremulous, clumsy and talkative. He may run a high
temperature, and even collapse. Because of their action on
the brain, amphetamines have been used to treat depression,
to combat fatigue, and to depress the appetite in the obese,
but unfortunately they have proved to be drugs of addiction

upon which the susceptible can easily become dependent, and it is known that brain damage and madness can result from continued high doses. The use of amphetamines has therefore been discontinued in cases of obesity, fatigue, and to a great extent in depression, and the drugs are only used in cases of narcolepsy (q.v.), a rare condition, and in certain cases of epilepsy. Amphetamines cannot be bought without a doctor's prescription, and doctors are for the most part abandoning their use. It has recently been found that subjects who take amphetamines by intravenous injection are liable to develop a necrotizing form of arterial disease.

Ampicillin: a synthetic penicillin. The manufacture of artificial types of penicillin became possible in 1959, when the nucleus of penicillin was first made in the laboratory. Ampicillin is important because it is absorbed from the intestine, and can therefore be given by mouth, and because it is effective against some 'gram negative' bacteria. It has a wide range of activity, and is used in conditions as widely different as typhoid and chronic bronchitis. Side effects of its use can include sensitivity rashes and disturbances of the bowels, but often the slight degrees of nausea, heartburn or diarrhoea it causes are a small price to pay for its effectiveness.

Amputation: the removal of a part of the body, usually a limb. Many surgeons have given their names to special amputations, for in the past a good deal of surgery was concerned with saving life by removing gangrenous limbs. But today the operation is rare because antibiotics and chemotherapy have made it possible to treat conditions such as infected compound fractures which were formerly fatal unless the limb was cut off. Apart from injuries sustained in war and in accidents, amputations are necessary today in cases where the blood supply to the limb is so poor that it cannot live, generally as the result of sclerosis of the main arteries of the leg. Even in these cases, however, amputation is not carried out as frequently as it used to be.

Amylase: an enzyme concerned with the breakdown of starch. It is found in the salivary glands and in the pancreas; and in diseases which cause obstruction of the pancreatic duct (through which the enzymes pass to the duodenum) the amylase level rises in the serum and the urine.

Amyl Nitrite: an oily liquid which evaporates easily and has the effect of relieving spasms and dilating the blood vessels. It is used as an inhalation in capsule form for easing the pain of angina pectoris (q.v.).

Amyloid: in some patients with chronic tuberculosis, rheumatoid arthritis, syphilis, or osteomyelitis, a peculiar substance is deposited in the walls of the blood vessels and in connective tissue. The substance is called amyloid because it bears a superficial resemblance to starch; it interferes with the function of organs because it makes the connective tissue swell at the expense of the essential tissues or parenchyma, which the connective tissue normally supports.

Amytal: the trade name for amylobarbitone, a drug used as a sedative and as an aid to sleep. *See* Barbiturates.

Anabolic Drugs: one of the effects of the male hormone is to increase the weight and strength; a man is heavier and stronger than a woman. It has been argued therefore that patients who need building up should be given male hormones, but a drawback is that, whereas it is all very well for debilitated men to grow hair on their chests, it is not so good for ladies. Various compounds similar to male hormones, but without their virilizing effects, have been synthesized and are offered on the market for use in convalescence from severe illness and to increase growth and appetite, but there are differences of opinion about their value. They are called anabolic compounds because of their tissue-building properties. It is now illegal for athletes to use anabolic drugs, but there was a time when, it is said, female weightlifters found them useful.

Anaemia: there are many types of anaemia, but they all fall into two broad classes: (1) those in which the red blood cells are smaller than usual and contain less haemoglobin than they should; and (2) those in which the red blood cells are larger than normal and contain more haemoglobin than usual. In both types of anaemia the total number of red blood cells is reduced. The first type is called microcytic hypo-chromic anaemia, the second megaloblastic hyperchromic anaemia. Microcytic hypochromic anaemia, otherwise referred to as common or secondary anaemia, is caused by a variety of conditions involving loss of blood, inadequate in-take of iron or deficient absorption, and defective formation of red blood cells. Although 'anaemia' is often used as an explanation when an individual feels generally run-down, is nervous, has a poor appetite and so on, it leads to these symptoms much less frequently than is generally believed; in any case, anaemia can only be diagnosed with certainty by actually testing the blood, and the red cell count and haemo-globin levels have to be markedly low before a firm diagnosis is made. The mere fact that somebody looks pale is no proof that anaemia exists, and it is certainly no indication for self-treatment with an 'iron tonic', because iron is quite useless to those who are not lacking in it. Nor is it sensible to speak of 'a tendency to anaemia' or to continue for years taking iron mixtures or pills which can only have the effect of wasting money and upsetting the digestion. One either has anaemia to a measurable degree or one has not got anaemia; and it is no use continuing to take iron for uncomplicated secondary anaemia for more than six months. It is also a mistake to think that capsules or pills containing substances such as liver or stomach extract, vitamins etc., have any advantage over simple iron preparations. Some forms of iron are more elegant or disturb the digestion less than others, but addi-tional ingredients are useless. The common causes of secondary anaemia are: (1) loss of blood which may be sud-den, as in an operation, an accident, or childbirth, or sus-tained over some time, as in repeated heavy menstruation or bleeding from a peptic ulcer or haemorrhoids; (2) defec-tive blood formation after or during severe or chronic infec-tions or, more rarely, in chronic kidney disease; (3) lack of iron in the diet – an uncommon cause, for the necessary in-take of iron is small, being of the nature of 15–20 mg a day; (4) inadequate absorption of iron from the digestive tract in diseases of the intestine.

Definitive treatment of secondary anaemia is the treatment of the condition causing it, and subsequent administration of iron. *See* Pernicious Anaemia, Sickle-cell Anaemia, Thalassaemia.

Anaesthesia: the primary meaning is a loss of feeling (particularly of the senses of touch and pain), found in organic diseases where damage to the sensory nerves or their centres has occurred, or in certain psychological states. More generally, it is applied to the deliberate induction of partial or total insensibility for the purpose of performing surgical operations.

In ancient times opium, hemp and alcohol were variously used to produce partial anaesthesia for surgery, but none of these drugs could do more than reduce the pain. Surgery was a bloody and brutal business up to the introduction of modern anaesthetics about 130 years ago, and the rapid advances made by surgery in the last hundred years are due as much to the discovery and refinement of anaesthesia as to increased understanding of physiology and pathology. In 1785 Dr Pearson, an English physician, suggested the use of ether for asthmatic attacks and in 1800 Sir Humphry Davy observed the anaesthetic effects of nitrous oxide (laughing gas). He proposed the use of nitrous oxide in surgical operations, and in 1818 Faraday and several American physicians noted the anaesthetic effects of ether, but it was left to the American dentist Horace Wells of Hartford, Connecticut, to use nitrous oxide as an anaesthetic in 1844, and another American dentist, Dr Morton of Boston, to use ether in 1846. In the same year Liston carried out the first operation in Britain under ether anaesthesia, and during 1847, J. Y. Simpson of Edinburgh used ether in childbirth for the first time. Simpson discovered the use of chloroform a few months later. Until recent times, ether, chloroform, gas, ethyl chloride and trichlorethylene were the main general anaesthetic drugs. They were all given by inhalation, and this made them moderately unpleasant to the patient; but nowadays intravenous barbiturates such as pentothal are commonly used to induce anaesthesia much more agreeably. The modern anaesthetist has a number of new drugs at his disposal to produce unconsciousness, relaxation of the muscles and variation of blood pressure, but nitrous oxide is still used in dental anaesthetics a century and a quarter since its introduction, and ether continues to be a useful drug for the occasional anaesthetist who wishes to be above all safe. Chloroform has been abandoned because it can cause arrest of the heart and poison the liver, and its place has been taken by halothane (q.v.).

A modern general anaesthetic starts with the injection of premedication in the ward. This is usually a dose of morphine or pethidine (demerol) to make the patient sleepy, combined with atropine or scopolamine to dry up the secretions of the lungs, which can otherwise cause trouble. In the anaesthetic room the anaesthetist injects a barbiturate – thiopentone (Pentothal), for example, or methohexitone (Brietal, Brevital) – into a vein, and when the patient has fallen asleep he prepares to pass a tube through the nose or mouth into the trachea. This is made easier if the patient is given a muscle-relaxing drug such as suxamethonium chloride (Scoline).

Once the anaesthetist has passed the tube successfully, he can control the patient's breathing, and he now continues the anaesthetic with drugs chosen according to the requirements of the operation. If necessary, he will fix a needle into a vein so that he can set up an intravenous drip easily, for the anaesthetist is responsible for the patient's general condition during the operation. After the operation the anaesthetist continues to keep an eye on the patient, and prescribes post-operative drugs to relieve pain, anxiety or nausea when the patient has regained consciousness.

Partial anaesthesia is produced by local anaesthetics, which are applied to the surface of the body or injected into the skin or the sensory nerves. Cocaine can be instilled into the eye or into the nose to make the membranes insensitive and to stop bleeding (the only use for pure cocaine in medicine, for it is a drug of addiction), but in general, local anaesthetics are synthetic compounds such as amethocaine (which replaces cocaine), procaine and lignocaine. Procaine is used in weak solutions 0·5–2% and to it is added adrenaline, for on its own procaine dilates blood vessels and promotes bleeding. Lignocaine is used in slightly weaker concentrations 0·25–1%, except where it is applied directly to mucous membranes or the skin, when concentrations of 2–4% are useful. A common use of lignocaine is in the urethra, before passing a cystoscope or other instrument. Infiltration of the skin to anaesthetize the nerve endings at the site of operation is called field block, and injection of the sensory nerves that supply a particular area, for example the brachial plexus for the arm, is called regional nerve-block. Local anaesthetics

39

can sometimes usefully be combined with a light general anaesthetic.

Anaesthesia of the lower part of the body can be produced by injection of local anaesthetics into the fluid in the space round the spinal cord and the nerves which issue from it, a technique called spinal anaesthesia, or into the space just outside the dura mater which envelops the spinal cord (epidural anaesthesia). For the anatomy of these techniques *see* Spinal Cord.

Finally, you need not worry about giving away important secrets under anaesthesia – nobody ever does.

Analgesia: the relief of pain in the conscious patient. Various drugs may be described as analgesics, from aspirin to morphine, and inhalation anaesthetics, for example nitrous oxide and trilene, can be used in childbirth and dentistry to produce an analgesic effect short of unconsciousness.

Anaphylaxis: an antibody-antigen reaction (*see* Allergy). The word is used to describe the condition produced in laboratory animals by the injection of a foreign protein, commonly horse serum. A second injection of the same protein triggers off a severe reaction. In human beings anaphylaxis can be an untoward result of serum therapy, as in passive immunization against tetanus and gas gangrene; the patient reacts to the serum either because he has had it injected more than ten days previously or because he is naturally sensitive to horse serum. The reaction, called anaphylactic shock, comes on within half an hour, and the patient collapses with increasing circulatory failure and difficulty in breathing. The condition may be desperate.

Adrenaline or, perhaps better, hydrocortisone is given intravenously in large doses until the patient recovers. Tracheotomy with suction may be necessary; half-measures or indecision are likely to be fatal. Luckily the condition is very rare, and sensitivity to injections is usually shown by milder reactions, but it is sensible to ask all patients who have injections likely to produce reactions to remain under observation for half an hour until the absence of sensitivity has been established. Sensitivity can often be demonstrated by using small test doses, but in anaphylactic shock the test dose itself can trigger the reaction. The use of anti-tetanus serum can be avoided if patients are actively immunized against tetanus; the present writer, who has seen a friend killed by anaphylactic shock after an injection of anti-tetanus serum for a scratch received while playing football, cannot advise his readers strongly enough to have themselves and their children actively immunized against tetanus.

Anastomosis: a communication between two hollow organs or vessels. Communication between blood vessels is a feature of normal anatomy, but anastomotic communication between two hollow organs, for example between the stomach and small intestine to bypass the duodenum, are made artificially by the surgeon, or, more rarely, follow disease. *See* Fistula.

Anatomy: the study of the structure of the body and its parts. In ancient times physicians and surgeons could only make a superficial study of human anatomy (possibly on the battlefield), and based many of their ideas on the examination of animals. It was, for example, believed that the uterus was double as in the sow. Not until the Renaissance did scholars begin to study human anatomy in detail, but even then, for many years, their difficulties were made greater by the attitude of the Church. Few bodies were available; dissection had to be carried out quickly because means of preserving bodies were lacking. Students of anatomy attended demonstrations held in anatomy theatres, but they did not have the chance of dissecting bodies for themselves. In recent times things have changed for the better and all students now dissect the body in detail. The provision of bodies for dissection has always been difficult, and even to-day the supply is often unequal to the demand. It is therefore sensible to consider leaving one's body for anatomical study, and those who wish to do so are advised to consult the Professor of Anatomy in the nearest University or Medical School.

Androgen: a substance which causes masculinization. The testes secrete the hormone testosterone, which is partially responsible for male sexual development, and is the chief androgen. Used in the treatment of male castration and in retarded development of the male sexual characteristics, it is given either by injection as testosterone propionate, or by mouth as the synthetic compound methyl testosterone. Testosterone is useless in the treatment of impotence (q.v.) and both useless and dangerous as an aphrodisiac. Androgens have the effect of increasing the size of the muscles and the use of protein in the body. They are therefore sometimes used when these effects are wanted, as after severe operations, but this use is limited because of their virilizing action in women. *See* Anabolic Drugs.

Aneurin: thiamine, one of the B complex of vitamins (q.v.).

Aneurysm: a swelling upon the wall of an artery or vein which is filled with blood. Aneurysms are formed in consequence of damage or congenital deficiency of the vessel walls, and fall into several classes. In a true aneurysm, the inner lining of the vessel wall has given way and the swelling is still covered by the blown-up outer walls; in a false aneurysm, the whole of the vessel wall has split and the blood is contained in fibrous tissue. Aneurysms may be congenital or acquired, the acquired type being caused by injury or disease – commonly atherosclerosis or syphilis. Disease can lead to the formation of a dissecting aneurysm, in which the blood tracks between the layers of the vessel wall and in the end bursts out. Dissecting aneurysms are prone to occur in the aorta of people with high blood pressure.

Aneurysms are classified also according to their shape – fusiform, saccular, berry, serpentine – and according to where they occur. One of the commonest sites for an aneurysm is in the skull, where they form on the arteries that supply the brain.

SYMPTOMS: these vary according to the site and type of aneurysm. Sometimes the swelling is painless but can be seen, for example the rider's aneurysm behind the knee, or the serpentine or cirsoid type that forms on the scalp. In the abdomen, where they form on the aorta, they can be painless and unsuspected, or they can cause discomfort, or interfere with the blood supply to the intestines or the kidneys. Aneurysms on the arteries of the brain can press on neighbouring structures, for example the optic nerves, and so cause blindness or paralysis. The bursting of an aneurysm is accompanied by dramatic and often fatal illness. Dissecting aneurysm of the aorta causes great pain and collapse, and is at first sometimes confused with perforation of an ulcer, but as the dissection spreads the diagnosis becomes clear. Rupture of an aneurysm inside the skull produces subarachnoid haemorrhage – a sudden bleed causes a blinding headache and unconsciousness; a slow leak causes headache and signs of irritation of the meninges.

TREATMENT: is difficult and uncertain. In the abdomen it is possible to cut away the damaged part of the aorta and substitute a plastic graft, but in the case of a leaking or dissecting aneurysm the operation is severe and often unsuccessful. Some surgeons believe that an aneurysm discovered before it has given rise to symptoms should be cut out and grafted, because the condition is so dangerous, but each surgeon and patient must make up his own mind. As for aneurysms inside the skull, many cases have been successfully operated on and the burst or leaking aneurysm tied off.

Angina: originally meaning choking or suffocating pain, the word is now applied to the disease causing this sort of pain. The two common sorts of angina are Vincent's angina, an infection of the mouth and throat which may make breathing difficult, and angina pectoris, a heart disease described below.

Angina Pectoris: patients with disease of the coronary arteries of the heart may suffer from characteristic pain which is brought on by effort, particularly at the beginning of the day, after large meals and in cold weather. The pain is suffocating, and is often described as gripping or pressing. It is felt behind the breastbone and it spreads into the neck, into both sides of the chest, into the left arm and down over the upper part of the abdomen. It may be very severe, but it is not usually sharp – sharp pains in the chest are more often due to indigestion than to heart disease. Anginal pain is caused by reduced blood supply to the heart muscle, which sends out distress signals when the circulation is too poor to cope with the work the heart is required to do. The pain produced stops the patient in his tracks – a particularly effective alarm system, for when the patient rests the heart stops being under load, the poor circulation becomes just adequate, and

43

the pain goes. Anginal pain that persists when the patient is at rest is a sign of serious disease. The diagnosis is made on the basis of the characteristic nature of the pain, and the results of an electrocardiogram (q.v.).

TREATMENT: obviously calls for rest and relief of anxiety and fear, and the patient must learn to live inside the 'envelope of performance' defined by the pain. Smoking ought to be stopped, but there is no objection to alcohol in moderation. Many doctors advise a diet low in cholesterol (q.v.), and the use of vegetable oils which lower the blood cholesterol levels, because there is some evidence suggesting that high blood cholesterol levels and the incidence of coronary disease are linked; the matter is still a subject for argument, but there is no doubt that a diet designed to reduce the patient's weight is certain to reduce his symptoms as well. The most effective drugs are nitroglycerin and amyl nitrite, which dilate blood vessels; they help in two ways – by dilating the coronary arteries themselves, so that more blood can flow through them, and by dilating the vessels of the rest of the body so that less resistance is offered to the passage of blood and less work has to be done by the heart in pumping the blood around the body.

In exceptional cases, when the pain does not improve with medical treatment, the nerves which carry pain impulses from the heart can be cut by the surgeon or interrupted by injection. Other surgical operations have been carried out with the aim of increasing the blood supply to the heart, but the results are uncertain. An ingenious and sometimes effective treatment is reduction of the basal metabolic rate (q.v.), which decreases the demand for oxygen and therefore the load on the heart. The patient is given radioactive iodine, which concentrates in the thyroid gland and diminishes the secretion of thyroxin. *See* Coronary Disease.

Angiography: radio-opaque substances injected into the blood vessels make them show up on X-ray plates. The resulting angiograms demonstrate the outline and course of the vessels so that abnormalities and displacements can be seen.

Angioma: a tumour or swelling made up of a cluster of abnormal blood vessels. Angiomas may occur in the internal organs, especially in the brain where they may bleed dangerously, or on the surface of the skin in the form of 'naevi' or birthmarks. Treatment is indicated when they are inconvenient or ugly; small angiomas can be cauterized with the electric needle, larger ones removed under local or general anaesthetic. Angiomas are not malignant or cancerous. *See* Birthmark.

Angioneurotic Edema: also called giant urticaria, this produces large swellings of the subcutaneous tissues, particularly of the face or hands. Occasionally the swelling involves the air passages of the nasopharynx or the larynx so that there is obstruction to the breathing. This condition, like that of common urticaria, may follow a general antibody-antigen reaction (*see* Allergy). It can be the result of infection with worms, or it may follow a meal of shellfish or strawberries. Some families are particularly prone to the condition.

Diagnosis is made on the family history, on the fact that young people are commonly affected, often ones of a sensitive and nervous disposition (the condition sometimes appears after emotional stress), and on the appearance of the swellings. A full diagnosis should include identification of precipitating stimuli.

TREATMENT: is by antihistamines in most cases, a reliable drug being chlorpheniramine (Piriton or Chlor-trimeton). In acute cases in which the swelling is causing difficulty in breathing adrenaline is injected, and the patient is put to bed.

Aniline Poisoning: aniline is amino-benzene, and the term 'aniline poisoning' is taken to include poisoning with nitro- as well as amino-compounds of benzene and chlorbenzene, for example nitro-benzene and tri-nitro-toluene (T.N.T.). The substances are absorbed through the skin or through the mouth.

SYMPTOMS: dizziness, headache, nausea and difficulty in breathing. The patient may go blue. Jaundice may follow because of liver damage, especially with T.N.T.

DIAGNOSIS: in acute cases this may be easy, because the patient is known to have been in contact with aniline, but in chronic cases where the poison has been slowly absorbed the diagnosis can be difficult. In chronic poisoning, the patient feels

45

weak and tired, and he gets out of breath easily. He may complain of indigestion, and may become jaundiced.

TREATMENT: in acute cases the whole body must be washed, and if there is much difficulty in breathing the patient may need oxygen. He must be put to bed; alcohol is dangerous and must not be given. During convalescence many patients need iron, because they tend to develop anaemia (q.v.). There is no special antidote to aniline poisoning.

Ankylosis: fixation or near-fixation of a joint which is normally freely movable, brought about by disease, injury or the surgeon. Common diseases causing ankylosis are tuberculosis, rheumatoid arthritis or septic arthritis; in these conditions the bones are fixed together by scar tissue. Joint deformities caused by fractures result in ankylosis, and fixation of a joint can follow if a normal joint is kept still for a long time, as when the treatment of a fracture makes it necessary to immobilize neighbouring joints in plaster. Ankylosis of a joint can be achieved by gross hysterics who maintain that a joint is paralysed, or by mystics who hold a limb for years in the same position as part of their religious devotions. Sometimes the surgeon deliberately causes complete ankylosis in a painful joint with restricted movement in order to relieve chronic pain. Ankylosing spondylitis is a disease of unknown cause afflicting young adults, usually male, which results in the stiffening and eventual fixation of the spine. It is also known as bamboo spine.

Ankylostoma: the hookworm, a parasite found in the tropics, parts of Western Europe and the Southern States of the U.S.A. In temperate lands it is usually found in damp and insanitary places like sewers and tunnels. *See* Hookworm, Worms.

Anopheles: a genus of mosquito, some species of which can carry from man to man the parasites of malaria (q.v.). The emale anophelene mosquito bites an infected person and takes up from the blood the sexually differentiated forms of the malaria parasite. These couple in the mosquito and produce many hundred asexual parasites, which the mosquito passes on to the next person it bites. The female Anopheles is identified by its position at rest; its body makes an angle with the surface on which it rests, whereas the culicine mosquitoes, which do not transmit malaria, rest with their bodies parallel to the surface.

Anorexia Nervosa: a nervous condition confined mainly to young women who refuse to eat, sleep very little, and yet remain very active. Sometimes the state begins with an obsession that the person concerned is becoming overweight, appetite being at first restricted by deliberate intent and then being genuinely lost. Emaciation may become severe and even result in death, the patient often deceiving her attendants as to the amount of food she has taken. Treatment is psychological but, of course, in severe cases the first thing to do is to ensure adequate intake of food by compulsion if necessary. Psychiatric advice should always be sought.

Anosmia: absence of the sense of smell.

Anoxia: lack of oxygen, which may be relative or absolute.

Antabuse: a proprietary name for disulfiram. *See* Alcoholism.

Antacids: medicines for counteracting gastric acidity. *See* Alkalies.

Anthelmintics: drugs for causing the expulsion of parasite worms. The most commonly used are piperazine, which is active against roundworms and threadworms (pinworms); bephenium hydroxynaphthoate in cases of infection with hookworm and roundworm; thiabendazole for infection with Strongyloides stercoralis; and viprynium or pyrvinium pamaote (Povan) in cases with threadworm (pinworm) infection. *See* Worms.

Anthracosis: the greyish-pink or black changes in colour found in the lungs of miners, and found in varying degrees in most city-dwellers due to the inhalation of coal-dust or soot. There is no evidence that it leads to any harm. *See* Pneumoconiosis.

Anthrax: an infectious disease caught from animals. Farmers, veterinary surgeons and butchers are liable to contract

47

anthrax, which is also known as woolsorter's disease, rag-picker's disease, and malignant pustule. Workers in industries dealing with bones, hides, hair and bristles are at risk. The disease is caused by a bacillus, Bacillus anthracis, and is most common in Australia, Russia and South America.

SYMPTOMS: there are two types of anthrax, external and internal. The external type can occur by infection through cracks and cuts even from hides long removed from the animal; a 'boil' appears on the area, often the face, neck or arm, and the inflamed area spreads until a small area of pus appears in the middle which bursts to produce a black scab about half an inch in diameter. In the internal type, caused by breathing in the spores of the bacillus (mainly from infected wool), or eating infected flesh, acute pneumonia or gastro-enteritis develops.

DIAGNOSIS: this is suggested by the patient's trade, and is confirmed by finding the anthrax bacillus in scrapings from the sore in the external type. The diagnosis of the internal type is far more difficult and may prove impossible.

TREATMENT: fortunately the anthrax bacillus is sensitive to antibiotics; the drug of choice is benzylpenicillin. Prevention includes destruction by burning of all hides and bodies thought to be infected, disinfection of premises, and prevention of grazing in the infected area. Free ventilation of factories will stop the spread of respiratory and gastro-intestinal anthrax, and protective clothes should be worn by workers. It is now possible to immunize with safety against anthrax.

Antibiotic: a collective name for any substance produced by micro-organisms or fungi which is capable of destroying or stopping the growth of pathogenic organisms, i.e. organisms which cause disease. Penicillin, streptomycin and aureomycin are well-known antibiotics; the list grows every year, but as each new antibiotic comes into general use it stimulates the growth of resistant organisms. The problem of resistance has been made more difficult by the indiscriminate use of antibiotics. They should not be employed in trivial illnesses; instead, their use should be confined to infections in which the organism has been identified and shown to be sensitive. Antibiotics must be used in adequate doses for at least five days.

Antibody: *see* Allergy.

Anticoagulants: drugs which reduce the clotting-power of the blood. They are used to prevent the extension of clotting in the veins in cases where it is known that clots are forming in deep vessels, in vascular surgery and in dialysis of the blood. Some physicians use anticoagulants following coronary thrombosis but not all agree that the effort spent in controlling the dose – for continual laboratory tests are needed to assess the effect of the drugs – is worth the probable result.

The main drugs used to prevent clotting are heparin, which is prepared from liver and acts quickly when injected into the veins (the antagonist which restores the clotting power of the blood is protamine sulphate injection); and warfarin, the name of which is taken from the Wisconsin Alumni Research Foundation. Warfarin is given by mouth, and the antagonist is Vitamin K_1 (phytomenadione injection). Patients who are taking anticoagulants should carry with them a card giving the name of the drug and the dose. Warfarin has been used widely as rat poison. Diptran is used to prevent the clotting which occurs in thrombotic thrombocytopenia.

Antidotes: a substance given to counteract the effects of poison. There are very few specific antidotes, and they are only to be used after general measures to get rid of the poison and support life have been started.

Arsenic. The antidote is ferric hydrate, which can be made by mixing 30 ml of 15% solution of ferric chloride with 30 g sodium bicarbonate in 120 ml water.

Cyanide. Amyl nitrite capsules are inhaled, and sodium nitrite given intravenously.

Phenol. White of egg.

Aspirin, Iron tablets. Sodium bicarbonate taken by mouth or used as 1% stomach washout.

Mercury. Raw eggs in milk.

Acids. Give milk of magnesia, washing soda or toothpaste by mouth.

Alkalies. Vinegar, one third strength, by mouth. If in doubt, give white of egg and encourage vomiting. *See* Poisons.

Antigen: *see* Allergy.

Antihistamines: histamine is one of the substances liberated from the cells of the body in cases of allergy (q.v.); it produces the symptoms of various allergic diseases. Antihistamines are drugs which counteract the effects of histamine. They are most effective in preventing the onset of an allergic reaction, and they will control hay fever, urticaria and angioneurotic edema (q.v.). They are not very useful in asthma. There are a number of antihistamines, and it is worth trying several in order to find one which suits a particular person best. Antihistamines produce drowsiness, a property which is useful when a sedative is needed, but dangerous to those who have to keep alert in order to work machinery or drive vehicles. Alcohol intensifies this effect.

Antimony: a metal similar in its effects to arsenic. It used to be employed in the treatment of fever and bronchitis, and in the form of tartar emetic as an emetic (for which it is not to be recommended). It is very poisonous to protozoa, and is therefore used in the treatment of some tropical diseases. It is still probably the best drug, as antimony sodium tartrate, for use in bilharzia, although it is not free from side-effects, and it is used in the treatment of Leishmaniasis or kala-azar, as a pentavalent compound.

Antiphlogistics: substances used as poultices in the treatment of inflammation on the surface of the body, the most familiar being the kaolin poultice. This is much the best form of applying heat to infected areas as it does not make the skin wet and sodden like boric lint, but rather absorbs liquid and retains heat for longer periods. The poultice may be prepared by placing the tin of kaolin in water and boiling (taking care not to let the water into the kaolin), then spreading the kaolin on lint and carefully applying it to the skin as hot as possible without burning or causing discomfort. An alternative method is to spread the kaolin cold on the lint and heat it under a toasting grill.

Antipyretic: a substance or method of treatment which reduces fever.

Antiseptic: strictly speaking a substance that destroys or arrests the development of the germs which cause putrefaction. A disinfectant destroys the germs causing disease; but the two terms have been so often confused, that they have become virtually synonymous. Although Louis Pasteur (1822–95) first discovered the fact that germs could cause disease, the Hungarian Semmelweiss had demonstrated their function in producing wound infection and sepsis in 1847. Semmelweiss tried to make his colleagues understand his discovery that childbed fever was caused by infection, but they would believe neither him nor Oliver Wendell Holmes of Boston, who had maintained that puerperal fever was contagious in 1843. It was left to Lord Lister (1827–1912) to introduce antisepsis into surgery. Lister had the operating theatre sprayed with carbolic during operations, and he used carbolic acid on his dressings.

Gradually antisepsis in surgery was abandoned in favour of asepsis (q.v.), in which everything used in an operation is sterile, so that germs are kept away rather than killed on arrival. Nowadays antiseptics are used only to clean the skin or to clean dirty wounds. They have to be used carefully because they tend to delay healing; many surgeons believe that the best and mildest antiseptic is soap and water. Household antiseptics are better used on drains and lavatory pans than on cuts and abrasions.

Antiserum: serum from an animal that has been infected with a disease naturally or artificially and has formed antibodies which are contained in the serum. The use of serum to prevent development of a disease, notably diphtheria and tetanus, is not without danger (*see* Serum Sickness, Anaphylaxis), and although the risks of these diseases outweigh the risks of giving the serum, it is better to be immunized actively when possible. *See* Immunization.

Antispasmodics: drugs that counteract spasm occurring in various hollow organs and structures such as the stomach, or the ureter, which can be extremely painful. Atropine and Hyoscine are the most commonly used antispasmodics.

Antitoxin: an antibody formed in the blood which reacts with the toxin of a micro-organism to neutralize it.

Antivenin: an antiserum produced by injecting increasing

ANTRUM

doses of snake venom into animals, usually horses, used in
cases of snake-bite. Antivenins should be specific to the snake,
and should be given within twelve hours of the bite. For some
snakes, e.g. the coral snake and some sea-snakes, no effective
antivenin is available.

Antrum: used in anatomy to mean a cavity, especially inside
a bone. The maxillary antrum lies in the upper jaw-bone
between the palate and the socket of the eye, and the mastoid
antrum lies behind the ear.

Anuria: a condition in which no urine is produced from the
body. It can be caused by failure of the kidneys, low pressure
in the renal arteries, or blockage of the ureters.

Anus: the end of the alimentary canal, where the rectum
opens to the exterior. It is formed by two sphincters or rings
of muscle.

Anxiety: *see* Neurosis.

A.P.C.: abbreviation for aspirin, phenacetin and caffeine
compounded as an analgesic tablet.

Aorta: the main artery of the body. Beginning at the left
ventricle of the heart, it curves over and down to pass through
the chest, pierce the diaphragm, and enter the abdomen,
where it ends opposite the fourth lumbar vertebra. It has
numerous branches through which the whole body is supplied with arterial blood.

Aperients: *see* Constipation.

Aphasia: loss of the power of speech or the understanding of
speech caused by damage to the parts of the brain concerned
with these functions. Dysphasia is a lesser degree of the same
defect. Theoretically aphasia can be sensory or motor, for the
main parts of the brain concerned with speech are divided
into the afferent or sensory side, and the efferent or motor
side. The sensory side is in the upper part of the temporal
lobe, and it is responsible for the understanding of words both
written and spoken. The motor area is in the lower rear part

of the frontal lobe above the sensory area, and in front of it. The 'speech centre' is present on the dominant side of the brain – that is, on the left side in right-handed people, and on the right in those who are left-handed. Again in theory, damage to the surface of the brain in these areas could produce word deafness, where words cannot be understood although the power of hearing is intact, word blindness where the patient is not blind but cannot read written words, motor aphasia where he can make noises but not words, and agraphia where the function of the hand is apparently normal but the patient cannot write. In practice, word deafness or blindness affects the power of speech, for if the subject cannot hear himself talk his speech soon relapses into nonsense; moreover, injuries and diseases of the brain nearly always affect a mixed area and produce mixed symptoms. Because we think largely in words, serious aphasia may lead to a degree of confusion.

Aphonia: loss of voice. This may be partial or complete, and is caused by disease or trauma of the nerves controlling the muscles of speech, infection of the throat and larynx, or by neurosis. Hysterical aphonia is brought about by an unconscious desire not to speak at all, or not to speak in a particular situation. Aphonia clericorum is an occupational disease, clergyman's sore throat.

Aphrodisiac: a substance which gives rise to sexual desire or increases the potency. Unhappily genuine aphrodisiacs have so far defied detection; but much practical research has been pursued in the matter. *See* Cantharides, Impotence.

Apical Abscess: an abscess forming at the tip of the root of a tooth as a result of disease in the tooth. The abscess may extend through the bone in one of several directions and cause the face to swell. It may present itself as a localized swelling in the mouth – a gum boil. Treatment usually involves extraction of the tooth and a course of antibiotics.

Apollonia, St: the patron saint of dentists. She was burned at the stake after having her teeth struck out.

Apomorphine: a drug derived from morphine, used as an

53

emetic when given by injection. Its action is violent and most disagreeable.

Apoplexy: a stroke. The condition is caused by an acute accident (haemorrhage, thrombosis or embolism) occurring in a diseased blood vessel responsible for part of the blood supply of the brain resulting in loss of consciousness, paralysis or death.

SYMPTOMS: strokes are not uncommon. If a patient suddenly becomes unconsious and lapses into a coma, the chances are that he has had a stroke; the smell of alcohol on his breath can be confusing, but must not be misleading. Strokes usually occur in the middle-aged or elderly, but if the apoplexy is caused by a burst aneurysm (q.v.), it can happen to younger people. Sometimes warning signs go before a stroke, especially when clotting begins in a small branch and spreads back into the main artery; tingling or clumsiness in a limb may be followed by paralysis and coma. If the stroke is due to clotting in the internal carotid artery (the main artery supplying the brain, which runs up the neck) there may have been previou- attacks of weakness, difficulty in speech or confusion. Somse times a severe headache gives warning of an impending haemorrhage. Strokes following embolism (the blocking of an artery by a clot formed elsewhere) are quite sudden.

TREATMENT: the immediate treatment is to make sure that the patient can breathe freely and easily and is kept warm. Do not try to give him alcohol, or indeed any food or drink. Patients who are going to recover begin to regain conscious- ness within a day or two, being at first confused and restless. As they become more aware of their surroundings it becomes possible to tell how much paralysis the stroke has caused. The danger now is from pneumonia and bedsores, and the nursing is hard work. Over the weeks recovery begins to take place, but unless the paralysed limbs are moved through their full range by the attendants at least four times a day they will stiffen irrevocably and become painful. The limbs must not be allowed to contract, and splints must be worn as the muscles become spastic and tend to bend the limbs at the joints. Convalescence is long and hard, especially if the patient is left with difficulty of speech and comprehension, and demands courage from the sick man and determination and patience from his attendants. The only sort of apoplexy which is likely to respond to active treatment in the early stages is that due to bleeding from an aneurysm, but occasionally a large clot is left in the brain after a haemorrhage which can with advantage be taken away by the surgeon. Both these conditions are revealed by angiography (q.v.).

Apothecaries' Weights: now obsolete, but once used in compounding remedies.

20 grains or minims	= 1 scruple
3 scruples	= 1 drachm
8 drachms	= 1 ounce
12 ounces	= 1 pound

Apothecaries' liquid measure was:

60 minims	= 1 fluid drachm
8 fluid drachms	= 1 fluid ounce
20 fluid ounces	= 1 pint

Appendicitis: inflammation of the vermiform appendix, a vestigial structure attached to the caecum at the place where the small intestine joins the large intestine. A bacterial infection, appendicitis is not caused by swallowing fruit stones, an idea produced by the concretions (faecaliths) looking like fruit stones that are often found in a diseased appendix. Although appendicitis now accounts for about half the acute abdominal emergencies occurring between the ages of 10 and 30, it was not recognized before the last quarter of the nineteenth century. Inflammation of this part of the gut was called perityphlitis, which means inflammation about the caecum. One of the first operations for appendicitis was carried out on King Edward VII in 1902, and after this it became fashionable. Appendicitis is more often found in 'developed' than 'underdeveloped' countries.

SYMPTOMS: pain is felt at first round the navel; it later travels to the right lower part of the abdomen. The pain may be preceded by general discomfort in the abdomen, indigestion, diarrhoea or constipation. Nausea is common, and the patient may vomit once or twice. The tongue and mouth are dry, and there is loss of appetite.

DIAGNOSIS: the abdomen is tender, especially in the right lower part. There may be a slight rise of temperature or none at all. Internal rectal examination discloses tenderness in the pelvis, and is very important. If the appendix perforates, then all the signs are intensified; there is great tenderness with rigidity of the muscles of the abdominal wall, the temperature rises, and the patient becomes shocked, pale and clammy as peritonitis spreads.

If the infection spreading from the ruptured appendix is successfully localized by natural processes an appendix abscess may be formed.

TREATMENT: the best treatment for an inflamed appendix is removal as soon as possible. Only if removal is impossible should the patient be treated conservatively by rest in bed, antibiotics, e.g. ampicillin, tetracycline, cephaloridine, and a liquid diet.

Peritonitis calls for urgent operation, but if an abscess is forming it is important to let it localize properly before trying to drain it.

Chronic or 'grumbling' appendix: recurrent pain in the right lower abdomen with constipation, loss of appetite and mild nausea is sometimes diagnosed as chronic appendicitis. Although there is no doubt that a patient may suffer from recurrent mild attacks of acute appendicitis, only to be terminated by removal of the organ, many surgeons doubt the existence of grumbling or chronic appendicitis. In any case it is only to be diagnosed when a diligent search has failed to demonstrate any other cause for pain in the right lower abdomen.

Areola: a round coloured area surrounding a raised centre, e.g. the area round a pustule. The areola of the breast is the pink area surrounding the nipple which becomes brown in women who have borne children.

Argyll-Robertson Pupil: a condition in which the pupil of the eye does not contract when a light is shone into it, but does contract on accommodation; that is, when the patient is asked to look at something far away and then something very near.

The affected pupil is small and irregular. Argyll-Robertson pupil is characteristic of syphilitic infection of the central nervous system.

Arrhythmia: a term which describes any abnormality of the rhythm of the heartbeat.

Arsenic: a metallic substance which when given in big enough doses irritates the stomach and intestines. It is not now used in medicine to any extent, although small doses are said to revive the appetite and make the hair shine. However, before penicillin, it was universally used in the treatment of syphilis in the form of Salvarsan. It is a traditional poison, and the symptoms are nausea and faintness, followed by violent vomiting and diarrhoea, cramps, convulsions and coma. Although it is easily available, the criminal is advised not to use it, for it is readily identified. The treatment for arsenic poisoning is a mixture of ferric chloride solution 15% with sodium bicarbonate in water and stomach washout. Dimercaprol, or B.A.L., which was originally invented to counteract the effects of the arsenical war gas, Lewisite, is also used in the treatment. It is possible to build up an immunity to the effects of arsenic; the arsenic eaters of Styria took doses which would kill several normal men. Clare Booth Luce developed poisoning from paint flaking from the ceiling of her Italian villa.

Arsine Poisoning: arsine is arseniuretted hydrogen and is a cause of industrial poisoning. It may affect chemists or workers in any industry where interaction can take place between metals which contain arsenic and acids. It can cause sudden death.

SYMPTOMS: faintness, weakness and nausea, and severe headache, followed by abdominal pain, pain in the muscles and shivering. These symptoms often develop some hours after exposure to arsine, and they are followed by jaundice, passage of blood pigment in the urine, and then anaemia and suppression of urine.

DIAGNOSIS: if any worker liable to come into contact with arsine falls ill suddenly at work or at home, the diagnosis must be suspected and the man at once sent to hospital.

TREATMENT: this must be carried out in hospital. In the meantime the patient should be kept warm and comfortable, given alkalies by mouth, and encouraged to drink as much fluid as possible. If it is available, he should inhale oxygen. In hospital treatment may include massive transfusions and use of the artificial kidney.

Arterial Disease: because the arteries are solely responsible for bringing to the vital organs and other parts of the body oxygen and nourishment without which they die, death and disease are often determined by the state of the arteries. The commonest cause of death in men over 40 is insufficient circulation to the brain or to the heart caused usually by atherosclerosis. In this condition the lining of the artery, called the intima, becomes thick and fibrous, and a fatty substance is deposited in its inner layers; passage of blood through the artery becomes less and less easy, for the elastic properties of the vessel wall are lost and the opening of the artery is narrowed.

SYMPTOMS: the symptoms of arterial disease depend on the part of the body supplied by the diseased arteries. If the blood supply to the brain becomes insufficient, the patient shows mental symptoms; if the heart is affected, he may develop angina pectoris (q.v.). Haemorrhages from diseased arteries, thrombosis and embolism are mechanisms which produce apoplexy (q.v.). Many of the changes normally found in old age are caused by disease of the arteries.

TREATMENT: in general directed to the alleviation of symptoms rather than the improvement of the underlying condition. Drugs, including alcohol, which dilate normal arteries are useful; although they may not have much effect on badly diseased arteries they may improve circulation through anastomoses (*see* Arteries). Some authorities recommend special diets low in cholesterol, for one of the main constituents of the atheromatous deposits in atherosclerosis is cholesterol, and rabbits fed with cholesterol develop atheroma. Treatment must also be directed towards any other condition, such as diabetes, which may make the arterial disease worse. Patients with arterial diseases should invariably stop smoking.

Arteries: the arteries are tubes with muscular walls which convey oxygenated blood from the heart to the rest of the body. As the arterial system splits into ever smaller branches, the resistance to the passage of blood increases; in a normal man it needs a pressure of 120 mm of mercury to ensure that the circulation is properly maintained, so that if you cut an artery, you are left in no doubt of the fact – the blood will spurt out. The very small terminal branches of the arteries are called arterioles, and they are continuous through the capillaries with the venous system. The arterial system has many anastomotic connections between its branches, so that interruption of one artery does not mean that all blood supply to the part is cut off; the circulation can be carried on through various anastomoses (q.v.). *See* Circulation of the Blood.

Arthritis: inflammation of a joint or joints. *See* Rheumatism.

Arthrodesis: surgical abolition of movement in a joint in order to stop pain or make the joint stable. *See* Ankylosis.

Arthroplasty: the opposite of arthrodesis; the surgical formation of moving joints.

Artificial Insemination: the introduction of semen into the uterus by artificial means. This procedure has been used for years in animal breeding, and it is available for families in which the husband is unable to impregnate his wife in the ordinary way because there is some impediment to intercourse. His semen is injected by a syringe into the womb, a method known as A.I.H. (artificial insemination by the husband). If the husband is sterile it is possible to obtain semen from an anonymous man (known to the doctor) and inject that into the wife's womb. This is called A.I.D. (artificial insemination by the donor) and is regarded as morally wrong by most religious bodies. It is specifically forbidden by the Roman Catholic Church, and the legitimacy of the child conceived by A.I.D. has been questioned.

Artificial Kidney: the function of the kidney (q.v.) is to filter the products of metabolism from the blood and to keep the chemical balance of the blood within normal limits. In severe kidney disease the kidney fails to do this and the patient becomes very ill; he may eventually die from accumulation of waste products and disturbance of the blood chemistry. It is now possible to withdraw blood from the body, remove the waste products from it and return it to the body again by using an artificial kidney. The principle is that the blood is passed over a membrane on the other side of which is a specially formulated solution. Waste products pass across the membrane, so that the composition of the blood is gradually rectified. The process has to be carried out frequently, but

59

by its use patients otherwise doomed can be kept alive indefinitely.

Artificial Respiration: before you can introduce air into a patient's lungs the airway (q.v.) must be clear, and the first step in reviving the apparently drowned is to get all the obstructions out of the mouth and throat, pull the tongue well forward and the head well back. Then pinch the patient's nose with the left hand, keep his jaw up with the right and blow into his mouth until you see the chest wall rise. Let the air come out of the lungs by itself before you blow again. The rate of artificial respiration should be between twelve and twenty times a minute, and it should be carried on until the patient starts breathing or is obviously dead. In cases of electrocution artificial respiration should go on for 2 hours before hope is abandoned. Some people may find mouth-to-mouth artificial respiration (the kiss of life) aesthetically unattractive, but it is possible to carry it out satisfactorily through a handkerchief put over the patient's mouth and nose. Other more modern techniques of artificial respiration – see II Kings iv, 34 – are the Holger-Nielsen method and Eve's rocking method. In the Holger-Nielsen technique the patient is laid flat on the ground face downwards with false teeth and anything obstructing the mouth and throat removed. The arms are placed forwards on each side of the head and the elbows bent outwards so that the hands lying palm downwards, one on top of the other, are beneath the forehead. The back is then smacked hard to bring the tongue forward. The operator kneels on his right knee in line with the patient's head and facing his back, the left leg being placed with the heel near the patient's right elbow. The hands are placed on the patient's shoulderblades and the operator leans forward until his straight arms are vertical, causing the patient to force air out of his chest. This takes $2\frac{1}{2}$ seconds and the hands are then moved along the arms until the patient's elbows are reached; done slowly and deliberately this should take 1 second. The arms and shoulders of the patient are then lifted upwards until the weight of the chest is felt but without moving either chest or head and this causes inspiration lasting a further $2\frac{1}{2}$ seconds. The elbows are then lowered and the operator's hands move back to the shoulderblades to repeat the cycle. In Eve's rocking method the patient is rocked up and down while lying tied to a stretcher, the tilt of the rocker extending 45° from the horizontal. This is carried out 10 times per minute and has the advantage of stimulating the circulation as well as the respiration. Nevertheless, the best method is without much doubt the kiss of life. In some cases the heart has stopped beating, or is beating so feebly that the pulse cannot be felt. If this is so, carry out cardiac massage by pushing hard on the breastbone about once a second – give about eight pushes, then inflate the lungs. The main thing is speed in starting artificial respiration and cardiac massage. Don't wait – get on with it. *See* Cardiac Massage.

Asbestosis: the lungs of workers in the asbestos industry are liable to react to inhaled asbestos dust by becoming fibrous. The symptoms produced are breathlessness, cough, and loss of appetite and weight. These symptoms, which may develop quite quickly, may become worse in established cases because of added tuberculous infection or cancerous change which is particularly liable to occur in asbestosis. Treatment is not effective, except for the cases in which tuberculosis or cancer develops, when treatment of the secondary disease is possible. The only real treatment is preventive. *See* Pneumoconiosis.

Ascaris: the roundworm, in appearance very like a large earthworm, which is a parasite in the intestines of people and horses. *See* Worms.

Ascites: accumulation of fluid inside the peritoneal cavity of the abdomen. It makes the abdomen swell in conditions such as heart, kidney and liver diseases which bring about exudation of fluid from the blood vessels. If the accumulation of fluid becomes very large it can be drawn off by a needle passed under local anaesthetic through the abdominal wall, an operation called paracentesis abdominis.

Ascorbic Acid: the chemical name of Vitamin C.

Asepsis: in modern surgery, infection is prevented by excluding germs from the operation wound rather than destroying them after they have gained entry (*see* Antiseptic). In theory the operating theatre is sterile, but everybody who works there is, of course, covered with germs. All staff in operating theatres should change their clothes before they go in; if this is not possible, they must at least cover their clothes up with a gown and discard their outdoor shoes. Masks must cover the mouth to catch infected droplets from the nose and throat and caps must completely cover the hair. The surgeon washes his hands thoroughly and wears sterile gloves; he is careful not to touch anything that has not been sterilized, and he even avoids touching things he knows to be sterile – his gown or instruments – more than he must. Everyone who enters an operating theatre must submit to the discipline of asepsis; there is no room for carelessness or sloppiness.

Asphyxia: suffocation. It can be brought about by obstruction to the air passages or by lack of oxygen in the air, or by gases which interfere with the use of oxygen by the body. An example of this is the gas carbon monoxide – it has no colour, smell or visible vapour, and it is rapidly absorbed by the lungs. It has 200 times more combining power with the blood than has oxygen so that it soon swamps the circulation. People asphyxiated by obstruction to their breathing or by lack of oxygen go blue, but victims of carbon monoxide poisoning retain the red colour of their cheeks and lips. Sometimes the problem of rescuing those overcome by asphyxia is very difficult, and it may be hard to remember that two casualties are far worse than one. If a fresh-air respirator or oxygen apparatus is not to be obtained, then at least the rescuer should have a rope tied round him in case he is overcome. Coal gas is lighter than air, so that where coal gas is known to be present there may be fresher air near the floor.

TREATMENT: make sure the airway (q.v.) is clear and that the patient can breathe freely. If necessary give artificial respiration, and where possible give oxygen.

Aspiration: withdrawal of fluid from the body, for example, from the joint in the case of an effusion into the knee.

Aspirin: trade name invented by the Bayer Drug Company for acetylsalicylic acid (the German name for salicylic acid is *Spirsäure*). It is a mild analgesic, it lowers body temperature raised by disease, and it has an important effect in reducing the swelling which accompanies inflammation. It is extremely useful in the treatment of rheumatic fever, in which it is used in large doses for a long time. Unfortunately, aspirin has a tendency to irritate the stomach and cause bleeding, but soluble calcium aspirin is less irritant than pure aspirin. The signs of over-dosage are headache, ringing in the ears, confusion and sleepiness. In more severe poisoning the patient vomits and may become delirious. Other harmful effects of aspirin include urticaria (q.v.) in sensitive people, and, particularly in those who suffer from asthma, spasm of the air passages of the lung. *See* Salicylates.

Asthenia: debility, or loss of strength.

Asthma: a disease of the respiratory system which produces difficulty in breathing. The difficulty is not in breathing in, but breathing out, and it is caused by spasm of the smaller air passages in the lung. The effect is to blow the lungs up, because the patient cannot drive the air properly out of his lungs before he has to take another breath. Attacks may last an hour or, in 'status asthmaticus', for days, and the disease is found in children as well as adults.

CAUSE: Allergy (q.v.), infection of the lung, and emotional factors. Patients often know what will bring on an attack: for example, cats in the house, wool or feathers. Dust can be a precipitating factor, particularly house dust containing a mite called Dermatophagoides culinae. Unfortunately attempts to desensitize patients are not often successful, possibly because asthma is caused by a combination of factors. Although it is uncommon for asthma to be caused by psychological reasons alone, it is a matter of common observation that emotional tension, particularly involving anxiety or frustration, can start off an attack. Infection is very important in asthma; many people develop the disease after a severe infection, and most asthmatics are prone to recurrent attacks of bronchitis which may become chronic.

SYMPTOMS: attacks of breathlessness which often occur at night. The patient has to sit up, and the attack may last for a short or long while. As the difficulty in breathing gets worse the patient develops a cough, and the condition may become very distressing. Children may vomit during an attack. The most obvious features to the bystander are the wheezing, coughing and anxiety which accompany the attacks.

The only other common condition which produces attacks of breathlessness at night is heart failure.

TREATMENT: for an acute attack this is by drugs which dilate the air passages of the lungs. There are a number of drugs which have this effect, and the most commonly used are ephedrine and isoprenaline. Ephedrine is given in tablet form, and isoprenaline as an aerosol; sometimes it is compounded with atropine to make its action last longer. A severe attack of asthma may require an injection of adrenaline. The drug used ought to be taken as quickly as possible – as soon, in fact, as the patient suspects that an attack is about to develop. It may be possible to prevent attacks coming on during the night by taking promethazine hydrochloride (Phenergan) an hour before going to bed. If it is known that the patient is sensitive to a particular stimulus, a course of desensitizing injections can be tried (*see* Allergy); if the attacks are determined more by emotional factors, psychiatric treatment may help. The treatment of chronic cases is not straightforward. Infection plays a larger part than in 'episodic' asthma, and although the object of treatment is the same, that is to keep the air passages dilated, drugs which dilate the bronchi have less effect after damage by chronic infection, so that while isoprenaline is still effective, there is a natural tendency to increase the dose to excess. Infections are treated as they arise, but they may be severe and require a prolonged course of antibiotics. If all else fails and asthma is making the patient's life miserable, then corticosteroids (q.v.) may be used, although the treatment carries various risks. Once it has been established corticosteroid therapy has to be carried on for a very long time – it may be for life. Recently the substance disodium cromoglycate (Intal) has been introduced; it prevents asthma by interfering with allergic reactions in the lungs, and is taken by inhalation. Disodium cromoglycate treatment may be combined with other forms of therapy.

Astigmatism: if the refracting surfaces of the lens and cornea of the eye are not truly spherical, objects seen will be distorted in one axis (a circle for example, will look oval). Glasses which have a cylindrical lens are prescribed to correct the abnormality.

Astragalus: or Talus. The bone of the ankle that forms the link between the bones of the foot and the bones of the leg, the tibia and fibula.

Astringents: these cause contraction of mucous surfaces and therefore stop bleeding or discharge of moderate degree. Examples are tannic acid, witch-hazel (hamamelis) and alum (aluminium and potassium or aluminium and ammonium sulphate).

Ataractic Drugs: these produce a calm mind without clouding the consciousness. *See* Tranquillizers.

Ataxia: inability to co-ordinate movements of the muscles. It is due to a defect in the part of the sensory system normally concerned with detecting and signalling the position of the muscles and joints.

Atelectasis: collapse of part of the lung or failure to expand at birth.

Atheroma: a disease of the arterial wall in which there is thickening of the inner layer with deposition of fatty matter in the thickened part. The deposited fatty patches can be seen as light areas. *See* Arterial Disease.

Athlete's Foot: ringworm of the feet. The disease is caused by a fungus which lives in the horny, or keratinous, layer of the skin. Because it likes wet and warm places it is found in the clefts between the toes, usually the fourth.
SYMPTOMS: itching and discomfort may lead to the discovery of sodden white dead skin in the toe cleft, or the fungus infection may give rise to an acute attack of eczema bad enough to put the patient to bed.
TREATMENT: if there is eczema or added infection of the skin this is treated first, but it is sensible to avoid antibiotics as the infecting fungus may make the patient sensitive. In the chronic phase the disease is almost impossible to eradicate, but it can be kept under control by keeping the feet dry, clean and cool, using dusting powder and some application to kill the fungus such as Whitfield's ointment or undecylenic acid (Desenex). The infection spreads easily and is caught by

walking in an infected place in bare feet, especially around swimming pools.

Atomic Radiation: nuclear weapons produce a large area of devastation and death by blast and burning, and to this they add the harmful effects of atomic radiation. These effects are produced by gamma-rays, which are electromagnetic radiations very much like X-rays, and neutrons – slow neutrons are not important, but fast neutrons have high energy and penetration. In addition the bombs can give rise to danger from the fallout of radioactive isotopes (q.v.) such as ^{113}I, ^{90}Sn and ^{137}Cs, which contaminate food and air. Natural sources of radiation are small (one source of radiation is granite), but medical and industrial sources are considerable. Apart from the study of the victims of the two bombs exploded over Japan in 1945, and those involved in various accidents, most of our knowledge of the effects of radiation is derived from the observation of patients exposed to radiotherapy.

Effects of excessive exposure to radiation

SYMPTOMS: Acute; very high doses produce damage to the brain. This is fatal, and shows itself within a few hours; the victim develops nausea and vomiting, and then tremors, unsteadiness and convulsions. Lower doses damage the stomach and intestines, and the patient suffers from nausea, vomiting and severe diarrhoea coming on a few days after exposure. Still lower doses may produce vomiting and nausea without diarrhoea. If the victim survives these illnesses, he may after a few weeks start to show the effects of damage to the bone marrow. The formation of blood cells is disturbed; at first the white cells become fewer (*see* Agranulocytosis) and then the red cells disappear so that the patient develops severe anaemia and, possibly, fatal bacterial infection. Transfusions, meticulous nursing and treatment with antibiotics may be successful in preventing death.

LONG-TERM EFFECTS: cataracts (q.v.) may develop after exposure, and it is common knowledge that leukaemia may ensue years after a damaging dose. Various cancers are also known to occur after radiation. Although nobody can avoid the conclusions from evidence of animal observations that radiation must produce genetic damage, it has so far been impossible to demonstrate harmful mutations in man.

Sterility following exposure to radiation may be reversible. *See* Ionizing Radiation.

Atresia: incomplete development, resulting in the lack of an opening in structures normally perforated, for example the anus, the oesophagus.

Atria: the two smaller cavities of the heart which receive the blood from the veins and pump it into the ventricles. Often called the auricle, but this is, properly speaking, only an appendage of the atrium, not the whole chamber.

Atrophy: wasting away or shrivelling up of a part of the body as the result of lack of nutrition or use.

Atropine: an alkaloid found in the plant deadly nightshade. It dilates and paralyses the pupil of the eye, dries up the secretions of the mouth and the air passages of the lungs, and relaxes the muscle of the gut and the ureters. It is frequently used in the examination by ophthalmoscopy of the back of the eye, or in treating eye conditions where it is necessary to dilate and paralyse the pupil, but the action of atropine on the eye lasts for several days and the similar but shorter action of homatropine may be preferred. As a premedication before anaesthesia atropine has much to commend it, and it is useful in the treatment of gastric and duodenal ulcers and of renal and biliary colic. Atropine poisoning causes restlessness, convulsions, coma and paralysis of the muscles of respiration. Atropine is the specific antidote to poisonous organo-phosphorus compounds used as insecticides (T.E.P.P., H.E.T.P., Parathion).

Audiogram: an audiogram is a record of the examination of the power of hearing by audiometry. Each ear is tested in turn through earphones. The subject is asked to listen to pure tones of different frequencies, and the intensity is altered to find the quietest sound that can be heard. The frequencies are altered to cover the range normally heard by the human ear, and the results are plotted as an audiogram, which shows the sensitivity of the ear tested compared to the sensitivity of a normal ear.

67

Aura: sensation felt by a subject who is about to have an epileptic attack.

Aureomycin: trade name of chlortetracycline. *See* Tetracyclines.

Auricle: *see* Atria.

Auscultation: method of examining the body by listening. Mostly used in the chest, where the doctor can listen to the sounds made by the heart and by the air passing through the lungs. In ancient times the ear was applied directly to the chest wall, but at the beginning of the nineteenth century the Frenchman Laënnec invented the stethoscope. This was at first a rolled-up piece of paper, and then a wooden cylinder; gradually the modern binaural instrument was evolved with two ear-pieces and a separate chestpiece, connected by rubber tubing.
Many signs of disease in the heart and lung can be picked up by the educated ear, as well as certain conditions of the abdomen and even of the skull and brain.

Autoclave: in the autoclave steam under pressure sterilizes instruments, dressings, etc. to be used in surgery. A valve regulates the pressure of the steam and therefore the height of the temperature just as it does in a domestic pressure cooker.

Autogenous: applied usually to vaccines prepared from organisms found in the patient's own body (for example in boils or bronchitis) and used in treating his disease.

Autoimmune Diseases: individuals normally react to the introduction of foreign tissues or proteins into the body (*see* Allergy). In some cases, it seems probable that individuals produce an immune reaction to one of their own tissues in consequence of changes which are not understood. The resulting antibodies set up inflammation which causes disease of the organ or tissue concerned. Diseases which are thought to be produced by autoimmunity occur in the thyroid gland, the suprarenal bodies, and the thymus; myasthenia gravis (q.v.), rheumatoid arthritis, lupus erythematosus, some kinds of blood disorder, and the complications of orchitis or encephalitis following mumps are other possible manifestations of this important and dangerous abnormality.

Autointoxication: self-poisoning thought to be brought about by an area of sepsis somewhere in the body, for example infection in a tooth socket or in the sinuses, which some believe causes arthritis. As a term for the alleged results of constipation the word is now out of date, for nobody who is qualified to know thinks that constipation leads to 'poisoning of the bloodstream' or indeed any evil consequences except a feeling of fullness in the lower abdomen. There is little evidence that septic foci do in fact produce disease elsewhere in the body.

Autonomic Nervous System: that part of the nervous system which regulates those aspects of body function which are not under conscious control, for example the heartbeat, movements of the intestines, size of the pupil of the eye and, to some extent, the chemistry of the blood. It has two divisions, the sympathetic and parasympathetic, whose actions are opposed to each other; roughly speaking the sympathetic prepares the body for action, the parasympathetic for rest. *See* Nervous System.

Autopsy: examination of the dead, made so that physicians may see for themselves the effects of injury or disease upon the vital processes, arrive at a true diagnosis and gather new observations for use in the future.

Avascular Necrosis: fracture or other injury to a bone may disrupt an artery so that the blood supply to one fragment is cut off and the cells die. One of the bones most liable to this process is the femur, and fracture of the neck of this bone, a common accident in the elderly, may lead to avascular necrosis of the head of the bone.

Avomine: proprietary name for promethazine theoclate, which is effective in the prevention of travel sickness. Avomine causes sleepiness and increases susceptibility to alcohol.

Axon: the long extension from a nerve cell along which nerve impulses run. A nerve is made up of a bundle of axons.

Azotaemia: the presence of nitrogen which is not bound up in a protein in the blood. It may occur in kidney failure or as the result of abnormal blood chemistry. *See* Uraemia.

B

Babinski Reflex: if the outer part of the sole of the foot is firmly stroked the toes normally 'clench' – the great toe goes down and the other toes curl. Before an infant starts to walk, and when the nerve tracts that connect the brain with the motor nerves (the corticospinal tracts) are damaged, the response is altered, and the great toe goes up while the other toes fan out. This abnormal response is called Babinski's sign or reflex.

Bacillus: a name used originally in bacteriology to mean a rod-shaped as opposed to a round micro-organism. It is now properly used only to denote one genus, of which Bacillus anthracis is the sole organism harmful to man, but old usage dies hard.

Bacitracin: an antibiotic active against staphylococci. It was originally isolated from a culture of Bacillus subtilis taken from the leg infection of a little girl of 7 called Margaret Tracey, when she was a patient in the Presbyterian Hospital, New York. It is too toxic to be given by injection, but in combination with other antibiotics it can be applied externally to wounds, abscesses or burns. It can also be taken by mouth.

Backache: is a symptom of many conditions. It may arise from the bones of the vertebral column or the pelvis and the muscles associated with them, or from organs some way away. Conditions localized in the back which produce pain are fibrositis, prolapsed intervertebral disc, muscular strains, or the strain of exercise involving muscles not ordinarily used. Osteoarthritis of the spine may cause pain in older people, and disease of the bones or joints can cause pain at any age. Kidney disease or disease of the ureters produces pain in the loin, and low back pain often accompanies disease of the ovaries or of the womb or menstrual disorders. Pain under the right shoulderblade is felt in gall-bladder disease, and peptic ulcers may cause pain on

71

the left side of the back at the level of the twelfth rib. The pain of pleurisy may be felt in the back and in influenza there is often backache. A bad posture is a common cause of backache, as also are psychological conditions associated with emotional stress which bring about spasm of the muscles.

Bacteraemia: the condition of having bacteria in the bloodstream.

Bacteria: members of the kingdom Protista, which includes animals and plants made up of one cell. Bacteria are smaller than yeasts but larger than viruses. Some produce disease, some are harmless, some are actively useful: for example, the nitrogenous bacteria of the soil. They can be classified by their shape: cocci are round, bacilli are like rods, vibrios are curved like a comma, and the spirilla is wavy. Staphylococci are cocci arranged in bunches, streptococci are arranged in chains, diplococci in pairs. Spirochaetes and Rickettsiae are other Protista of interest in medicine but they are not properly to be called bacteria. A further classification of bacteria is founded on their reaction to a method of staining invented by the Danish physician Gram; bacteria are said to be Gram-negative or Gram-positive. *See* Gram's Stain.

Bagassosis: a disease of the lungs similar to farmer's lung caused by inhaling a mould growing on bagasse, which is broken sugar cane left after the extraction of sugar. Bagasse is used in making artificial boards.

B.A.L.: this stands for British Anti-Lewisite, a substance called dimercaprol discovered in World War 2 by Professor R. A. Peters of Oxford, originally as an antidote to Lewisite poisoning (q.v.). It was found to be a useful treatment for poisoning with some of the heavy metals – lead, arsenic, antimony, gold and mercury.

Balanitis: inflammation of the parts beneath the foreskin.

Baldness: the hair may be lost after acute fevers, in thyroid disease, secondary syphilis or tuberculosis, but it grows again in most cases when the disease is cured. The baldness which comes on with advancing age cannot be cured. It is hereditary and is apparently determined by hormone balance, for it is not seen in eunuchs. In men it affects the whole head, but in women it only affects the crown of the head and never leads to complete loss of hair. Alopecia areata (q.v.) is a condition in which bald patches appear which may progress to involve the whole scalp. Nervous strain or shock rarely has anything to do with the loss of hair.

Ballismus: violent involuntary throwing about of the limbs. It may affect only one half of the body, when it is known as hemiballismus. It is caused by damage to a nucleus called the corpus Luysii below the thalamus in the midbrain.

Balsam: vegetable resin combined with oil, for example Canada balsam, which comes from the balsam fir of North America; or balsam of Gilead, still made from a tree which grows by the Red Sea.

Bamboo Spine: (Ankylosing Spondylitis). A disease of unknown cause belonging to the rheumatoid group of afflictions affecting young people between the ages of 14 and 40, in which the ligaments of the spine become calcified and are changed into bone, so that the spine is completely stiff, resembling a length of bamboo.

Bandage: a piece of material used for binding wounds or keeping dressings and splints in place. Roller bandages are made of long strips of fabric wound into a firm roll, but they are now only used in special cases, such as where the patient is sensitive to adhesives or, as in the case of the lower jaw, where adhesive bandages are not practical. Otherwise plain roller bandages have been supplanted by adhesive bandages, or by seamless tubular gauze made in various sizes and marketed under the name Tubegauz. Roller bandages made of crêpe are still used, particularly on the leg for support and pressure over injured knees or ankles.

Barber's Itch: *see* Sycosis Barbae.

Barbiturates: derivatives of malonylurea or barbituric

73

acid. A group of drugs used for their depressant action on the central nervous system; they produce sedation, sleep or anaesthesia. They may be divided into three groups according to the length of their action.

Group 1. Thiopentone (Pentothal), methohexitone (Brietal, Brevital), thialbarbitone. Action: very short. Group 1 barbiturates are therefore used as intravenous anaesthetics. *Group 2.* Pentobarbitone (Nembutal), quinalbarbitone (Seconal), cyclobarbitone (Phanodorm), amylobarbitone (Amytal), butobarbitone (Soneryl). Action: a dose of 100 mg produces about six hours sleep. Group 2 barbiturates are used as hypnotics. *Group 3.* Barbitone (Veronal), phenobarbitone (Gardenal or Luminal), diallybarbituric acid. Action: slow. Not generally used as hypnotics. Phenobarbitone is used for its action against epilepsy and for mild sedation.

All barbiturates are dangerous and must not be used except under medical advice, and they must be locked up where they cannot easily be got at if they are kept in a house where there are children. Doctors are very careful about prescribing barbiturates for various reasons: they can produce dependence or even addiction; they are often used for suicide; they produce confusion in the elderly; and patients are quite frequently sensitive to them. Alcohol should never be taken with barbiturates as together they make a particularly dangerous mixture; an ordinary dose of barbiturate used as a sleeping pill may when taken with alcohol produce coma or severe depression of respiration. Patients taking barbiturates must be careful that they do not keep the bottle by their bed at night, for it is possible for the drug to produce a state in which the patient takes several consecutive doses without knowing that he has taken more than one.

Barium: barium sulphate is insoluble in water and is radio-opaque – that is, it shows up on X-ray plates because radiations do not pass through barium. It is therefore made up into mixtures which are taken by mouth to outline the shape of the stomach or given by rectal enema to show the form of the lower intestines.

Barotrauma: injury caused by pressure. The term is used to describe injury to the eardrum in aviators caused by a difference between the pressure in the middle ear and the pressure of the atmosphere. Similarly, if there is any swelling of the mucous membrane at the openings of the sinuses (q.v.) this may block free passage between the inside of the sinus and the nose, and damage may result from difference in pressure inside the sinus and in the nose. People with bad colds which may give rise to inflammation and swelling at the lower end of the Eustachian tubes or at the openings of the nasal sinuses and thus lead to the risk of barotrauma are advised not to fly without a decongestant.

Bartholin's Gland: Bartholin was a Danish anatomist who gave his name to a pair of glands lying on each side of the opening of the vagina. They sometimes become infected and cause a painful abscess.

Basal Metabolic Rate: the output of energy at rest is about the same for all mammals if it is expressed not per unit of weight but per unit of body surface area. The B.M.R. is measured by finding the amount of pure oxygen a patient takes up in 3 or 5 minutes from a closed circuit and comparing his mean oxygen consumption with the normal level. His surface area is calculated from his height and weight. The Basal Metabolic Rate is increased in overactivity of the thyroid gland, and diminished when the gland is functioning below the normal level as in myxoedema. *See* Goitre.

Basophil: a white blood cell which stains with basic dyes. (In chemistry a *base* is a substance which will combine with acids to form salts.)

B.C.G. Vaccine: a vaccine introduced in France about 1908 by Calmette and Guérin. The Calmette-Guérin bacillus used is a live attenuated strain of the Mycobacterium tuberculosis. It may be given to infants who are especially exposed to the risk of tuberculous infection and to young people who are shown by the tuberculin test to have no natural immunity to the disease. It may be given to all medical students, veterinary students and nurses who have no natural immunity and come into contact with tuberculosis. It is not used in the United States because chemical means of prevention are considered more effective without interfering with the skin test used in epidemiology and private practice as a single means to test incidence of infection in the population.

Beat Elbow, Hand or Knee: a term applied by miners to swelling and inflammation of the joints arising from constant pressure and ingrained particles of dirt.

Bed Bug: a wingless blood-sucking insect known scientifically as Cimex lectularius. It hides by day in cracks in walls or floors, or in grooves in beds, and feeds on man at night.

Bedsores: form in those confined to bed who cannot change their position often and regularly. They are most common over the heels and the sacrum, for here pressure on the skin quickly interferes with the blood supply and causes necrosis or death of the tissues. Bedsores also form on the shoulders, the elbows and the ankles. The affected part at first goes blue and then ulcerates to form a black slough which comes off to leave an open sore likely to get bigger. The most important measure in treatment is prevention. Two-hourly changes of position and a dry skin are essential and should be ensured in all bedridden people, not only the old, thin, debilitated or paralysed. The skin must be washed at least once a day, dried carefully, rubbed with spirit and dusted over with powder. When an area becomes red or bluish it should be padded with cotton wool and an air-ring or air bed used. Treatment of established bedsores is a matter for the surgeon.

Bed Wetting: children normally learn to control the passage of urine by day during the second year, and by night during the third year. Bed wetting may go on until the fourth or even fifth year without the child being abnormal. About one in ten children who wet the bed after they are five have some disease which can account for the trouble; the rest are found to be suffering from an emotional disturbance, commonly lack of security.
Punishment plays no part in the successful treatment of the condition.

Belladonna: a preparation of Atropa belladonna, or

deadly nightshade, used to relieve spasm of the stomach, and involuntary muscle spasm in general, because it contains atropine. One of the actions of atropine is to dilate the pupil of the eye, and a widely dilated pupil is or was thought by some to be an attractive attribute of a beautiful lady. Belladonna can therefore produce beauty not only in the eye of the beholder; but unfortunately it produces blurred vision as well as that faraway look.

Bell's Palsy: the commonest cause of paralysis of the face. The facial nerve enters the face just below the ear, having passed through a canal in the bone related to the ear and the mastoid air cells. The cause of Bell's palsy is not known, but the facial nerve becomes inflamed inside the canal and is unable to transmit impulses. The condition is benign and usually recovers of itself after a few weeks.

SYMPTOMS: one side of the face is paralysed, so that tears flow from the eye and the mouth dribbles. Food may collect in the palsied cheek.

DIAGNOSIS: the sudden onset may be confused with a stroke, but the difference is soon obvious. Facial paralysis can also be caused by injury to the skull which compresses or tears the nerve in its canal.

TREATMENT: in three-quarters of the cases no treatment is needed, for recovery is spontaneous, but until the patient can close his eye properly it is best to cover it up for protection against dust. A wire splint can be arranged to hold up the corner of the mouth. Corticotrophin as soon as the diagnosis is made is said to be beneficial, as it may prevent the nerve swelling too greatly in the bony canal.

Operations have been carried out to decompress the nerve by removing part of the wall of the canal, but the necessity for this is not universally accepted. If no recovery of the paralysis takes place plastic operations can improve the appearance of the paralysed half of the face.

Benadryl: proprietary name for diphenhydramine, an antihistamine (q.v.).

Bends: *see* Caisson Disease.

Benzene Poisoning: benzene, not to be confused with

77

benzine, is used in industry as a solvent. Acute poisoning by benzene causes headache, giddiness and restlessness, sometimes confusion, muscular twitching and occasionally convulsions. Chronic benzene poisoning which results from exposure over a number of years causes aplastic anaemia and agranulocytosis (q.v.), because the bone marrow, which makes the blood cells, is destroyed.

Benzocaine: a rather weak substitute for cocaine, made up into lozenges to ease pain in the throat, or into ointment to relieve itching of the skin round the anus.

Berger Rhythm: in 1924 Hans Berger, a neurologist in Jena, described electrical activity in the brain showing itself as a wave rhythm between 8 and 13 times a second in the electroencephalogram (q.v.). To this day the source of the rhythmic electric activity is unknown, but it is a matter of observation that the rhythm only occurs in healthy subjects when they close their eyes.

Beri-Beri: a vitamin deficiency disease at one time prevalent in the rice-eating countries of the East, but never very common in Europe. There are two main types, the 'wet' and the 'dry'. In the wet type, the heart muscle becomes flabby and the patient weak and oedematous (i.e. with swelling of the legs and abdomen due to excess fluid leakage into the tissues), and in the dry the main damage is to the nerves supplying the limbs so that the patient is unable to walk properly. Beri-beri is caused by lack of Vitamin B_1, or thiamine, and it used to occur among people who lived on polished rice – the husk with the vitamin-containing embryo having been removed in the milling process – and those who drank spirits to excess so that they developed a gastritis which not only interfered with the absorption of vitamins but also took the appetite away. It was common in the Japanese prison camps of World War 2. The treatment is to give thiamine, and the results are dramatic. The total daily requirements of thiamine are about 1.5 mg a day. It is found in all living cells, and therefore in most natural foods.

Beryllium Poisoning: workers in industries that use beryllium, especially beryllium oxide, may find their eyes irritated and weeping, and develop a severe cough and sore throat. If they are removed from exposure to the metal the lung irritation recovers in a matter of weeks. There is no specific treatment, but in cases where recovery is delayed treatment with corticosteroids may be advised. Another reaction to beryllium produces dermatitis and ulcers on the skin, which are probably due to sensitivity rather than poisoning.

Bicarbonate of Soda: (baking soda). *See* Alkalies.

Biceps: the biceps muscle, which stands out between the shoulder and the elbow at the front of the upper arm, takes its name from the two 'heads' which arise in the region of the shoulder. The belly of the muscle lies in the front part of the upper arm, and the tendon runs across the elbow joint to be fixed into the radius and into the connective tissue covering the muscle of the forearm. The biceps plays a big part in flexing the elbow; it also is used to supinate the forearm – that is to say, it helps turn the screwdriver.

Bile: a greenish-brown fluid secreted by the liver; it is a watery solution of glucose, urea, and complicated substances such as bile salts, cholesterol, and bilirubin, with some protein. The bile duct runs from the liver to the duodenum, and the bile can run straight from the liver into the small intestine, but normally it is diverted through the cystic duct into the gall-bladder where it is concentrated and stored. Bile in the gall-bladder has more mucus in it than when it is secreted by the liver, and it contains a greater concentration of cholesterol, bile pigment and calcium. This sometimes results in the formation of gallstones in the gall-bladder. Bile is partly a secretion which helps in the digestion of fats, and partly an excretion of substances which result from the destruction of old red blood cells. Many substances excreted in the bile are reabsorbed from the gut, and again excreted in the bile, circulating from the liver to the intestine and back again. Blockage of the bile ducts can cause jaundice, and interfere with the digestion and absorption of fat from the intestine. 'Biliousness' and 'liverishness', thought to arise from disorder of the bile, are largely imaginary diseases popular among those who have been in the East; they are polite names for the results of eating or drinking too much. The vomiting of bile is popularly considered to have a sinister significance, but any attacks of repeated vomiting may result in discoloration of the vomit with bile whether the cause be trivial or serious. *See* Gall-bladder.

Bilharzia: a disease found in Africa, South America and in the East, affecting the bladder and intestine.

CAUSE: a fluke, Schistosoma haematobium, picked up by man from infected water, either by bathing or wading in the water or by drinking it. The parasites enter the bloodstream and travel to the portal vein (which carries blood from the intestines to the liver) where they stay for six weeks and become mature adults. The male and female copulate in the portal vein; the female then goes off to lay her eggs in the mucous membrane of the bladder, rectum or lower colon. The eggs leave the body in the urine or faeces, and if one drops into water it changes into a miracidium, in which form it can swim. The miracidia search out a water-snail, for it is only in such a creature that the flukes can develop into the next stage, the cercaria. The cercariae live in the water until the next unwary man comes along, and the cycle starts again.

SYMPTOMS: the eggs in the bladder or rectum cause irritation and bleeding. In the case of the bladder, blood is passed in the urine. Chronic inflammation produces pain, frequency of urination, stones, and possibly cancer. Eggs in the rectum create the symptoms of dysentery; enlargement of the liver and spleen may produce discomfort in the upper abdomen.

DIAGNOSIS: the diagnosis is made on the symptoms and on the discovery of eggs in the urine or faeces.

TREATMENT: antimony compounds destroy the parasite, and the most effective drug is sodium antimony tartrate (tartar emetic), given intravenously. Fouadin given intramuscularly is used in some cases, and another drug which can be given by intravenous injection is Triostam. Miracil D has recently been introduced as a remedy to be taken by mouth, and another oral preparation is niridazole. All these drugs produce side effects, ranging from abdominal pain and nausea to heart failure or temporary madness. There is as yet no harmless remedy that can be taken by mouth. Local damage caused by the parasite in the bladder, rectum and liver may call for surgical treatment.

PREVENTION: without water-snails the disease cannot occur. Control of snails is therefore the obvious way of preventing infection. Apart from this, a great deal can be achieved by simple measures, as with nearly every tropical disease. Proper sanitation, the disposal of excreta without fouling water supplies, and stopping people wading and bathing in infected water will go a long way towards cutting down bilharzia, which is one of the great plagues of the world. *See* Flukes.

Binet-Simon Test: the earliest form of intelligence test devised in 1904 by the Frenchman Alfred Binet in collaboration with Théophile Simon. Items such as 'point to nose, eyes, and mouth' (for age 3) and 'repeat months of the year' (one of the questions at age 10) were standardized for children of various age-groups according to the average performance of the group in the population as a whole. When a child of 7 passed all the tests for age 7 his mental age was said to be 7 and his Intelligence Quotient (mental age divided by chronological age × 100) was said to be 100; if his real age was 8 years 6 months and he could only pass a test for 88 months his I.Q. would be 88/102 or 86. In the form revised by Terman this test is still in use for the younger age-groups. An I.Q. of at least 120 is necessary before an individual would have much chance of passing into a university, or an equivalent institution, and profiting therefrom.

Bioassay: the biological effect of an unknown drug, or of a known drug in unknown concentration, when compared with the effect of a standard solution enables the pharmacologist to identify the drug and measure the strength of a solution.

Biochemistry: the chemistry of living things.

Biopsy: examination of fragments of tissue taken from a living creature. Usually applied to the microscopical examination of fragments of tumour tissue taken from patients to determine the nature of a growth.

Biotin: a member of the Vitamin B group, an essential constituent of the diet of men and animals.

Bird Breeder's Lung: an allergic reaction taking place in the lung after inhalation of the dried droppings of birds. *See* Farmer's Lung.

Birth: the average child weighs 7 lb (3.2 kg) at birth. A still-born child is 'any child which has issued from its mother after the 28th week of pregnancy and which did not at any time after being completely expelled from its mother breathe or show any other signs of life'. Premature birth is one which takes place before the natural time but in which the child is capable of surviving. A birth which takes place so prematurely that the child must necessarily die is known as an abortion or miscarriage.

Birth Control: *see* Contraception.

Birthmark: the commonest kind of birthmark is a benign tumour called a haemangioma, which grows rapidly in the first year of the child's life. It is made up of many small blood vessels and blood spaces and is red or purple. Usually only slightly raised above the surface of the skin, it may sometimes be heaped up – the 'strawberry' birthmark. The best treatment is watchful waiting, for in time the haemangioma stops growing, a pale mark appears at the centre, and over the course of a few years the blemish entirely disappears. Another type of birthmark is the well-known port-wine stain, which does not disappear spontaneously and is best treated by the application of diathermy. Ugly hairy moles should be removed surgically after the 5th birthday.

Bismuth: a metal used in the treatment of amoebic dysentery as emetine bismuth iodide or compounded with arsenic to form glycobiarsol. It is also used as bismuth subgallate in the treatment of piles, but is no longer used in the treatment of syphilis.

Bistoury: a type of knife once used in surgery. It was long and narrow, and could have a straight or curved blade.

Bites and Stings: *Dog-bites:* are only serious if the dog has rabies.

TREATMENT: if the dog is healthy, the wound is treated like any other; it is cleaned and dressed, while precautions are taken against tetanus. If the dog is likely to have rabies more elaborate treatment is needed (*see* Rabies).

Snake-bites: in Europe, only the adder or viper is poisonous, and death from snake-bite is very uncommon; estimates vary between two and twenty in a year.

In North America, there are more poisonous snakes: rattlesnake, water moccasin, copperhead, and in parts of the South, coral snake; and between 1950 and 1959, 138 people in the United States died of snake-bites.

In India, between 20,000 and 30,000 people every year die of the bites of cobras, kraits, vipers and sea-snakes.

In Africa, the snakes include cobras, some of which are able to spit a jet of venom into a man's eye, green and black mambas, and the ugly and excessively venomous gaboon viper.

In Australia, the dangerous snakes are the death adder, tiger snake, copperhead, brown snake and black snake. There are also vicious snakes called taipans.

SYMPTOMS: a man who thinks he has been bitten by a snake is with very few exceptions frightened, and the first thing is to quieten him down, and remember that he may complain of all sorts of symptoms which only confuse the issue. In general, snake venom falls into two classes: one attacks the nervous system, and is called neurotoxic; and the other, cytotoxic, attacks the cells both of fixed tissues and of the blood. One paralyses the prey while it is eaten, the other helps the snake by pre-digesting his prey.

Rattlesnakes, adders and vipers secrete toxins which are mainly cytotoxic, that is, poisonous to cells both of fixed tissues and of the blood. Pain and marked reaction at the site of the bite is characteristic of a viper bite; rattlesnake bites may produce local gangrene. A severe bite will cause blood staining of the urine and the motions. Nose bleeding and vomiting of blood may occur, for the venom diminishes the clotting power of the blood.

Cobras, kraits and mambas are among the snakes with predominantly neurotoxic venom; there is less pain at the site of the bite, and less local reaction. The main effect is paralysis of the nervous system, with spreading numbness, difficulty in speaking, disturbance of vision, nausea and vomiting and great anxiety. The patient may become unsteady on his feet, and the breathing may be depressed.

TREATMENT: kill the snake and keep it so that it can be identified. Send for help and keep still. If you have to move, move slowly. Suck the wound, if it is accessible, but do not cut it. Wash it well. If the bite is on a limb, splint the limb so that it cannot move, and tighten a tourniquet between the heart and the wound. This must be loosened every 30 minutes for 1 minute.

Opinion is against the use of antivenom in Europe, for it is made from horse serum and the risk of anaphylactic shock (q.v.) is probably greater than the risk from the snake-bite. Where snakes are very venomous, however, it is a different matter, and antivenom is injected both locally around the bite and intravenously. If there is a severe reaction adrenaline and antihistamines are used. Antibiotics should be given, for all snakes have pathogenic bacteria in their mouths, and precautions should be taken against tetanus. The most important single thing to remember about snakebite is: *keep still.*

Spider-bites: the Black Widow spider is found in America, and there are other poisonous species in Europe, India, Russia and Australia.

SYMPTOMS: the Black Widow lays its eggs near latrines, and the consequence is that the victim is often bitten in the rear. About half an hour after the bite, which may not be noticed, the venom causes the muscles to contract, and cramping pain is felt all over the body. If the cramp is very marked in the muscles of the abdomen the condition may be mistaken for an 'acute abdomen'. It is said that the soles of the feet burn after a spider-bite.

TREATMENT: the injection of atropine and morphine, and intravenous calcium gluconate. The brown recluse spider in the southern area of the United States is an aggressive arachnid which causes a necrotizing ulcer at the site of its bite.

The only biting spider likely to be found in Great Britain is a large one called Phoneutria fera, imported in bunches of bananas. It is not very dangerous.

Scorpions: the sting of a scorpion is very painful but rarely fatal, and the treatment is the same as for spider-bites.

Bee and wasp stings: these can cause a great deal of trouble, especially if the victim is sensitive to them; swelling of the bitten part, general urticaria and even anaphylactic shock with coma and death can follow a bee sting.

TREATMENT: the bee leaves the sting in the wound, and it should be taken out – better by scraping than squeezing, for it has a venom sac still attached to it. Weak alkalies such as ammonia or baking soda take away some of the pain, but antihistamine creams are disappointing. In the case of wasp stings weak acids (vinegar, lemon juice) are soothing.

Blackheads: *see* Acne.

Black Motions: known medically as melaena, black motions are caused by the presence of iron taken for anaemia, or of altered blood from bleeding peptic ulcers or disease of the intestine. Black motions can also be caused by drinking heavy red wine.

Blackwater Fever: a condition occurring in those suffering from malignant tertian (falciparum) malaria, who have had several attacks treated unsuccessfully with quinine.

CAUSE: not properly understood. The symptoms are brought on by a sudden breakdown of red blood corpuscles and the escape of the pigment they contain.

SYMPTOMS: blackwater fever begins in the same way as an attack of malaria, but the urine is dark red, and may look black. There is severe headache, pain in the back and abdomen, fever and vomiting; in fatal cases the kidneys fail and the secretion of urine dries up. The skin becomes yellow.

TREATMENT: absolute rest. If the kidneys fail, the only hope is an artificial kidney. Corticosteroids are used to diminish the rate of breakdown of the red blood cells, and anaemia is treated by the infusion of packed red cells. The accompanying malaria is controlled by any antimalarial drug except quinine. If the patient recovers he must be very careful to take one of the modern antimalarial drugs regularly if he is exposed to the possibility of further infection with falciparum malaria.

Bladder, Urinary (for Gall-bladder *see* below). The

bladder lies in the pelvis, guarded in front by bone – the symphysis pubis. In the male, the rectum lies behind the bladder, and the prostate gland below it; in the female the vagina and the neck of the womb lie behind the bladder. The womb in its normal position is separated from the upper surface of the bladder by a pouch of peritoneum in which may lie intestine. In the normal living male the bladder holds about 300 ml of urine, which enters the bladder from the kidneys by way of two tubes called ureters passing through the muscular wall of the bladder at its base; near them, in the mid-line, the urethra leaves the bladder to take the urine to the exterior. The wall of the bladder is muscular, for it has to be able to expel the urine by contracting, and the muscle has the property when relaxed of being able to expand more if the bladder is distended slowly than if it is blown up quickly. Sudden distension of the bladder quickly produces the urge to urinate. A nervous reflex controls the mechanism of passing urine, which can normally be over-ridden by the conscious mind; the reflex is set in motion by distension of the bladder or by irritation of its most sensitive part, the triangle at the base where the two ureters enter and the urethra leaves. The nerves concerned in the reflex are the sympathetic and the parasympathetic fibres which reach the muscle of the bladder through the pelvic plexus and the pelvic splanchnic nerves, and the pudendal nerves which supply the muscles which close the urethra and have to relax to let the urine pass. The centre for the reflex is in the sacral segments of the spinal cord, and conscious impulses to control the reflex travel through the spinal cord from the brain. All these structures have to be intact for the act of passing water to be carried out normally.

Bladder Disease: *Congenital deformity.* (*a*) Ectopia vesicae: a condition in which the front wall of the bladder and the lower abdomen have failed to close, so that the child suffers from continual leaking of urine from the opening.
TREATMENT: surgical removal of the ureters from the bladder to the lower bowel, so that the urine is discharged into the colon and rectum, and plastic repair of the defect in the abdominal wall. Commonly a defect of formation of the penis called hypospadias is found with ectopia vesicae, and this deformity can be repaired at the same time. The

operation is carried out after the child is 4 years old.

(*b*) Rarely urine escapes from the umbilicus because the urachus, the duct which joins the bladder and the umbilical cord in the embryo, fails to close properly.

TREATMENT: surgical closure.

Inflammation. This is very common, and is described under the heading Cystitis. *See also* Bilharzia.

Tumours. May be benign or malignant.

SYMPTOMS: the first symptom is usually. painless passage of blood in the urine. If the tumour is malignant, pain will follow, with frequent passing of water.

TREATMENT: this depends on the nature of the tumour, which is determined by microscopic examination of the urine, special X-ray examination (*see* Pyelography), and examination of the inside of the bladder through the cystoscope. Benign tumours, called papillomata, can be controlled by diathermy treatment through the operating cystoscope, but other tumours may have to be cut out with a varying amount of the wall of the bladder. Treatment either by diathermy or surgical removal may be combined with radiation therapy.

Infection is always liable to occur in the presence of tumours of the bladder, and it is treated as it arises.

Injury. Uncommon, but can occur with fracture of the pelvis or penetrating wounds of the lower abdomen. The danger is from leakage of urine into the peritoneal cavity or the tissues of the pelvis, and the treatment is drainage of the bladder.

Foreign bodies. The commonest foreign bodies found in the bladder are stones, which usually form as the result of inflammation but occur more commonly in men than women. Foreign bodies ranging from lead pencils to hairpins are occasionally found in the bladder, having been introduced through the urethra.

TREATMENT: unfortunately – and contrary to popular belief – there are no drugs which can dissolve stones found in the bladder. The surgeon can, however, sometimes crush the stones with an instrument called a lithotrite, which is passed into the bladder through the urethra, and wash the fragments out. Often it is necessary to open the bladder through the abdominal wall in order to remove stones (or other foreign bodies). The operation of cutting for the stone is one of considerable antiquity, which used to be carried out through the perineum without anaesthetic.

Obstruction. Usually caused by enlargement of the prostate gland in men; may be caused in women by tumours of the uterus, or by pregnancy occurring in a retroverted uterus.

TREATMENT: *see* Prostate.

Associated with disease of the nervous system. The nervous control of the bladder is complicated, and normal passage of water depends on an intact nervous system. Damage to various parts of the controlling mechanism will have different results.

1. Damage to the upper part of the spinal cord: voluntary control of the bladder is lost, and the passage of water in time becomes automatic.

2. Damage to the sacral segments of the spinal cord: reflex control is lost, and the bladder muscle contracts by itself from time to time, but not very powerfully. In the end the bladder becomes full of urine, small quantities of which are voided frequently.

3. Damage to the nerves which supply the muscles at the neck of the bladder. Here there is no control of the outlet of the bladder, and the paralysis allows urine to dribble away as it comes down from the kidneys, the bladder remaining empty.

4. Sudden injury to any part of the spinal cord, or the nerves of the cauda equina (q.v.): acute retention of urine follows, with inability to pass urine even though the bladder becomes grossly distended.

TREATMENT: varies according to the problem, but in general the bladder is kept drained and clean until the cause of the trouble can be dealt with. If this is impossible, the first aim is to set up automatic voiding of urine; if this cannot be achieved, then a system of drainage has to be used. The great danger is urinary infection.

Blastomyces: types of yeast which can cause disease in man. North American blastomycosis is caused by infection with Blastomyces dermatitidis; the organism enters by the lungs, where it produces many small abscesses, and may spread to other organs and tissues, especially the skin, where it causes pustules and ulcers.

Bleeding Time: the length of time needed for a small wound (pinprick) to stop bleeding, Normal, 0–7 minutes; prolonged in diseases which produce abnormality of the blood platelets (q.v.).

Blepharitis: inflammation of the eyelids, from infection with staphylococcus, in which small abscesses develop in the hair follicles of the eyelids, especially in children – the common name for these is styes – which are painful and cause the eyelids to swell. Application of simple antiseptic ointment is the preferred treatment. Antibiotic ointments are liable to produce scaliness and swelling of the eyelids as well as sensitivity to future doses of the drug. Frequent hot bathing of the eye is recommended.

Blindness: may be congenital or acquired, the result of abnormality, disease or injury affecting any of the structures in the 'visual pathway' – the eye, the optic nerves, their connections in the brain, or the visual cortex. In the United Kingdom a blind person is defined by the National Assistance Act of 1948 as one 'so blind as to be unable to perform any work for which eyesight is essential'. In the case of children the term includes not only the totally blind but those who cannot be taught by visual methods, even by the use of large print, blackboard writing, or lenses for magnifying ordinary print. *See* Eye, Cataract, Glaucoma.

Blisters and Counter-irritants: in former days actual blistering of the skin was produced by instruments like small branding-irons and by cauterizing substances, but counter-irritation is nowadays brought about by gentler methods. The reasons for wanting to produce counter-irritation are: (1) to distract attention from an already existing pain by producing other irritation in the area; (2) to increase the flow of blood and so improve the local circulation The commonest uses for counter-irritants are in rheumatic pain, strains and muscle injuries; some still employ them in sciatica and lumbago, and apply them to the chest in bronchitis, pneumonia and pleurisy, but it is doubtful whether they are useful in such complaints. Commonly used proprietary preparations are Algipan, Cremalgin and Transvasin. Methyl salicylate is often used by athletes.

Blood: a fluid composed of plasma, a pale, slightly yellow liquid, and white and red cells which separate from the plasma on standing. The cells are present in the blood in constant quantities and any variation is a sign of illness. There are normally between 4.5 million and 5.5 million red cells per cubic millimetre, between 4,000 and 10,000 white cells per cubic millimetre, and 150,000 to 400,000 platelets (q.v.). The white cells are subdivided according to appearance and staining characteristics; a differential count gives: Polymorphs: Neutrophil 40–75%, Basophil 0–1%, Eosinophil 1–6%.

Monocytes: 2–10%.

Lymphocytes: 20–45%.

(All these cells are described elsewhere; *see* Leucocytes.)

Many chemical determinations and analyses can be carried out on the blood which give an accurate picture of the state of the individual in health and disease. The blood circulates through the body in arteries, veins and capillary vessels, being pumped by the heart. The functions of the blood are:

1. Transport of oxygen, which is carried in combination with the haemoglobin of the red blood cells.

2. Removal from the cells of carbon dioxide, formed as the cells use oxygen.

3. Transport of food substances to the cells and the removal of waste products.

4. Heat exchange; the blood removes excess heat from deep structures and carries it to the surface where it can be dissipated.

5. Control of many vital processes by the transport of hormones and other chemical substances.

6. Defence of the body against infection by the transport of antitoxins, antibodies and white cells to the infected part.

The amount of blood circulating in health in the normal adult is about 5,000 ml per minute at rest. Normal blood volume in the adult is 4 to 5 litres.

Blood Disease: *see* Anaemia, Leukaemia, Hodgkin's Disease, Purpura, Hemophilia, Agranulocytosis, Christmas Disease, Hemolytic Disease of the Newborn, Polycythemia, Thalassaemia, Thrombocytopenic Purpura, Sickle-cell Anaemia.

Blood Groups: early attempts to transfuse blood from one man to another were sometimes successful, but often ended in death. The reasons were not understood until 1901 when the Austrian biologist Landsteiner, working in the U.S.A., discovered the blood groups. All human beings of whatever race belong, in respect of their blood, to one of several groups classified according to the power of the serum of one person's blood to agglutinate or clump the red cells of another. The reaction depends on the presence of antibodies called agglutinins in the serum and antigens called agglutinogens on the surface of the red blood corpuscles. The make-up of the blood is inherited. Although there are nine blood group systems, only two are of importance in clinical medicine: the ABO and the Rh systems. Landsteiner showed that people could be divided into four groups, A, B, AB, and O. The antigens are A, B, and AB; people in group O have no antigen. The antibodies in the serum are anti-A, anti-B, and anti-A and B. Those in group A have the antigen A, the antibody anti-B; those in group B, the antigen B, antibody anti-A; those in group AB neither antibody; those in group O, no antigen, but both anti-A and B antibody. Blood can only be given to another person of the same group – although in very grave emergency group O blood can be given to any patient, for there is no antigen in the corpuscles and they will not agglutinate. Normally, blood for transfusion is carefully grouped, and then cross-matched; the serum of the patient who is to receive the blood is mixed with red cells of the donor's blood. If the blood is compatible, the red cells will be unharmed. If the cells clump together in the laboratory, they will do so inside the patient and possibly kill him.

The Rh (Rhesus) system was discovered by Landsteiner and Weiner in 1940. They found that they could prepare an antibody in the serum of a rabbit by using the red cells of a rhesus monkey as the antigen. This antiserum reacted with over 80% of human red blood cells; they called the group of people whose cells were agglutinated by the rabbit anti-rhesus serum 'Rh positive'. Those with cells that did not react were called Rh negative. It is very uncommon to find the antibody to the Rhesus cell occurring naturally in human beings, but it can be acquired by Rhesus negative people after an Rh positive blood transfusion or, in the case of a woman, by an Rh negative pregnant mother who is carrying a Rhesus positive child. The importance of the Rh factor is that if a mother acquires the Rh antibody in this way, or after a transfusion, further pregnancies with an Rh positive child may result in haemolytic disease of the newborn, worse in subsequent pregnancies (*see* Haemolytic Disease of the Newborn). No woman of childbearing age, and no young girl, should be given a blood transfusion without the Rh reaction being known.

Blood Poisoning: terms used to signify the presence of bacteria, their toxins, or infected matter.

CAUSE: bacterial infection virulent enough to invade the bloodstream (bacteraemia): the presence of bacteria multiplying and releasing toxins in the bloodstream (septicaemia); or the release of fragments of infected clot or pus into the bloodstream (pyaemia).

SYMPTOMS: there may be a bright red rash, spikes of temperature with shivering, increased heart rate, deterioration in general condition, and collapse. In pyaemia small abscesses may form in many places in the body.

TREATMENT: antibiotics according to the infection. It is probable that in many severe diseases bacteria are present in the bloodstream; recovery takes place because the powers of the blood to kill bacteria are considerable. Septicaemia, with its innumerable multiplying bacteria and circulating toxins, is more serious, and pyaemia has the risk of abscesses forming in the lungs and the brain. Nevertheless, blood poisoning is no longer the almost invariably fatal condition that it was not so long ago.

Blood Pressure: the blood is driven through the arteries by the heart under considerable pressure – if there were no blood pressure, there would be no circulation. It is highest when the heart contracts (systole) and lowest when it relaxes (diastole). In a healthy young adult the systolic or highest pressure is 120 mm of mercury, and the diastolic or lowest pressure 80 mm of mercury. This is expressed as a blood pressure of 120/80; the difference between the pressures is the 'pulse pressure'. The blood pressure tends to increase with age, and certain diseases cause an increase of blood pressure (*see* Hypertension).

Blood Spitting (Haemoptysis). This may be a symptom of a number of diseases – or it may mean nothing at all. It may, for example, be produced by bleeding gums, or a nose-bleed, or more seriously by disease of the lungs. It should always be regarded seriously until the doctor has found the cause, and it is sensible to ask his advice even when the reason seems obvious and trivial.

Blue Baby: *see* Fallot's Tetralogy.

Boils: (Furuncles). These are infections of the sweat glands or hair follicles of the skin.
CAUSE: infection with staphylococcus, which enters the sweat glands or hair follicles where the clothes rub on the skin: for example, at the wrists or at the back of the neck, in the armpits or on the buttocks.
SYMPTOMS: a painful red nodule appears, which grows bigger and then breaks down in the middle for pus to collect and show yellow under the skin. Crops of boils may appear simultaneously, or a succession of single boils may follow each other.
TREATMENT: never squeeze a boil, or interfere with it at all except by applying a dressing and keeping the surrounding skin clean. It is too easy to spread the infection and produce cellulitis or worse. A kaolin poultice may be useful if the site of the boil is suitable, but do not let the skin get soggy.
Long-term treatment includes the use of special antiseptics such as hexachlorophane on the skin and in the soap, scrupulous cleanliness and a good varied diet. The urine must be tested, for boils are frequently associated with diabetes. Antibiotics are not recommended except in the case of severe or spreading infection, for they often prolong the time needed for the boil to clear up.

Bone Disease: *see* Osteitis, Periostitis, Osteomyelitis, Osteosarcoma, Fibrocystic Disease, Paget's Disease, Rickets, Osteomalacia, Tuberculosis.

Bones: the bones support and protect the soft tissues, and by acting as levers make it possible for the individual to move about. The bones are made of varying amounts of soft tissue and a hard crystalline mineral called calcium apatite. A child's bones contain nearly two-thirds of fibrous tissue, whereas the bones of an old man are two-thirds mineral; it is easy to see why the child's bones may bend while the old man's brittle bones break.

Bones can be classified according to their shape as long, flat, irregular and short.

Long bones: these have a tubular shaft and two ends made of cancellous, or spongy, bone. The plates of thin bone which go to make up the spongy structure are developed according to the mechanical strain put on them, and are covered by a layer of compact hard bone. The limb bones are long bones.

Flat bones: for example, the bones of the skull. They are composed of inner and outer plates, or tables, of compact hard bone with a sandwich of spongy bone between them.

Irregular bones: for example, the vertebrae. These also contain spongy bone and are covered by compact hard bone.

Short bones: these have the same structure as the long bones.

The bones are covered by a membrane called the periosteum, and are pierced by small holes for the passage of blood vessels to the interior. After growth has stopped, a further supply of blood is derived from the periosteum. At birth the marrow of all the bones is red, because it is a factory for the production of blood cells, but gradually the active marrow recedes until in the adult most marrow is fatty and yellow, and red active marrow is confined to the vertebrae, the skull, the pelvis, ribs, and breastbone, although the marrow of the long bones remains capable of making blood cells in a crisis – for example, after severe haemorrhage.

DEVELOPMENT AND GROWTH: the bones develop from membranes or from cartilage, which persists throughout the period of growth as a plate at the end of the growing bone called the epiphyseal plate. In the case of the long bones there are epiphyseal plates at each end of the shaft, and they go on producing bone until the growth of the skeleton stops. Bones are shaped during growth by two sorts of special cells – osteoclasts, which can absorb bone, and osteoblasts which form the fibrous framework upon which the mineral content is laid down. In childhood and adolescence more bone is laid down than is absorbed; the adult keeps the amount of bone constant, although there is continual absorption and deposition of bone so that a complete change has occurred in 20 years; and in old age there is more

BOTULISM

absorption than deposition of bone. This leads to rarefaction of the bone, a condition called osteoporosis which can produce fracture or collapse of the bones.

Boracic or Boric Acid: a mild antiseptic prepared from borax, used in dusting-powders, eye lotions, or on lint as a fomentation. Sodium perborate is a useful mouth-wash.

Bornholm Disease: (The Devil's Grip). A disease originally described as occurring on the Danish island of Bornholm.
CAUSE: infection with a virus of the Coxsackie B group.
SYMPTOMS: fever, headache, sometimes cough and characteristic gripping pain round the base of the chest. Occurs in epidemics during the summer months, particularly in young people.
TREATMENT: no specific treatment. The condition is self-limiting and never fatal.

Botulism: a very rare form of food poisoning.
CAUSE: the bacterium Clostridium botulinum elaborates a very powerful toxin in contaminated food. This organism grows without oxygen at low temperatures; its spores are resistant to boiling and heat.
SYMPTOMS: the toxin is absorbed by the gut and taken up by the central nervous system, where it produces drooping of the eyelids, double vision, dilatation of the pupils, paralysis of the face, difficulty in swallowing, and eventually paralysis of the muscles used in breathing and arrest of the heart. More than half the cases are fatal.
TREATMENT: because the damage is done not by the bacteria but by the toxins they elaborate in the food, it is no use giving antibiotics. The only treatment likely to be helpful is the giving of emetics and, if possible, antitoxin; and speedy removal to hospital. Prevention is the best safeguard, and commercial interests are continually on their guard against the possibility of contamination of food with Cl. botulinum. The occurrence of botulism from commercially prepared food is almost unknown; faulty preparation and preservation in the home are the cause of the rare cases that are reported. Boiling destroys the toxin and thus poisoning may be

95

prevented by not tasting home canned products before reheating. The food usually smells spoiled.

Bougie: instrument made to insert into the urethra, rectum or other body opening.

Bowels: the intestines.

Bow Legs: (Genu varum). Formerly a consequence of rickets, it is now in Western countries more commonly found in children without obvious cause. It tends in such cases to be self-correcting. Bow legs can be acquired by people who spend enough time on horses.

Brachial: pertaining to the arm.

Brachycephalic: short-headed. A term applied by anthropologists to those races with skulls the breadth of which is at least four-fifths of the length. (Cf. dolichocephalic, where the breadth of the skull is less than four-fifths of the length.)

Brachydactyly: term applied to conditions in which the fingers and toes are abnormally short.

Bradycardia: slow pulse (i.e. below 60 a minute).

Branchial Arches: at an early stage in the development of the human embryo six 'visceral arches' form just below the head. The first arch corresponds to the lower jaw of the fish, the second to the gill cover, and the last four, which are called the branchial arches, to the arches of the gills. Between the arches are clefts, and from the arches and the clefts develop the structures of the neck and the lower jaw as well as part of the ear. All vertebrate embryos go through the stage of development where they have 'gills', but only in the fish do these structures go on to form part of the breathing apparatus. Sometimes in human beings the final development of the branchial arches is abnormal, and cysts or slits, like rudimentary gills, persist in the neck.

Breast Diseases: the breast may be the site of cancer, benign tumours, cysts and inflammation. *Cancer of the breast:*

cause unknown, although there is some indication that it may run in families and may be less common in mothers who have suckled their children. It is a common cancer in women, and not entirely unknown in men. About 8,000 women die of cancer of the breast every year in England and Wales.

SYMPTOMS: a hard lump in the breast, which may be tender or painless, or the discharge of bloody or clear fluid at the nipple are the classical symptoms. Enlargement of the lymph glands in the armpit on the same side or puckering of the skin over the tumour may occur. One form of cancer looks at first like eczema of the nipple. Except in rare fulminating cases the growth enlarges fairly slowly, but sooner or later if left the cancer spreads through the lymphatic system and the bloodstream to other parts of the body, particularly the bones of the vertebral column and the pelvis, where the deposits give rise to symptoms not immediately obvious as part of the disease.

TREATMENT: this depends on the state of the disease. If it has been detected quickly, the surgeon will remove the breast after he has satisfied himself that he is dealing with a malignant growth by removing a small part of it for biopsy. If the lymph glands in the armpit are affected – and they very often are – they may be removed along with the breast and the muscle upon which it lies. The surgeon may advise that a course of radiotherapy should follow the operation, and he will in any case wish to see the patient at intervals for many years after the operation to be sure of recognizing any signs of recurrence of the tumour in time to deal with them. It may be that by the time the patient first comes to the surgeon secondary deposits have already begun to grow; in this case he may only carry out a local removal of the breast, and rely on radiotherapy for the main line of treatment. Some tumours can be affected by the use of hormones, and some respond to the removal of the ovaries or the adrenal glands, but as yet there is no way of telling which tumours will respond. Some good results have been obtained by removal of the pituitary gland or its destruction by the placing of radioactive yttrium in its substance. Nothing is as important in treatment as speed; any lump in the breast must be seen by a doctor at once.

Benign tumours: the commonest benign tumour is the

fibroadenoma, which is composed of fibrous tissue with a variable amount of gland tissue.

SYMPTOMS: the tumour presents as a firm lump in the breast.

DIAGNOSIS: this is made certain by biopsy, q.v.

TREATMENT: simple surgical removal of the tumour.

Duct papilloma: a simple tumour arising from the tissue lining a milk duct.

SYMPTOMS: bleeding from the nipple.

TREATMENT: biopsy and removal.

Lipoma: this is a fatty tumour which is not very common in the breast. In common with other benign tumours of the breast, it may easily be removed by the surgeon.

Acute inflammation of the breast: abscess of the breast is a complication of the lying-in period.

CAUSE: it is associated with cracked or depressed nipples. The infecting organism is usually Staphylococcus aureus.

SYMPTOMS: tenderness and redness of the infected area, fever and constitutional upset.

TREATMENT: the breasts are emptied by hand, and breast feeding is stopped. Antibiotics are used to control the infection and if the inflammation goes on to form an abscess it must be incised and drained.

Cysts of the breast: these are commonly associated with a condition often called chronic mastitis, which is not in fact anything to do with inflammation but is probably dependent on hormone balance, for it occurs during the child-bearing period of life and produces symptoms which vary with the menstrual cycle.

SYMPTOMS: pain and a feeling of tension in the breasts, worst before the period starts. Collections of small lumps are felt in the breast, sometimes with discrete larger cysts.

TREATMENT: if necessary, biopsy and surgical removal, especially of the larger cysts or any separate swellings. In cases with any sort of swelling or hardness in the breast a surgeon's advice is essential, even if in his opinion there is no tumour and no operation is advised. Although it is far from true that all lumps in the breast are dangerous, they may be due to cancer – which is much more likely to be cured if it is treated immediately.

Breasts: the mammary glands are typical of a group of highly developed animals which suckle their young and are known as mammals. In the adult human female there are usually two breasts.

Structure: each breast is divided into 12–20 compartments containing systems of branching tubes lined by cells that secrete milk. In each compartment the tubes join together to form a single duct which opens on the surface of the nipple. There are therefore 12–20 openings; the tissue intervening between the tubes is filled with muscle fibres, fibrous strands and fat.

The nipple: lies usually in the lower outer quadrant of the breast near the centre, and it is surrounded by an area of darker skin called the areola. In fair-skinned pregnant women the areola darkens from pink to brown.

Function: the size of the breast is no indication of its efficiency in producing milk – in fact small breasts are often more productive than large ones. The activity and size of the breasts are controlled by hormones produced by the pituitary gland at the base of the brain. Milk is secreted on the third day after the baby is born; before that the breast secretes a small amount of clear fluid called colostrum. The exact factors involved in the secretion of human milk are not yet fully understood, but it is known that beside the ovaries and the pituitary gland it is essential that the adrenals and thyroid glands should be functioning normally, and that the suckling of the baby is itself a powerful stimulus to milk production, so that it will continue for as long as the child is at the breast. In the West, babies are weaned from the breast in a few months, but it is quite common for the mothers of Asia and Africa to suckle their children for up to three years. Conception of another child is less likely to happen in a nursing mother, although suckling is a very imperfect form of birth control. The average yield of human milk is just under a litre a day.

Abnormalities: accessory breasts may develop anywhere along a diagonal line running from the armpit to the lower abdomen (the milk line). If they are unsightly or embarrassing they can easily be removed. In certain circumstances men can develop swelling of the breasts. In puberty there may be undue sensitivity to hormones circulating in the blood, and the enlargement, which is usually slight, one-sided and often only noticeable to the patient, in time diminishes. Men working with oestrogens are liable to develop swelling of the breasts, and so are those who are being given oestrogens for medical reasons such as enlargement of the prostate. Only very rarely is swelling of the breast in men or youths associated with testicular insufficiency.

Breath, Bad: (Halitosis). This is common in many people at all times and in all people some of the time, and if it is often the case that the sufferer is unaware of the discomfort he (or she) causes to others it is equally often possible to find those who worry unnecessarily about more or less imaginary halitosis which upsets nobody. The common causes of halitosis are any conditions of the nose, mouth, respiratory tract, or stomach which are associated with chronic infection or local upsets of one sort or another, for example, bad teeth in which decaying food may lodge, infections of the gums (as in Vincent's angina or chronic pyorrhoea), chronic tonsillitis, lung diseases such as chronic bronchitis and bronchiectasis (in the latter the breath may be exceedingly foul), chronic gastritis, and diseases of the nose or sinuses which cause a discharge at the back of the throat. Constipation, except insofar as it is associated with chronic gastritis, is not in itself a cause of halitosis whatever the patent medicine advertisements may say. The treatment depends upon the cause, but in the absence of any symptoms relating to the chest or stomach the first thing to do is to see a dentist who will treat the tooth or gum infection which is the most usual cause of the trouble; if nothing abnormal is found, the tonsils and nose and throat generally may need attention. The bad breath of a hangover is caused by gastritis brought about by strong drink taken the night before, but there are very few people, drunk or sober, who do not have bad breath in the morning. Assuming that no disease is found to account for the condition, antiseptic toothpastes or mouth-washes may be used. In some instances those who are unduly concerned about halitosis are suffering basically from a sense of inferiority and guilt which causes them to haunt the doctor's surgery in the conviction that their breath, urine or other bodily excretions smell foul.

Breathalyser: a device used at the roadside to estimate the amount of alcohol in the breath of a suspected drunken driver. In the United Kingdom it is used by the police, who have the power to ask any driver to take a breath test at any time. The police officer must be in uniform when he asks the driver to take the test. If the test shows that the driver probably has an amount of alcohol in his blood exceeding 80 mg per cent, the police officer will ask him to go to the police station to have another breath test. The test consists of breathing through a tube of bichromate crystals into a bag with a capacity of 100 cc until the bag is full. The crystals will change colour from yellow to blue-green as they are reduced by alcohol, and the colour change is in direct proportion to the amount of alcohol in the breath. The change of colour starts at the mouthpiece and if the change reaches beyond a mark on the tube then there is an excess of alcohol in the blood.

Alcohol stays in the mouth for about twenty minutes after it has been drunk, so that there may be a positive first test followed by a negative test at the police station. It is an offence to drink more alcohol after being stopped by a police officer. If the second test is positive, the suspect is asked to provide two specimens of urine within the next hour or to allow a doctor to take blood for analysis. Refusal to do this is an offence with automatic conviction. The tubes of the breath-testing apparatus are not kept for evidence, but thrown away as soon as the driver has been charged, because in time the colour change extends throughout the crystals.

The Road Safety Act of 1967 made it an offence to be driving a motor vehicle with a blood alcohol level above 80 mg per cent, or with 107 mg alcohol by weight in 100 ml of urine by volume, or more. For the first time in the laws of Great Britain this Act made it an offence to withhold evidence that might be self-incriminating.

Breathlessness: may occur in any condition in which there is deficiency of oxygen in the blood or an excess of waste products. It may therefore result from deficiency of oxygen in the inspired air, obstruction to the air passages, diminution in the areas of lung tissue able to carry out exchange of oxygen and carbon dioxide between the blood and the air, diseases of the heart which prevent efficient circulation of the blood, or diseases of the blood in which its capacity to carry oxygen is reduced.

Bright's Disease: *see* Nephritis.

Bromides: the salts of bromine were up to recently used as sedatives, but there is really little place for them in modern medicine although when they were introduced well over a hundred years ago they were a decided advance in the production of a sedative which was effective, fairly safe, and less habit-forming than opium. Unfortunately, bromides have objectionable features: rashes develop in those who are sensitive, and the taking of bromides over a long period of time results in mental dullness and sometimes even confusion. There is, however, no foundation of truth for the belief prevalent in the British Army that bromides are put into soldiers' tea.

Bromidrosis: the secretion of bad-smelling sweat. *See* Perspiration.

Bronchiectasis: abnormal permanent dilation of the bronchi or breathing-tubes.
CAUSE: babies may be born with congenitally dilated bronchi, or bronchiectasis may be acquired in later life after infection, such as an attack of measles, influenza or pneumonia. Anything which obstructs the bronchus may lead to the development of bronchiectasis – a cancer of the lung, or a group of tuberculous glands. Asthma and chronic bronchitis are associated with bronchiectasis because of the intermittent obstruction and infection.
SYMPTOMS: cough, with a great deal of foul-smelling sputum. The patient may spit blood and suffer from chronic low-grade fever with sweating, quick pulse and general malaise, breathlessness and even blueness (cyanosis). The cough is usually at its worst in the morning.
DIAGNOSIS: if the physician is in doubt, a bronchogram (q.v.) will demostrate the dilatation of the air passages in the lung.
TREATMENT: the milder cases are treated with antibiotics and postural drainage. This means that the patient uses the force of gravity to help him cough up the sputum. Various parts of the lung may be affected by bronchiectasis, and the

posture to be adopted depends on the site of the disease. If the upper lobes are affected, drainage naturally occurs when the patient stands up; but if the lower lobes are at fault he should lie face down with his head hanging over the side of the bed, supporting himself with his hands and coughing in order to bring up the sputum. Postural drainage should be continued for as much as twenty minutes twice a day, and in this way the vicious circle by which pus retention leads to further infection may be broken or at any rate alleviated. In selected suitable cases, especially in children, the best treatment is surgical removal of the diseased lung or part of the lung.

Bronchitis: inflammation of the bronchi or air passages of the lung. It may be acute or chronic, and can be caused by various bacteria.

Acute bronchitis

CAUSE: acute bronchitis very often occurs as the sequel of a common cold – the cold 'going down to the chest' – or as the result of an attack of influenza. First the trachea, or wind-pipe, is infected, then the infection spreads into the bronchi, the smaller bronchioles, and even into the lung substance to produce bronchopneumonia. There is no hard and fast line between these states, and the severity of the disease depends on the extent of the spread of infection which is assisted by exposure to cold, damp and smoke. Bronchitis may be acquired as a complication of measles.

SYMPTOMS: at first a painful unproductive cough, aching in the muscles, depression and lack of energy. There may be a slight temperature. After a day or two the patient begins to bring up sputum and the pain of the cough subsides.

DIAGNOSIS: commonly this presents little difficulty.

TREATMENT: bed and warmth, hot drinks, inhalations of steam or special preparations. There must be no smoking in the room, nor cold draughts, for cold air sets off fits of coughing. In cases where they are indicated the doctor will prescribe antibiotics. An attack of acute bronchitis that does not clear up after treatment has to be investigated to see if there is any underlying disease of the lung.

Chronic bronchitis

A common disease in England, it affects mainly the middle-aged and old, may run in families, and may lead to emphysema (q.v.) and heart disease.

CAUSE: exposure to cold, damp, dust, fumes and smoke – including tobacco smoke. The linings of the bronchi are irritated, and recurring infections (possibly several attacks of acute bronchitis) produce a state of progressive slow destruction of lung tissue by excessive secretion of mucus and scarring.

SYMPTOMS: shortness of breath, at first on exercise and finally at rest. Cough, particularly at night. Wheezing and difficulty in breathing resembling asthma, which may complicate chronic bronchitis or may itself lead to chronic bronchitis.

DIAGNOSIS: a diagnosis of chronic bronchitis is not made until it has been demonstrated that there are no underlying conditions such as cancer of the lung or tuberculosis.

TREATMENT: this is difficult. First, all patients must stop smoking, for the benefit they will feel from this simple measure is difficult to exaggerate. Breathing exercises are good, and the patient working in dusty conditions must try to change his job. Fogs and smoke outdoors must be avoided like the plague; although it is not possible for many people to live outside towns, if they can do so they should move into a country district. From time to time those with chronic bronchitis will develop acute infections of the lungs leading to acute bronchitis, bronchopneumonia or pneumonia. Antibiotics are used in full doses as soon as acute infection is suspected, and are continued until the acute infection has been controlled. The most commonly used antibiotics are tetracycline and ampicillin. Morning coughing and wheezing can be helped by hot drinks and drugs such as isoprenaline (q.v.), or sometimes by postural drainage (*see* Bronchiectasis). Inhalation from a steam kettle will often loosen obstinate plugs of mucus.

Bronchogram: an outline of the bronchial tree made by injecting a radio-opaque substance into the trachea (windpipe) and taking an X-ray of the lungs.

Bronchopneumonia: extension of infection from the bronchi to the substance of the lung results in combined inflammation of the lung and the air passages. *See* Pneumonia.

Bronchoscope: an instrument for the examination of the air passages. It is based on the principle of the telescope, and carries a source of illumination which lights up the interior of the bronchi. It is commonly used with the patient under local anaesthetic; the instrument is passed down the trachea between the vocal cords, and guided into the right and left main bronchi. The examination is uncomfortable but painless.

Bronchus: the trachea, the air passage in the neck, divides in the chest into two main bronchi – the air passages to the right and left lungs, which in turn divide into smaller branches. The smaller bronchi branch to form the bronchial tree, and when the branches are below about 0.2 mm in diameter they are called bronchioles. The bronchioles divide still further until they end in minute air-sacs called alveolar sacs, which are lined by the alveoli, small pockets in which the exchange of gases takes place between the blood and the air. *See* Lungs.

Brucellosis: *see* Undulant Fever.

Bruise: an escape of whole blood from damaged vessels into the surrounding tissues brings about discoloration of the skin, which at first goes red, then 'black and blue', and then as the blood pigments break down changes to yellow. Eventually the colour fades away. Usually bruises show in the area where the injury has been sustained, so that a blow in the eye leads to a black eye; but there are times when blood will track along muscles and the planes of connective tissue and show under the skin some way away from the injury. Bruises are sometimes painful, but if the pain is excessive the bruise is probably overlying a more important injury such as a fracture.

Bubo: swelling of a lymphatic gland or a group of lymphatic glands. It occurs particularly in the groin or armpit, as the result of inflammation. *See* Plague.

Bulbar Paralysis: the medulla oblongata, which is part of the brain stem, is sometimes called the spinal bulb, and paralysis of the motor cranial nerves which take their origin from nuclei in this neighbourhood is called bulbar palsy or paralysis. It brings about difficulty in speaking, coughing and swallowing, and sometimes in chewing.

Bunions: a common deformity of the foot is deviation of the great toe towards the outer side of the foot. This is called hallux valgus, and in this condition the joint between the deviated great toe and the first metatarsal bone of the foot becomes prominent. Pressure over this joint produces chronic irritation and inflammation of the overlying tissues with the formation of an adventitious bursa (q.v.) which in this situation is called a bunion. Treatment is to wear wide shoes which do not press on the prominent joint; if the bursa is painful it can be removed surgically. It may be necessary for the surgeon to treat the hallux valgus deformity which caused the bunion to form.

Burns and Scalds: scalds are caused by boiling water or steam, burns by dry heat, flames, electricity or chemicals. They are divided into classes according to the depth of tissue destroyed: (1) superficial, with reddening or blistering of the skin but no more; (2) partial thickness, where most of the skin is destroyed but small areas of skin cells survive from which the skin can grow again; (3) full thickness, in which the skin is entirely destroyed and the burn penetrates into the underlying structures. This classification depends on the extent of damage to the skin. The reason for this is that the danger of a burn varies according to the amount of skin destroyed. The burns of class (1) are rarely dangerous, although they can be painful; but burns of (2) and (3) which involve more than a third of the body surface are a serious danger to life, for a great deal of fluid leaks away from the burnt area and salts and water are lost. In addition to this there is shock and the risk of infection.

TREATMENT: first-aid treatment is to cover the burns with a sterile or clean cloth. Keep the injured man warm, give him hot drinks, and get him to hospital quickly. Nothing else in the way of dressings should at first be applied, but if help is not forthcoming then the cloths may be soaked in weak salt water and bound in place, or the patient may be put into a warm bath with one teaspoonful of salt to each pint of water. Minor burns are best treated by being covered with gauze. Do not interfere with blisters if they form. In hospital, serious burns are treated with intravenous fluids to counteract the loss of water and salts, and if more than one-fifth of the body surface is affected blood transfusions are given. Pain is best treated with morphia. The burns are cleaned by the surgeon, and if they are obviously full thickness they are grafted as soon as possible. Local treatment of the burnt areas varies, but all treatment is directed towards excluding infection and encouraging natural healing. In general there are two methods of treatment – occlusive dressings or exposure to the air. Each method has its place, and both are usually combined with the use of antibiotics. But no amount of antibiotic can take the place of complete cleanliness in dealing with burns; if you are faced with the prospect of dealing with bad burns without help or dressings, you will not go wrong if you leave the burns exposed to the air and take great pains to keep them clean.

Bursa: a natural space containing a little fluid situated in fibrous tissue at a point where there is constant pressure or friction. Sometimes bursae develop in areas where abnormal chronic pressure irritates the tissues, as in a bunion (q.v.), and sometimes they become inflamed as in housemaid's knee where a small natural bursa in front of the knee blows up and secretes excess fluid.

Butazolidine: proprietary name for phenylbutazone. This drug is a powerful analgesic, and has some action against inflammation. It is very useful in the treatment of arthritic conditions, particularly rheumatoid arthritis, spondylitis and gout, but it has side effects which include interference with blood cell formation and the exacerbation of peptic ulcers. It must therefore be used with discretion.

Byssinosis: a lung disease found in workers in the cotton industry.
CAUSE: exposure to fine dust containing vegetable matter, moulds and cotton fibres.
SYMPTOMS: cough, wheezing and breathlessness worst at the

beginning of the week (Monday fever), deteriorating over a period of years.

TREATMENT: the only treatment likely to help is removal from exposure to the dust, otherwise the condition will progress to chronic bronchitis and emphysema (q.v.).

C

Cachexia: the extreme debility produced by a serious chronic illness.

Cadaver: a corpse; used mostly to mean a preserved dead body used in the study of anatomy.

Cadmium Poisoning: acute poisoning is caused by the fumes arising from molten cadmium, which produces intense irritation of the lungs. Treatment is absolute rest, pure oxygen and the injection of atropine. Chronic poisoning results from exposure to cadmium fumes or dust for years and produces breathlessness, nasal discharge and anaemia. The kidneys are also damaged. Treatment is by sodium calcium-edetate.

Caduceus: the wand of Mercury, the messenger of the gods. Used as the symbol of the U.S. Army Medical Corps, it is to be distinguished from the staff of Aesculapius, which is the symbol of the medical profession. The winged staff of Mercury has two serpents twined round it; the staff of Aesculapius has only one serpent and is used, surrounded by a laurel wreath, as the badge of the Royal Army Medical Corps.

Caecum: the blind sac at the beginning of the large intestine where it joins the small intestine. The caecum may be affected by inflammation, ulceration or cancer. *See* Appendicitis.

Caesarean Section: the delivery of a child by an incision through the abdominal wall and womb from in front, named after Julius Caesar who, according to tradition, was delivered in this way. Previously a serious operation employed only when natural childbirth was impossible or the mother was dead, it is now done for a number of different conditions: for example small pelvis; disease or swellings in the womb which would make delivery difficult; cases where the placenta is placed right over the internal opening of the womb (placenta praevia); haemorrhage in the womb; some cases of heart disease or abnormal (breech) presentations in older women; toxaemia of pregnancy; inertia of the womb; or repeated difficult pregnancies. Thus today it does not necessarily signify any very grave condition; nor is the operation particularly difficult nor in the average case dangerous.

Caffeine: an alkaloid found in tea and coffee; cocoa contains the related alkaloid theobromine. Caffeine stimulates the central nervous system, counteracts tiredness and, it is said, increases the capacity for brain work. The dose is about 100 mg, or two cups of fresh-ground coffee. About twice this amount is needed to get the same effect from instant coffee. Caffeine acts on the kidneys, increasing the flow of urine, and on the heart, which it stimulates to the extent of producing palpitations after over-indulgence. It also increases gastric secretions and can induce gastritis and peptic ulcers. Caffeine was once popular with students who used it prior to university examinations, although it was more likely to produce an uncomfortable bladder than counteract the serious effects of not knowing enough. It has little place in modern medicine, but is still often combined with aspirin and phenacetin (a popular proprietary formula), where it is supposed to balance out the dulling effect of aspirin.

Caisson Disease: work in compressed-air chambers is a common feature of civil engineering works in water-bearing strata, or actually under water up to a depth of 60 ft. Caissons or diving-bells consist of a compressed-air chamber at a pressure of 1 atm for every 10 m of depth, with an air-lock in the shaft. A worker returned too quickly to normal air pressure may develop caisson disease.

CAUSE: when men are subjected to increased air pressure an increased amount of oxygen and nitrogen – the main constituents of the air – go into solution in the blood and so into solution in the tissue fluids. When the pressure drops too quickly, the gases come out of solution in the tissues and blood to form small bubbles. Oxygen is at once used up, but bubbles of the inert gas nitrogen may remain for hours.

SYMPTOMS: 'the bends' – pain in the joints due to bubbles

forming in the joint space. May not develop for an hour or two. 'The chokes' – tightness in the chest and breathlessness due to bubbles in the blood vessels of the lungs. 'The staggers' – bubbles of nitrogen in the vessels of the brain may bring on giddiness, double vision and dimness of vision, and even convulsions. Bubbles of gas in the spinal cord may paralyse the legs. There may also be pain in the abdomen, with nausea and vomiting, deafness and 'the itch' – irritating red patches on the skin.

TREATMENT: the patient is recompressed in a recompression chamber to the same pressure as that at which he was working, and slowly decompressed over a period of about six hours, or even more.

Calamine: calamine lotion is mildly astringent and soothing to an inflamed and irritating skin. If 1% phenol is added to the lotion its soothing and anti-irritant properties are intensified.

Calcaneum: heel bone or os calcis.

Calciferol: a form of Vitamin D_2, made by irradiating ergosterol, a sterol found in yeast and fungi. Vitamin D occurs naturally in milk, butter, cheese, eggs and liver, particularly fish-liver. Lack of Vitamin D produces rickets, a disease of the poor and of sunless cities, for Vitamin D can be produced in nature by the irradiating action of sunlight on naturally occurring sterol in the skin. Overdose of Vitamin D is dangerous for it can lead to high levels of calcium in the blood and abnormal formation of bone.

Calcification: the deposition of calcium salts in the tissues, for example in the scars left by tuberculosis in the lungs.

Calcium: a metal which is essential to life. It is absorbed from the intestines, a process for which Vitamin D is essential, and is used to make the bones. The adult human skeleton contains something like 1.25 kg of calcium, which is supplied chiefly in bread and milk. Calcium is essential for proper blood clotting, for the functioning of muscle and nerve, and for the efficient action of the heart. The balance of calcium in the body tissues and its absorption and excretion are regulated by the hormone of the parathyroid glands (q.v.). Lack of calcium leads to malformation of bone (*see* Rickets, Osteomalacia) and a low level of calcium in the blood produces tetany (involuntary contraction of the muscles caused by high irritability of the muscular tissue, not to be confused with tetanus). Chronic low levels of calcium in the blood may produce brittle ridged nails, dry hair, eczema of the skin, mental disturbances and even fits. Levels of calcium in the blood which are too high produce mental changes, loss of appetite, thirst, vomiting and weakness. Calcium deposits may be laid down in abnormal places, such as the kidneys, the blood vessels and the cornea of the eye.

Calculus: hard, stony concretion, formed usually as the result of bacterial infection in the bladder, kidneys or the gall-bladder. Calculi are named 'stones' in English.

Caldwell-Luc: the name for a successful operation designed by these two surgeons to drain the maxillary antrum or sinus permanently by making an artificial opening into the sinus through the upper jaw opposite the second molar tooth.

Calipers: used in orthopaedics, they are external metal splints designed to take a great deal of the weight of the body off a diseased or fractured leg-bone when the patient stands and walks. The word also means compasses with curved legs which are used for measuring diameters and the distances between points, principally in medicine by obstetricians estimating the size of the pelvis.

Callosity: an area of thickening of the horny layer of the skin caused by chronic pressure or friction. *See also* Corns.

Callus: when a bone is broken blood collects between the broken ends. In this collection of blood osteoblasts or bone-forming cells multiply, and a lump of irregular or 'woven' bone is formed which knits the two ends of the fracture together. This is the callus, and its size depends on the size of the original collection of blood and the degree of splintering of the bone. Calcification of the callus takes about four weeks, after which it becomes tougher and begins to take on the structure of formed bone, until in time the swelling decreases and the fracture is firmly united.

Calomel: mercurous chloride. Formerly used as a purgative and to stimulate the flow of bile, it was often taken by those whose livers were damaged. Mercury is a poison which accumulates especially in the liver, so that calomel, far from helping the patient to health, thrusts him farther into his illness.

Calorie: a unit of energy used in physics and dietetics. For the former purpose the small, gram or standard calorie is used which is defined as the amount of heat required to raise 1 g of water 1 °C in temperature; the large or kilogram calorie used in dietetics is the amount of heat required to raise 1 kg of water 1 °C in temperature.

Cancer: general name for malignant tumours. The characteristics of malignant tumours are: (1) They have no capsule or limiting membrane. They therefore invade and destroy the tissues in which they arise. (2) They reproduce their cells in a disorderly and uncontrolled way. (3) The cells are of a more primitive type than the originating tissue. (4) The rate of growth is unusually rapid. (5) They are capable of producing secondary growths in parts of the body remote from the original tumour. (6) They are usually fatal because of the destruction of the tissues into which the primary and secondary tumours grow. The opposite to a malignant growth is a benign tumour. The characteristics of a benign tumour are: (1) It has a capsule of fibrous tissue and does not invade normal tissue. (2) It reproduces its cells in an orderly way. (3) The cells resemble those of the tissue in which the tumour originates. (4) The rate of growth is slow, and may stop spontaneously. (5) They do not spread except by direct extension. (6) They are not fatal (except in the skull), and only produce ill effects by taking up room and pressing on adjacent normal tissue. The greatest difficulty in treating cancer is posed by its ability to spread both by local invasion, with no obvious border between it and normal tissue, and by metastasis, or the formation of new tumour deposits at a distance.

Metastasis: cancer spreads mainly through the lymphatic

system, passing along the lymphatic vessels and into the glands where it often begins to grow as a secondary tumour. Less commonly cancer spreads by invading the bloodstream and setting up secondary growths in bones, lungs and particularly the liver; cancers of the intestines especially spread to the liver through the portal system of vessels (*see* Veins). Cancers arising in the brain do not metastasize, but cancers arising elsewhere metastasize to the brain.

CAUSE OF CANCER: there are a number of factors which are known to play a part in the growth of a cancer, but the prime cause of cancer is not known. It is thought that cancer is a reaction occurring in the tissues as a response to various different stimuli, rather as the process of inflammation can occur in response to infection by all sorts of bacteria, or in response to various injuries. The following factors are known to affect the growth of cancer: (1) *Chemical carcinogens*. The mechanism is not understood, but since 1775 when the London surgeon Percival Potts attributed cancer of the scrotum in chimney sweeps to irritation from soot on the skin, several chemical agents have been identified. Some of them are:

(*a*) Hydrocarbons. Cancers of the skin affect workers handling tar and oil derived by the application of heat from coal, shale and mineral oil. The substance responsible has been found to be 3:4-benzpyrene, which produces cancers when painted on to the skin of mice; 3:4-benzpyrene is found in tobacco smoke and in diesel oil fumes. Other carcinogenic hydrocarbons are the derivatives of 1:2-benzanthracene.

(*b*) Organic amino compounds. Workers in some branches of the dye industry develop cancer of the bladder. The compounds found to be responsible are 2-naphthylamine and benzidine. The dye Butter Yellow will produce cancer of the liver in rats and mice, and some animals develop tumours after a dose of dimethyl nitrosamine.

(*c*) Arsenites and arsenious oxide may produce cancer of the skin if applied over a period of time.

(2) *Viruses*. There is no doubt that a number of malignancies found in animals are transmitted by viruses. Examples are the Shope papilloma in rabbits, the Rous fowl sarcoma, and leukaemias in birds and mice. There is a tumour found in children in Africa (called the Burkitt lymphoma after the

surgeon who discovered it) which is thought to be due to infection by a virus. (3) *Ionizing radiation*. Many of the pioneers working with X-rays developed cancers of the skin, and those exposed to radiation may develop leukaemia. Ultraviolet radiation may in certain circumstances cause cancer of the skin. (4) *Continued irritation*. The sharp edges of broken teeth may in time produce cancer of the edge of the tongue. There was a time when men would develop cancer of the lower lip after smoking clay pipes for many years. In ulcerative colitis (q.v.) malignant change may occur. Some of the cancers of the lung which are associated with smoking may be due to incessant irritation of the lining membranes of the air passages or bronchi. Cancer of the bladder may develop in people suffering from bilharzia (q.v.). (5) Genetic. It is thought, but far from proved, that inherited characteristics may make cells more likely to develop malignant change. (6) Age. The majority of cancers occur in the age group 50–60. (7) Sex. Sex affects the site of growth rather than the incidence of growth. In men, cancer is commonly found in the intestines, the prostate and the lungs, whereas in women the site is commonly the breast or uterus, gall-bladder or thyroid.

SYMPTOMS: the symptoms of cancer vary according to the site of the growth. In general, the following symptoms indicate the need for consultation with a doctor, although they are by no means to be interpreted as certain signs of cancer.

Blood in the sputum, motions or urine.

Changes in the menstrual periods, especially flooding or bleeding between periods.

A mole present for years changing appearance, size or colour, or bleeding.

Any sore, particularly on the face, which will not heal in a reasonable time.

Any persistent swelling on the surface of the body or in the breast, or swelling of a single limb.

Difficulty in passing water.

A persistent dry cough.

Unexplained loss of weight.

Indigestion occurring for the first time in later life; changes in bowel habits – constipation, chronic diarrhoea or loose stools.

If you think you have cancer, go to the doctor. Do not delay, because success in treatment depends on speed.

TREATMENT: this varies according to the site and nature of the cancer. In general, a combination of surgical removal and application of X-rays is most effective, but each case will be treated by the surgeon on its merits. There is no universal cure for cancer. A number of chemical compounds have been found which help, but none are yet used as a first-line method of treatment. These chemical substances have an effect upon dividing cells, and can be given by local injection, intravenously, or by perfusion through the arteries. Some can be given by mouth. The obvious difficulty is in finding a substance and dose which is poisonous to the dividing cells of the cancer but not to the dividing cells of normal tissue. Some cancers, such as cancer of the prostate, breast and thyroid, may be sensitive to certain hormones. *See* separate entries.

Candida: Candida albicans is a fungus commonly present in the mouth in health, which can, in run-down children, old people, and those treated for a long time with antibiotics, produce the disease called thrush (q.v.). The treatment is the drug nystatin, which is dissolved in the mouth. Candida can also give rise to inflammation of the vulva and vagina in women; the symptoms are itching and white discharge, the treatment nystatin pessaries.

Cannabis Indica: Indian hemp, hashish, bhang or gunjah, marihuana or pot, is derived from the flowers and leaves of the plant Cannabis indica which flourishes in Asia and America. Together with opium, hashish is one of the oldest known drugs and was used in early medicine to produce drowsiness and relative insensitivity in the treatment of pain and the performance of surgical operations. It has no medical use today, but is illegally taken in the form of cigarettes, when it leads to a gay and cheerful mood with a sense of exhilaration without delirium or excessive excitement. Visual hallucinations may occur, but the most typical results of marihuana are prolongation of the senses of space and time; because of the latter effect it is used by performers of popular music, for it appears to improve the control of rhythm. The limbs may feel heavy and the eyes look bright; there is no hangover effect although a feeling of unreality

CARBOLIC ACID

may persist for some hours. Like any form of narcotic, hashish is best avoided, although it comparatively rarely leads to addiction or any other ill effects in normal people. Possibly its worst effect is the sort of company into which its use may lead.

Cantharides: a powder made of the dried bodies of the beetle Cantharis vesicatoria, or Spanish fly. It contains an active principle, cantharidin, which has a powerful blistering action on the skin, and was used at one time as a counter-irritant. Together with bay rum, cantharides is still used as a hair tonic. It has had since ancient times a reputation as an aphrodisiac, founded on the fact that if it is taken internally and excreted in the urine it irritates the urethra so badly that it produces priapism (q.v.). As the kidneys may be permanently damaged, and the irritation of the urethra greatly exceeds any advantage gained in the sexual field, it is perhaps safest for the impotent to see a psychiatrist.

Capillary: the smallest blood vessels in the circulation are called capillaries, although their size is considerably less than a hair. They join the arterioles and the venules, and in fact have about the same diameter as a red blood cell; it is in the capillaries that the blood and the tissue fluids exchange gases, food and waste products, and heat. Red blood cells remain inside the capillaries, but white cells can pass through their walls.

Carbohydrate: a substance with a formula including carbon, oxygen and hydrogen, the oxygen and hydrogen being in the proportions 2 of hydrogen to 1 of oxygen – the proportion which forms water. There are many carbohydrates, and the chemical formula is CH_2O_n. The word carbohydrate is used in dietetics to mean the sugars and starchy elements of a diet.

Carbolic Acid: one of the first antiseptics introduced by Lord Lister in 1867 (*see* Antiseptic), carbolic acid is still used as the standard by which to test other germicides. Apart from this use and its employment on drains and bedpans, it has no application in modern medicine.

Carbon Dioxide: when oxygen is burned by the body carbon dioxide is formed in the tissues. It is removed in the blood and excreted from the lungs in the air breathed out. In anaesthetics carbon dioxide may be used in combination with oxygen to stimulate respiration, for the body detects the presence of excess carbon dioxide and speeds up the breathing in an effort to get rid of it and maintain a normal balance between oxygen and carbon dioxide in the blood. Carbon dioxide is also used in medicine in its frozen form as carbon dioxide snow, which forms when the gas under pressure is allowed to expand quickly, and is used to burn off warts.

Carbon Monoxide: a very deadly gas which has many sources, including town gas (a mixture of coal gas and water gas) and motor-car exhaust fumes. Its deadliness arises from the fact that it combines with the haemoglobin of the blood 200 times more readily than oxygen, and moreover impedes the giving up of oxygen to the tissues, so that any appreciable amount of carbon monoxide in the air leads to a concentration in the blood, and chemical asphyxia; 0.2% is dangerous, 0.4% fatal in under an hour. Poisoning by this gas is insidious, for it may not be detected in time if it comes from, for example, a faulty geyser in a small bathroom or incomplete burning of Calor gas. A brazier of coke has on occasion proved fatal to a watchman on a cold night. It is important to be sure that a rescue can safely be carried out before you rush into a room or a confined space where the victim of carbon monoxide poison is lying, for you, too, can be overcome quite quickly and sometimes the use of the legs is lost before unconsciousness supervenes – there may be little warning. Town gas is lighter than air, so there may be purer air near the floor. Do not go without help into a confined unventilated space where a person has already been overcome. Treatment of carbon monoxide poisoning is inhalation of oxygen preferably with 5% carbon dioxide. Make sure the airway is clear, and until the oxygen arrives use mouth-to-mouth artificial respiration. Carbon monoxide must not be confused with carbon dioxide. (*See* above.)

Carbon Tetrachloride: a volatile solvent used in industry, in fire extinguishers, and as a dry cleaner in the home. Its vapour is readily given off and is poisonous. It produces abdominal pain, but its most dangerous effect is damage to the kidneys leading to acute failure. If it is used as a fire extinguisher and comes into contact with a hot surface various gases, including phosgene (q.v.), are formed. Its toxic properties are increased by alcohol.

Carbuncle: a large boil with several openings and a tendency to spread, commonly occurring on the back of the neck. It is usually caused by infection with Staphylococcus aureus, and it is particularly prone to arise in diabetics. Treatment is by antibiotics; the urine must be examined for sugar in all cases.

Carcinoma: a malignant tumour arising from epithelial cells. *See* Cancer, Epithelium.

Cardiac: pertaining to the heart. A 'cardiac heart', like a 'gastric stomach', is a tautology, but not a cause of ill health.

Cardiac Massage: if the heart stops suddenly in an otherwise healthy person, it may be worth starting heart massage. You have 3 minutes in which to act. Lay the patient flat, face upwards on the floor, note the time, call for help, and kneel down. Put the heel of one hand on the lower part of the breastbone, the other hand on top of it, and press straight down using all your weight so that the breastbone gives. Then release the pressure and let the breastbone come up. Do this 6o times a minute. If possible get an assistant to start mouth-to-mouth artificial respiration – one breath for every five to eight pressures over the heart – but if you are by yourself, start the pressure on the chest before you stop it every eight to ten pressures to blow up the lungs. Keep it up for as long as you can; a patient has recovered after an hour of cardiac massage. *See also* Artificial Respiration.

Cardiogram: a tracing made by a cardiograph, an instrument for recording the action of the heart. *See* Electrocardiogram.

Caries: decay and death of a bone, usually applied to the teeth.

Carminatives: drugs (usually the essential oils and spices) which allegedly aid digestion, relieve spasm or colic, and expel flatulence. Among these are: cloves, nutmeg, cinnamon, lemon, pepper, ginger, cardamoms, oil of lavender, peppermint, aniseed, coriander, dill and gentian. There is no evidence that anything 'aids' digestion unless something is lacking in the first place, for example hydrochloric acid or enzymes; there is little evidence that these particular substances relieve to any significant extent colic or spasm; nor, since flatulence of the stomach is the result of swallowing air, is there much likelihood that carminatives can help it. However, it is quite likely that the pleasant taste or smell of most of these condiments may make one feel hungry.

Carotid Artery: the great artery of the neck, which supplies the head and brain with blood. It arises in the chest as the common carotid artery, and divides in the neck into the internal branch, which goes to the brain, and the external which goes to the outside of the skull. Disease of the carotid artery may make it increasingly narrow (carotid stenosis) and so decrease the flow of blood to the brain that cerebral function is impaired. The narrowing of the artery may be associated with a clot, which may throw off small pieces into the circulation of the brain and cause a stroke. It is possible in some cases to remove the clot from the diseased carotid artery at operation.

Carotid Sinus and Carotid Body: just above the division of the common carotid artery into internal and external branches there is a slight swelling of the wall of the internal branch called the carotid sinus, and between the two branches of the artery lies a small structure called the carotid body. The carotid body is concerned with the chemical balance of the blood, and the carotid sinus with maintenance of the blood pressure. They both derive their nerve supply from the glossopharyngeal and vagus nerves.

Carpal Tunnel Syndrome: the median nerve, which runs down the forearm to the hand, passes across the front of the wrist joint. Under certain circumstances it may become irritated or compressed in its passage through the 'carpal tunnel', formed by the transverse ligament and the underlying bones of the wrist.

CAUSE: arthritis, or old fracture, pregnancy, acromegaly (q.v.), and myxoedema (q.v.).

SYMPTOMS: tingling in the pulp at the tip of the index and middle fingers. Pain in the wrist and arm, followed by muscular weakness of the thumb with wasting of the outer part of the ball of the thumb.

DIAGNOSIS: the condition has to be differentiated from the results of pressure on the nerve roots in the neck.

TREATMENT: the condition may be temporarily treated by the local injection of hydrocortisone under the compressing transverse ligament of the wrist. If this gives relief, then the ligament should be divided surgically. The operation is not serious and the results are good.

Carpus: the wrist.

Carrier: a person who unknowingly carries with him the germs of a disease without developing the symptoms of the disease. People may carry with them, for example, the germs of diphtheria, meningitis, scarlet fever and typhoid, or the staphylococci which cause boils and infections of wounds. The organisms are commonly carried in the nose and throat, except for typhoid germs which are carried in the gall-bladder, the intestines and the urine.

Cartilage: a special type of supporting tissue which with bone makes up the skeleton. The bony skeleton is originally formed in cartilage, and as the foetus develops the process of ossification (q.v.) takes place until the only cartilage left is at the ends of the bones, where it forms the epiphyseal plate (*see* Epiphysis), and the articular surfaces of the joints. Cartilage in the joints has a very slippery surface – more slippery than ice. The only parts of the skeleton made of cartilage in adult life are the ends of the ribs, where they join the breastbone; it also forms the rings of the trachea (the windpipe) and the framework of the external ear.

Cascara: Cascara sagrada or 'sacred bark' is the bark of the California buckthorn, used in liquid or solid form as a purgative (cathartic). The active principle of the drug is absorbed into the bloodstream, and acts upon the large bowel about ten hours later.

Caseation: a process found principally in tuberculosis in which the dead central part of a chronically infected area instead of turning into pus to form an abscess changes into a cheesy mass which may later be replaced by fibrous tissue or undergo calcification and turn into chalk.

Castor Oil: oil squeezed from the seeds of the Indian castor oil plant, Ricinus communis. The seeds themselves are a deadly poison, but castor oil is soothing when applied to the skin (as in zinc and castor oil paste). When it is taken by mouth it is changed by digestion into ricinoleic acid which is a violently irritating purgative, and it acts with fairly explosive effect within three or four hours. It has been given medicinally when a single rapid purgation is required, but it is difficult to see why anyone should want to use it.

Castration: the removal of the testicles (sometimes applied also to removal of the ovaries in women). This is generally done for local disease of the organs, but occasionally for cancer of the prostate gland which is less quick to progress in the absence of the hormone secreted by the testis (testosterone). Castration leads to results which vary with the age at which it is done. Thus before puberty the operation leads to failure of development of the male sexual characteristics: the voice remains high-pitched, the figure becomes feminine in shape, and the beard does not grow. After puberty there are few physiological changes and such as they are these are likely to be very gradual; but complete sterility develops, although not necessarily impotence as occurs in prepubertal cases. 'Pharmacological' castration can be produced by the administration of stilboestrol, the synthetic female sex hormones; it leads to the same results. Among the past and present reasons for castration are: (1) in animals it is done in order to make the beast more placid and put on more flesh; (2) in sexual perversions and homosexuality either surgical or pharmacological castration (depending upon the law of the land' is sometimes performed to reduce the sexual impulse and keep the individual out of trouble; (3) in some countries the mentally defective or seriously mentally ill are castrated in order to prevent procreation and the handing on of a hereditary defect; (4) in women the ovaries are removed either for local disease or to prevent conception where this would be dangerous to the individual or bad for the community; (5) during the seventeenth century the Sistine Chapel in Rome substituted 'castrati' for the imported male sopranos or 'falsettists' of Spain, and such singers were much in favour during the seventeenth and eighteenth centuries in Europe, the most celebrated of all castrati being Farinelli – the voice is not quite the same as a boy's treble or a woman's soprano, but has a quality most closely resembling a contralto; (6) in the East castration was performed upon male slaves whose function it was to guard the harem or seraglio.

Catalepsy: an old-fashioned word used to describe any form of suspended animation characterized by immobility and lack of movement. It is a symptom of gross hysteria and somewhat rare since hysteria became unfashionable, but it may be found in advanced schizophrenia.

Cataplasm: poultice.

Cataract: an opacity in the lens of the eye which obscures the vision.
CAUSE: in childhood it may occur without obvious cause, it may be associated with a defect of calcium metabolism in the mother, such as may occur in parathyroid disease, or it may follow syphilis or an attack of German measles during pregnancy. It is often found in association with other defects in the eye. In later age, usually after 50, it develops as an extension of the process whereby most people undergo an increasing hardening of the lens which leads to difficulty in focusing on near objects as the years go by. In cataract more pronounced hardening and consequent shrinking occurring near the centre lead to 'splintering' of the lenses and opacity. Senile cataract of this type has nothing to do with the general health or even with the health of the rest of the eye. Other causes of cataract are diabetes, injury, prolonged exposure

to heat as with glassworkers, and exposure to ionizing radiations.

SYMPTOMS: (1) An appearance of spots before the eyes which; unlike those seen by perfectly normal people when they pay attention to them, do not move; (2) bright lights are sometimes seen double (for example street lamps seen at a distance in the dark); (3) short sight, at first helped by glasses; (4) gradually increasing blindness – at first vision in twilight may be better than in full daylight since light is admitted round the more widely dilated pupil in the dark; (5) in the final stages an obvious greyish-white discoloration in the pupil.

TREATMENT: the only possible treatment is by operation. Unscrupulous people may sell salves to 'dissolve cataract'; these often contain atropine, which dilates the pupil with the effect mentioned above (see 4); although vision may improve for a matter of hours no lasting cure will result. The operation is carried out under general or local anaesthesia, and the surgeon removes the opaque lens from its capsule. It is an operation of great antiquity; the results are very good, and no visible scar is left. Obviously patients have to wear glasses after the operation, for they have no lens of their own.

Catarrh: an Hippocratic word meaning discharge from an inflamed mucous membrane, particularly from the membranes lining the air sinuses of the head and the air passages of the nose and throat. As a diagnosis 'catarrh' has rightly almost disappeared, for it is entirely unspecific; as the name for a symptom it tends to linger.

Catatonia: in some types of schizophrenia the patient may show a disturbance of movement. He may be immobile, and stay where he is put or where and how he is told to stand, sit or lie – a state of automatic obedience. He may imitate exactly the movements of someone else; but he may also suddenly break out into wild excitement, and become violent and destructive and dangerous. He is confused and hallucinated, but the condition is not permanent and there is a good possibility of recovery from a catatonic state. It may recur.

Catgut: catgut is made not from the guts of a cat but from the intestines of sheep. The fibrous tissue is split up into threads and then woven to give various thicknesses and strengths; it can be treated with chromic acid to make chromic catgut, which stays intact in the tissues for up to three weeks instead of being absorbed like ordinary catgut in a week. It is used by the surgeon to tie off vessels and to stitch in places where there is a risk of infection or where it is better that the stitch should be absorbed. It is not normally used to stitch skin, for skin stitches can be removed at will, and silk and nylon are stronger, create less reaction, and are easier to use for this purpose.

Cathartics: purgatives.

Catheter: a tube for introduction into the cavities of the body to draw off fluid, especially one for passing through the urethra into the bladder. Catheters were originally made of metal, but the introduction of rubber and later plastics revolutionized their use. Modern catheters are made in all manner of shapes, sizes and materials, and with the introduction of disposable ready-sterilized catheters in flexible materials it once again becomes possible to follow our great-grandfathers' example and carry a catheter coiled up in one's hat.

Cat-scratch Fever: a disease in which there is fever and swelling of the local lymphatic glands after superficial damage to the skin.
CAUSE: it is thought that the infective agent is a virus. The disease often, although not necessarily, follows a scratch or bite from a cat, but no infective agent has been identified in cats from which the disease has been acquired.
SYMPTOMS: 7 to 21 days after a small wound in the skin has been sustained the lymph glands draining the part become enlarged and may even break down to form an abscess. There is a raised temperature and the patient feels ill, but the disease is self-limiting. It runs its course in a matter of weeks.
DIAGNOSIS: this is made by using a skin test. The importance of the condition is that it may resemble more serious diseases that cause enlargement of the lymph glands.
TREATMENT: there is no specific treatment.

Cauda Equina: the spinal cord is one-third shorter than the vertebral column in which it lies, but the nerves that come from the cord run out one by one between the vertebrae. The consequence is that the nerves in the neck run out almost straight from the cord to the spaces between the vertebrae, but as the discrepancy in length becomes greater the nerves take on a more slanting course, until the spinal cord ends opposite the second lumbar vertebra. By then it has given off the nerves that are going to go through the spaces between the lower lumbar and the sacral vertebrae, and they continue vertically downwards as a leash of nerves which is called the cauda equina, the horse's tail.

Cauliflower Ear: a blow on the ear may cause bleeding between the cartilage of the ear and its lining membrane, the perichondrium. If the blood is left it may not in the normal course of events be absorbed, because there is no pressure on the ear and no movement to break up the clot. In consequence it may become fibrous, so that the ear is distorted as scar tissue forms and contracts. The result is called a cauliflower ear from its resemblance to the vegetable. TREATMENT: in an established case a plastic surgeon may be able to help. The best treatment is prevention, and after an injury the blood should be let out while it is still liquid. If it has clotted it should be removed through a surgical incision. A pressure dressing is used to prevent the blood collecting again.

Causalgia: a very severe burning pain which may develop after injury to a nerve.
CAUSE: incomplete division of a nerve is most likely to lead to this distressing complication, and the nerves most commonly affected are the median nerve in the arm, the sciatic nerve in the leg, and the brachial plexus, the collection of nerves which supplies the arm. It is thought that the burning sensation is the result of impulses spreading abnormally at the site of injury between sympathetic and sensory nerve fibres.
SYMPTOMS: a few weeks after the injury the patient notices that his hand or his foot or leg is beginning to tingle, and then the sensation turns into a burning pain which is set off by various stimuli, some quite slight. The affected area

turns red and sometimes moist. The patient's whole life is eventually governed by the pain.

TREATMENT: fortunately for most of us the condition is rare, so that there is no unanimity about treatment. It is possible to operate on the sympathetic nervous system (*see* Nervous System) or to make injections into it, or to explore the damaged nerve and rejoin the ends. It is said by some that the condition given time will disappear by itself; others say that it gets worse and that operation should be carried out early. One thing is certain, that no habit-forming drugs ought to be used to control the pain.

Cautery: either the process of killing tissues by the application of heat or chemical substances, or the instrument – a hot iron, for example, or electrical apparatus – by which the heat is engendered or applied.

Cell: the unit of which the body is made. Some primitive organisms are made up of one cell, but the most complicated animals, the mammals, are made up of many million cells of many different types. Study of the cell is basic to an understanding of the function and chemistry of living creatures, and it has been carried on ever since optical microscopes were invented; the electron microscope has recently given an enormous impetus to the work. The cells found in man are of all sizes and shapes, from the cells of the nervous system that may give off processes which extend for two or three feet to the smallest cell of all – the red blood cell which has a diameter of 0.007 mm.

The cell usually includes the following structures: outer limiting membrane, cytoplasm and nucleus. The nucleus consists of the envelope, nucleoplasm, the nucleolus and the sex chromatin. The cytoplasm consists of a matrix, endoplasmic reticulum, the mitochondria, lysosomes, Golgi apparatus, ribosomes and centrioles. The cell membrane is made of protein, carbohydrate and fatty molecules, and in life is in incessant motion. It regulates the passage into and out of the cell of chemical substances, and carries antigens on its outer surface which identify it (*see* Allergy). The cytoplasm is the name given to all the material inside the cell except the nucleus, and it is seen by the electron microscope to be organized into many definite tubes, circles and other structures, called the endoplasmic reticulum. Parts of the endoplasmic reticulum have been named – the Golgi bodies, whose function is uncertain, the ribosomes which contain RNA, the substance concerned in the synthesis of proteins, mitochondria where metabolism takes place, lysosomes of doubtful function, and centrioles which are to do with cell division. The nucleus inside the cell is contained in a membrane of its own, the nuclear membrane, formed from the endoplasmic reticulum. Inside the nuclear membrane is the nucleoplasm, and in it there is a concentration of RNA called the nucleolus. The rest of the nucleus is made up of DNA, the substance which holds the key to the re-duplication of cells and therefore of the whole individual. Each type of cell is different, and each has special features which vary according to function. Study of cell structure and function is especially valuable in the understanding of cancer (q.v.). For example, one of the properties of normal cells which would seem to be lacking in the cancer cell is the ability to stick together, which might explain the diffuse and invasive nature of a cancer.

Cellulitis: inflammation which is not localized by the reaction of the infected tissues may spread into the surrounding connective tissue, usually that just under the skin. This is shown by a spreading area of red, swollen, painful skin, with red lines where the infecting organisms have invaded the lymphatic vessels leading to the regional lymph glands. Treatment must be quick and adequate, for cellulitis may lead to septicaemia, and multiplication of bacteria and toxins in the bloodstream, which is sometimes fatal. Medical advice is essential.

Cellulose: a carbohydrate which forms the skeleton of most plants, cellulose is not digested by human beings. It therefore provides the bulky part of the intestinal contents, and plays a part in the treatment of cases of constipation where it is thought that an increase in the volume of the contents of the large bowel might help evacuation. As methyl cellulose it has been used in the treatment of obesity, for taken with water it swells up in the stomach and so quells the pangs of hunger. Its advantage is that it has no action whatever either as drug or nourishment; its disadvantage is that people often imagine that they have to take it in addition to their normal daily intake of food.

Cephaloridine: scientists have obtained antibiotics from all sorts of unlikely places: oxytetracycline has the proprietary name Terramycin because it was obtained from an earth mould; bacitracin came from a culture taken from a leg infection in a little girl called Margaret Tracey; and, as everybody knows, penicillin came from a piece of mould blown from the dust of a London street to enter a window of Sir Alexander Fleming's laboratory and contaminate one of his culture plates. Cephaloridine, or rather cephalosporium, the mould from which it came, was picked up by Professor Brotzu of Sardinia at the seaward end of a sewage pipe. The Professor had his reasons for looking in this unsalubrious spot, for he thought rightly that sewage, which contains a deal of excrement, might be associated with something which could attack the organisms of intestinal disease. Cephaloridine (Ceporin, Loridine) is similar in structure to penicillin, but it can be used against organisms which do not respond to penicillin therapy. It cannot be taken by mouth.

Cerebellum: the part of the brain which occupies the lower rearmost part of the skull. *See* Nervous System.

Cerebro-spinal Fever: *see* Meningitis.

Cerebro-spinal Fluid: the fluid in which the central nervous system lies, contained within the meningeal membranes. Abbreviation 'C.S.F.' *See* Nervous System.

Cerebrum: the main, and largest, part of the brain, lying within the upper part of the skull. It is divided into two cerebral hemispheres. *See* Nervous System.

Cerumen: waxy secretion normally found in the human ear which in excess may cause blockage and temporary deafness. It is easily removed by the doctor, but it is dangerous for uninformed people to try to get it out, for the eardrum is easily damaged.

Cervical: concerned with the neck, as in cervical vertebrae or cervical nerves. Also concerned with the cervix, the neck or entrance to the womb.

Cervical Intervertebral Disc Disease: the discs of elastic and fibrous connective tissue that separate the bodies of the vertebrae are sometimes the seat of degenerative disease. The ring of fibrous tissue that encloses the elastic centre of the disc may give way and allow the disc centre to protrude, or prolapse, so that it presses against the spinal cord or the nerve roots where they emerge from between the vertebrae. The part of the spine most commonly affected is the small of the back, but it can occur in the neck.

SYMPTOMS: sudden pain in the neck, stiff neck, pain going down the arm; weakness or even paralysis of the legs, retention of or difficulty in passing urine, or difficulty in controlling it. Later, if the disease progresses, various symptoms of nerve compression may develop in the arm, and symptoms of compression of the spinal cord may develop at a level below the protrusion.

DIAGNOSIS: this is a matter for a neurologist, who will distinguish the condition from similar conditions caused by cervical spondylosis (*see* below), spinal tumour or disseminated sclerosis. Prolapse of a cervical disc is not as common as cervical spondylosis, and is often associated with it.

TREATMENT: massage and manipulation may help, and traction on the neck, either intermittent or continuous, is used. A high collar or even a plaster cast keeps the neck still and prevents further irritation of nerve roots. If there are signs of acute compression of the spinal cord – a developing paralysis of the legs and arms with disturbance of the bladder – an operation may be performed to relieve the pressure. It is dangerous to try to remove the disc itself.

Cervical Rib: normally the first vertebra to bear a rib is the first thoracic, but on occasion the lower vertebrae of the neck, commonly the seventh but sometimes also the sixth, may bear a rib or the rudiment of a rib. This may show itself by pressing on the subclavian artery or the brachial plexus and producing symptoms in the arm. *See* Thoracic Inlet Syndrome.

Cervical Spondylosis: spondylosis of the spine is an arthritic process involving the vertebrae, and is often associated with osteoarthritis in the rest of the skeleton. Because it commonly follows repeated minor injury, it occurs in the movable parts of the spine – the neck and the lower back. It may follow an injury sustained many years before, particularly the 'whiplash' injury of the neck which may occur in a motor-car accident. There is often some disc disease involving a degree of prolapse, and the X-ray shows a narrowed space between the vertebral bodies. It also shows the essential feature of the condition, spiky small outgrowths of bone round the edge of the vertebral bodies and the edges of the spaces by which the nerves leave the spinal column. These outgrowths of bone which press upon the nerve roots and upon the spinal cord are called osteophytes.

SYMPTOMS: the same as those found in association with a prolapsed intervertebral disc, with the addition of headache felt over the back of the head. The trouble is worst when the neck is moved, and is relieved by rest.

TREATMENT: the same as for cervical intervertebral disc disease (q.v.). General treatment for osteoarthritis such as aspirin or phenylbutazone may be useful.

Cervicitis: inflammation of the cervix, the neck of the womb.

CAUSE: may follow childbirth or gonorrhoea, or prolapse of the uterus.

SYMPTOMS: a discharge, pain on intercourse, frequency of urination. May continue and become chronic, and may lead to erosion of the cervix (q.v.).

TREATMENT: treatment of any associated infection. Cautery of the cervix, which may be carried out under general anaesthetic but can be done without, by electric cautery or diathermy, or by chemical cautery with zinc chloride.

Cestodiasis: tapeworm infection. *See* Worms.

Cetrimide: proprietary names Cetavlon, Cetavlex; this is a mixture of alkyl ammonium bromides in the form of liquid, powder or cream. It is used in 1% solution for cleaning the skin in acne and seborrhoea, or for cleaning wounds.

Chalazion: a small round swelling of the eyelid, caused by blockage of the duct of one of the sebaceous glands (Meibomian glands) with consequent formation of a retention cyst.

Chancre: the early ulcer or sore of syphilis or chancroid; the former feels hard, the latter soft (hence the name 'soft sore'). The chancre develops on that area where inoculation took place, usually the genitals but occasionally round the mouth or elsewhere. *See* Syphilis, Chancroid.

Chancroid: a venereal disease found mainly but not exclusively in tropical and subtropical countries.
CAUSE: infection with Ducrey's bacillus.
SYMPTOMS: painful soft ulceration of the genitals beginning a few days after infection. The lymph glands of the groin are enlarged and form a bubo; if the condition is allowed to progress not only is there much pain but skin may be lost from the genitals.
TREATMENT: sulphonamides are the first choice; if they fail, which is rare, then streptomycin or tetracycline may be used. Penicillin is worse than useless, for it may obscure syphilis acquired at the same time. The condition leaves scars, but does not progress to secondary or tertiary stages like syphilis.

Change of Life: *see* Menopause.

Chapped Hands: *see* Chilblains.

Chaulmoogra Oil: a volatile oil obtained from an Asiatic shrub (Taraktogenos kurzii) by pressing the seeds; it was used internally and externally in the treatment of leprosy but has been replaced by the sulphones.

Cheiropompholyx: a condition of the skin of the hands and sometimes of the feet in which tiny blisters appear along the sides of, and between, the fingers. There may be intense itching. The rash may be a reaction to irritants, it may develop in association with eczema, or it may be part of a sensitivity reaction to fungus infection in another part of the body. Attacks of athlete's foot (q.v.) are often the exciting cause. The itching and any secondary infection following rupture of the tiny blisters may be treated by corticosteroid ointments with neomycin added.

Cheloid: an overgrowth of scar tissue at the site of an old cut or burn. It occurs in some races more than others and is particularly common among some Negro peoples, although it is by no means confined to them. The scar instead of disappearing spreads and sends out offshoots like claws which pucker up the surrounding skin, usually where it is stretched, for example on the front of the chest. Treatment includes plastic surgery, although clearly the site of the plastic operation may be subject to cheloid formation, and the local injection of triamcinolone. Cheloid is also spelt keloid.

Chemotherapy: the treatment of infections by chemical agents which deal with specific organisms. The first such agent was quinine, which deals specifically with the parasite of malaria; this was followed many years later by the discovery by Ehrlich in 1910 of his 'magic bullet' – Salvarsan, or arsphenamine, which was fatal to the organisms of syphilis. The difficulty is, of course, to find compounds which kill bacteria without killing their host, but many chemotherapeutic agents have been discovered since Ehrlich showed the way, notably the sulphonamides.

Chest, Diseases of: the main organs in the chest are the lungs and the heart, and the main symptoms affecting the chest are associated with these organs. In general, pain in the chest can come from the ribs, the muscles between the ribs, the pleura – the membrane lining the lungs – and the heart. It can also arise because of disease of the vertebrae affecting the nerves of the upper part of the spinal column. The only pain brought about by heart disease is that felt as the result of poor blood supply to the heart muscle (*see* Angina Pectoris); a great number of patients who think that they have heart disease are in fact suffering from indigestion. Other symptoms that are brought about by disease in the chest include cough, breathlessness and blueness (cyanosis) of the skin. *See* Lungs, Heart, Aneurysm, Angina Pectoris and Coronary Thrombosis, Pleurisy,

Pneumonia, Bronchitis, Tuberculosis, Bornholm Disease etc.

Cheyne-Stokes Breathing: a type of breathing found in those in deep coma or dying. The breathing rhythm is in cycles, starting with shallow breaths, which gradually increase until having reached a peak they die away again. The breathing may stop altogether between cycles. Also called periodic respiration.

Chickenpox: (Varicella). A common infectious disease of children.

CAUSE: a virus related to that of herpes zoster (shingles).

SYMPTOMS: incubation period 14–21 days. On the first day the rash appears; it begins as tiny red spots in the area covered by the vest and spreads outwards to the limbs, unlike smallpox which starts on the limbs and moves inwards. The spots turn into blisters which finally become pustules and form scabs. The child may have a headache, be irritable and have a slight temperature.

TREATMENT: if the child feels ill then he should be put to bed and perhaps given aspirin, but there is no reason why all cases should be put to bed. Calamine lotion, to which up to 1% phenol may be added to stop irritation, will help if the rash is very uncomfortable, but if the rash in its later stages becomes infected medical attention is essential. It is important to keep the rash clean and to try to avoid secondary bacterial infection, for it is this which produces scars. The child should be encouraged not to scratch.

Complications are very rare in children. The infective period extends from 5 days before the rash to 1 week after the eruptions first appear. There is no reason why other members of the family should not be exposed to a harmless infection which confers immunity for life, but other people's children are another matter.

Chilblains: (Erythema pernio). An inflamed condition of the skin of the hands, feet and sometimes the ears and nose which is related to poor circulation and cold weather and seen most often in young people. The backs of the fingers and toes, and especially of the little finger and little toe, are affected.

SYMPTOMS: the skin becomes purple and starts to burn and itch, and then often forms blisters which can be very painful. These may break open and leave a sore which takes a long time to heal.

TREATMENT: those liable to chilblains should wear thick boots, gloves and stockings when they go out, and when they come in from the cold it is important that the heating indoors should be at a reasonable level. Various proprietary preparations are said to improve the circulation, but none takes the place of warm clothes. One treatment formerly recommended was taking exercise, a hot bath and a cold shower.

Chill: a meaningless term better avoided.

Chimney Sweep's Cancer: cancer of the scrotum. *See* Cancer.

Chiropractic: a system of medicine founded on the dubious belief that disease is caused by abnormal function of the nervous system; manipulation, particularly of the spine, is said to restore the nerves to their normal condition.

Chloral Hydrate: this substance depresses the central nervous system and is, like the barbiturates, a sedative; it is mostly used to send the old and the young to sleep. Although it is safe it has an unpleasant taste and is inclined to irritate the stomach. A dose of 1 g sends the average person to sleep in about half an hour for up to six hours. There is little or no hangover.

Chloramphenicol: (Chloromycetin). An antibiotic originally prepared from a sample of soil collected in Venezuela in 1947. It has a wide range of action, but unfortunately it has been found to interfere in some cases with the function of bone marrow so as to cause aplastic anaemia – anaemia occurring because no blood cells are being made – and its use is therefore dangerous. There are, however, infections in which its value is greater than its danger, such as fulminating enteric fever, meningitis caused by infection with Haemophilus influenzae, and other infections where

135

bacteriological sensitivity tests show that chloramphenicol is the antibiotic of choice.

Chlorhexidine: (Hibitane). An antiseptic, used as a cream in midwifery and as a solution on the skin for general antisepsis. It may be used on superficial skin wounds.

Chlorine: this gas, contained in compounds like sodium hypochlorite which release it, kills bacteria, fungi and viruses. Chlorine is cheap and easily produced, and it is therefore widely used in disinfecting water for drinking. It is also used in swimming-baths. In the form of eusol, which contains hypochlorous acid, chlorine is used to disinfect chronic ulcers, but its use is limited because its action is stopped by the presence of too much organic matter. The fumes of chlorine are poisonous because they are very irritating (indeed, an overchlorinated swimming-pool will soon bring complaints of sore eyes), and after a patient has apparently recovered from exposure to chlorine gas he may develop oedema, or wet swelling, of the lungs and become seriously ill; the appropriate treatment is administration of oxygen. Chlorine is used for bleaching, and some household bleaches which contain hypochlorites give off chlorine to produce their effect. If they are swallowed the stomach, gullet and mouth can be dangerously irritated.

Chloroform: introduced as an anaesthetic agent in 1847, and used freely as a general anaesthetic until quite recent times, its use is now rare; it was found to act on heart muscle so as to produce irregular beating and a fall of blood pressure, sometimes fatal. It is also toxic to the liver. A great deal of chloroform, however, is still consumed in cough mixtures and in medicinal mixtures in general, particularly those intended to aid digestion. (Chloroform water is used to make up the bulk of mixtures.)

Chloromycetin: *see* Chloramphenicol.

Chlorophyll: the green colouring matter of plants; its structural formula is the same as that of haemoglobin with the iron component replaced by magnesium. Although it has been taken internally as a medicine, there is no reason to suppose that it has any action in man except to provide minute amounts of magnesium. Local application is said to reduce bad smells, and tablets dissolved in the mouth are widely advertised to cure bad breath. However this may be, there is no evidence to encourage the belief that when taken in tablet form it prevents what is known to the advertising trade as body odour.

Chloroquine: (Nivaquine). This is one of the most powerful drugs known for suppressing malaria, as a dose of as little as 300 mg weekly will protect against most Plasmodia. Unfortunately, resistant strains of Plasmodium falciparum, the organism responsible for malignant malaria, have developed, so that chloroquine prophylaxis cannot entirely be trusted. Although the use of chloroquine was once recommended in active rheumatism its early promise has not been sustained, and it is now rarely used; however, in liver abscess caused by Entamoeba histolytica, chloroquine is still the drug generally preferred. It has no action on intestinal amoebic dysentery.

Chlorpromazine: (Largactil or Thorazine). This drug is chemically related to the antihistamine drug promethazine, and its use in mental disorders as a 'tranquillizer' is said to have been suggested by the observation that the giving of allergy-suppressing drugs to the mentally ill was often accompanied by a sedative effect and an improvement of mental symptoms. Another version has it that the sedative effect was noticed in experimental animals; however, chlorpromazine has been used with great success on patients seriously ill with schizophrenia, mania and depression. It was once used on patients showing anxiety, but other drugs have since proved more useful in neurotic states. Chlorpromazine is used as a premedication before anaesthetics, for it potentiates the action both of analgesics and anaesthetics, and reduces vomiting. It is also said to have the specific action of terminating the effects of the drug L.S.D.

Chlortetracycline: Aureomycin. *See* Tetracyclines.

Choanae: the posterior nasal apertures, by which the nasal cavity communicates with the upper part of the pharynx. They are divided by the bony part of the nasal septum.

Choking: the gullet and the windpipe divide in the upper part of the throat behind the tongue, and there is a mechanism to shut off the windpipe when food is being swallowed. If this mechanism fails, either because of paralysis of the muscles concerned, as can happen in bulbar paralysis (q.v.), or because the individual is laughing or talking or taking a breath at the same time as he is trying to swallow, food or drink or other things such as chewing-gum can 'go down the wrong way'. An involuntary gasp may have the same effect. TREATMENT: try to dislodge the obstruction by slapping the victim hard on the back in time with his coughing. If it is a child that is choking, turn him upside down – an obvious measure that can save a great deal of distress. If the obstruction cannot be dislodged by simple means, and the patient goes on choking (he may start to turn blue) call for help, and try to hook out the fragment of food from the area immediately behind the tongue with your finger. It has been known for elderly people to collapse and die inside five minutes from the effects of choking on a gobbet of food.

Cholagogues: drugs said to stimulate a flow of bile. The only true cholagogues are bile and bile salts, but they are rarely used.

Cholangiogram: an X-ray picture of the biliary apparatus, which can be outlined by radio-opaque substances either taken by mouth, injected into the veins, or introduced directly into the bile ducts at operation.

Cholangitis: inflammation of the bile ducts.
CAUSE: infection due to blockage by stones, tumour, or resulting from operations on the bile ducts.
SYMPTOMS: jaundice, vomiting, pain in the upper right part of the abdomen due to an enlarged tender liver, dark urine, pale motions, and intermittent fever, in which every day or two there is a severe short rise of temperature with sweating and shivering.
TREATMENT: the infection is first brought under control with antibiotics, and as soon as possible an operation is

performed to free the bile ducts of any obstructions and if necessary to drain or remove the gall-bladder.

Cholecystitis: inflammation of the gall-bladder; acute or chronic.

(a) Acute

CAUSE: infection with such bacteria as streptococci, Escherichia coli, and sometimes the typhoid bacillus, usually in the presence of stones.

SYMPTOMS: acute pain felt in the upper part of the abdomen under the ribs, which can radiate through to the back and be felt under the right shoulderblade and even in the tip of the right shoulder. There is nausea and vomiting; the attack may come on after a long period during which the patient has suffered from indigestion and wind.

TREATMENT: at first conservative. The patient is put to bed, given antibiotics such as tetracycline, and only allowed fluids by mouth. All fats are forbidden. If there is no improvement, or the state gets worse, then operation has to be considered at once, but if all goes well and the patient responds to medical treatment operation for removal of the gall-bladder is performed about six weeks after the acute attack.

(b) Chronic

CAUSE: again, bacterial infection and stones.

SYMPTOMS: this condition tends to be found in women 'fair, fat and forty'. They may complain of indigestion and wind, which comes on after eating fatty food, or they may have recurrent pain under the ribs on the right which can travel up to the shoulderblade and tip of the right shoulder. The state of the gall-bladder is investigated by cholangiography (*see* Cholangiogram).

TREATMENT: low-fat diet, removal of the gall-bladder.

Cholelithiasis: stones in the gall-bladder and the bile ducts.

CAUSE: uncertain, but often associated with infection of the gall-bladder. There are three sorts of gall-stones: (1) mixed, made of bile pigments, calcium, cholesterol; (2) pure cholesterol; (3) bile pigments alone – a soft, rare stone.

SYMPTOMS: usually the patient has suffered from attacks of inflammation of the gall-bladder for some time, or gives a story of 'indigestion'; then suddenly he has an attack of biliary colic, a severe pain under the ribs on the right radiating up to the right shoulder. This lasts until the stone causing it passes out of the bile duct; if it does not do so, it may be caught where the bile duct joins the small intestine. A blockage of bile ensues, with more or less pain and increasing jaundice; but sometimes this type of blockage is painless. Obstruction to the bile ducts may cause cholangitis (q.v.) or empyema of the gall-bladder, when the gall-bladder is full of pus.

TREATMENT: the treatment of the acute phase is treatment of the pain by atropine, which relaxes the smooth muscle of the bile ducts, and perhaps morphine or pethidine. The patient is put to bed and allowed only fluids by mouth, but even if the symptoms subside under medical treatment stones can only be treated properly by operation. No drug is known that can 'dissolve' them. Often it is the small stones that give more trouble than really big ones, which stay in the gall-bladder without emerging to block the bile ducts.

Cholera: a disease originating in Bengal, in India. It spread from India during the nineteenth century in a series of epidemics along the trade routes. In 1817, it spread to Japan; in the same year it reached Astrakhan, in Russia; in 1826 it was in Moscow, in 1831 Berlin, and by 1832 it had reached Paris and London. From London it was taken to Canada by emigrants. Other devastating epidemics reached Europe in the years 1847–55, 1865 via the pilgrim route from India to Mecca, and 1885, but by 1895 cholera had almost disappeared from Europe. Its mortality had been terrifying – for example, in 1892 there were nearly 17,000 cases, more than half of which were fatal, in a single epidemic in Hamburg.

CAUSE: infection with the Cholera vibrio.

SYMPTOMS: incubation period 2–5 days. The greatest danger is loss of body fluids. There are three stages of the illness:

1. Mild diarrhoea and vomiting, which rapidly get worse until the motions contain no faecal matter and look like rice-water. Severe cramps begin in the muscles of the limbs and abdomen caused by lack of salts. The temperature is raised, but the skin is cold and blue, the pulse weak, and there is a terrible thirst which, when satisfied with water,

only makes the cramps worse by diluting the body salts still further. This 'stage of evacuation' lasts from 3 to 12 hours.

2. The stage of collapse. Now the body starts to become colder, the skin dry, wrinkled and purple, the voice weak and husky, the urine scanty and dark or altogether absent. The blood pressure falls to a very low level, so that the pulse can scarcely be felt, and the cramps are agonizing. It is in this 'algid' stage that the patient may die, as little as 24 hours after the onset of symptoms.

3. In favourable cases the third stage, the stage of recovery, follows when all the changes appear to reverse themselves, with fluid loss decreasing and the general condition improving; but even now relapses may occur, or the patient may sink into a condition resembling typhoid fever when he gradually deteriorates over a period of 2 or 3 weeks. During this 'stage of reaction' the temperature may be raised, and the patient may be in danger from pneumonia.

TREATMENT: this is directed from the first towards combating the loss of fluids and salts from the body, which can best be done by giving intravenous infusions of saline solution – the patients may need 5 litres or even 10 litres a day, although care is necessary to avoid waterlogging the patient through too enthusiastic treatment. Potassium may have to be added to the infused fluid. The intestines can be cleared of the cholera organisms by antibiotics, notably tetracycline, which is given for 5 days. The most important part of treatment is prevention. Cholera vaccine can be obtained which gives immunity for a few months, but it cannot take the place of extreme care in the preparation of food and water for drinking, and its protection against flies. All cases must be isolated and excreta, bedding and everything soiled by them sterilized. Cholera nowadays is only likely to spread when catastrophe disorganizes public health services, to whose work the disappearance of cholera from the West is due.

Cholesterol: a substance synthesized in the liver and supplied in the diet. It is a monatomic alcohol, and is found in fat and animal oils; it makes up a large proportion of gall-stones either by itself or more commonly mixed with bile pigments, and it is of importance in arterial disease (atheroma) including disease of the coronary arteries. The steroids, which include the sex hormones and the hormones of the adrenal glands, are made from cholesterol.

Choline: a substance found in egg-yolks, liver and meat; its absence from the diet of animals leads to fatty liver and cirrhosis, but attempts to cure the same condition in humans by giving choline have not been successful.

Chondroma: a benign and harmless, although sometimes inconvenient, tumour of cartilage.

Chordee: a condition in which the erect penis is bent. It may result from the congenital deformity hypospadias (q.v.) or gonorrheal infection.

Chordotomy: surgical division of the fibres in the spinal cord which carry pain impulses, sometimes carried out for the intractable pain of cancer. Also spelt Cordotomy. *See* Pain.

Chorea: a condition in which there is incessant involuntary jerky movement. There are two main varieties of chorea named after the physicians who described them – the Englishman Thomas Sydenham (1624–89), and the American George Huntingdon (1850–1916).
Sydenham's Chorea
CAUSE: inflammation of the brain associated with rheumatic fever.
SYMPTOMS: young children are affected, girls more than boys. The child becomes restless, irritable and tired. The involuntary movements at first are often thought to be clumsiness, but then the weakness which is a part of the disease and the incessant jerkiness and irregularity of the bodily movements are recognized for what they are. The face may be affected, so that the child grimaces and sticks its tongue out; the movements of the limbs may be confined to one half of the body.
TREATMENT: rest. The child must be put to bed in a quiet room without disturbances. Feeding may be difficult because of the movements and the grimacing, but the patient must be encouraged and helped to take a good varied diet. The main continuing danger is the development of rheu-

matic disease of the heart, for the chorea will pass but rheumatic heart disease leaves a permanently damaged heart. Treatment is given as for rheumatic fever (*see* Rheumatism), and the child kept in bed for up to 8 weeks, although the chorea may have passed off in 14 days.

Huntingdon's Chorea

CAUSE: an hereditary illness.

SYMPTOMS: continuous jerky movements are associated with progressive dementia. The disease shows itself in people of 40 or 50.

TREATMENT: there is no known cure; treatment has to be symptomatic. Largactil (Thorazine) is useful, and thiopropazate dihydrochloride (dartal) is used to quieten the movements.

Chorion: the outer of the two membranes enclosing the foetus. It may be the site of abnormal change, which at the expense of the foetus forms what is called a hydatidiform mole (q.v.). There may be very rarely a malignant change in the chorion following hydatidiform mole or even more rarely following a normal pregnancy. The malignant tumour that results is named Chorionepithelioma.

Choroid: (1) The middle pigmented and vascular coat of the eyeball (q.v.). (2) Choroid plexuses. Three plexuses of blood vessels, one lying in each lateral ventricle of the brain and one in the mid-line third ventricle, which secrete the cerebro-spinal fluid.

Christmas Disease: a blood disease similar to haemophilia in which coagulation is impaired and bleeding readily occurs which is difficult to control. Named after the surname of the first case reported in England, it is discovered in one in ten of the cases diagnosed clinically as haemophilia. It can only be distinguished by laboratory test.

Chromium: used in industry in making alloys, paints, ceramics, dyeing, tanning, in carrying out plating and producing aviation petrol, chromium and its salts can be poisonous.

SYMPTOMS: dermatitis, with or without ulceration of the skin. There may be swelling of the face and itching, and if ulcers form they tend to penetrate deeply into the skin and sub-cutaneous tissues. The septum of the nose may perforate. TREATMENT: the ulcers are treated with calcium E.D.T.A. ointment 10%. Prevention depends on maintaining proper ventilation to remove dust and vapour, in some cases the wearing of protective clothes, and frequent washing.

Chromosomes: the D.N.A., deoxyribonucleic acid, in mammalian cells is split up to form several rods or chromosomes, so called because of their staining reactions. Each species has a characteristic number of chromosomes: in man the number is 46. When cells divide, the chromosomes split, so that each cell still has 46 chromosomes. The chromosomes transmit inherited characteristics. *See* Cell, Mitosis, Meiosis, Heredity.

Chronic: lasting over a long period of time, as opposed to acute, which signifies something sudden.

Chrysotherapy: treatment with gold, usually in the form of its salts.

Chyle: the contents of the chief lymph vessel, the thoracic duct, which carries food substances absorbed from the intestine by the lymph vessels of the intestinal wall, the lacteals, to the jugular vein in the neck.

Chyme: the contents of the stomach – partly digested food.

Cicatrix: scar.

Cilia: the hairs growing on the eyelid; the eyelashes. Hence small processes like eyelashes which are present on the outer surface of some cells.

Cinchona: a genus of trees growing in South America in the bark of which is found quinine. It is known as Jesuit's bark, as it was the Spanish priests who first observed its use against malaria by the native people during the Spanish invasion of Central and South America. Cinchona itself is named after the wife of the Viceroy of Peru, the Countess of

Cinchon, who is said to have brought the substance from the New World to Europe in 1640.

Circulation of the Blood: the fact that the blood circulates through the body was demonstrated by the English physician William Harvey in 1628. He did not, however, understand how the blood flows from the arteries into the veins, and assumed that it must percolate through 'pores' in the flesh. This gap in knowledge was filled 30 years later by Malpighi, of Italy, who with the new microscope was able to find the minute capillary vessels which join the arterial and venous systems.

The course of the blood through the body is as follows: arterial blood comes from the lungs into the left side of the heart, enters the left atrium, and is pumped by the contraction of the atrium through the mitral valve into the left ventricle. The left ventricle contracts; the mitral valve closes, and the blood, which cannot run back into the atrium, is pumped through the aortic valve into the aorta, the great artery of the body. The arterial system branches into many separate arteries, and the blood is carried to all parts of the body. The arteries branch into smaller arterioles, which in turn branch into many capillary vessels. These are very small indeed – much smaller than the hairs after which they are named – and in them the bright arterial blood gives up its oxygen to the tissues, and becomes dark venous blood. This is carried back to the heart through the venous system, which includes a special arrangement (the portal system) by which blood from the intestines is carried to the liver through which it passes before joining the venous blood from the rest of the body. The dark venous blood, exhausted of oxygen, passes through the superior and inferior venae cavae to reach the right side of the heart. Entering the right atrium, the blood is pumped through the tricuspid valve into the right ventricle; from the right ventricle it is pumped through the pulmonary valve into the pulmonary artery, and so to the lungs. Here the vessels again branch into many progressively smaller channels until in the capillaries the venous blood is only separated from the air in the alveoli – the air sacs – by an extremely thin wall. The blood exchanges gases with the air, and leaves the lungs full of oxygen, to flow into the left side of the heart and to begin circulating through the arterial system again.

Circumcision: removal of the foreskin of the penis is carried out for two reasons, religious and medical.

Religious: circumcision is a religious rite of great antiquity. It is found in many parts of the world, and was practised among others by the ancient Egyptians, the Coptic branch of the Christian religion which copied it from the Egyptians, the primitive Arabs and the Aztecs of South America; it is obligatory among Moslems, Jews and the aborigines of Australia. Its religious significance is not clear, but presumably it was both a form of sacrifice and a distinctive tribal mark. Female circumcision involving the removal of the larger part of the external genitals is still practised by a few primitive peoples; unlike male circumcision, which is a trivial procedure medically, this is a cruel, barbaric and dangerous rite.

Medical: the operation of circumcision is performed in infancy in cases where the foreskin is allegedly so tight as to interfere with urination. That this is mechanically so is doubtful, and some psychiatrists believe that even at this early age the operation may leave scars upon the mind as well as the body. There are other indications for the operation in later life, but although it is known that women married to uncircumcised men are more likely to develop cancer of the cervix (the neck of the womb) and that uncircumcised men are more likely to develop cancer of the prostate gland, these facts have not yet been taken as reasons for advocating large-scale circumcision.

Cirrhosis: development of fibrous tissue in an organ with consequent scarring, hardening and loss of function. The term is nearly always used to mean cirrhosis of the liver, called 'hobnail liver'.

CAUSE: (1) In some cases cirrhosis of the liver is associated with a very poor diet; cirrhosis of this kind is found in tropical countries and in chronic drinkers whose diet is very often almost entirely alcoholic. In other cases the illness follows infective jaundice, and in yet other cases the causes have not been identified, although the illness is identical. (2) A different kind of cirrhosis may follow repeated infection of the biliary system (*see* Gall-bladder). (3) Cirrhosis can occur rarely in other conditions, such as bilharzia and syphilis.

SYMPTOMS: (1) There may be no symptoms, the condition being found at post-mortem, or on routine examination in life. Often, however, the patient complains of vague ill health, loss of appetite, perhaps nausea and even vomiting – which may, of course, be due to alcoholic gastritis – swelling of the ankles, impotence, and more spectacularly, vomiting blood. Jaundice is not a common or early part of cirrhosis except when it is due to infection of the biliary apparatus.

TREATMENT: no alcohol; a good diet, with enough protein, and treatment for gastritis if it is present. If the condition progresses so far that the blood pressure in the portal system (*see* Veins) is raised, special treatment for this and for associated complications will be needed.

SYMPTOMS: (2) Repeated attacks of infection of the gall-bladder and the bile ducts, with perhaps biliary colic, which may have led to an operation for gallstones. Fever, pain in the upper right side of the abdomen, and jaundice return, and eventually the jaundice in spite of treatment of the inflammatory condition of the biliary apparatus becomes permanent. Itching may be associated with the jaundice, and there is intermittent fever. In this type of cirrhosis the liver is enlarged and smooth.

TREATMENT: antibiotics are used to control infection, and an operation to explore the bile ducts for narrowing or obstruction is carried out. The surgeon may be able to relieve the obstruction and drain the infected bile ducts, or carry out a plastic operation to open up a scarred and narrow duct.

Cisternal Puncture: it is possible to introduce a needle through the back of the neck immediately below the lower margin of the skull into the collection of cerebro-spinal fluid contained in the cisterna magna – the great cistern, into which the fluid drains from the fourth ventricle (*see* Nervous System), and from which the fluid passes down over the surface of the spinal cord and upwards over the surface of the cerebellum. This is not an operation to be done without due care: the cistern is about 2 inches in from the skin surface, and at 2½ inches in the same direction lies the medulla oblongata which is full of structures essential to life.

Cisternal puncture is not often used, but it is sometimes essential.

Claudication: limping, from a Latin word (the Emperor Claudius was a cripple). Usually applied to a condition arising from bad circulation of blood in the legs, where a cramping pain attacks the patient when he walks for a certain distance (which varies from patient to patient) and causes him to limp and stop. Because the pain wears off at rest, the claudication is called 'intermittent'.

Claustrophobia: an irrational fear of enclosed spaces. It is a symptom of neurosis, but that does not mean that anything need necessarily be done about it as many otherwise normal people have this feeling and avoid it by avoiding the circumstances which bring it about. *See* Agoraphobia.

Clavicle: the collar bone, called clavicle for its resemblance to a little key (of a very old-fashioned pattern).

Claw-hand: a condition of the hand which follows when the muscles supplied by the ulnar nerve are paralysed as a result of injury, leprosy or syringomyelia. The wrist is flexed, the knuckle joint extended and the fingers flexed. It is also called 'main en griffe'.

Cleft Palate: the nose, upper lip and palate are formed in the embryo by the fusion of three separate blocks of tissue. Growing downwards from the region of the forehead is the fronto-nasal process, and growing towards the mid-line from each side are the right and left maxillary processes. The fronto-nasal process forms the middle of the upper lip, the nose and the forehead, and the very front part of the hard palate. The two maxillary processes form the cheeks, the two sides of the upper lip, and the rest of the hard and soft palate.

If the development is abnormal, the following deformities may be produced:

1. Cleft face, where one maxillary process fails to unite with the fronto-nasal process. There is a cleft in the face running from the inner angle of the eye to the side of the mouth.

2. Bilateral or unilateral cleft lip, or hare lip; here one or

both maxillary processes have failed to fuse with the fronto-nasal process below the nose, so that the outer part of the upper lip is separated from the middle part.

3. If the two parts of the maxillary processes that grow in towards each other to form the roof of the mouth fail to meet and join, a cleft palate is the result; the cleavage may be in the soft or the hard palate. If the failure extends to include failure of fusion with the fronto-nasal process, there is a complete cleft palate and hare lip on one or both sides. TREATMENT: plastic surgery. If the palate and the lip are cleft, the child cannot suck and growth is retarded. Surgery is more of a risk in the undernourished baby, and the repair is therefore commonly postponed until the infant is over a year old. It should be done before the child is 2, otherwise it may not be easy to teach him to speak.

If the deformity is confined to the lip, and the child can suck, the operation may be carried out after he is 3 years old.

Climacteric: *see* Menopause.

Climate: is obviously linked with health, but no precise relationship has been worked out beyond the obvious factors – in the delta of the river Niger, for example, one tends to be ill, and in the mountain resorts of Switzerland one tends to be well; in some climates the parasites of tropical diseases flourish and in some they cannot live. It is common for climatic conditions to have an effect on subjective feelings, but subjective feelings are not to be equated with health.

Clinitest: proprietary tablets used to estimate the amount of sugar in urine. At one time this estimation involved making solutions and heating the specimen, but in common with various other estimations of chemical substances in urine and blood, methods have been so simplified that tests which once needed a laboratory can now be carried out in the surgery or in the patient's home. Very accurate determinations still need laboratory facilities.

Clostridium: a member of a family of bacteria which are rod-shaped, live without oxygen, and form spores – inactive forms which lie dormant and can resist conditions which kill the active organisms. The family of Clostridia include the bacilli of gas gangrene (Clostridium welchii), tetanus (Cl. tetani) and botulism (Cl. botulinum); they are commonly found in soil and dust.

Clotting: *see* Coagulation.

Cloxacillin: (Orbenin). An expensive semi-synthetic penicillin which can be given by mouth. It is not affected by staphylococcal penicillinase, a substance elaborated by some staphylococci especially in hospitals, which makes them resistant to naturally occurring penicillin, and it is therefore best reserved for the treatment of serious staphylococcal infections by penicillinase-producing organisms.

Clubbing: in certain conditions which interfere with respiration, notably chronic diseases of the lungs, the soft tissues over the ends of the fingers and toes are the site of tissue overgrowth, so that the ends of the fingers become club-shaped, with the root of the nail lifted in a characteristic way.

Club-foot: talipes; a deformity of the ankle and the foot which renders the patient unable to stand with the sole of the foot flat on the ground.

CAUSE: congenital; rarely acquired through nervous or muscular disease, for example poliomyelitis, or scarring after severe injury.

DESCRIPTION: club-foot is classified by description of the deformity.

1. Talipes equinus: the heel is pulled up so that the patient walks on his toes like a horse.

2. Talipes calcaneus: the toes are pulled up so that he walks on his heel.

3. Talipes varus: the sole of the foot is turned inwards so that he walks on the outer edge of his foot.

4. Talipes valgus: the sole of the foot is pulled outwards so that he walks on the inner edge of his foot.

Combinations of these basic deformities are usually seen, and the commonest are talipes equino-varus, in which the toes are on the ground and the foot is twisted inwards, and talipes calcaneo-valgus, where the heel is on the ground and the foot is twisted outwards.

TREATMENT: surgical operation, manipulation, or surgical appliances.

Clyster: archaic name for enema. The phrase was to 'throw up a clyster'.

Coagulation of the Blood: a very complicated process. Essentially, a circulating substance called fibrinogen is converted into an insoluble substance, fibrin, which forms the framework of the clot. So far 13 factors in the production of a clot have been identified, and if all of them function properly a circulating factor, prothrombin, is changed by tissue juice liberated by injury, or thromboplastin, to the substance thrombin, which acts on fibrinogen to make it into fibrin. Calcium is necessary for the process, and the platelets of the blood play a large part. They collect at the site of an injury where the walls of the blood vessel are cut through or torn, and form a plug which may stop minor leaks. They liberate substances necessary for coagulation as they coalesce to form the plug. It is clear that once a clot begins to form, something must keep it within bounds, or else it might fill the whole of the vascular system; and in fact there is a substance in the blood called plasminogen which in the presence of damage to blood-vessel walls is changed into plasmin, an enzyme which can break up thrombin. As soon as a clot begins to form because of damage to a blood vessel it is attacked by plasmin produced by the same injury and kept under control, and during the course of the day many small reactions of this sort must occur in the body. In such a complicated mechanism there is room for many accidents and deficiencies, and there are a number of conditions in which the abnormalities produce symptoms. The best-known disease affecting the coagulation of the blood is haemophilia (q.v.).

Coal Gas: contains 4–9% carbon monoxide; town gas usually supplied for use in homes is a mixture of coal gas and water gas, and may contain up to 20% carbon monoxide (q.v.).

Coarctation: a condition of narrowing or stricture, the term being used of the aorta.

Cobalt 60: a radioactive isotope used in the radiation treatment of malignant disease.

Cocaine: an alkaloid, obtained from the leaves of the South American tree Erythroxylon coca.
ACTION: it stimulates the central nervous system and induces feelings of alertness, euphoria and loss of fatigue. An overdose produces symptoms of poisoning – confusion, excitement, headache, fever, rapid pulse, irregular respiration, sweating, collapse and sometimes convulsions. Cocaine is a local anaesthetic; when applied to mucous membranes it causes constriction of the blood vessels.
USE: rarely used in medicine because of its toxic effects and because it is a drug of addiction. Its application is confined to the surgery of the nose and throat, where superficial spraying of 1–5% solutions produces local anaesthesia, and by constricting the blood vessels cuts down bleeding.
MISUSE: as a drug of addiction, cocaine is less used than opium and its derivatives, but it is more likely to produce dependence than any drug except heroin. It is used in most cases in the form of snuff ('snow'), occasionally by injection, and is usually taken in combination with other drugs, such as morphine. The addict looks anxious, thin, depressed and irritable. He is often sexually impotent; the pupils of the eyes are dilated. Sometimes there are hallucinations, visual and auditory, and a feeling of insects creeping beneath the skin (the 'cocaine bug'). The septum of the nose is often ulcerated. If he takes a dose of cocaine the addict becomes cheerful, witty and inexhaustible, but the exhilaration is soon followed by depression. No physical disorder follows the withdrawal of cocaine, but the patient habituated to it and psychologically dependent upon it is not often cured.

Coccydnia: severe pain in the region of the coccyx, which is the small bone at the lower end of the spinal column.
CAUSE: a fall on the bottom, which breaks or bruises the coccyx, a kick, or damage during childbirth.
TREATMENT: injections of local anaesthetic, or rarely surgical removal.

Cochlea: the essential organ of hearing in which the pressure of the sound waves transmitted from the eardrum and through the middle ear by the ossicles is transformed into impulses in the auditory nerve. The cochlea is shaped like the cavity in a snail shell, and it has $2\frac{3}{4}$ turns. It lies in the petrous temporal bone. For full discussion *see* Ear.

Codeine: methyl morphine – that is, codeine – has the same formula as morphine except that a methyl group has been added; but from its actions one would not recognize it as so nearly related to morphine. Its action in relieving pain is insufficient in serious cases, but it has a constipating action and an action in suppressing coughs which are useful, and it can be used in quite large doses without the dangers of morphine. It is made up into tablets with aspirin and phenacetin and sold under a number of proprietary names, and is relatively harmless. Addiction is no problem with codeine, but the drug is no substitute for morphine.

Cod Liver Oil: a rich if nauseating source of Vitamins A and D, often given as an emulsion to infants and small children to ensure that they do not become rickety. The smaller the child the less he appears to dislike the taste. It is possible to give too much Vitamin D and produce toxic effects; the dose of cod liver oil emulsion should not exceed 5 ml a day (about 2.5 ml of cod liver oil).

Coeliac Disease: a condition in children in which the small intestine fails to absorb food, particularly fats.
CAUSE: sensitivity to gluten, a protein found in wheat and other grain.
SYMPTOMS: after the addition of cereals to the diet of an infant between 6 and 9 months old, a child previously healthy begins to lose weight, becomes irritable and passes large pale offensive motions. After a time the abdomen begins to protrude, the limbs waste and the child may even develop the deficiency diseases, anaemia and rickets.
TREATMENT: a gluten-free diet. All flour and food containing flour must be avoided. Special flour without gluten is on the market, and gluten-free bread can be bought already baked. This method of treatment is a case of good coming out of evil, for during World War 2 the Dutchmen Kamer and

Weijers noticed that children suffering from coeliac disease improved when bread became unobtainable. On this observation our understanding of coeliac disease is based. *See also* Steatorrhoea.

Coil: a name for one type of intrauterine contraceptive device. *See* Contraception.

Colchicum: Colchicum autumnale, the meadow saffron, yields from its bulb the alkaloid colchicine, which is an effective remedy for gout. Given in tablets – the dose is 1 mg followed by 0.5 mg two-hourly – it usually takes between 5 and 8 mg to relieve an attack. The side effect of colchicine may be a gastro-intestinal upset.

Cold, Common: (Acute rhinitis, acute coryza). An infection of the upper respiratory tract.

CAUSE: the viruses involved include influenza, para-influenza, adenoviruses, rhinoviruses and many others.

SYMPTOMS: in a mild case, sneezing, clear discharge from the nose becoming thicker, perhaps a slight cough. In worse cases there is a slight temperature, shivering and a feeling of being cold, and a bad headache. The nose begins to run, and the throat feels sore. The eyes are red and moist, for there is mild conjunctivitis. There is a cough, at first dry. Cold sores, or herpes labialis, may break out on the lips. In an uncomplicated case recovery takes about three days, or the inside of a week, but very often secondary infection affects the nasal sinuses, the middle ear, the bronchi or the lungs; the secondary invaders are staphylococci, streptococci, H. influenzae, and pneumococci, and they produce tracheitis, bronchitis, acute sinusitis, otitis media with earache, and rarely broncho-pneumonia.

TREATMENT: there is no specific treatment for the common cold. Symptomatic treatment with aspirin, Dover's powder, or similar remedies will bring down the temperature and ease the headache. A solution made of two soluble aspirins in water may with advantage be used as a gargle and swallowed three or four times hourly; a dose of whisky with or without lemon juice is undoubtedly medicinal. Inhalations of steam with menthol or eucalyptus help, and ephedrine drops clear the nose. Antibiotics cannot influence an uncomplicated cold, but are used if there are signs of secondary bacterial infection; the spread of infection in a known sufferer from bronchitis can be prevented by antibiotics (ampicillin, tetracycline). The patient who has a cold ought to be confined to his room for two days, for colds are very infectious, but most people persist in 'fighting' the cold, continue to go to work, and spread the infection freely. Vaccines made from bacteria and taken by mouth are not likely to be effective, but immunization against some types of influenza virus and some adenoviruses can be helpful. On the whole, however, immunity is so short and the number of viruses causing upper respiratory tract infection is so large that vaccination is a lottery.

'Cold' Abscess: tuberculous abscess. So called because it develops slowly, with little reaction of inflammation and hardly any redness or heat in the surrounding tissues.

Cold Injury: accidental exposure to cold (1) of babies, and (2) of the elderly, resulting in serious illness.
In babies
SYMPTOMS: cold injury may occur when the room temperature falls much below 18 °C. (64 °F.), and all babies are liable to be affected, although premature and weakly babies are the most likely to be injured. The affected infant becomes quiet, shows little sign of hunger, and feels cold. The colour is red, and if the condition is allowed to continue the fat under the skin becomes hard and thick especially over the cheeks and the posterior. At first the pulse is fast, but if the baby's temperature begins to fall seriously below normal, the heartbeat slows down.
TREATMENT: slow warming in an incubator in hospital. Infection is liable to occur and must be treated as it arises.
In the elderly
SYMPTOMS: the temperature of the patient is below 35 °C. (95 °F.), and the old person is confused and slow. The pulse is slow, perhaps irregular, the skin cold, the breathing slow, the blood pressure low. The patient may be exposed to cold low enough to produce this state in his own home, and the cold in the room will be obvious.
TREATMENT: patients must not be warmed too quickly, but nursed under one blanket in a warm room. It may be

necessary to put up an intravenous drip and give antibiotics to ward off possible infection. Clearly the patient should be admitted to hospital.

Note: the lethal effects of cold on the young and old are not universally recognized. Babies must not be kept in cold rooms; every winter in Britain and in other 'temperate' countries a number of babies die because the danger of cold is not understood. The temperature of the baby's room must be kept above 18 °C. (64 °F.) and the baby's rectal temperature must never be allowed to fall below 35 °C. (95 °F.). The mortality of cold injury in the newborn is about 25% – that is, one of every four babies affected dies. The susceptibility of the old to cold injury is often greater than one might expect, and the illnesses of the elderly – stroke, heart disease, myxoedema – render them all the more vulnerable. Warmth is essential for the aged.

Colectomy: surgical removal of part of the colon or large intestine (partial colectomy), half of the colon (hemicolectomy), or the whole of the colon (total colectomy). The operation is performed for the removal of tumours, and for the radical cure of ulcerative colitis.

Colic: characteristic pain felt in the abdomen as a result of complete or partial blockage of one of the hollow tubes – intestines, ureters and bile ducts. The muscles lining the tube contract in order to expel the contents, but cannot, and the resulting tension produces the pain. Tension and colic may be produced by irritation of the linings of the tubes, for example in inflammation of the colon after eating irritant or toxic food, or as a result of some poisons. Colic is commonly produced in the ureters or the bile ducts by stones which block the tubes and irritate them. The pain of colic is characteristically intermittent, rising to a peak and then dying away. The spasms may come at regular or irregular intervals, and are of great intensity. Colic is eased by atropine, which relaxes involuntary muscle, and by pethidine (demerol), but cannot be cured unless the cause is found and dealt with.

Colitis: *See* Ulcerative Colitis.

Collagen Diseases: a group of diseases characterized by changes in the collagen fibres which help to make up the fibrous supporting tissues of the body. These diseases affect the brain, heart, joints and subcutaneous connective tissue, and are polyarteritis nodosa, rheumatic fever, rheumatoid arthritis, lupus erythematosus, scleroderma and dermatomyositis. The cause of this group of diseases is unknown.

Collapse Therapy: at one time chronic pulmonary tuberculosis was treated by collapsing the lung, so that the diseased area was at rest. The introduction of drugs effective against tuberculosis has entirely changed the pattern of treatment so that collapse therapy has fallen into disuse, and artificial pneumothorax, the most common method of collapsing the lung, is hardly ever now performed.

Collar Bone: the clavicle, which keeps the shoulder propped out away from the rib cage, runs from the upper part of the breastbone to the outer part of the scapula or shoulderblade. It is the most commonly broken bone in the body – the collar bone of a steeplechase jockey feels like a row of beads. The usual fracturing injury is a fall on the shoulder, or on the outstretched hand, and the usual fracture is at the junction of the middle and outer thirds.

The immediate treatment is to tie a bandage round the wrist and then round the neck so that the wrist is kept as near to the neck as possible. The surgeon usually uses a figure-of-eight bandage passing round the front of each shoulder and crossing at the back to keep the shoulders well braced back while the fracture is healing. The arm is kept in a sling.

Colles' Fracture: a common type of fracture of the wrist which, like a fracture of the clavicle, is often caused by a fall on the outstretched hand. The radius – the outer bone of the forearm – is broken about 2 cm above the wrist joint, and the fragment is pushed backwards. The fracture is recognized by its appearance, which is described as a 'dinner fork' deformity.

Treatment includes X-ray and reduction under anaesthetic, followed by application of a light plaster cast for about one month. While the forearm and hand are in plaster the patient must be on guard against letting the shoulder become stiff, for once stiffness is established it is difficult to get rid of it; full movement of the shoulder may be permanently lost.

Collodion: a clear liquid which dries to leave a transparent film sticking to the skin. It is made of ether and alcohol in which pyroxylin is dissolved (pyroxylin is a substance made by the action of nitric and sulphuric acids on cotton). The addition of castor oil makes flexible collodion, the most useful form of collodion, which can be used with great advantage on the blisters of herbes zoster and simplex (q.v.). It can also be used as a protective covering for small cuts and wounds.

Colloids: literally, substances like glue. A colloid system consists of a dispersion medium throughout which matter, called the disperse phase, is distributed. In suspension colloids, the disperse phase is composed of insoluble matter – metal, for example – and the dispersion medium is a gas, liquid, or solid; in emulsion colloids the dispersion medium is liquid (usually water), and the disperse phase complicated organic matter such as glue.

Colon: the main part of the large intestine. Starting in the right iliac fossa – the right lower part of the abdominal cavity – where the small intestine joins the caecum at the ileocaecal junction, the ascending colon passes upwards. It then travels across the upper part of the abdominal cavity as the transverse colon, and bends downwards at the splenic flexure to become the descending colon, which passes down the left side of the abdominal cavity. In the pelvis it forms a loop called the sigmoid colon before it joins the rectum.

Colostomy: an artificial anus. A loop of colon (large intestine) is brought out through the abdominal wall, to which it is secured, and opened. A colostomy is used in cases of obstruction of the large intestine, or where some of the intestine is to be removed. It may be temporary or permanent, but even if it has to be permanent there is no reason why a colostomy should be more than a minor nuisance. The practical difficulty is in regulating the bowels, for the patient has no control over his evacuations; but simple methods have been worked out to lessen this handicap, for the number and timing of the motions is fundamentally controlled by the type of food the patient eats, and he can learn how to regulate his diet.

A colostomy need not prevent the patient leading a substantially normal life.

Colostrum: a clear fluid secreted by the breasts during the first two or three days after childbirth.

Colour Blindness: the theory of colour vision depends on the fact that any colour in the spectrum can be matched by a mixture of three pure spectral colours of variable intensity but fixed wavelength. If this is so, then the presence of three pigments in the eye will enable it to carry out the matching of any colour in the spectrum. The visual pigment rhodopsin, visual purple, has been identified in the rods of the retina, and its function is to do with the recognition of light, which bleaches it, but it does not play any part in colour vision; research has therefore been concentrated on finding three further pigments in the cones of the retina (*see* Eye). There are indications that such pigments are present, but the mechanism of colour vision is still far from clear. However, theory based on the hypothetical normal presence of three pigments accounts for the types of colour blindness that are found in the general population.

Colour blindness is quite common; commoner in men than in women. It is found in 0.4% of all women and 8% of all men, and is congenital. Complete absence of colour vision resulting from lack of cones in the retina is very rare, but it has been reported. The blindness that would result from the absence of two pigments and the presence of only one is extremely rare. Absence of one pigment leading to dichromatic vision – perception only of green and red, or more commonly blue and yellow – exists, but most common is the condition of anomalous trichromatopsia, where all three pigments are present but of an intensity different from normal. Anomalous trichromats see all the colours but have difficulty in distinguishing between red, green and yellow, or blue, green and yellow. The first is the red-green type of colour blindness, the second the blue-yellow type. Most colour-blind people are ignorant of their abnormality until it is demonstrated by special tests, but there are some situations in which it may be important to be able to distinguish special colours quickly so that for some jobs perfect colour vision is essential. *See* Ishihara Test.

Coma: a state of deep unconsciousness in which even the reflexes are abolished, for example the eyeball can be touched without making the patient blink. There is no response to the most painful stimuli and the patient cannot be roused. Some causes are: poisoning, perhaps by alcohol, apoplexy (q.v.), an overdose of insulin or not enough insulin (*see* Diabetes), the after-effects of an epileptic fit, and head injury. It is essential to make sure that the unconscious person is able to breathe easily through a clear airway (q.v.); turn the head to one side and make sure that the tongue has not fallen back in the throat.

Comminuted: broken into small pieces. Used to describe fractures in which part of the bone is in pieces.

Compensation Syndrome: some patients injured in industrial accidents, or other accidents for which financial compensation may be received, may make a recovery which is slower than usual, or even produce symptoms not strictly attributable to their injuries. This is most commonly found after head injuries, when the patient for example develops a headache which will not respond to treatment, or injuries to the back, which lead to continuing discomfort. The syndrome builds up in anxious people, and is a manifestation of hysteria. It will not improve before litigation is complete, and unfortunately it is not uncommon for the syndrome to continue after compensation has been paid.

Compositor's Disease: lead poisoning which is liable to affect those who handle lead type. *See* Lead.

Conchae: bony plates covered with mucous membrane which project from the lateral walls of the nasal cavity. There are three conchae, superior, medial and inferior, and they are called conchae because of their resemblance to shells. The other name for them is the turbinate bones.

Concussion: a violent shock, produced for example by an explosion, or a heavy blow, and by extension the state produced by such a blow especially on the head. In this sense concussion means a loss of consciousness partial or complete which recovers after a limited period, usually within 24 hours.

CAUSE: not properly understood. Any severe blow on the head probably does two things: (a) it accelerates the skull in relation to the brain, for the brain floats in water inside the skull; (b) it momentarily deforms the shape of the skull, for the bone is slightly elastic. In consequence of (a) the skull is moved away from the blow but the brain at first stays still, and then the brain moves away from the direction of the blow but may hit the wall of the skull on the side opposite the site of the injury, for the skull has stopped moving while the brain is still accelerating. In addition to this there may be twisting ('shear') forces applied to the brain. It follows that the brain is deformed and bruised twice – once on the side of the blow and again on the diametrically opposite side (contre-coup injury), and parts of the brain are moved in relation to each other by the twisting forces. In consequence of (b), there is a momentary wave of very high pressure inside the skull which is transmitted to the brain, and this is thought to produce many small pinpoint haemorrhages. It is assumed that this 'commotio cerebri' is enough to stop the higher centres of the brain working for a while, although the lower centres continue to function. It is probable that the injury to the brain in concussion differs in degree rather than kind from more severe injuries that lead to coma followed by confusion and cerebral irritation. *See* Head Injury.

SYMPTOMS: immediate loss of consciousness after a blow on the head commonly sustained without any wound of the scalp. It may be momentary or prolonged, and may be followed by a period of minor confusion and headache. No lasting damage ensues, and there should be no chronic headaches or other complications. If they occur they suggest a different diagnosis. There may, however, be a loss of memory for events leading directly up to the accident, which with the passage of time recovers to a certain extent, and sometimes even completely.

TREATMENT: everybody who loses consciousness after a blow

on the head ought to be kept in bed, preferably in hospital, for 24 hours. If he recovers consciousness before the period is out, the patient must be kept under observation, for in some cases there are sequels to the injury that only show themselves slowly. *See* Head Injury.

Condyloma: a warty proliferation of tissue near the anus or the vulva, found in secondary syphilis. Another variety called condyloma acuminatum is caused by a virus.

Congenital: a word meaning 'appearing with birth' which has become almost synonymous in popular usage with 'hereditary'. This is erroneous because an hereditary disease is one which has been handed on in the germ cells from parents to child, whereas congenital disease may arise in the womb after conception and before birth. Hereditary diseases are congenital; congenital diseases are not necessarily hereditary.

Conjunctiva: the thin transparent membrane covering the front of the eye.

Conjunctivitis: (Pink Eye). Inflammation of the conjunctiva. (Called 'Apollo eye' in Nigeria because of the coincidence of two large epidemic outbreaks with the flights of Apollo 11 and 12, which convinced some that the infection came from the moon.)
CAUSE: there are a number of different causes, but conjunctivitis is commonly due to bacterial infection, viruses, or mechanical irritation, for example by an eyelash growing inwards.
TREATMENT: in the case of mechanical irritation the cause is removed. If infection is present, the organism is identified, and drops of the appropriate drug instilled into the eye. The use of pads and bandages is not recommended; dark glasses are much better. If the infection has not spread to the other eye it is worth trying to keep it clean, but both eyes are usually infected at the same time. The eyelids are inclined to stick together, especially in the mornings, but this can be prevented by the use of a simple eye ointment. Bathing the eyes with lotion is soothing and in cases of minor infection may be all that is needed.

Constipation: infrequent or absent motions of the bowels.
CAUSE: absolute constipation may be caused by intestinal
obstruction; incomplete constipation in the same way, by
changes in diet, or by intestinal infections and upsets which
at first cause diarrhoea and then constipation. It is very
often the result of neglecting the urge to evacuate the bowels
regularly because of lack of time or opportunity, or because
of pain, for example when an anal fissure is present. In
children, it may be caused by Hirschsprung's disease (q.v.),
and in the old by general debility.

SYMPTOMS: no symptoms are produced by constipation itself,
although distension of the rectum can be uncomfortable.
Fifty years ago a generation of doctors had the idea that all
manner of illnesses followed constipation; they invented
'autointoxication', a gift the makers of proprietary laxatives
grasped with both hands. To this day notions of 'inner
cleanliness', 'regularity' and so on are the foundations of
considerable fortunes although the doctors have changed
their attitude completely. One might be led to believe that
only two days without defaecation will produce headaches
and ill-defined miseries, but in fact there is nothing wrong
with people who only open their bowels once a week, or
even once a month, providing that they do it regularly.

TREATMENT: regulation of the bowels is a matter of habit,
and proper training of children includes the establishment
of this habit. Constipation arising from neglect can only be
treated by return to the original habit (this often means
getting up five minutes earlier in the morning). Constipation
arising from megacolon, obstruction, or from painful
motions is treated by removal of the cause, and that arising
from change of diet by attention to the diet – usually more
liquids and more cellulose are needed. There is no reason
why one should not take almost any purgative occasionally,
but there is no reason why one should. There is every reason
why one should not take any purgative regularly, for this
depletes the pocket and irritates the gut. It may be important
to remember that the successful use of a purgative on
occasion will be followed by emptiness of the bowels for a
while afterwards, so that apparent constipation may ensue
and one may be tempted to take another dose of purgative
and so start a habit. Treatment of constipation in the old is
not easy, but depends on a number of factors such as diet,

habit and general health. Chronic constipation in the old
and in children may cause diarrhoea because the hard
retained motions irritate the rectum, a state not always
easy to recognize.

Contact Lens: a lens worn on the eyeball so that it is
almost invisible. The advantages are: many people do not
like to be seen wearing glasses, or find them tiresome;
contact lenses do not steam up in warm moist atmospheres;
they can be worn to play quite violent games; in certain
disturbances of vision they give better results than ordinary
lenses. Disadvantages are: many people find the process of
inserting and removing contact lenses unpleasant, and
some people find them too uncomfortable and irritating to
wear; they are not suitable for all visual disturbances. (It is
not possible, for example, to make bifocal contact lenses.)
The choice of contact lenses must be made with the advice
of an expert.

Contraception: the artificial prevention of pregnancy
following copulation. There are six main methods:
1. The use of chemicals in the form of foaming tablets,
capsules, pessaries, jelly or aerosol foam.
2. The use of mechanical means such as a sheath of rubber
used by the man or an occlusive diaphragm used by the
woman.
3. The use of permanent intra-uterine devices.
4. The use of douches after intercourse.
5. The use of sex hormones taken by mouth to suppress
ovulation.
6. The use of 'natural' means such as coitus interruptus
(premature withdrawal) or the 'safe period'.
Each method has its disadvantages and advantages:
1. *Chemical.* Theoretically not safe on its own, it is easy to
use and so may in some cases give better results than more
complicated but theoretically more effective methods.
Best preparations are foam, cream or synthetic gel. The
chemicals used kill the sperm before they can enter the
uterus, and must be introduced high up in the vagina, as
near the cervix, or neck of the womb, as possible, not more
than half an hour before intercourse.
2. *Mechanical.* The condom or sheath worn by the man

164

depends on its integrity for its effectiveness, and this cannot be guaranteed. Many authorities therefore recommend that a chemical method should be used as well as a sheath. The diaphragm worn by the woman similarly depends on its integrity for its effectiveness, and it also depends on being in the right place, upon the woman being instructed competently in its use, and upon it being the correct size. It is used with a chemical cream or jelly; theoretically it is very effective, but the correct use of a diaphragm is a little complicated.

3. *The permanent intra-uterine device* (I.U.C.D.). This method, which involves introducing a foreign body into the uterus, was invented more than forty years ago, but was largely abandoned because of the difficulty of finding an inert material which would not damage the uterus or lead to undesirable changes in the tissues, and because of the difficulty of fitting the device. About ten years ago intrauterine devices came back into use, now made of plastic materials which are inert, do not irritate the uterus, and are springy – so that they can be introduced much more easily, being straightened out in the introducer and springing back into shape once they are in the cavity of the womb. The best known devices are the loop and the spiral or coil, both named from their shape. The exact action of the I.U.C.D. in preventing pregnancy is still not understood, but the method is very effective and the only common reason for failure is that the device has been expelled without the fact being noticed. The I.U.C.D. is fitted by the doctor, who will explain how to check that it is in place and has not been lost. The disadvantages are that it may increase menstrual bleeding, and introduction may cause cramps and very rarely pelvic inflammation. The effectiveness of an I.U.C.D. is increased by combining it with a chemical method.

4. *Douching.* The use of douching after intercourse to prevent conception is mentioned only to be condemned. As one authority says, 'Douching is a tiresome way of becoming pregnant.'

5. *The use of sex hormones.* 'The Pill' has since its introduction gained much publicity both because of the ease and convenience in use of an oral contraceptive, and because there have been regular public warnings about its dangers. About fifteen years ago successful trials of a mixture of hormones,

oestrogen and progestogen, which were known to prevent ovulation (the liberation of the egg from the ovary), led to the widespread introduction of the method. It is possible to obtain the effect with oestrogen alone, but usually progestogen is added, if only during the last week before menstruation to control withdrawal bleeding. The combination of hormones is easy to take, for the pills are supplied in packets which carry precise instructions. Advantages of the method are reliability and simplicity; the menstrual period is completely predictable, dysmenorrhoea (q.v.) is helped, and in cases of excessive menstrual loss the condition is improved. Disadvantages are that some people put on weight, some are sensitive to the drugs and complain of headaches, sickness and general illness, some become excessively nervous and restless, and some may have discomfort in the breasts. The major drawbacks are an increased tendency to form blood clots in the vessels, and the risk of developing high blood pressure or jaundice. It is the increased tendency to form blood clots that regularly comes under public scrutiny, for in some cases fatal embolism (q.v.) follows. Surveys have been carried out both in the U.S.A. and in England and Wales, and they show evidence that oral contraceptives increase the risk of deep vein thrombosis with embolism by six or eight times. There is no evidence to suggest that oral contraceptives increase the risk of coronary thrombosis, but they do increase the risk of clotting in the blood vessels of the brain. It would appear that the greater the dose of oestrogen, the greater the risk; preparations are therefore recommended which have the lowest effective dose of oestrogen. Nevertheless, the danger of blood clotting must be put into perspective. Oestrogen and progestogen combined offer almost complete protection against unwanted pregnancy, and it is roughly true that the risks of dying of thromboembolism as a result of taking oral contraceptives for one year is about the same as the risk of dying from thromboembolism as the result of bearing a child.
6. '*Natural*' *means*. Coitus interruptus, or premature withdrawal, is unsafe and psychologically unsettling. The 'safe period' is badly named, for it is nothing of the sort. Avoidance of the mid-period decreases the risk of pregnancy but by no means precludes it, for conception can take place at any time during the menstrual cycle.

Information about contraception and the best methods for use in individual cases should always be obtained from the doctor or the birth control clinic. On the whole it may be said that the safest method is the combined use of mechanical (occlusive diaphragm) and chemical techniques, but reliability demands great care. The easiest method is the oral contraceptive, but it is not without risk. The newest method is the I.U.C.D. *See* Sterilization.

Contre-coup: *see* Concussion.

Convulsions: these commonly occur in children.
CAUSE: infections of the central nervous system and the meninges, generalized infections with fever, high temperatures associated with infection of the middle ear or tonsils, tumours of the brain, injury particularly at birth, various metabolic disorders including lack of oxygen, and epilepsy (q.v.).
SYMPTOMS: the child twitches and jerks, and becomes unconscious. The convulsions last for a variable time, and when they finish the child usually recovers consciousness, cries and goes to sleep.
TREATMENT: convulsions are symptoms of underlying disease, and basically treatment must be directed towards the underlying cause. Immediate treatment to stop the convulsions includes the intramuscular injection of paraldehyde or sodium phenobarbitone. Before the doctor comes the parents can help by making sure that the airway is clear so that the child can breathe properly, and by controlling the temperature by sponging the child's skin with tepid water. *See* Airway.

Cordotomy: *see* Chordotomy.

Cornea: the transparent part of the eyeball which lies over the pupil and iris, through which we see.

Corneal Graft: if the cornea is scarred by injury or disease the vision is disturbed or lost, although the eye may otherwise be intact. It is possible to graft part of another cornea into the eye after cutting out the scar because the cornea has very few blood vessels, and immunological reactions leading to rejection of the graft are therefore weak or absent. The graft can be taken from an eye removed at operation or from an eye taken from a dead body within six hours of death. As long as the eye is taken with full aseptic precautions, the cornea can be stored in a 'bank' until it is needed. It is possible to leave one's eyes for use in this way, but strictly speaking this is no more than a wish and if surviving relatives or the person who is legally in charge of the body objects, the eyes will not be used. It is important to know that the eyes of old people are entirely suitable for use in corneal grafting; indeed they are more suitable than the eyes of the young.

Corns: a corn is a localized thickening of the skin shaped like a pyramid with the apex pointing inwards. Thickening of the skin over a larger area is called a callosity, and is usually protective, whereas a corn is relatively small and painful. Both callosities and corns are produced by local pressure; corns are particularly liable to be formed on the feet as a result of badly fitting shoes. They are best treated by a chiropodist, for picking at corns at home never did any good, nor is there any point in doing anything to a corn while the shoes that caused it are still being worn. Verrucas, painful and infective warts that occur on the soles of the feet, may be mistaken for corns.

Coronary Disease and Thrombosis: disease and blockage by clot of the arteries that supply blood to the heart muscle.
CAUSE: atherosclerosis of the coronary arteries (*see* Arterial Disease). There are two main coronary arteries, the right and the left, which take origin from the aorta at the top of the heart. The left divides into an anterior interventricular branch, which as its name suggests passes downwards between the ventricles to the apex of the heart, and a left circumflex branch which runs round between the left atrium and the ventricle and then descends on the rearward surface of the heart. The right coronary artery runs round between the right atrium and ventricle, and supplies the right ventricle. It also supplies the sinuatrial node, the pacemaker

of the heart. Any disease process, and the process is almost invariably atherosclerosis, which narrows the lumen – the hole in the middle – of a coronary artery by a half, produces symptoms. The worse the narrowing, the worse the state of the patient. Narrowing by two-thirds may lead to complete blockage by clot. The commonest site for disease to affect the coronary system is in the first part of the descending branch of the left artery, the next most common the first part of the right coronary artery, and in about a quarter of the cases the first part of the left circumflex branch is affected. The symptoms of coronary disease are produced by ischaemia – deficient blood supply – of the heart muscle, which means that waste products, or metabolites, are not removed from the cells. As the metabolites accumulate so pain is produced, and when they are removed in the blood the pain diminishes. If the blood supply is totally cut off from the heart muscle then where the blood supply is not sufficient to nourish it the muscle dies. The branches of the coronary arteries form limited anastomoses (q.v.), and the pattern of anastomosis varies; the more the branches of the coronary arteries mingle, the less likely sluggish flow or blockage in one of them is to produce symptoms.

Coronary artery disease is commoner in men than women between the ages of 40 and 60; over 60 the proportion of attacks in men and women approaches unity, so that it appears that women up to the menopause are in some way protected from the disease.

SYMPTOMS: pain is the chief symptom produced by disease of the coronary arteries, and the sudden blockage of an artery by thrombosis causes intense pain unrelieved by rest or glyceryl trinitrate, unlike the pain of angina pectoris (q.v.). The pain is felt in the left side of the chest and down the left arm, and it runs up the left side of the neck into the lower jaw. The patient is shocked, and becomes pale. The skin is cold and sweaty, the pulse weak, the breathing often fast and gasping; the outcome is always uncertain, but about three-quarters of all cases of coronary thrombosis admitted to hospital recover. The pain may last for one or two days, and the breathlessness longer.

TREATMENT: (of the acute attack). The pain is relieved by morphia, which also calms the patient, who is in great fear of death. Oxygen is useful if available, and should be given

CORONARY DISEASE AND THROMBOSIS

at a rate of 10 litres per minute through a face mask. The patient should lie flat. Hospital treatment usually offers the best prospect of recovery, although it may only be a few days before the patient is ready to continue treatment at home (*see* Heart Failure).

Outlook and long-term treatment: the heart commonly goes into failure of greater or lesser degree, and according to the site of the blockage, various parts of the heart become affected. For example, blockage of the branch supplying blood to the pacemaker area will upset the heart rate, and interference with the structures that conduct the impulses from the pacemaker area to the rest of the heart will result in 'heart block'. The part of the heart muscle supplied by the blocked artery dies, softens and eventually forms a scar. Treatment is directed towards combating heart failure, correcting abnormalities of rhythm, and preventing the spread of the clot. It must also prevent too much strain being put on the heart muscle while the scar is forming. The most important part of the treatment is complete rest – no visitors, no telephones, no work. It will be 3 to 6 weeks before the patient can leave his bed for even short periods. Although he should stop smoking and perhaps cut down his weight, there is no reason why the patient should give up alcohol, particularly if he has been used to it. Anticoagulant drugs are often used to try to prevent the clot from spreading.

Convalescence must be slow, but a good number of patients find it too slow for their liking; nevertheless, they must agree that it is only common sense to try to stay inside the bounds of what is known to be safe rather than test out the limits of their individual performances. Generally speaking the length of convalescence is proportional to the severity of the original attack, and a return to normal life is dependent on the residual damage to the heart.

GENERAL COMMENT: it is often thought that the incidence of coronary thrombosis is increasing because of 'the strains of modern life'. Apart from the fact that life has always been a strain, it is more likely that people are now living to an age when coronary thrombosis becomes important and that the diagnosis is being made more often. It is also true that a diet rich in cholesterol (q.v.) is associated with arterial disease; so that it may be the case that if you eat well and believe all you see in the newspapers and on television you will get a coronary thrombosis. The disease is the most common cause of sudden death – the figures vary between 40% and 50% for the number of fatal attacks – and those who have once had an attack are more liable to have subsequent attacks. Coronary disease without other illness has been taken as an indication for attempting heart transplant operations; other less drastic surgical treatment has included the grafting of arteries. Nevertheless, surgery is not yet fully developed. We look forward to the possibility that the surgeon may one day be able to remove clots from the coronary arteries and restore them to their original dimensions.

Coroner: (in Scotland, Procurator Fiscal). An official who has the task of holding inquests, or inquiries, into unexplained, sudden or violent deaths. The Registrar of Deaths is chiefly responsible for reporting deaths to the Coroner, but usually the doctor, if he is in doubt about the need for an inquest, will consult the Coroner or his Officer himself. In some cases of unexplained death, the Coroner may order a post-mortem examination and if he is satisfied with the result may not hold a formal inquest. It should be remembered that the object of a Coroner's inquest into cases dying under medical care, for example after an operation, is to make sure that all the relevant facts are examined in public so that all may be satisfied, or if they are not, may voice their dissatisfaction in public and have their questions answered. If any member of the public thinks that there has been an unnatural or unexplained death he is advised to see the Coroner's Officer at the local Coroner's Court. Although increasing numbers of Coroners are men with double qualifications as lawyers and doctors, there is no legal requirement that says they must have more than one qualification.

In the United States, all death certificates must be signed by a physician who has attended the patient within a reasonable period preceding death. The mortician may not proceed with embalming and interment until he has recorded the death certificate and sent it to the Registrar of Vital Statistics. It is reviewed by the Coroner, whose qualifications vary according to the law of the state. Some states require a physician, but others permit non-professional persons to be appointed to this post. In any instance of suspicious or unknown cause of death, the Coroner may order post-mortem examination to be done.

Corpuscle: a small body or cell, generally used to mean the red blood cells or R.B.C.s, the smallest cells in the body.

Corpus Luteum: the yellow mass of cells that fills the ovarian follicle after the ovum itself has been expelled (*see* Ovary). In pregnancy it persists for a time, and its hormones, oestrogen and progesterone, assist in preparing a bed for the fertilized ovum in the uterus. Although these hormones suppress ovulation, and are therefore used in oral contraceptive pills, once ovulation has occurred they are essential for the maintenance of pregnancy.

Cortex: the outer layer of an organ or other structure such as the brain, kidney, suprarenal body or bone. The inner part is called the medulla.

Corticosteroids: aldosterone and cortisol (hydro-cortisone), steroid substances of physiological significance produced by the cortex of the suprarenal glands. They are made from cholesterol, and their action is essential to life.
Cortisol: influences the formation of glucose from substances that are not carbohydrates; because amino acids are used in the process, cortisol in this connection encourages the breakdown of proteins and discourages their synthesis. This action is reversed in the liver, where cortisol encourages the formation of protein from amino acids. The hormone causes fat to be released from some areas of the body and deposited in others, and plays a part in the regulation of the salt balance of the body and in the water balance of the tissues. It helps to maintain the blood pressure, and is essential for the formation of red blood cells, and maintenance of the strength of muscles. It has other actions which are not properly understood, including reduction of the normal level of allergic and inflammatory reactions. It is known that increased stress produces an increase in the secretion of cortisol, and sometimes patients who have diminished power to make cortisol because of disease of the suprarenal cortex will lead a normal life until they have an

accident or an operation, but then die unless they are given extra cortisol.

Aldosterone: is concerned with the balance of sodium and potassium in the cells and the fluids of the body.

Medical uses of corticosteroids: the first and obvious use is in Addison's disease (q.v.), which is caused by absence of the secretions of the adrenal glands. Corticosteroids are given to make up the deficiency.

When corticosteroids first came on the market, they were thought to have a remarkable effect on rheumatoid arthritis. It had always been known that this disease improves during pregnancy, a state in which there is an increased secretion of steroid hormones, and corticosteroids were therefore given to patients with the complaint. Unfortunately the early promise of successful treatment has not been fulfilled, and now the dangers of cortisone treatment in rheumatoid arthritis are thought to outweigh the benefits except in certain cases which do not respond to other treatment. There are some cases of surgical shock which do not respond to simple measures, and these may respond to corticosteroids. The most general use of the compounds is in cases where allergic and inflammatory reactions are excessive or harmful. In most instances these reactions are essential for the maintenance of health, and treatment is directed towards helping and encouraging them; but in asthma, for example, allergic reactions produce the disease and must be controlled. The same is true of anaphylactic shock and angioneurotic oedema, where the use of corticosteroids may be lifesaving. Certain skin conditions are controlled by the use of corticosteroids as an ointment or cream, but it is not sensible to apply more than the bare minimum of ointment for there is a risk of absorbing the drug and producing side effects. It must not be used as a routine.

Dangers of corticosteroids: the action of these compounds has been found to vary according to minor changes in the molecule, and synthetic preparations have been designed to cut down undesirable side effects while increasing the curative activity. Nevertheless, the side effects are serious: (1) Exaggeration of normal action. This produces high blood pressure, muscular weakness, loss of potassium from the tissues and retention of sodium and water with oedema. In children growth is retarded, and in adults the muscles eventually waste and the bones become soft (osteoporosis), so that the vertebrae may collapse. The requirements of insulin are altered because of the action of corticosteroids on carbohydrate metabolism, and on occasion patients develop diabetes. The face swells and becomes round, and there are profound mental changes that range from over-cheerfulness to depression and even paranoia (q.v.). Suicidal tendencies are in some cases dangerous. (2) The healing of ulcers is delayed, the time that wounds take to knit is lengthened, and the body's reactions to infection are altered so that severe disease may escape diagnosis. (3) The most serious consequence of prolonged treatment with corticosteroids is diminution of the activity of the suprarenal glands, for when the blood levels of corticosteroids are kept artificially high, natural secretion of corticosteroids stops. This state of affairs continues for months or even years after corticosteroid treatment is discontinued, and during this period the patient is at risk. Corticosteroids must be withdrawn slowly, and all patients under prolonged treatment with these drugs must carry a card stating the fact to warn doctors who do not know them – who may be responsible for them after an accident, for example – that they will need very careful treatment to tide them over acute illnesses or injuries.

Corticotrophin: the activity of the cortex of the suprarenal glands depends upon the hormones of the pituitary gland at the base of the brain. If the pituitary gland is removed, the suprarenal cortex withers, and it is possible to isolate from the pituitary hormones a substance called A.C.T.H. or adrenocorticotrophic hormone, without which the suprarenal cannot secrete corticosteroids (*see* above). This substance is also called corticotrophin.

Coryza: the common cold (q.v.).

Cough: the air passages of the lungs are lined with cells secreting mucus, which normally traps particles of dust. When the membranes are infected and inflamed, the secretion of mucus increases and the lining of the air passages is irritated; coughing is the action by which excess mucus is driven out. A complicated reflex produces the cough through the vagus nerve. First the man who is going to cough draws a deep breath in; he then closes his glottis (q.v.) and contracts his muscles so that pressure builds up in the chest; then he suddenly opens his glottis so that there is an explosive discharge of air which sweeps through the air passages and carries with it the excess secretions or, in some cases, foreign matter which has irritated the larynx, trachea or bronchi. Medicines which are supposed to loosen the sputum are called expectorants, but although there are a number of traditional remedies the modern belief is that a hot drink is as good as anything. Linctuses are given to suppress coughs. One of the most effective is honey and lemon juice in hot water, but more complicated and impressive mixtures are commonly prescribed.

Counter-irritants: *see* Blisters.

Cowpox: pox of cow's udders caused by a modified form of the virus responsible for smallpox. The causal organism of cowpox is used in vaccination of human beings against smallpox.

Coxalgia: pain in the hip-joint.

Coxa Vara: a deformity of the femur or thighbone in which the angle between the neck of the bone and shaft is decreased. CAUSE: congenital deformity, congenital dislocation of the hip, old fracture, Perthes' disease, slipped epiphysis, rickets, Paget's disease, osteomalacia.
SYMPTOMS: lameness, pain in the hip, shortening of the leg, inability to abduct the hip joint (raise the leg sideways).
TREATMENT: the treatment is first the treatment of the underlying condition, if it is recognized in time. If arthritis of the hip has resulted and is very painful it may be necessary to carry out an arthrodesis (q.v.).

Coxsackie Virus: originally isolated from patients in a place of this name in New York State, these viruses are found commonly in the gut. They are divided into two groups, A and B; the A group can produce upper respiratory disease and virus meningitis, and the B group pleurodynia or Bornholm disease (q.v.).

175

Cramp: a painful spasmodic contraction of muscles either in the limbs or in certain internal organs (when it is usually described as colic).

CAUSE: (1) Poor blood supply to the muscles due to arterial disease. (2) In swimmers, etc., poor blood supply due to exhaustion and cold, and sometimes minor injuries to the muscles, for example torn fibres, which irritate the muscle and cause it to contract uncontrollably. (3) In heat cramps, loss of salt from the body in excessive sweating. (4) In certain intestinal diseases such as cholera, excessive salt is lost from the gut and cramps are the result. (5) Colic is usually caused by blockage of hollow tubes such as the ureters or the bile ducts (*see* under Colic). (6) Occupational cramp occurs in people who carry out repetitive and fairly delicate movements of the hands and fingers, such as writers, violinists, tailors, typists and a host of other workers. It is thought that there is a psychological basis for this condition, for it is typical that occupational cramp (*a*) stops the sufferer from doing his job, (*b*) is not associated with any organic or bodily disease, and (*c*) rarely prevents the sufferer from doing other things. Thus the man with writer's cramp can use a knife and fork to eat his meals unless he has taken as much distaste to his food as he has to his job.

TREATMENT: (1) drugs are available which dilate the arteries and improve the blood supply to the muscles unless the arterial disease is spread too wide. This type of cramp is particularly likely to occur in old age, and useful drugs include inoxitol nicotinate (Hexopal) and tolazoline hydrochloride (Priscol or Priscoline). (2) Training, and the avoidance of eating before athletic effort, for after a meal blood is diverted from the limb muscles to the intestines. (3) Administration of salt; heat cramps can be avoided if salt tablets are taken with the drinking water. (4) Administration of salt by mouth or by intravenous infusion. (5) Atropine and the treatment of the underlying condition (*see* Colic). (6) A holiday.

Cranial Nerves: 12 nerves which arise from the brain and brain stem inside the skull. They are usually denoted by Roman numerals: I. *Olfactory nerve*, the nerve of smell through which impulses run from the nose to the brain. II. *Optic nerve*, which conducts impulses from the eye to the brain and through which we see. III. *Oculomotor nerve*; supplies muscles which move the eyeball, control the pupil, alter the shape of the lens (ciliary muscle) and lift the upper lid. IV. *Trochlear nerve*; this leaves the back of the brain stem and runs round it to pass forward and supply the muscle which moves the eyeball downwards and outwards (superior oblique muscle). V. *Trigeminal nerve*, which is mostly sensory but has a small motor part. The sensory root has three branches: first, which supplies the upper part of the head – eye, nose, forehead and scalp up to a line joining the ears; second, which supplies the upper lid, the cheek, the upper teeth and the roof of the mouth; third, which supplies the lower lip, the chin, the temple, the lower teeth and the floor of the mouth. The motor part supplies the muscles used in chewing. VI. *Abducent nerve*, which supplies the muscle that turns the eyeball outwards (the external rectus muscle). VII. *Facial nerve*, which supplies the muscles of the face. VIII. *Auditory nerve*, which carries to the brain impulses from the ear. It has two parts; one carries impulses from the organ of hearing, the other impulses from the organ of balance. IX. *Glossopharyngeal nerve*. This nerve carries sensory fibres from the middle ear, the Eustachian tube, the back of the tongue, the tonsil and side of the throat and the side of the soft palate. It also supplies branches to the parotid gland and the small mucous secreting glands of the tongue and part of the throat. X. *Vagus nerve*, called the 'wanderer' because it travels a long way. It sends branches to the pharynx, the larynx, the muscles moving the vocal cords, and brings parasympathetic fibres (*see* Nervous System) to the heart, the stomach and the lower part of the oesophagus, the whole of the small intestine and half the large intestine. XI. *Accessory nerve*. It gives a branch to the vagus nerve, and then leaves the skull to supply two muscles in the neck – the sternomastoid and the trapezius. XII. *Hypoglossal nerve*, which supplies the muscles of the tongue and the muscles which act on the tongue although they are separate from it.

Craniotomy: the operation of opening the skull.

Cretin: deficiency in the secretions of the thyroid gland, thyroxine and tri-iodo-thyronine in the newborn results in cretinism – stunted growth and mental deficiency.

SYMPTOMS: the infant does not feed properly and tends to be constipated, but at first it looks normal. If the condition is allowed to progress the appearance gradually becomes characteristic; a cretin looks stunted, thickset, with dry skin, coarse features and a disproportionately large tongue with deep fissures which sticks out of his mouth. The mental age of a cretin is that of an infant.

TREATMENT: as soon as the condition is recognized the child is given thyroxine, and administration of the hormone must continue for the whole of his life. If treatment is started before the child is six months old, mental development is usually normal, as is growth, but the later in life treatment starts, the worse the results will be. The state which results from lack of thyroid hormone starting during adult life is myxoedema (*see* Goitre).

Crisis: apart from its ordinary use implying a state of emergency, in medicine the word may be used to mean (1) a sudden paroxysm of pain in certain diseases, for example tabetic crisis in tabes dorsalis; (2) a state now rarely seen, in which a disease, for example lobar pneumonia, resolves suddenly by a rapid fall of temperature to normal. It only occurs if the disease is allowed to run its normal course; the introduction of sulphonamides and antibiotics has made this very unlikely.

Cross-Infection: infection of patients in hospital by organisms derived from other patients. This should not be a problem, but unfortunately it is; moreover the introduction of antibiotics, instead of lessening the difficulties, has increased them, because increasing reliance on antibiotics to control infection has tended to result in a drop in standards of asepsis in the wards and operating theatres, while at the same time unrestrained use of antibiotics has encouraged the growth of resistant strains of bacteria.

The only ways to minimize hospital infection, particularly of clean operation wounds, are strict adherence to the principles of asepsis and a continual lookout for sources of infection – discharging noses, minor boils, the patient with pulmonary infection who coughs all over the place, sloppy technique in dressing wounds and in the operating theatre. The sooner a patient can leave hospital and be nursed at home, the less likely he is to suffer cross-infection.

Cross-match: the process of ensuring before transfusion that the blood of the donor and the blood of the recipient are of the same blood group and are compatible (*see* Blood Groups).

Croup: occurring mostly in children, croup is caused by an obstruction in the larynx. There is a cough and difficulty in drawing breath; the underlying disease is commonly a virus infection of the larynx, trachea and bronchi. Diphtheria used to be a common cause of croup, but it is rarely seen now because of the success of modern methods of immunization.

Crural: to do with the leg.

Crush Syndrome: during World War 2 in Europe, it was observed that casualties who had suffered from injuries involving crushing of the muscles sometimes developed kidney failure. The condition was thought to be due to the kidneys being damaged by material released from the crushed muscle, but there is now some doubt whether the real cause was not profound surgical shock (q.v.), which is liable to follow any severe injury and can produce kidney failure.

Cryotherapy: (alternative spelling crymotherapy). Treatment by the physical agent, cold. In surgery patients are sometimes cooled (hypothermia) because the need of the tissues for oxygen is reduced by a drop in temperature and prolonged surgery is less dangerous; the technique can also be used locally where the blood supply to a part is reduced, as in arterial disease when gangrene threatens a leg. Warts can be removed by the application of carbon dioxide snow, and it is possible to make selected surgical lesions in the brain by the use of cold instruments.

Cryptorchism: imperfect descent of the testicle, so that the organ remains hidden in the abdomen.
CAUSE: the testicle develops near the kidneys in the embryo, and descends to the scrotum during the last months before

179

birth. The descent may be held up anywhere along the route, so that the testicle may lie in the abdominal cavity, at the internal opening of the inguinal canal in the groin, in the canal itself or at the external opening of the canal. The condition may affect one or both testicles.

TREATMENT: if the testicle can be drawn down into the bottom of the scrotum it will descend in time to the normal place. If it is not to be felt it may be in the inguinal canal, and an operation will bring it down into the proper place; the operation should be carried out when the boy is about five years old, and if there is an associated rupture in the groin (hernia), it can be dealt with at the same time. If the testicle has remained inside the abdomen it must be taken away, for it will be sterile and there is a risk of malignant growth developing in it. A certain type of case – the fat boy with small genitals and undescended testicles – may at puberty be successfully treated by hormones.

C.S.S.D.: (Central Sterile Supply Department). Modern hospitals have their materials sterilized in a central department for distribution to the wards. This makes the incidence of cross-infection less likely. Many instruments, such as syringes and needles, are used only once and then discarded.

Culicine Mosquitoes: the culicine tribe of mosquitoes are important carriers of disease. They do not transmit malaria, but are responsible for the spread of yellow fever, filariasis, dengue fever and various types of encephalitis. Culicine mosquitoes at rest hold their bodies parallel to the surface on which they are resting, unlike anopheline mosquitoes (responsible for the spread of malaria) which incline their bodies to the surface. The most important culicine mosquito is Aedes aegypti, which spreads yellow fever and dengue fever. It is a black mosquito with silver markings and it lives near houses.

Culture: the process of growing micro-organisms or other living cells on suitable material, such as agar mixed with blood or beef broth. 'Culture' is also used of a growing colony of cells or organisms contained in a dish, test-tube or flask.

Cupping: a technique once, but no longer, popular, in which diseases thought to be characterized by the congestion of underlying tissues were treated by measures designed to draw blood to the surface. A piece of cotton wool soaked in methylated spirits was lit on the skin and a cup clapped over it at once, so that as the wool burnt a partial vacuum was formed and the blood was drawn to the surface away from the congested deeper parts. In wet cupping the skin was first scratched to increase the flow of blood and lymph.

Curare: 'Indian arrow poison' – a substance made in South America from various species of strychnos which when injected paralyses the muscles. Its action is upon the junction between motor nerves and muscle fibres, where it interferes with the function of acetylcholine (q.v.). The most important active agent isolated from curare is tubocurarine, and this drug is used by anaesthetists to produce relaxation of the muscles when the patient is under general anaesthesia. It can also be used to reduce the spasms of tetanus.

Curette: an instrument for scraping the walls of a body cavity in order to remove unwanted material, growths or specimens for biopsy. Also used to refer to the act of using such an instrument. The most common operation carried out with the curette – the operation is called curettage – is performed on the interior of the uterus or womb. It is usually combined with dilatation of the neck of the uterus, and the operation is known as D. & C. (dilatation and curettage).

Curie: a unit used to measure radioactivity, named after the Nobel Prize winners Marie and Pierre Curie, pioneer workers on the phenomena of radiation.

Cyanides: the salts of hydrocyanic acid, used in industry for various processes including the manufacture of plastics and dyeing. Hydrogen cyanide is a very poisonous liquid – colourless, volatile, with the smell of bitter almonds, it is often encountered in detective stories, but poisoning is more likely to occur in industrial life from breathing hydrocyanic acid gas. If the gas is present in high concentrations it may at once be lethal.

SYMPTOMS: sore throat, weeping eyes and running nose, a

feeling of breathlessness, headache, sickness, giddiness and weakness of the arms and legs. This may get worse until the patient becomes very shocked, and he may stop breathing or become unconscious and start convulsing; the heart may stop.

TREATMENT: removal from the poisoned atmosphere, oxygen, artificial respiration. Capsules of amyl nitrite are broken and the vapour inhaled for a few seconds every minute for 5 minutes; sodium nitrite 3% and sodium thiosulphate 50% are given intravenously. Hydrocyanic acid is used for executions in the California gas chamber.

Cyanosis: blueness of the skin and mucous membranes. It is the blood that gives pink skin its colour, and normally the circulating blood is red. If the circulating blood is carrying less oxygen than it should it becomes blue, the colour it normally is in the veins, and the skin takes on a bluish tinge. Cyanosis is found in respiratory diseases in which the function of the lungs is depressed, so that the blood cannot take up the normal amount of oxygen, and in heart disease when the circulation is impaired and the amount of blood passing through the lungs is less than normal. If the circulation to a particular part is stopped or impeded in any way the part will become blue as the blood gives up its oxygen.

Cyclamates: chemical substances used for sweetening food and drink instead of sugar, now banned in many countries because of experiments said to show that cyclamates are liable to produce cancer in animals.

Cyclical Vomiting: periodic attacks of vomiting that affect children.

CAUSE: unknown.

SYMPTOMS: after the age of 3 the child falls victim to attacks of vomiting which may be preceded by headache or stomach ache, and last for 1 or 2 days. The vomiting is severe and is accompanied by abdominal pain.

TREATMENT: as soon as the vomiting stops recovery is quick, but while it lasts the child can keep nothing down. He must be put to bed and given frequent small drinks of water or whatever fluids he will take, if possible containing glucose.

It may be necessary to use the drug chlorpromazine either by mouth, or, if the vomiting makes this impractical, by injection. In very severe cases an intravenous infusion of glucose and saline may be required.

Obviously this cause of vomiting is only diagnosed when more dangerous causes have been considered and rejected, and even when a firm diagnosis has been made it is dangerous to take it for granted that every time the child develops an abdominal pain and starts to vomit the cause is always cyclical vomiting. The condition disappears at the time of puberty, but is sometimes succeeded by migraine.

Cyclopropane: an anaesthetic gas. It has no colour, but has a sweet smell; it is explosive when mixed with oxygen. Because it is expensive and explosive, it is used in a closed rebreathing circuit. Its value lies in the fact that it acts quickly, is quickly excreted, can be mixed with large concentrations of oxygen without losing its anaesthetic properties, and is non-irritating.

Cyst: a hollow swelling containing fluid, In general, cysts fall into the following categories. (1) Congenital: a developmental fault, commonly in the ovary or kidney, sometimes in the lung, shuts off groups of cells which proliferate and form fluid. (2) Retention; as when a gland that usually opens to the exterior is blocked and the secretions collect in the blocked duct and form a swelling – examples occur in the skin, where sebaceous cysts are formed from blocked sweat glands, and in the breast when milk ducts become blocked. (3) Cysts formed by parasites: hydatid cysts are produced by the larval stage of a tapeworm mainly in the liver and the lungs, although they can also occur in the brain or in any organ. (4) Cysts may form in tumours, either because the tumour is made up of tissue that secretes fluid, or because the inside of the tumour breaks down and becomes fluid. The treatment varies with the cause, but is surgical.

Cysticercosis: the tapeworm Taenia solium has a life-cycle involving the pig, and if infected pork is not sufficiently cooked, man can become infected by the worm. Larval cysts are present in the muscles of the pig, and when a man eats them they develop into the adult form of the worm in the intestines. It can sometimes happen later on that a man harbouring the worm infects himself by transferring the tapeworm's eggs on to his food, perhaps with his hands, and he then becomes infected not with the adult worms but with their larval cysts – a condition named cysticercosis, which may lead to serious consequences, for cysts form not only in the muscles but also in the brain, where they may set up epileptic attacks. There is no specific treatment.

Cystitis: inflammation of the bladder.

CAUSE: the organisms that infect the bladder are commonly Escherichia coli, staphylococci and streptococci; infections may include other organisms such as Bacillus proteus or B. pyocyaneus. Women are particularly prone to develop cystitis because infection occurs in pregnancy and gynaecological disorders such as prolapse of the uterus, and because the urethra is short. Rarely cystitis is brought about by tuberculous infection – it was much more common before effective drugs came into use for the treatment of tuberculosis – and in countries where bilharzia (q.v.) is found Schistosoma haematobium causes chronic cystitis. Recurrent attacks of cystitis are often associated with stones, enlargement of the prostate in men, or tumours.

SYMPTOMS: frequency of passing water, pain felt low in the abdomen and on passing water, and the constant desire to pass water. The urine may smell offensive and be bloodstained. Infection may be accompanied by fever and sweating.

TREATMENT: potassium citrate mixture is given in sufficient quantities to render the urine alkaline, and the patient must drink as much fluid as possible. Alcohol is avoided, for it irritates the bladder. A specimen of urine is tested and a culture made to identify the organisms present and establish drug sensitivity. Very often the organisms are not sensitive to penicillin, but there is a wide choice of alternative drugs including sulphadimidine, ampicillin, nalidixic acid (Negram) and nitrofurantoin (Furadantin). When the infection has been brought under control the condition of the urinary tract must be fully investigated to uncover any underlying disease of the bladder or the kidneys, which is treated as necessary. Tuberculous infection may be masked by infection with commoner organisms, but the diagnosis of bilharzia will usually be obvious in the countries where it is prevalent. The main object in treating cystitis is the prevention of damage not to the bladder but to the kidneys, for infection of one part of the urinary tract means infection of the whole tract. Infection from the bladder ascends to the kidneys, and what at first appears to be a mild attack of cystitis in a young woman can lead to a life crippled by chronic pyelonephritis (q.v.).

Cystoscope: an instrument passed up the urethra with a light at the end and an optical system which enables the surgeon to examine the inside of the bladder and perform various manoeuvres. He can, for example, pass thin catheters up the ureters into the pelvis or the kidney so that specimens may be taken and radio-opaque substances injected for X-ray examination, or he can remove small pieces of tumours for microscopy, and treat tumours by fulguration (coagulation with electrical diathermy).

Cystotomy: cutting into the bladder. This operation is performed by opening the abdominal wall above the pubic symphysis (the bone in the lowest central part of the abdomen), and is usually called suprapubic cystotomy. It is carried out under local or general anaesthetic for conditions in which the bladder has to be drained for a while, or in which there is an obstruction to the passage of urine which cannot be satisfactorily relieved by a catheter passed through the urethra. After the bladder has been opened a self-retaining catheter is passed into the cavity and the abdominal wall is closed around it.

Cytology: the study of the structure and function of cells.

Cytotoxic Agents: although cancer cells are remarkably like normal cells in their vital processes, there are small differences which make it possible to hope that drugs will be found to kill cancer cells while leaving normal cells intact. At present results are disappointing, and 'cytotoxic' drugs take third place in treatment to surgery and radiotherapy except in cases where it is obvious that the surgeon and the radiotherapist have nothing to offer. Research into the chemotherapy of malignant disease is being carried out unceasingly in many centres.

D

Dacryocystitis: inflammation of the tear-sac at the inner angle of the eye. Tears are formed by the lacrimal gland which is at the outer angle of the eye in the upper part of the orbit or eyesocket, and they reach the conjunctiva covering the front of the eyeball through about twelve small ducts. The tears then pass across the eye towards the nose, and are collected through very tiny holes in the inner angles of the upper and lower eyelids – the lacrimal punctae – and drain into the lacrimal tear sac. From there they go down the nasolacrimal duct into the lower part of the nose, where they are lost with the nasal secretions. (It is a matter of common observation that in crying we usually sniff.) Inflammation of the lacrimal sac may follow infection spreading from the conjunctiva or from the nose.

D.A.H.: disordered action of the heart, or effort syndrome; this condition is described under the latter heading.

Dandruff: *see* Seborrhoea.

Dangerous Drugs: the sale of drugs to the public in Great Britain is controlled by law. Poisons are listed under the Pharmacy and Poisons Act of 1933 and the Poisons Rules of 1964, with subsequent amendments. The list of poisons is divided into first and second parts, and substances in Part I can only be sold by qualified pharmacists. Those in Part II can be sold by listed sellers of poisons. Poisonous drugs, most of which are in Part I, the first list, are further divided into four Schedules. Substances in Schedule I may be sold without a prescription provided that the seller knows the buyer, and the buyer signs a poisons book. Schedule IV, which is divided into two parts, is a list of poisonous drugs that can only be sold on prescription. There are also Dangerous Drugs Acts which are concerned with drugs of addiction, and control their import, manufacture and distribution in co-operation with the World Health Organization. In the United States a federal agency called the Food and Drug

Administration is responsible for controlling which drugs may be sold freely and which can be issued only by doctor's prescription. A doctor may dispense drugs directly to a patient, but the pharmacist is held liable to legal action if he gives a restricted medicine without a physician's order.

Dapsone: (Avlosulphon). Used in the specific treatment of leprosy (q.v.). Reactions are rare provided that the drug is taken carefully in small doses – 25 mg weekly for 4 weeks, 50 mg weekly for 4 weeks, and then 100 mg to 300 mg weekly for 2, 3 or 4 years according to the type and progress of the disease.

Daraprim: (Pyrimethamine). Given in doses of 25 mg once a week to suppress malaria. Daraprim kills the asexual parasites as they divide in the red blood cells (*see* Malaria), and also has an effect on the parasites in the tissues. It prevents the parasites from developing in the mosquito and is therefore particularly useful in controlling the disease, but resistant strains of Plasmodium falciparum (the plasmodium which causes malignant malaria) have been found.

D. & C.: dilatation and curettage. *See* Curette.

D.D.T.: (Dicophane; Dichlorodiphenyltrichlorethane). First synthesized in 1874, its insecticidal properties were not discovered until 1940. It owes its undoubted efficiency to the fact that it is chemically stable and physically inert, so that it has considerable residual properties. Although this has made it a great blessing to people who live in countries infested by mosquitoes, lice, flies, fleas, bed bugs, and all the host of insects that carry crippling if not fatal diseases such as plague, malaria, typhus, cholera and enteric fevers, the fact that D.D.T. persists unchanged has meant that in the end it has figured involuntarily in the diet of men. If taken in large doses D.D.T. affects the nervous system, producing tremor, convulsions and even paralysis; and because it is found widely in the body fat of people, birds, fish, cows, pigs, sheep, and even penguins, it has been argued that in time D.D.T. and similar insecticides will poison the world, and various countries are considering banning the use of it completely. However, the mammalian liver is able to break D.D.T. down and excrete it well before toxic levels are reached, so that it might be argued that the risk to human life from the use of D.D.T. has been a little exaggerated.

Deafness: inability to hear.

MECHANISM OF HEARING: the ear is divided into three parts, and deafness may be caused by damage or disease in any one of the three parts as well as by interference with the function of the auditory nerve which carries impulses from the ear to the brain. The anatomy of the ear is described in more detail under the heading Ear, but in essentials it is as follows.

The outer ear: this includes the pinna, which is what is meant in common parlance by ear, and the external acoustic meatu., which is the canal leading from the external ear to the eardrum.

The middle ear: this includes the eardrum, the little bones or ossicles which pick up the movements of the drum and conduct them to the inner ear, the cavity in which the bones lie, and the communication of that cavity with the air cells in the mastoid part of the temporal bone. The middle ear communicates with the throat through the Eustachian (auditory) tube.

The inner ear: this consists of the bony labyrinth, a system of canals in the petrous part of the temporal bone, and the membranous labyrinth which lies inside it. The labyrinthine system has two functions: it contains the organ of balance as well as the organ of hearing. Impulses from the eardrum are relayed to the organ of hearing by the ossicles of the middle ear, which move a membrane in the 'oval window' of the inner ear. Between the eardrum, to which is attached the bone called the malleus, and the membrane of the oval window, to which is attached the bone called the stapes, there is a 20:1 increase in power and a corresponding 20:1 decrease in amplitude of movement. Inside the inner ear the sound waves are turned into impulses in the auditory nerve.

DISTURBANCES OF HEARING: (*a*) *Outer ear.* Blockage of the external acoustic meatus either by a foreign body (in children or mental defectives) or by wax. (*b*) *Middle ear.* Infection of the middle ear can lead to damage to the drum or to the ossicles and the joints between them, so that the drum does not vibrate properly and the ossicles being fixed together or having insufficiently free movement cannot transmit the sound waves to the inner ear. The same result, inability of the ossicles to transmit sound waves, comes about if the stapes, which fits into the oval window, is fixed rigidly to it by otosclerosis, a condition in which there is abnormal formation of bony tissue in the inner ear. Chronic inflammation and suppuration may disorganize the ossicles and scar the eardrum. The function of the Eustachian tube, by which the cavity of the middle ear communicates with the throat and so with the atmosphere, is to equalize pressures and keep the pressure inside the middle ear at the same level as the atmosphere outside. A difference in pressures leads to deafness and in extreme circumstances pain, and it is a common experience among air travellers that descent may be accompanied by deafness and perhaps discomfort. This can be helped by swallowing, for the lower part of the Eustachian tube acts as a valve which allows air to pass out of the middle ear but tends to stop it passing in, and the acts of swallowing and yawning open the end of the tube. If the difference in pressures is extreme, as it may be with a blow on the ear or a loud explosion nearby, the drum may rupture, but this does not of itself make a man deaf. Infections of the nose and throat, such as the common cold, may make the mucuous membrane swell and prevent the Eustachian tube from functioning properly, and so produce some temporary deafness. (c) *Inner ear*. Disorders of the inner ear lead to 'nerve deafness' as opposed to conduction deafness.

TREATMENT: skilled examination is necessary for the type of deafness to be identified, and treatment obviously varies a great deal according to the cause. The examiner will make tests with tuning forks, and may use audiometry, which measures the sensitivity of the ear and helps distinguish between nerve deafness and conduction deafness.

Death: it has up to the present time been accepted that a man is not dead until he stops breathing and his heart is still. However, it is now possible to use machines to take over the function of breathing when nature has given up, and in cases where patients have suffered brain damage through accidents, tumours, haemorrhages, an overdose of drugs or an electrical shock, the heart may continue to beat strongly after breathing has begun to fail. Because it is not possible to tell at once whether damage to the brain is irreversible these patients are often connected to an artificial breathing machine which keeps the blood full of oxygen. If the heart continues to beat and the circulation is maintained all the other organs of the body will continue to live until it is clear whether the brain is going to recover or not. It is at this point that confusion arises, for it is not necessarily easy to accept the concept of 'brain death'. If the patient shows no response to stimuli – if the pupils of the eye are dilated and fixed and do not react to light, if electro-encephalography (q.v.) produces no sign of activity, if angiography (q.v.) shows that there is no cerebral circulation – then when the breathing machine is disconnected the patient will not breathe spontaneously and the heart will stop. In such a case, death may be equated with irreversible damage to the brain resulting in permanent deep coma, paralysis of the muscles of respiration, and cessation of cerebral circulation and electrical activity; although breathing machines may keep the patient's blood full of oxygen and his heart may therefore still be beating, the patient is regarded as dead. This explains the uproar about dramatic heart transplant operations, for whereas most journalists decided that death was marked by the stopping of the heart, the surgical teams believed that it was marked by the death of the brain. The tissues of the body do not live for very long without oxygen, and soon suffer permanent damage if the blood supply is cut off. The brain suffers irreversible damage after 5 minutes of anoxia, and neither the liver nor kidney survive for much longer. This means that they have to be taken from the donor as quickly as possible after death, and it has been argued, particularly in the case of heart transplants, that as long as the brain is dead there is no point in waiting until the circulation ceases; in some centres the 'beating heart' has been removed for transfer. This routine is clearly likely to stir up differences of opinion, and surgeons are divided on the matter. You will notice that it is assumed in the medical profession that the seat of the 'soul' is in the brain, if any such metaphysical question is considered. Other people consider the heart to be the seat of the emotions and the soul; not so long ago the liver was thought to be the seat of life. Strictly materialistic views on death agree that it is proper to remove a beating heart for transplantation in cases where the brain is dead. Those who believe in the existence of things that cannot be measured find it harder to be dogmatic and assured.

Debility: or weakness; this is a symptom of many diseases or none at all. From the strictly medical point of view the diseases in which debility is a striking factor are certain types of pulmonary tuberculosis and cases of Addison's disease (q.v.) or pernicious anaemia (q.v.). These are rare compared with the number of people who complain of debility and the number of patent medicines which mention the word on their wrappings. It is clear that anyone who feels weak is either (*a*) suffering from some specific illness which must be diagnosed and treated appropriately, or (*b*) simply 'feels' weak without any specific organic disease being present. The latter case is typical of many neurotic conditions. It is notable that those who are extremely ill with a serious physical disease do not, on the whole, frequently complain of weakness as a main symptom. When one is feeling ill in a non-specific way (which is what debility is usually taken to mean), it is important to have a proper medical check-up before resorting to 'tonics' which are for the most part valueless. *See* Tonics.

Decompression: 1. Any surgical operation or manoeuvre designed to release or relieve pressure in or upon an organ. Often applied to operations in which part of the bone of the skull is removed in order to relieve pressure inside the head caused by tumours which cannot be removed, and to operations designed to relieve pressure on the spinal cord caused by a fractured spine.
2. The gradual lessening of pressure on divers as they ascend from the deep, and on aviators as they ascend into the sky. Also part of the treatment for caisson disease (q.v.) when the diver is re-compressed and then slowly decompressed again.

Defibrillation: fibrillation is a condition occurring in muscle when the constituent fibres contract singly or in small groups instead of together. The muscle as a whole does not contract, but parts of it twitch very rapidly. It can occur in heart muscle, and when it does it can affect the atria (q.v.) or the ventricles. If the ventricles start to fibrillate no co-ordinated contraction can take place and the heart stops beating; a very fine shimmering can be seen as the fibres of the ventricular muscle contract. The condition, which is obviously rapidly fatal, is most commonly the result of existing heart disease, coronary artery insufficiency or the use of certain drugs including anaesthetics. If help is at hand, as it will be in the operating theatre for instance, cardiac massage will keep the circulation going but will not restore the heartbeat. To do this the fibrillation has to be stopped with a defibrillator, an electric machine which delivers shocks to the heart through electrodes placed on the chest wall. The current is in the first instance 100 volts for one twenty-fifth to one tenth of a second; if this fails the voltage may be increased to 250. If no defibrillator is at hand, and the heart will not start with cardiac massage (which makes it likely that the ventricles are fibrillating), an electric shock may be tried at mains voltage A.C. delivered through chest electrodes over the heart. It is important to keep the respiration going, if possible with oxygen, if not by mouth to mouth ventilation of the lungs, while efforts are being made to stop fibrillation.

Deformities: distortions of the normal shape of the body or its parts, occurring congenitally or acquired by accident or disease.

Degrees and Diplomas: in the United Kingdom medical degrees are given by universities, and diplomas are granted by the Royal Colleges of Physicians and Surgeons of England, Scotland and Ireland, and the Apothecaries Company in London. These can legally be registered and enable the holder to sign prescriptions for dangerous drugs and poisons and to sign death certificates. In the United States, medical degrees are given by Universities and diplomas, or Board certification, by specialty Boards. A medical degree entitles the physician to apply for a licence to practise medicine in the state of his choice. In most states, he must pass examinations designed to ensure competence before he is given a licence. The licence entitles him to write prescriptions for dangerous drugs, treat individuals seeking his services as a physician, and to sign death certificates. The diploma is earned by post-graduate training and examinations in the specialty branch of medicine wherein the doctor wishes to devote himself. There are numerous Boards, ranging from Allergy to the various subdivisions of surgery.

A physician may practise a specialty without a Board diploma; his state licence allows the individual doctor to limit his practice as he thinks appropriate.

Dehydration: lack of water in the body.

CAUSE: starvation, as after shipwreck. Abnormal loss of fluids without replacement as in sicknesses which cause vomiting and diarrhoea, for example cholera. Excessive sweating (which may go unnoticed).

SYMPTOMS: in the infant, the lips, tongue and mouth become dry. The child is restless, and although it may be vomiting is thirsty. The anterior fontanelle (q.v.) is depressed, and as the condition progresses the skin becomes blue because the circulation collapses and the child feels cold to the touch. If the child becomes difficult to rouse, intravenous infusion is the only thing that can save it.

The adult suffering from heat exhaustion has great thirst, his temperature is raised, he may be giddy. He feels exhausted, and if he has accompanying salt loss he may suffer from muscle cramps and nausea. In cholera, the skin and mouth dry up, there is intense thirst, muscular cramp, and progressive circulatory collapse with suppression of urine.

TREATMENT: in infants, the effects of dehydration are quick and dangerous; if an infant has severe diarrhoea and vomiting its condition as it loses water and salts can deteriorate almost visibly, and it must have intravenous fluid if it cannot stop vomiting. Sodium and potassium are lost as well as water, and must be replaced in the intravenous infusion. Adults are liable to become dehydrated after operations, especially when the function of the intestines or stomach is upset, and intravenous fluids may be needed in the first day or two. Diseases of the intestines such as cholera produce their worst effects by bringing about an excessive loss of water and salts, and can be treated effectively only by close attention to fluid and electrolyte replacement by mouth or through the veins. Excessive sweating in hot conditions results in heat exhaustion if the loss of water is not made good; it may be coupled with salt depletion, and treatment must take notice of this.

PREVENTION: the urinary output ought to be between 1,200 ml and 1,500 ml a day in the adult, and in a temperate climate the loss by insensible perspiration and from the lungs is about 1,000 ml. There is variable loss from the faeces. The smallest amount of fluid intake which will keep a reasonable fluid balance going is 2,500 ml a day. If the supply of water is strictly limited, then a man can live on 500 ml a day taken in three portions; if conditions are desperate, he has a good chance of survival on half that amount. Despite some opinions to the contrary, sea water is dangerous to drink and may prejudice chances of survival. It is not recommended even in the most severe conditions.

Delhi Boil: dermal Leishmaniasis, Oriental sore, Baghdad sore, Aleppo sore.

CAUSE: infection with Leishmania (q.v.).

SYMPTOMS: found in tropical and subtropical countries. Starts as a small papule which itches, and is usually scratched until it ulcerates. Left alone it heals by itself after 6 months or a year and leaves a scar. One sore will produce immunity to subsequent infection.

TREATMENT: the sore must be cleaned, and secondary infection controlled if necessary with penicillin or other antibiotics. Leishmania tropica which causes cutaneous sores responds to injections of sodium stibogluconate (Pentostam). Unsightly sores on the face may be prevented by vaccination with live L. tropica on the leg.

Delirium: a Latin word meaning 'off the track'. It signifies confusion and excitement combined with hallucinations, illusions and delusions.

CAUSES: intoxication with various drugs, severe diseases, heat exhaustion, high fever. Examples of agents producing delirium are meningitis, heart failure, alcohol, typhoid fever. As delirium is not in itself a disease but a mental symptom it may be found in many physical disturbances.

SYMPTOMS: restlessness, excitement, inability to make correct deductions from what is seen to be happening in the surroundings, with consequent confusion, suspiciousness,

195

hallucinations, delusions, anxiety, and feelings of persecution. The state of consciousness, that is apparent awareness of the surroundings and of other people, varies from time to time.

TREATMENT: quietness, careful nursing, a good diet, and treatment of the underlying disease if possible. The best sedative is paraldehyde (q.v.), for barbiturates may increase the delirium. Alcoholic delirium (delirium tremens) is self-limiting, and stops after a few days, usually inside a week; in these cases a good diet is particularly important because there is nearly always a vitamin deficiency, and the delirium may have followed the complete loss of appetite that alcoholics sometimes show. Extra doses of Vitamin B should be given. It may be remembered that 'D.T.s' is sometimes caused by complete withdrawal of alcohol, so that a certain amount must be allowed.

Delta Waves: abnormally slow waves seen in the electro-encephalogram (q.v.) in cases of disease of the brain, for example some sorts of epilepsy, deep brain tumours.

Delusions: are false beliefs or judgments usually taken to be a sign of serious mental illness. However, a little thought will make it evident that we should be very cautious in ascribing them to this cause even if it is true that they do so occur; thus a person may exaggerate the significance of a true belief (such as that his body odour is objectionable), by supposing that everyone notices it (which may not be true at all), without being insane. Similarly, a delusion must be taken in its social and cultural context, for example a native of East Africa who thinks that he is being poisoned by a witch-doctor may have a belief which, although untrue, is quite usual in the circumstances, whereas a European with a good education who thought the same would probably be deluded in the sense of being mentally ill. There are people who believe the earth to be flat; the fact that they have formed a society to propagate this belief is, on the whole, a sign of relative normality since insane people do not ordinarily form societies. Delusions should not be confused with hallucinations, which are not false *beliefs* but false *sense-impressions*, i.e. seeing, hearing, feeling, or more rarely smelling, what is not there. But even here other factors

196

must be taken into account such as the individual's beliefs and cultural background. *See* Hallucinations, Mental Illness.

Dementia: is a symptom in mental illness the typical feature of which is regression, i.e. a return to more primitive forms of behaviour. It occurs in serious physical diseases of the brain where a large number of nerve cells are destroyed (for example, chronic alcoholism and drug addiction, syphilis and other infections of the brain, arteriosclerosis); in old age, to varying degrees; in the delirium of fevers; and in the functional psychoses such as schizophrenia. Its main features are poor memory, rambling talk, indifference to the feelings of others or unawareness of their disapproval of certain behaviour, sometimes incontinence of urine and faeces – 'second childishness and mere oblivion'. The outlook depends upon the cause, since the functional psychoses sometimes recover with treatment and temporary states of delirium recover with their accompanying disease, whereas in old age and long-drawn-out physical disorders of the brain where structural changes to the arteries or nerve cells have occurred the outlook is poor. *See* Mental Illness.

Dengue: an acute fever occurring in tropical and in subtropical countries.
CAUSE: a virus (B group arbovirus) transmitted by the bite of the mosquitoes Aedes aegypti,. the yellow fever mosquito, and A. albopictus. Incubation period about a week.
SYMPTOMS: sudden attack of fever with reddening of the skin and the eyes, headache and sore throat, and pain in the joints and bones which gives dengue its popular name, breakbone fever. These pains may be remarkably severe. After a day or two the fever abates and the patient feels better, but in about twenty-four hours the temperature rises again and the pain comes back. There may at this stage be a rash that looks like measles.
TREATMENT: pain is treated by aspirin, and the patient is kept quietly in bed. There is no specific treatment, but in some very severe cases in which there is a haemorrhagic rash and the patient is very ill it may be thought best to use steroids. The disease lasts a short time – it is usually over in a week – and it is very rarely fatal. Like other virus diseases,

dengue may be followed by a period of mental depression which may need treatment.

Depression: *See* Mental Illness.

Dermatitis: inflammation of the skin. The dividing line between dermatitis and eczema is not clearly drawn. It has been suggested that 'dermatitis' should be used to describe cases where inflammation of the skin is caused by an agent that is known; it has also been said that 'eczema' should be used to mean reaction of the epidermis (*see* Skin) as opposed to dermis. In general terms it appears that 'dermatitis' and 'eczema' are synonymous.

CAUSES: There are almost as many possible external causes of dermatitis as there are substances which can touch the skin, and it would not be sensible to try to set them all down here. They can be separated into groups:

Physical irritants. Detergents, strong acids and alkalies, oil, soap, antiseptics, etc.

Allergic irritants. Penicillin, flowers, various sorts of cloth used to make clothes, nickel (in clips, fastenings, etc.), cosmetics, dyes, etc. Allergic irritants may cause eruptions in areas of skin well away from the place of contact, and it is possible for the secondary eruptions to overshadow the primary dermatitis so that it is overlooked.

TREATMENT: identification and removal of the irritant. If it turns out that the irritant is a substance the patient encounters at work (industrial dermatitis) it may mean that he has to change his job. In time the skin eruptions of dermatitis often become infected and angry, because they are scratched or otherwise interfered with, and anti-infective preparations have to be used. A certain care is necessary, for these anti-infective substances themselves can cause dermatitis. The simplest preparations are often the best, such as gentian violet or clioquinol, and a good skin antiseptic is hexachlorophane; but the infection may require treatment with antibiotics such as tetracycline either locally or by mouth. Neomycin and bacitracin are only to be used locally. Anti-infective agents are commonly prescribed with corticosteroids as a cream or ointment, for the corticosteroids are a very effective treatment for dermatitis. In the most severe cases it may even be necessary to use corticosteroids by mouth, but this is only done in cases which will not respond to anything else. In general the patient should rest and should restrict his intake of alcohol. If he is emotionally disturbed it may be necessary to use a mildly sedative drug, usually one of the antihistamines.

Dermoid Cyst: a cyst, usually quite small, lying under the skin, which may arise in one of two ways.
1. *Congenital:* the cyst is found in a place where fusion of tissues takes place during development, such as at the outer angle of the eye.
2. *Acquired:* dermoid cysts sometimes form from a little piece of skin driven under the surface either by injury or during the course of an operation. These are called 'implantation' or 'sequestration' dermoids.
TREATMENT: surgical removal.

Desensitization: *see* Allergy.

Desoxycorticosterone: a steroid nearly identical with corticosterone. *See* Corticosteroids.

Dexamphetamine: (Dexedrine). *See* Amphetamine.

Dextran: substances (polymers of glucose) produced by the fermentation of sucrose by the bacterium Leuconostoc mesenteroides. Different preparations can be made which have different molecular weights, and these are given by intravenous infusion as substitutes for plasma in the treatment of surgical shock or burns.

Dextrocardia: a congenital anomaly in which the heart is on the right side of the chest. It may be associated with a similar abnormal position of the abdominal organs named situs inversus.

Dextrose: a substance obtained by the hydrolysis of starch, used in intravenous infusions to supply calories.

DFP: a gaseous organophosphorus compound, which is very poisonous; it works by interfering with the action of acetylcholinesterase in breaking down acetylcholine (q.v.).

If it is inhaled the effects are those of overdosage with acetylcholine – slow pulse, nausea, dizziness, headache, colic, sweating, salivation; later there is muscular weakness, which can progress to paralysis of the breathing muscles, and constriction of the pupils which prevents the eye focusing on near objects. Convulsions and coma may lead to death in very severe cases.

TREATMENT: atropine by injection into the muscles or the veins, and a substance named pralidoxime which is given in a dose of 1–2 g intravenously. It is available from special centres.

Dhobie Itch: a contact dermatitis caused by the marking ink used by native laundrymen in India. Sometimes used to mean tinea cruris. *See* Ringworm.

Diabetes: *Diabetes insipidus.* A condition in which the patient passes large quantities of dilute urine.

CAUSE: deficiency in the hormone vasopressin, the antidiuretic hormone, secreted normally by the posterior part of the pituitary gland (q.v.).

TREATMENT: replacement therapy by injections of vasopressin, or the use of snuff containing the hormone. The dosage is increased until the required effect is achieved. (Alcohol produces its diuretic effect by suppressing the secretion of vasopressin.)

Diabetes mellitus. The well-known 'sugar diabetes'.

CAUSE: lack of the pancreatic hormone insulin. The existence of insulin, or rather the fact that removal of the pancreas led to the development of diabetes mellitus in dogs, was discovered in 1889 in Germany, but the hormone was 'not isolated until 1922, when Banting, Best and Macleod working in Canada made an active extract of insulin from the islet cells of the pancreas and won a Nobel prize.

SYMPTOMS: the disease may occur for the first time in middle age, when it is relatively mild. It may be discovered on routine examination, particularly if the patient has been suffering from recurrent infections such as boils; it is also associated with arterial disease. Women may suffer from irritation of the private parts (pruritus vulvae). It is common in the obese.

If the disease comes on earlier in life it is usually more severe. The patient complains of increasing thirst, weakness, and loss of weight, and he passes small quantities of urine frequently. Women cease to have their periods, and may be troubled by pruritus vulvae, and men may become impotent. The tongue is often smooth, the gums tend to be inflamed and patients are prone to suffer from boils, cramps in the legs at night, and pins and needles or numbness in the hands and feet. The urine is found to be full of sugar, and if the disease is severe the breath may smell of acetone. If the patient is not treated he may become unconscious and die in a diabetic coma. A full examination is always carried out on diabetic patients because the disease may be associated with another chronic complaint such as pulmonary tuberculosis.

TREATMENT: this is a matter for the specialist. It may be enough to keep to a diet; the diet may be combined with an anti-diabetic drug taken by mouth; or the diet may have to be combined in the more severe cases with insulin, which is given by injection. There are many preparations of insulin, all of which have definite indications, and when a particular preparation and dosage has been recommended it must not be changed without consultation with the doctor. A diabetic patient will be taught how to test his urine and regulate his treatment, but in severe cases there is always a danger of coma due generally to low blood sugar, but sometimes to high blood sugar and ketones – diabetic coma.

1. *Hypoglycaemic coma*

CAUSE: low blood sugar through overdose of insulin, or through missing a meal, or taking strenuous exercise.

SYMPTOMS: sudden onset in a patient previously well is characteristic, and the warning signs are restlessness, faintness, palpitations, cold sweating, and hunger. The patient gets to know the symptoms and can usually cut short the attack by taking sugar, but if he does not he becomes confused and unsteady on his feet. He may cry out and appear to be drunk, and may eventually lapse into coma.

TREATMENT: diabetics must carry sugar with them if they are taking insulin, and they ought to have a card on them which says that they are diabetic and tells a helper where to find the sugar. If there is sufficient warning the patient can take the sugar himself, but if he is overtaken by confusion and unconsciousness and cannot swallow, the matter becomes more difficult. Injection of adrenalin 0.6 ml beneath the skin elevates the blood sugar and may make the patient conscious enough to swallow; an intravenous injection of concentrated glucose will bring him round but is less likely to be at hand. A way of getting sugar into the bloodstream via the stomach is to use a stomach tube, but it is essential not to allow anything to go 'down the wrong way' into the lungs in an unconscious patient. If it is possible an injection of glucagon (q.v.) is the best treatment, for it is quite safe. It can be supplied in ampoules which are mixed with a special fluid, also supplied in an ampoule, and it is safe for any intelligent person to make it up and inject it because it does not matter if it is given under the skin, into the muscle or into a blood vessel.

2. *Diabetic coma*

CAUSE: too much sugar and the presence of ketones in the blood. In known cases of diabetes, the omission of a dose of insulin, too little insulin, acute infection or emotional upset brings this about, and it occurs in untreated cases.

SYMPTOMS: this condition comes on slowly. The patient loses his appetite, becomes nauseated and may start to vomit. There may be pain in the abdomen and drowsiness. The skin becomes dry, the mouth dry and foul, the blood pressure falls and the pulse becomes rapid and weak. The breathing is deep.

TREATMENT: patients are admitted to hospital as soon as possible, for although the principle of treatment is simple – the administration of insulin – the detail is complicated and laboratory tests are needed.

It will be seen that there are great differences in the two types of coma associated with diabetes; the more common type is (1), the hypoglycaemic coma, and if there is reason to suppose that an unconscious patient has diabetes and is therefore ill, then he should be treated by the administration of sugar or glucagon in the first instance.

Complications of diabetes mellitus: the most common are blurring of vision and neuritis, which leads to alteration of sensation especially in the feet and legs.

Diagnosis: the determination of the nature of a disease in a given case.

Dialysis: the process (used in the artificial kidney) whereby colloids and crystalloids in a solution are separated by their different rates of passage through a semi-permeable membrane.

Diaper Rash: *see* Napkin Rash.

Diaphoretics: it used to be thought that in certain cases of fever it was a good thing to promote a flow of perspiration, and substances like aspirin and quinine which were used for the purpose were called diaphoretics. Nobody nowadays finds much virtue in this method of treatment.

Diaphragm: the muscular partition between the abdominal and thoracic cavities. The fleshy outer part of the diaphragm takes its origin from the lower six ribs and their cartilages, the lowest part of the breastbone in front and the upper lumbar vertebrae behind. The central part of the diaphragm is tendinous, and to it is fastened the outer muscular part. The general shape of the diaphragm is like a dome, and when the outer muscle contracts it pulls the dome downwards and flattens it so that the volume of the thoracic cavity is increased at the expense of the abdominal cavity, and the lungs expand provided that the ribs are fixed or raised. The nerve supply of the diaphragm is the phrenic nerve, which comes down from the neck (the reason is developmental); damage caused to the spinal cord in the neck through disease or accident can paralyse the diaphragm and so interfere with the breathing. There are large openings in the diaphragm through which pass the oesophagus, the aorta and thoracic duct, and the vena cava, and two small openings in front through which go the superior epigastric arteries. It is possible for the stomach to herniate upwards through the opening which normally transmits the oesophagus. *See* hiatus hernia in Hernia.

Diarrhoea: frequent passage of loose motions.
CAUSE: there are many causes of diarrhoea, and it helps to divide the cases into acute and chronic.
Acute. The commonest cause of acute diarrhoea is food poisoned or contaminated by organisms of the Salmonella group. Diarrhoea suffered by travellers is sometimes due to

food poisoning, but it may occur because the organisms in the bowel change. The new organisms may not normally produce disease but they may irritate the bowel while the body is getting used to them. Bacterial dysentery (*see* Dysentery) has a less sudden onset than food poisoning, and is caused by organisms of the Shigella, Flexner and Sonne groups. It is common in hot countries, but may be found in temperate climates, particularly in institutions, where outbreaks can be quite serious. Diarrhoea is severe in cholera (q.v.).

TREATMENT: for food poisoning and travellers' diarrhoea this is symptomatic; the best medicine for quietening the bowels is a mixture of chalk and opium or kaolin and morphine. In bacterial dysentery the organism should be cultured and tested for sensitivity to antibiotics, but cases in which this is not possible usually respond to tetracycline. The organisms of dysentery are increasingly resistant to sulphonamides, which used to be the great stand-by. Rest is important; the disease may be severe, particularly in Shiga infections, and measures may have to be taken to combat dehydration especially in children. In mild diarrhoea in small children no specific treatment may be necessary, and in infants the best treatment is often to stop all solid food for a day and give only sugar-water. In more severe cases neomycin is given.

Chronic. Chronic diarrhoea is a symptom of many diseases, not all centred in the alimentary canal. They include: tumours of the gut, infections with amoebae, infestations with worms, coeliac disease in children, ulcerative colitis, 'nervous diarrhoea' and 'irritable colon', Graves' disease, poisoning, and reaction to treatment with various antibiotics. The treatment of chronic diarrhoea is the treatment of the underlying condition, particularly in cases of nervous diarrhoea and irritable colon in which diagnosis may be difficult. Some people poison themselves with purgatives under the impression that if they do not keep their bowels on the verge of diarrhoea they are going to suffer from the dreadful (but imaginary) consequences of constipation; others use their bowels as the mirror of their emotions.

Diastase: an enzyme found in malt which is capable of converting starches into sugars.

Diastole: the part of the heart's cycle when the chambers dilate, as opposed to systole when they contract. It is applied particularly to ventricular dilatation.

Diathermy: if a rapidly oscillating current is passed through the tissues they heat up because of the resistance they offer to its passage. This effect can be used in surgery, where an indifferent electrode of large area is fastened to the leg, and the other electrode is a needle point or the points of a pair of forceps. The tissues in contact with the needle or forceps will be heated enough to make the needle cut or an artery caught in the forceps coagulate. A dampened oscillating current is used for coagulating, an undampened current for cutting soft tissues. In physiotherapy diathermy is used to engender heat in deep tissues, but insufficient energy is used to heat to the point of harm. Shortwave diathermy is the use of short waves of 30 m to 10 m to heat the tissues; if the wavelength is less than 10 m the process is called ultra-shortwave diathermy.

Dick Test: a skin test that was formerly used to indicate an individual's susceptibility to scarlet fever before penicillin was introduced. As penicillin is so successful in destroying the organisms of scarlet fever (Streptococcus pyogenes) the Dick test has fallen into disuse.

Dicoumarol: an anti-coagulant drug, a derivative of coumarin, which acts by interfering with the synthesis in the liver of prothrombin (*see* Coagulation of the Blood). It is not now commonly used; warfarin (q.v.) is the drug of choice among the oral anti-coagulants.

Dieldrin: a chlorinated hydrocarbon used as a rapidly acting insecticide with a wider range than D.D.T. It is poisonous to man and to animals and its use is restricted. The symptoms of Dieldrin poisoning are: clumsiness, headache, nausea, muscle twitching and convulsions. Treatment is to clean the skin, control the fits if present and keep the patient quiet.

Diet: food is one of those things we either accept as being simply a part of living which may be arranged pleasantly or unpleasantly, or consider to be a matter of the utmost importance (which it is), containing the key to all disease and health (which it does not). It may be said at once that a normal individual taking the kind of food in the kind of quantities usual in Western Europe and the U.S.A. has no need to worry about his food except for the reason that, as he gets older, he may have to reduce its amount. Dietetics, except of the most ordinary and commonsense kind, plays little part in the treatment of disease. It would be difficult to think of more than half a dozen or so important diseases which need dietetic advice of any specialized sort. Conflicts rage in the background of people's minds when they talk about food, although it is a matter perfectly susceptible to scientific study. The non-scientific attitude is well illustrated by the remarks made to a medical committee by a presiding layman who announced that his cure for a cold was to starve himself for 3 days and eat nothing but Vitamin C in the form of grapefruit 3 times a day. When it was pointed out to him that he could have obtained 100 times the amount of Vitamin C in the more concentrated form of tablets he was quite annoyed, yet it is obvious that he was making a number of absurd claims: (1) that he alone had discovered the cure for a cold; (2) that grapefruit, and not oranges or lemons or pills which also contain Vitamin C, was a necessity for the cure, thereby implying either that Vitamin C was not the curing agent, or that it took a different form in the other fruit and in the pills, or that a mysterious 'something else' undiscovered by chemists and capable of curing colds lurked in the grapefruit; (3) that feeling better is a criterion of cure in a disease when it has been known from the earliest times that entirely inert substances (such as the 'tonics' given with such good effect by doctors) can make people feel better and even cure them if they have sufficient confidence; (4) that colds, apart from complications, last longer than three days. Most of the curious diets that people go in for have no firmer basis than this: they simply state that a certain food is better without saying why, or without saying so in a way that science can accept, and they assume that feeling better is the same as being better. We need have no doubt that many businessmen and professional men would be the better for a couple of weeks on nothing but orange juice – but why orange juice rather than water? If the answer is that oranges contain sugar, then by all means give them sugar and water; if it is that they contain Vitamin C then one has to ask, why bother about Vitamin C and not Vitamins A, B and D? But perhaps the treatment would not attract so many people if the diet was vitamin soup and a little sugar.

In order to be adequate any diet must first of all supply enough energy, which is measured in calories (q.v.). Thus a 140-lb (63.5-kg) man leading a moderately active life will require about 3,000 calories daily in order to avoid living on his internal resources. The number of calories needed varies with age, size, and the amount of work done, from 1,500 calories for the lightweight sedentary worker to three or more times that amount for the heavy manual worker. Now, in theory, this could be supplied by sugar, starch, or fats alone since calories are merely a measure of energy which could be supplied by any food. But, in practice, an individual who tried such a diet would not live long because he needs for body maintenance certain kinds of food in correct proportions. Just as one cannot run a car on petrol alone and ignore lubricating oil or water for the cooling system, so the body cannot be run simply by taking in calories. There must be adequate quantities of the three basic foodstuffs: carbohydrates (the fuel); fats and oils (for insulation and other purposes); and proteins (for body-building purposes). Proteins are necessary to replace the cells of the body when they become worn out, and whereas fats and sugars can be transformed into each other as the obesity produced by eating too many sweets shows, they cannot produce protein which contains nitrogen. We could live on a diet of protein but not on a purely fat or carbohydrate one. The following foods are classified according to the predominating basic foodstuff they contain:

1. *Carbohydrates*. Bread, sugar, and all starchy or sweet things such as confectionery, pastries (which are also rich in fat), puddings either of the sponge or custard variety, cakes, certain fruits such as bananas, and root vegetables such as potatoes, swedes, parsnips and carrots.

2. *Fats*. Animal fats such as fat meat, lard, dripping, anything fried, and butter or anything containing it; vegetable or fish oils such as margarine, olive oil, peanut butter, nuts and olives, and certain fish which contain more fat than

DIGESTIVE SYSTEM

others, e.g. herring in its various forms.
3. *Proteins*. Lean meat, cheese, steamed, boiled or grilled
fish, eggs, oatmeal, soya bean, and to some extent milk and
wholemeal bread. Most fruits do not contain any significant
amount of protein but they do contain upwards of 90% of
water with vitamins and a little sugar; they are therefore
not usually excessively fattening.
In addition to these basic foods the body requires vitamins
in proper amounts (unless an actual deficiency exists,
vitamins taken over and above the normal amounts in the
food have no effect), and certain minerals such as iron,
manganese, calcium, copper, sodium and potassium. Water,
of course, is also necessary, but it is rubbish to suppose that
large amounts have any special virtue in 'cleaning out the
inside', although it is true that too little water can cause
constipation. It does not seem to matter in what form the
food substances are taken, except that vegetarians who are
strictly vegetarian are likely to have difficulty in ingesting
adequate supplies of protein, which is why cows spend all
day eating.

Digestive System: the digestive system begins at the
mouth and ends at the anus where the waste products are
excreted. Food taken in at the mouth is moistened by saliva
secreted by the salivary glands, the parotid in front of the ear,
the submaxillary under the angle of the jaw, and the sublingual under the tongue. Saliva contains an enzyme called
ptyalin which, while the teeth are cutting and grinding the
food into a pulp which can be easily swallowed, mixes with
the mass and begins the process of digestion by turning some
of the starch into sugars. This process is not of major importance; the main function of saliva is to lubricate the food
on its way down. Since 'the stimulus to the secretion of
saliva is basically psychological through the senses of sight,
smell and taste, or even through expectation, the importance
of food looking and smelling appetizing will be appreciated,
for without saliva, i.e. when the mouth is dry, food cannot
be properly chewed or swallowed. This happens when such
emotions as fear, anxiety or disgust inhibit the flow or when
the individual is preoccupied with something else, for example reading the papers or watching TV. The food passes
from the mouth into the oesophagus while a reflex action

normally closes the glottis to prevent it finding its way into the windpipe or the lungs; when someone is suffering from certain diseases of the nervous system, is laughing and eating at the same time, or unconscious, the failure of this reflex causes food or drink to 'go down the wrong way'. (This is one of the reasons for not giving drink to an unconscious person.) The oesophagus is about 10 in (250 mm) long and passes the food on to the stomach by a series of rhythmic movements which make it quite possible for someone to drink while standing on his head. The gastric juice of the stomach is acid because of the presence of hydrochloric acid which helps the action of the enzymes carrying out the actual process of digestion. Although it is usual to blame an excess of this acid for various types of dyspepsia, and in cases of peptic ulcer the acid content of the stomach is usually raised, it must be remembered that (a) some people suffer from severe dyspepsia in the total absence of hydrochloric acid, and (b) that it is by no means proved that it is the raised acid content which causes pain in ordinary indigestion. There are drugs such as belladonna which relieve indigestion without affecting the acid content of the stomach. The main enzyme (q.v.) in the gastric juice is pepsin, which digests proteins into their constituent parts. As the stomach finishes its work, the semi-liquid food is passed through a valve at the end of the stomach known as the pylorus into the duodenum, the beginning of the small intestine, where it comes under the influence of the alkaline intestinal juices with their enzymes which help in the breakdown of protein into amino acids, act upon complex sugars (disaccharides) such as sucrose and maltose to convert them into the mono-saccharide glucose, and split fats into fatty acids and glycerine. Other factors concerned with the digestion of food in the small intestine are: (1) the bile, which helps in the breakdown of fats and is collected from the liver and gall-bladder into the common bile-duct which, together with the duct from the pancreas, enters the duodenum shortly after its beginning; (2) the pancreatic juice which contains the enzymes lipase to break down fats, amylase which completes the digestion of starch, trypsin which completes the breakdown of proteins begun in the stomach, and a milk-curdling substance; (3) the bacteria of the lower part of the small intestine. Only one substance is absorbed directly from the stomach, i.e. alcohol, but by the time the food has reached the end of the small intestine everything eaten, no matter how complex, has been broken down into a few simple chemicals – the proteins into amino acids, the fats into fatty acids and glycerin, and the starches and sugars into glucose. It is probably the fact that glucose is the end-product of carbohydrate digestion and therefore easily and rapidly absorbed that has provided its quite unjustified reputation as an energy-provider with some sort of scientific basis. Of course, glucose is absorbed quickly and does supply energy, but the fallacy attaching to its use by normal people is that they are not normally suffering from lack of energy but rather from the psychological inability to put their energy to work. The duodenum is about 10 in (250 mm) long, and is continuous with the jejunum and the ileum which together measure after death about 20 ft (6 m), but whose length in life depends upon the tone of the muscle in their walls, and may be as little as 10 ft (3 m). At the end of the ileum the small intestine joins the large intestine or colon, which begins in the right lower part of the abdominal cavity and is continuous with the caecum and the appendix. The colon travels up as the ascending colon on the right side of the abdomen, crosses to the left (the transverse colon), and on the left forms the descending colon which joins the sigmoid colon and then the 6-in (150-mm) rectum, the anal canal and the anus through which waste matter is discharged. The large gut absorbs only water, but the walls of the small intestine absorb broken-down fats, bile salts, amino acids and glucose. The broken-down fats enter the lymph vessels of the intestinal villi, and then pass into the lymphatic system draining the gut, and so into the thoracic duct and the venous blood. The bile salts and the amino acids and glucose pass through the portal system of veins into the liver. The rate at which food passes down the alimentary tract varies; it appears that the stomach is empty about two or three hours after a meal, and the small intestine after about four hours. About twenty-four hours after a meal has been eaten the remnants are in the rectum ready to be evacuated. The food is moved along the alimentary canal by a com-bination of contraction and relaxation of the muscular walls, which in the small intestine is organized into three types of movement: peristalsis, which is a slow wave move-

ment passing along the gut wall; segmentation, in which
there is alternate relaxation and constriction of the gut; and
pendular movements which mix up the food as they pass
to and fro along the length of the gut. In the large intestine
the movements resemble segmentation and peristalsis but
are slower than in the small intestine. The rectum is normally
empty except just before the passage of the motions.

Digitalis: extract of the leaf of the foxglove (Digitalis
purpurea) used in the treatment of heart disease. The use of
this substance has been known for hundreds of years, and it
is still the most valuable drug available to improve the action
of failing heart muscle. Digitalis itself is a preparation of the
dried leaf of the foxglove, and the strength of different
preparations varies, so that chemically pure component
principles of the crude drug are usually used; their names
are digoxin and digitoxin, and lanatoside (cedilanid).
(Ouabain and strophanthin have identical chemical
formulae but come from different plants.) Digoxin is the
most widely used substance, and like the other drugs its
action is upon the heart muscle; the power of the muscle to
contract is increased, and the rate is slowed down so that the
contractions are more effective. The drug is given by mouth
in large doses to start with, for example 0.5 mg every six
hours for about two days. The dose is then dropped to 0.5
to 0.75 mg a day. The effective dose of digoxin is very near
the toxic dose, and it is important to know what the toxic
effects are. They include: loss of appetite; nausea and
vomiting; diarrhoea; headache; slow and irregular pulse.
If these symptoms occur digoxin is stopped for a time, and
potassium chloride tablets are given. Another useful drug
in these circumstances is propranolol (Inderal), which
controls pulse irregularities.

Digoxin: *see above* under Digitalis.

Dill: this is doubtless still being given to countless infants
for ailments of the digestive tract, but the only sensible
employment for dill almost precludes its prescription in the
disorders of childhood, for it is at its best when used in the
preparation of pickled cucumbers.

Dimercaprol: (B.A.L., British Anti-Lewisite). Invented during World War 2 as an antidote to Lewisite and similar arsenical gases, it is now used as an antidote to poisoning with arsenic, mercury, antimony, and gold. Combined with an arsenical preparation it forms Melarsoprol (Mel B), a drug active against trypanosomes (q.v.) both in the blood and in the nervous system.

Dindevan: (Danitone). *See* Phenindione.

Dinitro Compounds: dinitrophenol was once used as a slimming agent, but it proved fatal in a number of cases; dinitrocresol is used as a herbicide. The action of these compounds is to interfere with the metabolism of the cell so that it has to use up more energy, which means that it produces more heat. Symptoms of poisoning are a yellow discoloration of the whites of the eyes, tiredness allied with an inability to sleep, excessive sweating with increased thirst, loss of weight, anxiety, breathlessness, rapid pulse and a high temperature. Poisoning can be fatal, the patient dying in coma and heart failure.

TREATMENT: the patient must be removed from contamination, washed with spirit (alcohol) to remove the D.N.O.C., and given as much to drink as he can manage; if he is breathless he should be given oxygen. If he is suffering from a high temperature it should be reduced by the use of wet sheets and cold water.

Dinoseb: a dinitrocresol herbicide (*see* above).

Diphtheria: a severe infection most commonly affecting the upper respiratory passages.

CAUSE: the organism is Corynebacterium diphtheriae. This bacterium multiplies in the throat or nose and produces a powerful and dangerous toxin, which poisons surrounding structures and is carried in the bloodstream to other parts of the body.

SYMPTOMS: the toxin liberated in the throat by the bacteria kills the mucous membrane lining the pharynx and the upper air passages, so that a grey membrane sloughs off and the underlying tissues swell. The swelling and the membrane obstruct the larynx in cases where the infection is centred in that area (laryngeal diphtheria) and interfere with breathing, especially in small children. In other cases the infection is centred on the tonsils, and the membrane is seen on the surface of the tonsils where it does not obstruct the breathing. The child in these cases of tonsillar diphtheria looks pale and ill, and is fretful and poorly but may show little or no discomfort in the neck. If the infection spreads to the pharynx from the tonsil the diphtheria is called tonsillo-pharyngeal; the tissues at the back of the mouth swell, a dark bloody membrane may be formed, the glands of the neck become enlarged and the patient becomes very ill. Other forms of diphtheria are found in the nose, when the nose becomes sore and the mucous discharge may be stained with blood, and on the skin – this is particularly difficult to diagnose. From all these forms of infection the toxin spreads throughout the body, although the bacteria only multiply locally, and it poisons the heart and the nervous system. The pulse becomes weak, there may be pain in the chest and the heartbeat may show an increase of rate and irregularity. Damage to the heart is associated with vomiting, which is a grave sign in diphtheria. The heart may fail gradually or suddenly. In the nervous system neuritis may develop towards the end of the course of the disease, from which a complete recovery is possible; the damage done by the toxin may affect some of the cranial nerves (q.v.). In these cases the patient may develop paralysis of the palate, which alters the voice and allows food and drink to come up through the nose, palsy of the throat so that it is difficult to swallow and food may 'go down the wrong way', or weakness of the ciliary muscle of the eye so that it is difficult to read because accommodation (q.v.) is impossible. If the extrinsic eye muscles are involved the patient will complain of double vision.

TREATMENT: the main aim is to neutralize the toxin secreted by the C. diphtheriae as quickly as possible. This is done by injections of diphtheria anti-toxin serum, intramuscularly in mild cases but intravenously in severe cases when as much as 50,000 units, or even more, may have to be given. Penicillin is used to attack the bacteria, and the effect of the disease on the heart requires the patient to be confined to bed for the first week or 10 days. If the condition allows he is then gradually restored to normal activity, but it may take a few weeks before convalescence is complete.

CONTROL OF INFECTION: diphtheria has until recently been a great scourge, but in the last few decades the introduction of effective immunization has driven it out of Europe and the U.S.A. *See* Immunization. If a patient has been subject to infection with diphtheria it is very important to make sure that he is completely free of organisms at the end of the disease, for it is possible to carry C. diphtheriae in the nose or less commonly in the throat and be in good health. People who do so are called carriers, and they can spread the disease unless the organisms they carry are killed by adequate medical treatment. The incubation period of diphtheria is between 2 and 6 days, and the isolation period is 10 days, subject to negative cultures.

Diphyllobothrium latum: a very long tapeworm which lives in fish and in people who eat badly cooked fish. Treatment is by extract of male fern, niclosamide or dichlorophen; it cannot be said to be successful unless the head of the worm is expelled. *See* Worms.

Diplopia: (Double vision). This is caused by interference with the movements of the eyes in relation to each other, usually by inco-ordination or weakness of the muscles that move the eyeball, so that the image of an observed object does not fall upon corresponding parts of the two retinae. It may be transient and of no importance, but may be found as a symptom in various diseases.

Dipsomania: *see* Alcoholism.

Disinfection: the destruction of bacteria by antiseptics (q.v.).

Disinfestation: the destruction of parasites and pests that can spread disease, for example lice.

Dislocation: the displacement of a part from its normal position, used particularly when a bone is displaced from its normal relationship to another bone but is not necessarily broken.

Disorientation: difficulty in locating oneself correctly in space and time. A symptom of mental abnormality.

Dissection: cutting apart; used both of separating the tissues in the course of a surgical operation and of studying the structure of a dead body. A specimen which has been dissected to show some special feature is called a 'dissection'.

Disseminated Sclerosis: *see* Multiple Sclerosis.

Disulfiram: (Antabuse). A drug which interferes with the metabolism of alcohol so as to increase the level of acetaldehyde in the blood. A dose of 0.5 g taken in the morning will produce headaches, flushing, nausea and even vomiting if alcohol is drunk during the day.

Diuretics: drugs which increase the output of urine. They are used in heart failure, kidney and liver disease. The most commonly taken diuretic is alcohol, but it promotes a flow of dilute urine which is almost water, and a flow of salts as well as water is needed in the treatment of oedema (dropsy). There are a large number of diuretics which produce a flow of water and salts, most being preparations in the thiadiazine group such as chlorothiazide (Saluric or Diuril), or preparations with a similar chemical formula such as frusemide (Lasix). At one time a salt-free diet was commonly used in the treatment of oedema, but with modern diuretics the problem is rather different, for they may actually lead to excessive loss of salts, and it is good practice to guard against this by using potassium tablets such as Slow-K when a patient is being treated with frusemide.

Diverticulitis: inflammation of a diverticulum of the colon (*see* below).
SYMPTOMS: pain in the left lower side of the abdomen with diarrhoea or constipation. Attacks may recur over a long time. If the disease is severe the inflamed diverticulum may rupture and produce peritonitis (q.v.), but the rupture may not be into the general abdominal cavity; it is possible for inflammation to spread so that it only involves structures lying nearby, or the diverticulum may rupture through an area of inflammation into the bladder or into another part

of the gut and form a fistula (q.v.). Bleeding may occur into the bowel, and the inflamed diverticulum may attract a covering of omentum and form quite a large tumour. Confusion with a malignant growth is made more likely if there is obstruction of the gut, and the difference can sometimes only be established at operation.

TREATMENT: if an attack of diverticulitis can be diagnosed and there is no doubt that there is no malignancy the patient is put to bed, and given a fluid diet and antibiotics. If there is any doubt about the diagnosis, or the bowel becomes obstructed or a fistula forms, an operation is performed which usually involves a colostomy (q.v.).

Diverticulosis: a condition of the colon, usually involving the descending and pelvic parts, in which the muscular wall gives way in places and allows the mucous membrane lining the large intestine to form pouches which become filled with faecal material. It is usually a condition of middle and later age, and by itself is of no consequence. It happens sometimes, however, that diverticuli become inflamed – having no muscle in their walls they cannot empty themselves – and the condition of diverticulitis arises (*see* above).

Diverticulum: the pouch of mucous membrane formed when the muscular wall of a viscus, such as the colon, gives way. *See* Diverticulosis.

D.N.A.: (Deoxyribonucleic acid). An extremely long molecule made up of two strands wound in a double helix. It is the key to cellular reproduction, for it carries the information necessary to form proteins and enzymes and a duplicate copy of itself. The story of the recent discovery of the double helix of D.N.A. is fascinating but outside the scope of this book.

Dolichocephalic: long-headed. *See* Brachycephalic.

Douche: the treatment of any part of the body by a continuous flow of medicated water. The term is most commonly used in describing cleansing of the vagina.

Dover's Powder: a remedy composed of potassium sulphate with 10% each of powdered opium and ipecacuanha, once one of the most popular remedies in medicine. It was devised by the pirate Captain Thomas Dover, whose other claim to fame rests upon his rescue of Alexander Selkirk, the original Robinson Crusoe, from the desert island of Juan Fernandez. Dover's powder was used in the treatment of colds and fevers but has been replaced by the less swash-buckling remedy aspirin.

Dracunculus: the Guinea worm. Infestation by this long, thin worm is acquired by drinking water in which there are infected water fleas (the intermediate host). The adult worm makes its way through the tissues of the body and comes to the surface usually in the lower leg, whence it is extracted by being wound little by little over a period of days on to a stick. Niridazole (Ambilhar) is given by mouth for 10 days in a dose of 25 mg/kg body weight, the dose thus calculated being divided into two and taken twice a day. The drug makes it much easier to extract the worm cleanly in one piece, but if it should break an abscess may form and have to be opened by the surgeon.

Dramamine: (dimenhydrinate). An antihistamine pre-paration which is used to control travel-sickness, vertigo and migraine. It may make people feel sleepy, and it is not wise to drive after taking a dose.

Dressings: in general, dressings are applied to wounds to stop organisms from outside infecting a raw area, to absorb blood and discharge, and to protect the wound from contact with clothes, etc. A large number of wounds do not need to be dressed after they have been treated except for pro-tection, and they should be covered with as light a dressing as possible. It is sensible to cover up wounds that have just been inflicted; the dressing should be made of sterile gauze if possible, but if that is not to hand freshly laundered linen will do very well. Bind such dressings firmly in place, and if the bleeding shows through, do not remove the dressing but put on another tighter bandage. More dressings are used than are necessary, particularly those combined with adhesive tape. If you must cover up a cut, at least make sure that the skin does not become soggy and white from being

217

cut off from the air; and do not be surprised if the doctor
tells you to keep a wound uncovered.

Drop-foot: a condition in which the foot cannot be raised;
it hangs limp from the ankle joint. It is commonly caused by
paralysis of the muscles which normally flex the ankle joint
brought on by neuritis or other disease in the nerves which
supply them. The disease which used to cause severe drop-
foot is poliomyelitis, now not so common; causes of neuritis
are alcohol, typhoid fever, diphtheria, and vitamin deficiency; lead poisoning can cause drop-foot, and so of course
can injuries to the nerves. Treatment is directed to the cause
of the complaint, but it may be necessary to use a device to
keep the ankle flexed because drop-foot interferes badly with
walking.

Dropsy: technically known as oedema, this is an abnormal
accumulation of fluid in the body which may be localized
(as in some cases of allergy or interference with the local
circulation) or general (as in heart, kidney or liver disease).
Oedema occurs most frequently in heart or kidney disease,
and the treatment is that of the cause. In general it is true
to say that kidney disease causes oedema which is worse in
the mornings and is noticed first beneath the eyes and in the
face, whereas in heart disease the swelling tends to be worse
in the evenings and begins in the lower parts of the body such
as the ankles. In liver disease, which is often the result of
chronic alcoholism, the swelling is in the legs and abdomen.
It should be noted that (*a*) localized oedema with pain is
likely to be due to interference with the circulation whereas
when it is associated with itching allergy is likely to be the
cause; (*b*) that most normal people as they grow older have
some swelling of the ankles as the day wears on which is of
no significance whatsoever, and in hot weather everybody's
ankles are swollen. *See* Angioneurotic Edema, Heart
Nephritis, Cirrhosis, Allergy, Varicose Veins.

Drop-wrist: a similar state to drop-foot (q.v.) occurring
in the hand and wrist.

Drug Addiction: a person is regarded as a drug addict if
after taking a drug a number of times he becomes so de-

pendent on it that he has an uncontrollable urge to continue taking the drug. Drugs may produce physical dependence, psychic (mental) dependence or a mixture of the two. The types of dependence listed by the World Health Organization are:

1. Morphine, where the desire to take the drug is overpowering, and there is both psychic and physical dependence.

2. Barbiturate and alcohol, where the desire is strong; dependence is psychic and physical.

3. Cocaine, where the desire is overpowering, but there is only psychic dependence.

4. Amphetamine, where the desire is there but is not strong, and where the dependence is psychic although it may be slightly physical.

5. Hallucinogen (L.S.D.), where there is slight desire to repeat the dose, not present in all those who try it, and where such dependence as there is is mainly psychic.

6. Cannabis, where the same state of affairs exists – the desire to repeat the dose is present but not very strong, and there is no physical dependence.

The recognition of a drug addict is not easy, for he will try to hide what is happening and the signs may be slight. If addiction has followed medical treatment with the drug in question the doctor will usually spot the addict when the time comes to reduce or omit the dose of the drug. Moral delinquency very rarely gives the game away, although in severe cases the patient may be discovered if he has to lie or steal in order to obtain a dose. In general the patient becomes unreliable and lazy, and he may neglect his food and himself. The physical signs are small pupils in morphine addicts, tremor and possible neuritis (q.v.) in alcoholics, unsteadiness, trembling and confusion with barbiturates, and in those who inject the drug into themselves, the marks of the needle. The distribution of known addicts' ages shows that dependence on drugs is greatest in those under 35; more males than females are addicts; and in the United Kingdom the total number of addicts has increased enormously since 1960, although it still remains a very small proportion of the population. In 1960 the number of opiate addicts known to the Home Office was 437, and in 1968 it was 2,393. In 1968 the Dangerous Drugs (Notification of

Addicts) Regulations made it compulsory for doctors to notify the names of addicts to the Home Office, and doctors were forbidden to prescribe heroin and cocaine to addicts unless they had a special licence.

In the United States a physician may not administer or prescribe narcotics for an addict unless the patient has entered a recognized treatment facility, thus known to law enforcement agencies, and receives the drug as part of the medical management of his problem. They may, of course, prescribe these drugs for pain. For the actions of the drugs listed *see under* separate headings; *see also* Heroin, Opium, Pethidine, Tranquillizers, Smoking.

TREATMENT: this is a matter for specialists. Physical dependence, if present, means that withdrawal of the drug is followed by physical disorder – gooseflesh, feelings of coldness, muscular cramp, vomiting, diarrhoea and raised temperature in the case of morphine and heroin, delirium in the case of alcohol, and delirium and fits with barbiturates. These symptoms may be very distressing, but the drugs can in time be successfully withdrawn.

Psychic dependence is difficult to overcome, for a good half of the patients are suffering from psychopathic troubles, and the others tend to be anxious, hysterical or immature, so that treatment has to go far beyond the simple withdrawal of a drug. In all cases the most difficult time will be after the treatment has enabled the patient to give up a drug while in hospital, for he now has to establish a new pattern of life for himself. It is at this time that practical help is most important.

Drugs, the Commercial Aspect: a great deal has been said and implied about the conduct of manufacturers of what are described as 'ethical' preparations, i.e. those proprietary drugs which can only be obtained on prescription by a physician (in contrast to the 'patent medicines' which anyone can buy). Among the arguments brought against the drug firms are: (1) They make inordinate profits. (2) The cost of successful drugs is kept high. (3) Advertising to doctors is importunate, vulgar and meretricious. (4) The action of preparations is misleadingly described. (5) There is confusing and unnecessary proliferation of names – a simple drug may be described by as many names as there are drug firms selling it – to take an example, the substance paracetamol is sold under the following names beside its own: Calpol, Distalgesic, Eneril, Gerisom, Lobak, Norgesic, Panadeine, Panasorb, Panok, Panadol, Parafon, Paracodol, Sinulin, Tabalgin, Zactipar. (6) Some firms may not test a drug adequately before it is put on the market. The firms in question deny that their profits are inordinate, they point out that successful drugs have to bear the cost of research which produces unsuccessful as well as successful preparations, that their advertising is in line with modern advertising practice and that it works, that they are responsible people and describe their products in a responsible way, and that they must call their own product by distinctive brand names. The sixth argument is met by various government committees and agencies set up to control the marketing of drugs. In Great Britain the National Health Service keeps doctors well informed about the relative costs of drugs and the scientific merit of new preparations, and there is no doubt that by strict economy in prescribing doctors could save the N.H.S. some millions of pounds. In the United States, the Food and Drug Administration is responsible for evaluating the testing of new drugs by manufacturers, looking specifically for effectiveness and safety. Licences may be denied or withdrawn for products not meeting standards.

Ductless Glands: *see* Endocrine Glands.

Dumbness: the primary cause of dumbness from birth is deafness, for a child who cannot hear at all is unable to learn to speak even when his voice mechanism is normal. Some cases are due to defects in the mechanism of speaking or to mental deficiency and the inability to learn from experience. Diagnosis and treatment is a matter for the specialist. *See* Aphasia.

Duodenal Ulcer: *See* Stomach Disease.

Duodenum: the first part of the small intestine, which runs from the pylorus of the stomach to the jejunum. It is applied to the back wall of the abdominal cavity, is shaped like a C, and lies with the convexity of the C to the right of the middle line. In the concavity of the C lies the head of the pancreas, and into the duodenum are discharged bile and pancreatic secretions. The duodenum is about 25 cm long; it was named because the length is about equal to the breadth of 12 fingers. *See* Digestive System.

Dupuytren's Contracture: a condition in which the fibrous tissues of the palm of the hand gradually contract, pulling on the little and ring fingers so that they bend and cannot be straightened. The other fingers may in time be affected so that the whole hand becomes crippled. The contracture occurs in later life, and gripping tools may be a factor; but often it comes on with no apparent reason. The treatment is surgical.

Dura: the dura mater, the outermost of the membranes that cover the brain. *See* Meninges.

Dwarfism: the commonest type of dwarf is the achondroplasic (*see* Achondroplasia), but other forms of dwarfism include that associated with cretinism or deficiency of the thyroid gland, and pituitary dwarfism in which there is a deficiency of the growth hormone secreted by the anterior lobe of the pituitary gland. The pituitary dwarf is small because he grows at a reduced rate; he shows no deformity or mental deficiency. He may be underdeveloped sexually. A 'normal' or 'true' dwarf is a person who is strikingly undersized but otherwise quite normal.

Dysarthria: difficulty in speech, due to an impairment of articulation. The impairment may be due to disease of the muscles or nerves concerned with the mechanism of speech, to disease of the structures essential for speech or to disease of the central nervous system.

Dyscrasia: a state of abnormality brought about by lack of balance of essential factors. The word was once applied to states attributed to a 'bad condition of the essential humours'.

Dysentery: a condition in which there is diarrhoea with

the passage of mucus and blood, and pain or discomfort in the abdomen.

CAUSE: (1) Infection with bacteria of the Shigella genus, named after the Japanese bacteriologist Kiyoshi Shiga who first isolated the dysentery bacillus. Bacillary dysentery may be due to infection with Shigella dysenteriae, Sh. flexneri, Sh. sonnei, or Sh. boydii. Shigella dysenteriae is the most dangerous, Sh. flexner less so, and Sh. sonnei quite mild. (2) Infection with Entamoeba histolytica (amoebic dysentery).

SYMPTOMS: *Bacillary dysentery.* The onset is acute, about four days after infection, with a margin of three days on either side, and in a moderate attack there is colicky pain in the abdomen, diarrhoea, nausea, vomiting, and fever; the abdominal pain becomes worse, and there is tenesmus – straining to pass motions when there is nothing to pass. Mucus and blood constitute what motions there are. In severe infections with Sh. dysenteriae toxins are given off by the bacilli which may produce inflammation of the eye and neuritis (q.v.). There may also be effusions into the joints of the legs. Fatal cases are rare, but every case in a child or in an old person must be watched lest the patient loses too much fluid.

Amoebic dysentery. This disease is found in the tropics and subtropics; the onset is usually insidious, although it can be acute, and the character of the diarrhoea is different from that occurring in bacillary dysentery, being less marked although the motions are still mixed with mucus and blood. The pain in the abdomen varies a great deal and can be mistaken for peptic ulcers or appendicitis. Any patient who has been in the tropics and complains of vague ill-health with odd attacks of diarrhoea and constipation, perhaps associated with abdominal discomfort – a feeling of bruising rather than colic – must be investigated for the presence of amoebae in the motions. The danger of the disease lies in the formation of amoebic abscesses in the liver.

TREATMENT: *Bacillary dysentery.* Sulphonamides used to be the drugs of choice, but the bacilli have become resistant and if possible, particularly where the outbreak is in an institution, it is important to take bacteriological specimens and test for drug sensitivity before antibiotics, e.g. neomycin, are used. In mild infections, typically those due to Sh. sonnel, the best treatment is a mixture made up of chalk and opium, or one containing kaolin and morphine. If the infection is severe, treatment will include preventing excessive loss of water and salts.

Amoebic dysentery. The drug most active against the amoebae is emetine. In the acute stages of the disease it is given by injection as emetine hydrochloride or dehydroemetine hydrochloride (Mebadin), and the course of injections, which lasts a few days, is followed by a course of emetine bismuth iodine (E.B.I.). Emetine, given by injection, is toxic and patients under treatment with it must stay in bed. If the E.B.I. upsets the patient and makes him nauseated a dose of sedative given half an hour before the E.B.I. will often prevent vomiting. It is possible to treat amoebic dysentery with success by using antibiotics such as tetracycline, but the cure is not permanent, and such treatment is best used when there are no facilities for injecting emetine and keeping the patient in bed. Metronidazole (Flagyl) has given good results in doses of 400 mg to 800 mg three times a day for 5 to 10 days, and no serious toxic effects have at the time of writing been noted.

PREVENTION: dysentery is spread by poor standards of cleanliness, especially in cooking. The infection may reach food because flies have been able to settle on it after becoming contaminated with faeces, because people handling the food have the infection on their hands, or because infected dust is blown into the kitchen. Carriers may harbour bacilli or amoebae and pass them on without themselves being ill, and it is always necessary to search for a carrier if there is an outbreak of dysentery in an institution. Standards of hygiene must be kept high everywhere that food is handled; hands must be kept clean, flies and dust kept away and the food kept covered – and if possible refrigerated. The incidence of the disease in cities is growing.

Dysmenorrhoea: painful menstrual periods.

Dyspareunia: pain on sexual intercourse due either to physical or psychological causes.

Dyspepsia: this means quite simply discomfort in the process of digestion and may apply (*a*) to simple difficulty in the process (functional dyspepsia); (*b*) to actual physical changes in the stomach or duodenum such as ulceration; (c) to intestinal disease; (d) to 'nervous' complaints; (e) to temporary complaints. It is necessary to distinguish between the individual who has overindulged in food or drink the night before or may have a slight infection while not being prone to digestive disturbances, and the one who has frequently had such troubles. The former case is quite satisfied with a dose of alkali whereas the latter may need a more complex investigation. It is also necessary to be sure of the site of the trouble as a very great deal of indigestion is caused by intestinal disease, such as that brought about by excessive use of purgatives, subacute appendicitis or colitis; these will obviously not be helped by medicines containing alkalies since their cause has nothing to do with hyperacidity. Typical of gastric diseases or diseases of the duodenum is a regular pain after a specified period and in the same place, often $1\frac{1}{2}$–2 hours after eating, in the upper part of the abdomen on the right-hand side. The pain is relieved by taking more food or by alkalies. Nervous dyspepsia is accompanied by neurotic complaints such as flatulence or 'bringing up wind', which are pure neuroses and have no relationship to real disease (by and large it is found that the more dramatic the complaint the less the danger of trouble). The significance of abdominal pain is to be judged by whether it has been present before, how regular it is, how far it can be removed by ordinary remedies, how far it is accompanied by bizarre symptoms such as 'wind' or 'queer feelings' – the more specific the symptoms, the more real the disease, for example if someone says he has a pain just above the umbilicus which comes on at five in the evening one would in general believe him, but the man who has a 'terrible' pain 'all over the abdomen' which lasts 'all the time' is generally exaggerating. People with organic disease are very calm in describing symptoms which occur in a particular place at a particular time; they are specific symptoms, not just 'funny feelings', and they have no connection with conditions which one knows to be neurotic such as flatulence. Duodenal ulcers tend to occur in the thirties or forties, most commonly in men; they occur in ordinarily healthy people and those who have a particular type of character. The sufferer is the man who is 'lean and hungry, lives strenuously, driving mind and body hard', as one physician describes him. On the other hand the sufferer from gastric ulcer tends to be weak, older, with a poor appetite, bronchitic, and with too little rather than too much acid in the stomach. The fact is that some people can digest anything, chewing or no chewing, teeth or no teeth, while others can eat almost nothing without discomfort. *See* Stomach Diseases, Digestive System, Ulcerative Colitis.

Dysphagia: difficulty in swallowing.

Dysphasia: an impediment in speaking due to impairment of central function in the nervous system; a lesser degree of aphasia (q.v.).

Dyspnoea: difficulty in breathing. *See* Breathlessness.

Dystrophy: a condition brought about by defective nutrition.

Dysuria: pàin or difficulty in passing urine.

E

Ear: the ear is the organ of hearing and the organ of balance. It is divided into three parts: outer, middle and inner. The outer ear includes the visible ear, that is the pinna or skin-covered flap of cartilage whose function is to collect sounds, and the canal through which the sounds are conducted to the eardrum. This canal has an outer part of cartilage and an inner part which passes through bone, is lined with skin, and has hairs and glands which secrete wax in amounts that vary with the individual.

The middle ear is not visible as it lies behind the eardrum. It is a small cavity in the temporal bone which is continuous with the mastoid air cells; the cavity of the middle ear is 15 mm × about 5 mm × about 5 mm. The width is variable and irregular, narrowing from 5 or 6 mm at the top to about 4 mm at the bottom; it is only about 2 mm opposite the centre of the eardrum, which is drawn inwards, and set at an angle of about 55° to the external canal. The important contents of the middle ear are the ossicles – tiny bones that transmit the movements of the eardrum to the organ of hearing in the inner ear. There are three bones in the chain, the malleus (hammer), incus (anvil) and stapes (stirrup). They form joints with each other and are connected to the bone surrounding the middle ear by three ligaments, and are arranged so that there is a 20:1 increase in power and a 20:1 decrease in movement between the eardrum and the oval window where the footplate of the stapes connects with the inner ear. There are two muscles in the middle ear, tensor tympani, which as its name implies keeps the eardrum drawn inwards, and stapedius, which pulls the stapedius bone away from the oval window. These muscles, especially the stapedius, damp the oscillation of the ossicles so that they prevent very loud noises from hurting the ear. If the stapedius is damaged a loud noise is very uncomfortable to hear. The Eustachian (auditory) tube runs from the upper part of the throat to the middle ear in order to keep the pressure on both sides of the eardrum the same. The inner ear is made up of the organs of hearing and balance, which are systems of canals inside the hardest part of the temporal bone filled with fluid. There are two components of the system, the bony labyrinth and the membranous labyrinth lying inside; the fluid inside the membranous labyrinth is called endolymph, that between the bony and membranous labyrinths the perilymph. *The organ of hearing* is called the cochlea and is like a snail's shell. It contains a membrane called the basilar membrane which runs round inside the spiral and separates it into two spiral passages, upper and lower. The upper passage is again separated into two by another membrane, the vestibular membrane. Fluid filling the upper spiral passage, the scala vestibuli, is set in motion by movement of the stapes in the oval window, which is the lower termination of the scala vestibuli. The waves pass across the vestibular membrane into the cochlear duct, the middle spiral passage, and so reach the basilar membrane. Upon the basilar membrane is the organ of Corti, which consists of rows of cells carrying fine hairs covered by the membrana tectoria like a soft roof. The hair cells are connected to the fibres of the acoustic nerve through the spiral ganglia. When the sound vibrations carried from the eardrum by the ossicles of the middle ear to the oval window disturb the fluid in the cochlea, and so move the basilar membrane, the hair cells move against the tectorial membrane and impulses are set up in the auditory nerve and carried to the brain. Different parts of the spiral basilar membrane and the organ of Corti react to sounds of different pitches because of variation in resonance of the structures; presumably the pitch of a note is estimated in the brain according to which part of the organ of Corti is reacting most, and loudness will be signalled by the number of impulses set up. The sound waves are dissipated after they have set the basilar membrane in motion by the fluid in the scala tympani, the lowest spiral in the cochlea, which lies beneath the basilar membrane and opens into the middle ear at the round window, covered by a membrane free to vibrate.

The organ of balance is made up of three semicircular canals which lie in different planes of space. They arise from the central part of the labyrinthine system called the vestibule (from which on the other side the cochlea arises), and they each have an ampulla, or dilated sac in which there are hair cells. These sense the motion of the endolymphatic fluid in the semicircular canals and convey impulses to the brain through the vestibular part of the auditory nerve. In the vestibule lie two other structures, the saccule and the utricle, in which more hair cells detect gravitational forces. These hair cells carry on them otoliths, small deposits of calcium carbonate.

The central connections of the organ of balance include nerve fibres running to the nerve cells controlling the muscles that move the eyeball, which assist the eye to remain fixed on a still object although the head and neck may move. Disturbance of the semicircular canals results in giddiness, nausea and vomiting (*see* Motion Sickness). For diseases of the ear see under the appropriate headings.

Earache: *see* Otitis Externa and Media.

E.C.G.: *see* Electrocardiogram.

Eclampsia: fits or coma occurring in late pregnancy or in women who have just been delivered of a child, associated with high blood pressure, oedema and protein in the urine. The cause is unknown; the patient must be treated, if possible in hospital, with sedatives and must be kept quiet. If she is pregnant and does not go into labour, then labour must be induced or Caesarean section carried out. The condition is dangerous to both mother and child, but warning signs that it is developing can be detected by regular antenatal examination, and eclampsia can then be prevented.

Ectoderm: the embryo develops from three primary layers, the ectoderm, the mesoderm and the endoderm. The ectoderm gives rise to the skin, nervous system and organs of special sense.

Ectomorph: a type of bodily development in which ectodermal tissues predominate – there is a large surface area compared to the amount of muscle and bone, so that the figure is spare. *See* Endomorph, Mesomorph.

-ectomy: the suffix -ectomy is used to mean the cutting out of an organ or tissue, for example appendicectomy (appendectomy), or colectomy.

Ectopic Gestation: *see* Fallopian Tubes.

Ectropion: an eversion, or turning out, of the eyelid so that the conjunctiva is left exposed. *See* Entropion.

Eczema: a condition of the skin; the name is derived from a Greek word meaning 'to boil'.

CAUSE: irritating substances in contact with the skin; allergic reaction to irritants which have over the course of time provoked allergy in the patient – almost anything can be responsible from ointments to nail varnish, and direct irritation by the substance is sometimes added as with diesel oil; the eating of substances to which the patient is allergic; inhalation of such substances; the physical agents cold, heat, light; heredity; and in some cases emotional disturbances.

SYMPTOMS: the skin breaks out into very small blisters which burst and leave a red raw surface which dries and cracks and may heal or become thickened. At all stages the skin itches and in the wet stage it may become infected with bacteria. Healing of the condition is, of course, affected by scratching in response to the irritation, which not only spreads infection but lengthens the stage of dryness and scaling and encourages thickening of the skin.

TREATMENT: identification and removal of the irritant – a task which may be difficult and may involve extensive investigation into the patient's clothes, the substances used to wash them, materials encountered at work, the diet, and so on. The most effective ointments and creams for use on the skin contain corticosteroids and anti-infective agents. Of the older remedies coal tar is particularly useful and still has a place in the treatment of eczema after the acute stage, which may be treated by wet lotions such as calamine to which 1% phenol or other weak antiseptic may be added. Sedatives can be given by mouth, and aspirin and paracetamol help to deaden the itching. *See* Dermatitis.

Edema: swelling due to passage of fluid in excess through the walls of the blood or lymph vessels into the tissue spaces.

It is found in cases where the circulation is failing, and in cases where the composition of the blood is abnormal either because there is too much salt and water (nephritis) or because there is a depletion of protein (nephrotic syndrome).

E.E.G.: *See* Electroencephalography.

Effort Syndrome: the name given to a group of symptoms wrongly attributed by the patient to disease of the heart, for example palpitation, breathlessness, pain over the heart, etc. It is mainly associated with military life in which heart disease would, of course, be a serious drawback to further service and naturally the symptoms, which are emotionally caused, are not unrelated to this fact. However, it is quite common in civilian life to find people with similar symptoms, although in this case the patient is more willing to be re-assured that nothing is organically wrong. Treatment, after eliminating genuine heart disease, is to give plenty of exercise, which should be as violent as possible, and to ensure that the patient understands the nature of his condition.

Effusion: an outpouring of fluid into a tissue or a part of the body, for example an effusion into the knee joint, an effusion into the pleural space.

Elastic Stockings: used in cases of varicose veins during pregnancy, in the old, and after the deep veins of the leg have become obstructed by thrombosis. It is important that they fit properly and patients are advised to have them fitted by an expert.

Elbow: the joint formed by the bone of the upper arm, the humerus, and the two bones of the lower arm, the radius and ulna. It is a hinge joint; rotation of the radius on the ulna takes place between those two bones and is not part of the movement at the elbow joint, which is formed mainly by the hook-shaped olecranon process of the ulna and the pulley-shaped trochlear groove on the humerus. The facet upon the head of the radius rests in contact with the round capitulum of the humerus, and the radius is bound more strongly to the ulna than to the humerus. The bony points that can be felt through the skin are the inner and outer, or medial and lateral, condyles of the humerus and, behind the joint, the point of the elbow formed by the olecranon – the upper part of the ulna. The long axis of the upper arm is not in line with the long axis of the forearm when the elbow is extended and the palm of the hand open forwards because the transverse axis of the joint slopes downwards from outer to inner sides, but the bones come to lie in the same line when the palm of the hand is turned round so that it faces backwards with the elbow extended. The angle between the upper arm and the bones of the forearm with the palm forwards and the elbow extended is called the carrying angle, and it differs in the male and the female, being about 173° in men and 167° in women. This is held to account for the fact that women often have difficulty in throwing things accurately. The front of the elbow is protected by muscles and powerful ligaments.

Injuries to the elbow joint: the commonest dislocations are forwards and to the outer side – that is, so that the inner side of the joint is opened out. In the latter case the ligaments on the inner side of the joint are strong enough to tear away the inner bony part of the joint, and in the forward dislocations where the lower end of the humerus comes forwards out of the notch of the olecranon process it often breaks off the part of the notch called the coronoid process, so that both of the common dislocations are liable to be complicated by fractures.

Fractures of the elbow joint are sustained as the result of direct injury – for example the 'chauffeur's fracture', where the driver of a car has been conducting with his elbow propped up on the window-sill of the door so that the point is outside the line of the bodywork; in this position unexpected contact can be made with passing hard objects. The ulnar nerve passes behind the inner side of the elbow on its way from the upper arm to the forearm behind the inner condyle of the humerus, between the inner bony point that can be felt at the elbow and the point of the elbow. A sharp blow in this area impinges directly on the nerve, for there is nothing intervening between nerve and skin, so that the effects are considerable – a severe pain with pins and needles all the way down the forearm. The inner bony point of the elbow is therefore called the funny bone. Miner's elbow, 'beat' elbow, or bursitis of the elbow with pain and swelling over the point develops in those whose work entails resting on the point of the elbow – a condition similar to house-maid's knee and like it treated by rest and physiotherapy. Such a condition is liable to affect clerks and schoolchildren as well as miners. Tennis elbow is a condition which may occur in games players. It involves the outer part of the joint where considerable tenderness develops. The pain radiates down the forearm.

Electrical Injuries: these may be brought about by electrical currents or by lightning and the amount of damage produced varies greatly with a number of factors which are only partly dependent on the voltage of the current. Thus the amperage is more important than the voltage and alternating current more dangerous than direct current. A current received through dry clothing is less dangerous than one received through wet clothing or on the bare skin, and obviously all currents are more dangerous when the body is earthed, or grounded, than when insulation is provided by rubber-soled shoes. The most dangerous room in the house from the point of view of risk from electrical apparatus is the bathroom; for if a shock is received from a faulty switch or electric fire when the body is naked, wet, and earthed through the bath-tub, conditions are perfect for the passage of a current and such shocks are nearly always fatal. The effects of electric shock are both local and general. Spasm of the muscles may lead to fractured bones, and the flesh at the point of entry may be damaged to a degree which ranges from a mild burn to severe destruction of muscles and internal organs; these injuries take a long time to heal.

TREATMENT: sometimes muscular spasm makes it impossible for the victim to let go of the object producing the shock; remember it is essential to switch off the current before you pull him away. If you cannot switch the current off, make sure that your hands are dry and that you pad them with some dry material. If you find a person unconscious near a high-voltage line or a railway line make absolutely sure that he is not still in contact with the high voltage. If you are in doubt get hold of an electrical engineer, for there is no point in providing two victims instead of one, and dry or padded hands will not help here. If you are caught in a thunderstorm keep moving, because the column of warm air rising from you if you keep still can act as a lightning conductor. Keep away from rivers and ponds, trees standing by themselves, and isolated walls or fences. Do not carry steel-shafted golf clubs – come back for them afterwards. If the breathing stops after an electric shock or after a victim is struck by lightning artificial respiration (q.v.) must be started at once and kept up for hours if necessary. If the pulse cannot be felt start cardiac massage (q.v.). Whatever you do, do it quickly and do not wait until the patient has been carried from the scene of the accident or out of the rain. You only have a few minutes in which to act if you are going to save a life.

Electricity in Treatment: from the time of Galvani up to twenty or thirty years ago electricity was much used in medicine, especially in conditions which did not respond to other forms of treatment. But, like the use of water and ultra-violet rays, its range has been greatly reduced in the last two or three decades and really the only fields where electricity has much scope are in the use of diathermy for muscular pains, in shock treatment in psychiatry, and in defibrillation of the heart.

Electrocardiogram: an electrical record taken from the heart. When the heart muscle contracts and relaxes changes in potential are produced which can be picked up from the skin surface by electrodes applied to various parts of the body. The patient lies at rest and electrodes are fixed to his arms, legs and chest. The recorder traces the changes of potential on to a moving band of paper and the physician can change the leads as he wishes, for various combinations are used to elucidate various problems. A diagnosis is made from the shape of the tracing on the paper.

Electroconvulsant Therapy: a form of treatment in psychiatry devised by the Italian Cerletti to replace the use of drugs in convulsant therapy introduced in 1934 by von Meduna of Budapest. The history of the method is strange, for its original rationale was the belief (no longer held) of von Meduna that schizophrenia and epilepsy were antagonistic conditions such that one could not exist in the presence of the other. It was argued that the induction of artificial fits would have a beneficial effect in schizophrenia, and initially, as is so often the case, very good results were obtained. Later it was found that many of these cases relapsed and, although E.C.T. is still used discreetly in some types of schizophrenia, the main field of use for convulsant therapy is in depressive conditions for which it is almost specific, clearing up severe depressive states in 10 to 14 days. The main risk of E.C.T. was that fractures were sometimes produced by muscular spasms, but since the introduction of muscle relaxants and general anaesthesia during the treatment this risk has been removed.

Electroencephalography: electrodes applied to the surface of the scalp pick up changes of potential apparently arising from the activity of the brain. The precise processes underlying the production of these currents are not known, but the patterns are sufficiently distinctive to be used as aids to diagnosis, although first hopes that the E.E.G. would be the equal of or even supplant other methods of investigation have been disappointed. A basic rhythm is to be distinguished arising from the occipital, or rear, part of the brain when the eyes are closed, called the alpha rhythm; it has a period between 8 and 13 cycles a second, and is present in health. Other rhythms are to be distinguished in disease, for example the delta rhythm which is slow and seen in connection with some deep tumours of the brain and certain sorts of epilepsy. (The fact that electrical records can be picked up from the surface of the brain or the scalp is not to be taken as proof that 'the brain works by electricity'.)

Electrolyte: a solution through which electricity will pass because the current is conducted by the ions of salts. During the passage of the current from the anode, or positive terminal, to the cathode, or negative terminal, the electrolyte is decomposed and the products of decomposition are released at the electrodes.

Electromyography: when a muscle contracts changes of electrical potential are set up. These can be recorded by electrodes and the fluctuations inscribed on paper as an electromyogram.

235

Elephantiasis: gross swelling of the legs or genital organs caused by blockage of the lymphatic channels by small worms the size of fine catgut called filariae. There are a number of filarial worms of which Wuchereria bancrofti and Brugia malayi cause elephantiasis. *See* Filariasis.

Elixir: a sweet liquid containing some flavouring or medicinal substance made up with water and alcohol.

Embolism: the blocking of an artery by material carried in the bloodstream from another part of the body. The material may be a fragment of blood clot, perhaps from a diseased valve in the heart or a thrombosed vein in the leg, a piece of tumour, a mass of bacteria, globules of fat or bubbles of air. The immediate result is that the blood supply to a segment of tissue is cut off, so that the tissue dies and then softens; if the part affected is not essential to life, the patient survives with a scar forming to replace the dead tissue. The process of tissue death and softening in consequence of an embolism is called infarction, and the dead tissue is called an infarct. If the material forming the embolus contains bacteria an abscess will arise, and if it contains cancerous tissue a secondary tumour will grow. Fat embolism sometimes occurs after severe fractures, and air embolism can result from wounds of the veins of the neck and head sustained accidentally or at operation.

Embryo: in man, the developing organism from one week after conception to the end of the eighth week. Embryology is the study of the development of the embryo. *See* Fetus.

Emetics: drugs which cause vomiting. They are rarely used except in cases of suspected poisoning. They fall into two classes: (1) those which act by irritating the stomach, such as salt in warm water, or mustard in cold water; (2) those which act centrally on the vomiting centre in the brain such as apomorphine. By far the best and safest emetic is common salt in warm water; large amounts of water should be taken and the effect may if necessary be reinforced by tickling the back of the throat with the finger. Another popular emetic is syrup of ipecac.

Emetine: one of the active principles of ipecacuanha used in the treatment of amoebic dysentery. *See* Dysentery.

Emphysema: the abnormal presence of air in tissues of the body. Used in the main of a condition of the lungs in which the alveolar air spaces are grossly enlarged.

CAUSE: emphysema is frequently found in association with asthma and chronic bronchitis, so it is reasonable to assume that the main factors in the production of the disease are obstruction of the air passages and infection, which weakens the elastic tissues of the lungs.

SYMPTOMS: the main symptom is breathlessness which gets worse with the lapse of time – emphysema is essentially a chronic disease. Eventually the patient is breathless at rest, for the alveoli (q.v.) are so damaged that the exchange of gases between the blood and the air is much impaired. In addition to this, the chest itself becomes enlarged and the movement of the ribs diminished, so that the volume of air passed in and out of the lungs at each breath is very much less than normal.

TREATMENT: nothing can be done to improve the anatomical changes in the lung. The patient should stop smoking, he should if possible live in a place where air pollution is least, and the chronic bronchitis which is associated with emphysema must be kept as far as practicable under control. Breathing exercises can often teach a patient to make the best use of what he has, and inhalation of oxygen may make it possible for patients to move about more freely. Overweight patients will benefit from a reduction in the amount of body tissue. Emphysema is sometimes complicated by heart failure, and this must be treated as necessary.

Empyema: an internal abscess. Used to describe a collection of pus within one of the pleural cavities caused by the extension of an infection from elsewhere, for example following pneumonia, in chronic pulmonary tuberculosis, from septic wounds of the chest, tumours in the chest or abscesses in the lung. The treatment is surgical; if the pus is not too thick it can be drawn off by a needle and syringe, but more effective drainage may be necessary in which case a small part of the overlying rib is removed under general

237

or local anaesthetic. Antibiotics are used as indicated by the sensitivity of the infecting organisms.

Encephalitis: inflammation of the brain.

CAUSE: may be inflammation following bacterial infection, or the result of virus infection. If there is bacterial infection it usually becomes localized and forms a brain abscess, whereas viruses tend to produce diffuse inflammation. Many viruses can give rise to the condition, among them the viruses of mumps, herpes, measles, chickenpox, and cowpox. The infection is also produced by the arboviruses which are carried by mosquitoes or ticks, by the Coxsackie virus and ECHO viruses.

SYMPTOMS: fever, headaches, perhaps convulsions mark the onset of the disease, and the patient may complain of nausea and vomiting. Various paralyses of the eyes, face and throat as well as of the rest of the body may develop.

TREATMENT: there is no specific treatment for virus encephalitis, and the condition is treated symptomatically; antibiotics are used if the condition is known to arise because of bacterial infection. Brain abscess is treated surgically.

Encephalitis Lethargica: an encephalitis which spread in epidemics between the years 1915 and 1925; since that time it has become rare, although it is thought to occur sporadically. It is known as sleepy sickness (as opposed to sleeping sickness).

CAUSE: not known for sure, but thought to be a virus.

SYMPTOMS: fever, headache, irritability, rarely excitement; proceeding to lethargy, with various palsies as in other forms of encephalitis, and ending in some cases in coma. In cases which recover there are residual deficiencies which improve only slowly, and there may be permanent mental and neurological changes. The adult may become very slow in his mind, and the child victim may become unmanageable. In the years following an infection, some patients develop the condition of Parkinsonism (*see* Parkinson's Disease) which makes their limbs stiff in movement and shaky at rest.

TREATMENT: no specific treatment is known, and the condition has to be treated symptomatically. The mental changes may mean that the patient has to be admitted to an institution; the Parkinsonism is treated by drugs or operation.

Encephalography: examination of the contents of the skull by X-rays. It is not possible under normal circumstances to show the brain on a plain X-ray, but it is possible to introduce air (or gas, for example oxygen) into the space occupied by the cerebro-spinal fluid and so to show the outline of the cavities of the brain (the ventricles). An X-ray examination carried out usually under general anaesthetic after the injection of air into the subarachnoid space by lumbar puncture is called an air encephalogram or A.E.G. It shows up tumours in the brain because they deform the outline of the ventricles, and it shows the enlargement of the ventricles that accompanies cerebral arteriosclerosis and degeneration. Various other conditions may be demonstrated by air encephalography.

Encephalopathy: a condition resembling encephalitis, which may be caused by certain poisons including the heavy metals and some insecticides.

Endemic: adjective describing disease which is always present among the people.

Endocarditis: inflammation of the inside of the heart.
CAUSE: although normal hearts are almost immune to infection – they only develop endocarditis at the end of severe chronic diseases or in patients run down by drug addiction – infection is not uncommon in hearts which are abnormal. The cardiac defects may be the result of congenital deformity or such diseases as rheumatic fever, and the infecting organism is usually Streptococcus viridans, which produces a chronic type of inflammation.
SYMPTOMS: the disease has an insidious onset with a low fever and a general feeling of illness; as the patient is usually known to have an abnormal heart, the disease may be suspected if he has an intermittent obscure malaise and gradually becomes paler (the disease is accompanied by anaemia). In some cases the diagnosis is very difficult, because it may not be known that the patient has an abnormal heart and there may be no signs of it on examination.

239

The infected areas in the heart become covered with blood clot which crumbles so that little pieces break off and are carried round the circulation to cause small embolisms (q.v.). These show themselves by producing little areas of discoloration in the skin, or small subcutaneous nodules which may be tender. Red blood cells may be found in the urine after emboli have reached the kidneys.

TREATMENT: before antibiotics came into use this disease was fatal, but now it is possible to make a culture from the blood to identify the organism and determine its sensitivity so that antibiotics may be prescribed. Every patient known to have an abnormal heart as well as every patient with endocarditis must be examined periodically for foci of chronic infection; the most common finding is dental sepsis; and in these cases injections of penicillin have to be given before extractions can safely be carried out because they always result in a transient escape of bacteria into the bloodstream.

Endocrine Glands: glands which do not have a duct but secrete directly into the bloodstream are called endocrine or ductless glands, as opposed to those which have a duct and can secrete externally, the exocrine glands. The internal secretions of the ductless glands are called hormones, and they play a fundamental part in the control of growth, sexual development and function, metabolism, and intellectual and emotional development; a proper balance of hormones is essential for life. The main endocrine glands are: pituitary (anterior and posterior parts), thyroid, parathyroid, adrenal (cortex and medulla), kidneys, testes, ovaries, placenta, pancreas, stomach, duodenum, small intestine. (It will be seen that several organs have other important functions besides secreting hormones.) The thymus gland in the neck has until recently been a mystery, but it now appears that it produces both lymphocytes and a hormone which controls their formation in the rest of the body. The pineal gland in the brain has been called the 'third eye'; Descartes thought it was the seat of the soul, but modern work shows that it influences sexual development by secreting a hormone called melatonin – at any rate in rats.

For fuller discussion of the various glands see under their separate headings.

Endoderm: (Entoderm). The inner cell layer in the embryo from which grows the lining of the digestive and urinary tracts and the respiratory system. *See* Ectoderm, Mesoderm.

Endometriosis: a condition in which the kind of tissue which normally lines the uterus is found in abnormal places. CAUSE: various theories are current. One is that the tissue forms in response to abnormal hormonal stimulation of the sort of cells which originally gave rise to the uterus and Fallopian tubes (q.v.); another, that clumps of cells from the lining of the uterus may travel up the Fallopian tubes and implant themselves in abnormal places such as the surface of the ovaries and behave as a tissue culture. SYMPTOMS: the places where endometriosis may occur are:
1. On the surface of the ovaries.
2. At the umbilicus.
3. On the round ligament (q.v.).
4. In operation scars in the lower abdomen.
5. On the outer peritoneal surface of the bladder.
6. On the outer peritoneal surface of the pelvic colon.
7. In the tissue between the vagina and the rectum.
8. On the peritoneum lining the pelvis.
The disease does not usually occur before the age of 30, and it causes pain, dyspareunia (q.v.), dysmenorrhoea and, if it involves the bowel, obstruction of the intestine. TREATMENT: surgical removal. If this is impossible because of the extent or the site of the endometriosis, hormone treatment by the administration of progesterone may be employed.

Endometritis: inflammation of the lining of the uterus. It may follow abortion, criminal or otherwise, parturition, gonorrhoea, gynaecological operation, or may occur in old age when the vaginal acidity falls. The treatment is by antibiotics according to the infecting organism.

Endomorph: a type of bodily development in which endodermal tissues predominate – the body is round and soft. *See* Ectomorph, Mesomorph.

Endoscopy: examination through an optical instrument

ENDOTOXIN

of the interior of the body, usually of the bladder through a
cystoscope, the lower part of the gut through a proctoscope
or sigmoidoscope, the stomach through a gastroscope or the
trachea and bronchi through a bronchoscope. It is possible
to look into the peritoneal cavity through a peritoneoscope
introduced through the abdominal wall.

Endotoxin: a toxin present inside bacteria as opposed to
an exotoxin, found outside bacteria.

Endotracheal Tube: a tube passed into the trachea or
windpipe through the vocal cords during the administration
of a general anaesthetic in order to establish a clear airway
in an unconscious patient. It can be introduced through the
nose with the help of a laryngoscope, which gives the
anaesthetist a view of the vocal cords, or 'blindly' – that is
without looking at the cords. This latter technique can be
satisfactory, but it needs practice and is not always successful,
and the experienced anaesthetist keeps a laryngoscope
handy. The tube can if necessary be passed through the
mouth. An endotracheal tube commonly has a cuff round
its end which can be blown up. When this has been done the
trachea is sealed off and no foreign matter such as blood or
vomit can get down into the lungs while the cough reflex is
suppressed by the anaesthetic. The passage of an endotracheal tube is made easier by giving the patient a muscle-
relaxing drug.

Enema: the injection of special fluids into the lower bowel
via the anus for various purposes, e.g. as a purgative, as a
sedative, to supply nourishment when feeding by ordinary
means is not possible or advisable, to treat local diseases of
the bowel, or to deal with worms. It is true to say that apart
from those who are addicted to colonic lavage for the treatment of intestinal neuroses enemata are no longer as popular
as once they were because what they are capable of doing can
often be done with greater ease and efficiency in other ways.
There are, however, still cases in which they remain the
treatment of choice, such as overloading of the lower bowel
in the elderly.

Engagement: a term used in obstetrics to mean that the

head of the foetus, or if it is not a head presentation the presenting part, has entered the brim of the pelvis.

E.N.T.: abbreviation for ear, nose and throat.

Entamoeba histolytica: the amoeba found in the large intestine in cases of amoebic dysentery. During the course of the disease it may enter the liver and form an abscess there. It is a small amoeba, and when examined under the microscope usually contains red blood cells which it has eaten. It reproduces by splitting into two, and is able to form cysts if circumstances become unfavourable. The cysts remain alive for some weeks outside the body of the host providing that the temperature is about 5 °C. and that there is moisture in the environment. They are killed at temperatures of 50 °C. and by being dried. If another man eats the cyst as a contaminant of his food it passes through the stomach unchanged; it is not until it reaches the intestine that the cyst wall gives way and the enclosed amoeba escapes. The cysts contain four nuclei each, and the four nuclei split into eight, so that each cyst introduces eight amoebae into the host, which is usually man but may be monkey or ape. For amoebic dysentery, *see* Dysentery.

Enteric Fever: typhoid and paratyphoid fever.

Enteritis: inflammation of the intestine – usually the small intestine – caused generally but not always by bacteria.

Enterobiasis: infection with threadworms (pinworms), usually in children.
SYMPTOMS: itching round the anus at night. The female worms come out of the rectum, lay their eggs on the skin round the anus, and so set up the irritation.
TREATMENT: the drug viprynium (Povan in the United States), given in two doses, one 2 weeks after the other. Piperazine is also effective, and can be given in two large doses at an interval of a week. All the members of a family must be treated if one individual is found to harbour the worms.

Enterostomy: an artificial opening made into the

intestine. It may be made to open on to the surface of the abdominal wall, or may be used to connect the intestine with another part of the alimentary canal, as when a gastro-enterostomy is made to short-circuit the duodenum in some cases of scarring due to ulceration where a gastrectomy (q.v.) is not practicable. An enterostomy discharging on to the surface is used as a temporary measure in cases of intestinal obstruction or in some cases where it is desired to isolate the lower bowel. *See* Colostomy.

Enterotoxin: an exotoxin given off by some strains of Staphylococcus aureus which causes food poisoning, for it is possible for the staphylococci to contaminate food and grow in it. The colonies of staphylococci produce enterotoxin, and when the food is eaten acute poisoning ensues. The victim within a few hours develops vomiting, which gets worse, diarrhoea and faintness. The condition can be quite severe, but it is not an infection and the symptoms go within a day or so. The staphylococci themselves are not dangerous. Treatment is directed to relief of the symptoms – the patient is put to bed and kept as comfortable as possible.

Entropion: a condition in which the eyelid is turned in towards the eyeball as a result of scarring or disease. *See* Ectropion.

Enuresis: bed-wetting. If a child suffers from bed-wetting, it must be examined to make sure that the condition is not being caused by a disease such as diabetes, kidney disease or a defect in the nervous control of the bladder. If no abnormality is found, there may be a psychological basis for the trouble, but the main cause is usually found to be over-anxiousness on the part of the parents. It must not be forgotten that normal children cannot control their bladders consistently until they are over 18 months old, and that after they are 2 there can still be accidents which mean nothing. If the parents become upset every time the child wets his bed, then before long the situation can become difficult. In general it is true to say that the condition will respond to kindness and confidence and obvious measures such as cutting down drinks before bedtime.

Enzymes: biological catalysts responsible for most of the processes of metabolism both inside and outside cells. The enzymes are proteins, and are specific for one reaction or for a well-defined group of similar reactions. The speed of the reactions depends on the amount of enzyme present and the amount of the substance involved in the reaction, on temperature, the acid/base balance and a number of co-enzymes, inhibitors and activators. Many of the co-enzymes are related to vitamins, which explains why vitamin deficiencies alter metabolism so profoundly; but our knowledge of enzymes, although growing all the time, is far from complete. It is probable that as knowledge increases we shall be able to elucidate diseases at present obscure and improve treatment, for the organisms that produce disease in man depend on their enzymatic processes for life, and will prove vulnerable to new antibiotics when their metabolic processes are better understood.
(Catalyst: a substance in chemistry which changes the speed of a reaction without itself being part of the final product.)

Eosinophil: one of the white cells found in the blood which readily takes up the dye eosin when a blood film is stained with Leishman's stain, a mixture of methylene blue and eosin. Eosinophil cells are increased in allergic states and in infestation with some worms, and the state of having an increased number of eosinophil cells is called eosinophilia.

Epanutin: phenytoin sodium (mesantoin) (q.v.).

Ephedrine: an alkaloid isolated from the plant Ephedra equisetina, or Ma Huang, used in Chinese medicine for many hundreds of years, but known in the West only since the third decade of this century. It is a sympathomimetic drug, which means that it imitates the action of the sympathetic part of the autonomic nervous system. It raises the blood pressure, increases the heart rate, dilates the air passages and the pupil of the eye, and constricts the mucous membranes of the nose and throat. It is used in cases of asthma, but tends to keep patients awake and in elderly males to provoke retention of urine, and it is not safe to use it with isoprenaline (isuprel) (q.v.).

Epidemic: the occurrence of a number of cases of similar illnesses in excess of normal expectancy. The number of cases indicating the presence of an epidemic will vary according to the nature of the causative agent, the population exposed, and the time and place of occurrence. Thus epidemicity is relative to usual experience in a particular place, a specific population, and at the same season of the year. For example, the occurrence of even a few cases of locally transmitted malaria in London or in Washington D.C. could be considered epidemic, whereas hundreds of cases weekly is common in many areas of the world.

Epidermis: *see* Skin.

Epididymis: a structure lying on the rear aspect of the testis, consisting of a head, body and tail. It is formed from a thin duct about 6 m long coiled upon itself and connected to the back of the testis by 20 little ducts through which spermatozoa travel, for the epididymis stores the spermatozoa made in the testis. From the tail of the epididymis comes the ductus deferens through which the spermatozoa eventually reach the urethra and penis. It may be the seat of bacterial infection (epididymitis or epididymo-orchitis, when the infection involves the testis as well), or of tuberculosis. Cysts often form in the epididymis, especially in middle age.

Epigastrium: the upper part of the abdomen that lies within the angle of the ribs.

Epiglottis: the leaf-shaped piece of cartilage covered with mucous membrane that lies at the back of the tongue over the opening of the larynx, the entrance to the air passages. In the larynx is the glottis, the vocal apparatus – the cords and the opening between them. The epiglottis diverts food from the back of the tongue towards the oesophagus, or food passage, and helps to cover the entrance to the larynx during the act of swallowing. If a particle of food is inhaled, or there is anything wrong with the muscular co-ordination of the pharynx, the food 'goes down the wrong way', entering the glottis and irritating the vocal cords so that a paroxysm of coughing is set up usually with a spasm of the cords and consequent difficulty in breathing.

Epilepsy: the 'falling sickness', in which there is an abnormality of brain function which shows itself as periodic. paroxysmal activity resulting in momentary loss of attention or consciousness in the lesser form of the disease, 'petit mal', or prolonged loss of consciousness associated with convulsions in major epilepsy or grand mal.

CAUSE: no cause is known for idiopathic epilepsy; where a cause such as a tumour in the brain or injury is present the condition is called symptomatic epilepsy. All cases of epilepsy, in particular those in which the disease has shown itself in later life, must be fully investigated before they are labelled idiopathic (q.v.). Investigation includes full neurological examination, with special X-rays of the skull and an electroencephalogram.

SYMPTOMS: a typical fit is preceded in 50% of cases by an 'aura' or sensation which is peculiar to the individual (for example pain in a particular part of the body, strange tinglings, tremor, a mysterious smell or vision unrelated to anything in the surrounding environment, a feeling of panic). The patient then falls down unconscious, all the muscles of the body go into spasm and the breathing stops so that he is at first pale and then turns blue in the face. After about half a minute this 'tonic' phase is followed by a so-called clonic phase in which the limbs rhythmically contract and relax, the bladder or bowels may be emptied, and the tongue may be bitten. The contractions gradually cease and the patient lies still, breathing heavily, and remaining unconscious for a varying period of time. Sometimes he gets up almost at once and resumes what he was doing before, but in other cases a state of confusion may last for several hours. Obviously the danger from fits lies in the possibility that the patient may injure himself (for example by falling in the street, burning himself in the fireplace) and clearly epileptics should not drive a car or accept employment in any job where they would be in any danger should an attack come on suddenly. Death rarely occurs in a fit except in the comparatively rare status epilepticus, where one fit follows another with no return to consciousness in between. What has been described so far is what is known as grand mal or the great sickness, but there are two other types of epilepsy: petit mal (the little sickness) and Jacksonian epilepsy. In petit mal there is alteration of consciousness but no spasms and the individual may not even be noticed as he perhaps breaks off in the middle of a conversation and suddenly seems to be 'not there', returning to full consciousness after a brief period with or without some mental confusion. Sometimes he may stagger while walking, turn to one side or the other, grimace, and pay no attention to what is said to him. In Jacksonian epilepsy there is usually no loss of consciousness, but spasms occur in particular groups of muscles, for example beginning in the fingers and slowly passing up the arm, which writhes and becomes contorted as if it had a separate existence.

Epileptic fits may occur at any time of the day or night and be of any degree of frequency, but the pattern tends to be characteristic of the individual; they may occur only at night, in which case their existence may be unknown for many years, or daily, weekly or only once or twice in a lifetime. Sometimes they begin in early childhood (although they are not to be confused with the fits which may accompany high fever in almost any young child) and sometimes quite late in life. No physical handicap seems to accompany epilepsy and, apart from the fits, the individual remains in perfect health; in some cases there may appear to be some deterioration over the years, the patient becoming dull, irritable and impulsive, forgetful and self-centred. It is probable that this deterioration is basically due to the social situation the epileptic has to face. Thus it is often difficult for the epileptic to get a job – even one that is not a danger to himself – since many employers do not like the distress occasioned to other employees by an individual who may have fits during working hours. People tend to be afraid of an epileptic and he not unnaturally feels that he is shunned by society while being in all other respects a normal person. This, in part, may be a cause of the so-called epileptic personality, just as many of the symptoms of senility are caused by the social isolation of the old. One form of epilepsy which is of medico-legal importance is the attack which takes the form of extreme violence while the patient is in an altered state of consciousness; this is known as an epileptic equivalent or automatism and may take the place of a fit or follow one, so that the individual may carry out murderous attacks which are quite pointless without knowing what he is doing. Fortunately, however, these are not very common. Numerous great men have been epileptics and in many respects the novelist Dostoevsky, who was a sufferer, is typical of the epileptic character with its violence, its love of mysticism, its persecutory beliefs and impulsiveness.

TREATMENT: during a fit the patient should be laid down in an open space so that he cannot hurt himself in his convulsions. If it is not possible to remove all the obstacles he must be carefully restrained from knocking into them. A gag can be put into his mouth to prevent him biting his tongue – a rolled-up handkerchief will do – and his collar and tie can be undone. The fit looks very dramatic and if it is seen for the first time it is difficult to believe that the patient will recover unless something equally dramatic is done to him in the way of treatment, but in fact the best treatment is to restrain officious bystanders and to give the patient room to move about. There is no need to have the epileptic removed to hospital if he is adult, although it is important to take a child having a fit at once to the doctor or the hospital if there have been none before.

If the epilepsy is symptomatic, the basic treatment will be the treatment of the underlying condition if it is possible. The general treatment of epilepsy is by drugs. Phenobarbitone is the drug most commonly used because it is of low toxicity, and can be used in relatively large doses. Whatever drug is being used has to be given in a dose which will stop as many of the manifestations of epilepsy as possible without producing too much sleepiness and clumsiness, and a continual search goes on to find drugs which will control the paroxysms of cerebral overaction without clouding normal consciousness. Alternative drugs to phenobarbitone are phenytoin sodium (Epanutin or Mesantoin), primidone (Mysoline), sulthiame (Ospolot), and in the U.S.A. diphenylhydnatoin (Dilantin), and diazepam (Valisem): their effectiveness varies from patient to patient, all are to some degree toxic, and the only way of finding out which drug suits a given patient best is to try them for an adequate length of time – about three months in most cases. The drugs can be used in combination. Whichever drug is chosen must be taken consistently for a period of at least three years after the last fit, and it may be necessary for the patient to take

249

drugs for the whole of his life if fits continue, or if the electro-encephalogram remains grossly abnormal. Drugs suitable for the treatment of petit mal are ethosuximide (Zarontin) and troxidone (Tridione), and in most cases it is wise to give phenobarbitone as well.

Surgical treatment is sometimes considered in cases where there is evidence of a well-localized circumscribed area of abnormality, particularly in the temporal lobe; these cases are associated with disorders of behaviour, hallucinations and illusions, and the patients are sometimes confined to institutions. The treatment of symptomatic epilepsy often involves the neurosurgeon. People who are subject to fits must under no circumstances drive motor cars or other vehicles, or fly aircraft, or work at a height, or be in charge of heavy machinery. They must not swim without close supervision.

Marriage. Epilepsy can be hereditary, and a marriage of epileptics to each other should not be lightly undertaken nor should it result in issue if there is a history of epilepsy in their families. The marriage of one epileptic with no family history to a normal person is, however, no more likely to produce epileptic children than the marriage of two normal people. Symptomatic epilepsy cannot be passed on to the children.

Epinephrine: hormone produced by the medulla of the suprarenal glands. *See* Adrenaline.

Epiphysis: the end of a long bone, separated by a plate of growing cartilage from the shaft of the bone during the period of growth. It fuses with the shaft when the individual reaches the end of adolescence. *See* Bones.

Episiotomy: an incision made in the perineum during childbirth to prevent the mother being torn. An incision is under control, whereas a tear is not, and if it is necessary for the vaginal opening to be enlarged to allow the baby free passage an episiotomy can be made under general or local anaesthetic. The incision is made starting in the mid-line and travelling backwards to one or other side of the anus so that the rectum, anus and the muscles that control them are left intact. A tear sustained during childbirth often damages these structures and may leave the mother incontinent. The episiotomy is repaired as soon as the baby has been born.

Epispadias: a congenital deformity in which the urethra opens on the upper surface of the penis which is often split lengthways. In the worst form of the deformity there is a gutter running along the top of the penis where the urethra lies open, and there is a malformation of the bladder called ectopia vesicae (*see* Bladder Disease) in which the front wall of the bladder and the abdomen have failed to close. The pubic bones, which should join at the root of the penis in front of the bladder, fail to unite and are left separated. The treatment is surgical; when the defect is confined to the penis a plastic operation is carried out, but if the deformity includes the bladder, and there is no hope of providing proper storage and control of the passage of urine – in ectopia vesicae the urine escapes in dribbles all the time – the ureters are transplanted to the colon and the bladder removed.

Epistaxis: nose bleeding.
CAUSE: anything which causes inflammation of the nose, such as a common cold; picking the nose; small ulcers on the front part of the nasal septum; foreign bodies in the nose; injury, and in adults, tumours of the nose, and high blood pressure. Severe nose bleeding may occur with no obvious cause.
TREATMENT: cold compresses to the nose, and pinching the nostrils hard together for 10 minutes. A very cold compress or a piece of ice put on the bridge of the nose, and another on the nape of the neck, encourage constriction of the arteries. Obviously there must be no obstruction to the vessels of the neck which could lead to congestion – all clothing round the neck must be loose. If simple treatment has no effect (and often the most effective treatment is to make the patient lie down and stop blowing his nose) then the doctor may pack the nose with gauze. If bleeding still does not stop, the patient may have to go to hospital, particularly if he is elderly and has a high blood pressure, for it may need all the resources of the rhinologist to deal with what can be a very nasty and frightening emergency.

Epithelium: the tissue that lines the surfaces of the body is called epithelium. The cells making up the epithelium lie on a basement membrane, and stick to each other firmly. Epithelium is classified as simple where the layer of cells is one cell thick and stratified where it is more than one cell thick. The shape of the epithelial cells may be squamous – like a scale – cubical or columnar, and an epithelial layer may be made of cells of one type or of mixed types. If it is mixed it is called transitional epithelium. Transitional epithelium is found on surfaces which are in contact with urine, such as the linings of the ureters and bladders; squamous epithelium which is able to resist friction and which may be moist or dry, is found forming the skin and the linings of the mouth, the oesophagus, and the vagina; and columnar or cubical epithelium which is able to secrete and absorb various substances lines the intestines, makes up the linings of ducts in glands, and performs many other functions. Some columnar cells have hairs on them called cilia which beat rhythmically and move the fluid surrounding them, so that the ciliated columnar epithelium of the respiratory tract which lines the air passages is able to move sputum up from the lungs to the throat, and the ciliated columnar epithelium which lines the Fallopian tubes (q.v.) is able to move the ovum along from the ovary to the uterus. Epithelial cells which line the blood spaces of the liver and spleen, the blood and lymph vessels, and the bone marrow are able to eat up other cells and micro-organisms by the process of phagocytosis (*see* Phagocyte) and are called endothelial cells. With their basement membrane, they make up part of the reticulo-endothelial system (q.v.). The epithelial cells which line the peritoneal and the pleural cavities, in which lie the abdominal organs and the lungs, are of the simple squamous type and allow the lungs to slide in relation to the chest wall and the abdominal organs to move in relation to each other. This epithelium is also called mesothelium. Epithelial cells are able to reproduce themselves easily, for they are exposed to damage and wear; under some circumstances they fail to stick to each other, and invade surrounding tissues, and when they do this a malignant tumour or carcinoma is formed (*see* Cancer).

Equanil: *See* Meprobamate.

Ergosterol: this sterol is found in yeast and fungi (it was originally isolated from ergot, hence its name). If ergosterol is irradiated the substance calciferol is formed, which is Vitamin D_2. *See* Calciferol.

Ergot: the fungus, Claviceps purpurea. It attacks Secale cereale, which is edible rye, and in bygone times when the crop was badly infected bread made with it produced ergot poisoning in people who depended on rye bread for their staple diet. Ergot poisoning was called St Anthony's Fire; the limbs were afflicted with intolerable burning pain, became black and gangrenous and eventually fell off. Another form of ergot poisoning was called 'convulsive', as opposed to gangrenous. In the convulsive form the skin itched, there were feelings like insects crawling on the skin (formication), and pins and needles. Convulsions racked the body, and the victims might go blind or mad. During the nineteenth century the incidence of ergotism caused by bread made from infected rye declined because the crop was kept cleaner and the market for rye bread decreased, and ergot came into its own as a drug. It was first used to produce strong contractions of the uterus – an action that had been known for years to midwives – and it helped particularly in the delivery of the placenta in cases of bleeding after the birth of the child. Scientists started to investigate ergot, and it was found to be a source of many powerful alkaloids, all based on lysergic acid, which is not itself active but is when coupled with a base. The alkaloids derived from ergot that are used in medicine are ergometrine, ergotoxine, and ergotamine. Ergotamine is given in obstetrics either by injection or by mouth after the child is born to bring about contractions of the uterus in order to expel the placenta, especially when there is post-partum bleeding. Ergotamine is effective in the treatment of migraine, but it can produce the gangrenous type of ergotism if it is used to excess. The lysergic acid derivative methysergide is also effective in the treatment of migraine. This drug does not produce gangrene, but it can give rise to the formation of fibrous tissue behind the peritoneum which involves the ureters, and fibrosis in other areas such as the lung which may be mistaken for a malignant growth. In 1943, during investigation of the action on the uterus of derivatives of lysergic acid, a scientist

253

accidentally took a minute amount of lysergic acid diethyl-amide by mouth and became hallucinated – an experience which led to the discovery that this derivative of ergot is the most powerful drug known, for it acts in a dose of 1 μg per kilogram of body weight.

Ergotamine: *see* above.

Erosion: a condition affecting the neck (cervix) of the womb.

CAUSE: it is not as the name would suggest a wearing away of tissue, but rather the replacement by columnar epithelium of the normal stratified squamous epithelium which covers the vagina and the outside part of the neck of the womb as it projects into the upper part of the vagina (*see* Epithelium). When the cervix is seen through a vaginal speculum it looks as if the normal pink tissue has become reddened by chronic irritation, but although the change of colour suggests in-flammation or ulceration an erosion is associated with excessive alkaline discharge and overaction of the oestro-genic hormones. Cervical erosions are often found to be present after pregnancy.

SYMPTOMS: erosions are found on examination after preg-nancy, when they produce no symptoms, or on examination of patients complaining of vaginal discharge.

TREATMENT: if the erosion is found on post-partum examin-ation, no treatment is necessary unless the erosion persists after three months and causes a discharge. In such a case the neck of the womb is cauterized with an electric cautery, a minor operation that can be carried out without anaes-thetic if necessary. The same operation is carried out for erosions not associated with pregnancy.

Erysipelas: a streptococcal infection of the skin.

CAUSE: infection with Streptococcus pyogenes which may gain entrance through minor cuts or abrasions.

SYMPTOMS: a spreading reddening of the skin, raised up above the normal surface level, with pain, tenderness, fever and shivering. The edge of the inflamed area spreads rapidly, and as the infection covers a greater surface so the symptoms become worse until the patient may be delirious and very gravely ill. The infection may affect any part of the body, but is not uncommon on the face, where it spreads from the nostrils.

TREATMENT: antibiotics have completely altered the outlook in what used to be a dangerous disease; penicillin is given by injection for a period of 10 days.

Erysipeloid: a reddening of the skin a little like erysipelas but, unlike that condition, not accompanied by fever and constitutional upset.

CAUSE: an organism called Bacillus erysipelatus suis, which lives on some animals and fish.

SYMPTOMS: erysipeloid often attacks people who deal with meat and fish and are liable to be pricked perhaps by bones while they are in contact with the infected material. The skin on the hands is usually affected, and the colour of the infected skin is a darker red than true erysipelas; there is slight tenderness, and very little fever, if any.

TREATMENT: if left the condition is self-limiting and lasts about six weeks, but it responds to treatment with penicillin. It is not a dangerous disease.

Erythema: reddening of the skin. It is caused by dilatation of the blood vessels of the affected part by a number of different conditions, among them slight burns, excessive cold, abrasions, and various fevers and allergic reactions.

Erythrocyte: red blood cell. There are in health about five million red cells in each cubic millimetre of blood. They contain the chemical substance haemoglobin, which transports oxygen from the lungs to the tissues and takes back to the lungs the carbon dioxide released by the processes of cell metabolism. The normal content of haemoglobin in the blood is 14.5 g/100 ml, and each red cell is one-third haemoglobin. The red blood cell has a special shape which makes it easy for gases to diffuse to every part of the cell quickly, being biconcave – the sides of the round cell curve inwards. Red cells are made in the bone marrow, and the final cell has no nucleus, although its parent cells have large nuclei. When red cells are being made very quickly, as they may be after a haemorrhage, some appear in the circulation before the nucleus has entirely disappeared and when they are stained in a blood film the remains of the nucleus show up as a fine network. Such cells are called reticulocytes. The red blood cell is the smallest cell in the human body; its diameter is 7 μm. Red cells live for about a hundred days.

Erythromycin: an antibiotic used to treat infections with pneumococci, staphylococci or streptococci in people who are sensitive to penicillin, because sensitivity reactions are very rare with erythromycin and it is of low toxicity. Unfortunately, staphylococci often become resistant to erythromycin, and this restricts its use in hospital where organisms are much more likely to acquire a resistance to drugs than they are in the home.

Eserine: (Physostigmine). An alkaloid extracted from the Calabar bean. It acts by inhibiting the enzymes which break down acetylcholine, the substance by which impulses in the nervous system are passed from cell to cell, and which brings the parasympathetic nervous system into operation (*see* Acetylcholine). An overdose of eserine leads to over-action of acetylcholine, and the patient shows small pupils, sweating, weakness, slow pulse, difficulty in breathing, and he may go into convulsions and die. Eserine was first known as a poison in West Africa, but it is used now for its action in constricting the pupil of the eye. It is especially useful in the treatment of glaucoma (q.v.).

Esophagus: the gullet, a tube connecting the pharynx or throat with the stomach. It runs through the chest and the diaphragm; diseases affecting it are cancer, hiatus hernia (q.v.), stricture following injury, as in a case where a sword swallower made a slight mistake, or ingestion of corrosive poisons, spasm of the lower end, and venous varicosities in cases where the portal circulation is at a higher pressure than it should be, for example in cirrhosis of the liver. *See* Throat.

E.S.R.: (Erythrocyte Sedimentation Rate). If whole blood is mixed with a substance that prevents it from clotting, the red cells sink to the bottom of the fluid over a period of time which varies according to several factors, the most important of which are the number of red cells present and the concentration of proteins in the plasma. In a number of diseases plasma proteins are high, and this increases the rate at which the cells settle, so that the E.S.R. is raised in infections and in cancer. The E.S.R. is measured by drawing the blood mixed with citrate up into tubes 200 mm long, which are stood upright in a special stand. As the red cells sink they leave a clear column of plasma above them which is measured at the end of one and then two hours. The result is expressed as this distance in millimetres, for example, E.S.R. 5 mm in one hour. The normal rate is below 10 in one hour; it may be increased to 100 in some diseases. A normal E.S.R. does not exclude the presence of disease, but when the E.S.R. is increased although no specific physical signs can be found it means that there is disease hidden somewhere in the body. The E.S.R. is valuable in following the progress of treatment in a chronic disease.

Essential Hypertension: high blood pressure which is not secondary to some other disease. *See* Hypertension.

Estradiol: one of the hormones secreted by the ovaries; it is responsible for the development of the female sexual characteristics.

Estrogen: hormone secreted by the ovaries and capable in animals of producing the state of oestrus or heat. As the human female does not show a cyclical phase of sexual activity, it is applied to any hormone which will produce specific and characteristic changes in the human reproductive tract. The functions of the oestrogens are to regulate the development of the secondary sexual characteristics, to stimulate the tissues of the genital tract to hypertrophy, to play a part in the maintenance of salt and water balance, and to modify the action of other hormones.

Ether: a volatile liquid used as an anaesthetic, the correct chemical name being diethyl ether. It has been known since the sixteenth century, but was first used as an anaesthetic in the nineteenth century; the general use of it was started by William Morton in 1846 at the Massachusetts General Hospital. The introduction of ether was one of the inventions that made the development of modern surgery possible, for it proved to be safe in the hands of experienced people, which meant that general anaesthesia was quickly available in most hospitals. To this day it is the safest anaesthetic, although it has a number of disadvantages which mean that it is not often used by skilled anaesthetists. It irritates the air passages so that the patient is liable to hold his breath and cough when he first inhales the vapour, and the concentration has to be increased slowly to overcome this difficulty; but until the concentration is increased the patient will not relax properly and may not easily pass through the phase of excitement and confusion. The incidence of postoperative vomiting is high, and on the whole it is not very comfortable to be anaesthetized with ether. Nevertheless, it is safe and its use rarely leads to a fatal accident providing that it is fully understood by everyone in the operating theatre that ether is inflammable when mixed with air and explosive if mixed with oxygen.

Ethmoid: a small bone of irregular shape in the base of the skull. It helps to form the inner wall of the orbit, or eye socket, and the upper parts of the nose and the nasal septum, the partition which separates the two sides of the nose. Parts of the bone are filled with air cells which form the ethmoidal sinuses; they sometimes become infected. The middle part of the bone forming the roof of the nose has a large number of holes in it through which pass branches of the olfactory nerve, the nerve of smell, as they travel from the nose to the inside of the skull and the brain.

Ethyl Chloride: a volatile liquid used as a local anaesthetic (it acts by freezing the part by virtue of its rapid evaporation) and as a general anaesthetic, usually in the initial stages when anaesthesia is being induced. Neither use is nowadays common, for the drug has various disadvantages.

Ethylene Glycol: anti-freeze, which has been taken as an intoxicating liquor with fatal results. It damages the liver and the kidneys.

Eucalyptus: an oil obtained from the eucalyptus tree. It is a favourite popular remedy for coughs and colds applied externally as a rub or inhaled as a vapour, but there is little evidence that it has any marked curative effects although it may relieve the symptoms.

258

Eugenics: the study of conditions that may improve the hereditary qualities of a species, which largely originated with the work of Sir Francis Galton (1822–1911), a cousin of Charles Darwin. Today eugenics is viewed more critically, first because we no longer believe that heredity is all-powerful or our knowledge about it capable of giving accurate prediction, and secondly because of our unpleasant experience of the uses to which eugenics can be put in totalitarian countries. The same criticism applies to eugenics as to the concept of euthanasia (i.e. that once we accept the principle that we have the right to control inheritance or put some suffering individual to death there is no logical stopping-point and we may well end up making judgments as to who we think should breed or die). Certainly there are circumstances in which it is highly inadvisable that people should have children, and some diseases, such as haemophilia, are directly inherited, but it is easy to see that, if the eugenicists had had their way, many people who have contributed much to human progress and understanding would never have been born; for the incidence of insanity, neurosis, epilepsy and physical defects among geniuses has been quite high. It is generally accepted today that, certain diseases being transmissible, it is reasonable that in individual cases those who carry these diseases should be advised against having children or even (with their own consent) be sterilized. The real danger comes when scientists leave the field of physical disease and enter the psychological field to make judgments as to what sort of people are desirable, or when they want to apply positive eugenics in the form of selective breeding to human beings, a procedure which most people rightly view with disgust and which in any case is scientifically unjustified since human character is primarily a product of society and upbringing, not of heredity.

Eunuch: a man deprived of his testicles, usually in youth, to render him fit to take charge of the female part of the household. *See* Castration.

Eustachian Tube: the auditory tube, which connects the middle ear with the interior of the nasopharynx in order to equalize pressures in the atmosphere and the middle ear. *See* Ear.

Euthanasia: the recommendation that it should be legal to put to death those who are suffering from incurable, painful or distressing disease by some painless method. As noted in the case of eugenics, the most obvious danger of any such recommendation is that, once the principle is allowed, there is no knowing where it will end; there are very good medical reasons for treating human life as sacred. The main argument put forward by believers in euthanasia is that it is intolerable that people should be allowed to suffer needlessly when they are in any case doomed, but it is noteworthy that those who recommend it are not for the most part medical men who have seen much of death but laymen who are over-dramatizing the real state of affairs. In fact death is rarely accompanied by pains so severe that they cannot be controlled by drugs, and to put to death, even with his own permission, someone who is still in a clear state of mind is simply murder and should be regarded as such. Other reasons against euthanasia are that it would be intolerable should the general public come to associate the doctor with the role of public executioner instead of healer; that one has no right to perform euthanasia without the permission of the patient and no right to perform it with the permission of one who, by reason of suffering, is not in an unbiased state of mind and might well ask for something which in his normal state he would abhor; and, above all, that there are many diseases in which the general application of euthanasia would mean the complete cessation of any attempts to find a cure. Who, after all, is entitled to say that a disease is 'incurable' in view of the fact that it is not unknown for a patient to be found to be suffering from 'incurable cancer' and yet recover spontaneously without any treatment? Are we to put to death those who are suffering from leukaemia because it is regarded as incurable when there is every reason to believe that, like pernicious anaemia and diabetes which were once incurable and are now easily treated, leukaemia will be conquered also? When there are so many ways of relieving severe pain including, when necessary, the severing of the pain-bearing nerves, there seems to be little justification for euthanasia. Many who are not Catholic will agree with the position taken by the Roman Catholic Church that it is wrong to kill but, when a state is reached in which pain can only be relieved at the risk of the patient's life, that risk should be taken. Or, as a secular poet has it: 'Thou shalt not kill, but needst not strive officiously to keep alive.'

Exanthem: the skin eruption associated with some infective fevers.

Exercise: to the primitive man or even to the manual worker it must seem strange that exercise should present itself as a problem at all. Nevertheless, there exists in modern society a large number of people whose work is sedentary and who therefore feel a need for exercise or even a sense of duty in relation to it. But it is necessary to preserve a proper perspective since this is one of those subjects to which some people attach a quite disproportionate significance. The idea that, in general, exercise is not only a duty for the sedentary individual but that it has a remarkable effect on the health of the body is a reversal of the truth, which is that those who are healthy already will wish to take exercise from an overflow of physical energy, and many paralysed or otherwise immobilized individuals who are quite unable to walk have been noted for their longevity. For the normal person the best reason for taking exercise is to obtain pleasure, and compulsive exercising is a miserable and futile form of puritanism. There are two possible exceptions to this general rule: (1) it has been suggested in recent years that lack of exercise is associated with the risk of coronary thrombosis but few doctors accept this view without reservations (some groups of miners who obviously perform very heavy manual work have a high rate of coronary thrombosis); (2) specific types of exercise are necessary in certain ailments, for example breathing exercises are very important in certain types of chest disease, and wasted limbs need exercise to prevent further deterioration in the condition of the muscles. It will be noted that these cases have no bearing whatever on the general problem of exercise as the purpose of breathing exercises is basically to overcome bad habits of breathing, and the purpose of exercising the limbs is to prevent wasting; there is no vague idea that the exercises exert a magical tonic effect on the body as a whole. So far as the possible connection, dubious as it is, between lack of exercise and coronary thrombosis is concerned, it is quite sufficient if the individual walks for five or ten minutes on his way to and from work. Lastly, it should be pointed out that the effect of exercise on reducing weight has often been grossly exaggerated.

Exhibitionism: showing off the body in order to gain sexual attention; exhibitionism sometimes extends to a display of the sexual parts themselves.

Exophthalmos: *see* Goitre.

Exostosis: an abnormal outgrowth of bone.

Exotoxin: toxin liberated from bacteria which damages tissues at a distance from the organism. Exotoxins are usually specific for some special tissue, for example in tetanus the exotoxin affects the motor side of the nervous system. If exotoxins are mixed with formaldehyde and heated they lose their poisonous properties but keep their antigenic structure, so that active immunization is possible; the treated exotoxin, called a toxoid, is injected into the patient, who forms his own antitoxin. Once he has done this, providing that from time to time he has 'booster' doses of toxoid, an infection with the bacteria in question will stimulate the formation of antitoxins in time to prevent the appearance of the disease. If a patient contracts a disease produced by bacteria which form exotoxins against which he has not been immunized it is still possible to give him some degree of passive immunity by injecting antitoxins directly into him. The action of antitoxins produced in an animal (a horse) and injected into a man is effective, but not nearly as effective as the reaction of active immunization following the injection of toxoid. In addition there is a danger of anaphylactic reaction (*see* Anaphylaxis) from the horse serum in which the horse antibodies are contained. Important diseases produced by bacterial exotoxins are diphtheria, tetanus, botulism and gas gangrene; exotoxins, particularly the exotoxin of botulism, are among the most powerful poisons known.

Expectorants: substances used in cough mixtures which are supposed to liquify the sputum and make it easier for the patient to cough effectively. In general, they are substances which in larger doses have an emetic effect, such as ipeca-cuanha, tartar emetic and common salt, which in hot water is about the best expectorant of all.

To a certain extent inhalations of steam with or without Friar's balsam, menthol, eucalyptus, turpentine or Balsam of Tolu have an expectorant action.

Extradural Hemorrhage: the brain is covered by three membranes; the outer one is named the dura mater. It is closely applied to the inner surface of the skull, and in it run blood vessels, in particular the middle meningeal artery which is in the region of the temple. If the temple suffers a severe injury, or the skull is cracked and the fracture line runs across the temple, the middle meningeal artery may be torn so that blood escapes to form an ever-increasing swelling between the dura and the skull. It is possible for other vessels, usually venous, to be torn, but bleeding outside the dura from veins is not common, and the pressure of the escaping blood is nowhere near as high as the pressure of the blood escaping from an artery the size of the middle meningeal; venous bleeding inside the skull is usually inside the dura mater (*see* Subdural). The major cause of extradural bleeding is rupture of the middle meningeal artery.

SYMPTOMS: the classical story is that the patient regains consciousness after a blow on the head, and appears to have recovered; then after a period of time which may be hours, minutes, or rarely days, he goes into coma. This can mean that a patient is admitted to hospital because he has lost consciousness after a head injury, recovers, is discharged, goes home and then lapses into unconsciousness and dies. It can be even worse, for it has happened that a drunken man has been injured in this way as a result of his drunkenness, and has been returned to the custody of the police only to be discovered dead in his cell in the morning. Such accidents are very rare, for those in charge of casualty departments and head injury centres are well aware of the facts, and extradural haemorrhage is not common; but it is important to know that a doctor must be called at once if there is any suspicion of an alteration of consciousness after a head injury, even if the patient has been discharged from hospital as fit. Drunken people with head injuries must be treated with circumspection, and if there is any sort of doubt about the true state of affairs the advice of a doctor must be sought. Before the patient lapses into unconsciousness he often complains of severe headache, becomes restless and confused, and may act as if he were drunk; and if he has had a drink or two the diagnosis may not at once be apparent. In spite of what has been said about the lucid period – the time of apparent recovery from the first effects of the blow on the head – it is quite possible for a patient never to regain consciousness but pass into deepening coma from the time he sustained the injury. If it is not treated, an extradural haemorrhage is fatal.

TREATMENT: an operation must at once be carried out to demonstrate the collection of blood between the dura mater and the skull, and to release it when found. Often the pupil of the eye is dilated on the side of the haemorrhage; sometimes an X-ray shows a fracture of the skull on one side, or it is obvious which side of the head has been injured. The operation itself is quite simple, and consists only of making a hole through the bone of the skull, and if necessary enlarging it until the surgeon can see whether there is blood clot present. When he finds a clot, the surgeon removes it and finds the place where the artery is bleeding so that he can stop it. The main thing is to let the clot out before it presses on the brain so gravely that it can no longer function; after that the surgeon can take more time. The operation can be carried out under general or local anaesthetic.

Extrapyramidal System: the motor nerves – the nerves that make the muscles move – run for the most part from the cortex of the brain into the spinal cord and along it in well-defined bundles of nerve fibres called the corticospinal or pyramidal tracts, pyramidal because when the fibres pass through the medulla (q.v.) of the brain they raise the anterior surface into a pyramidal shape. But the pyramidal tracts are not the only pathway between the brain and the muscles; there are fibres which run from the cortex and relay in the basal parts of the brain and in the brain stem to other fibres which pass down to the muscles without passing through the pyramids. The motor fibres which do not travel in the pyramidal tracts are called the extrapyramidal system, and they have a slightly different function from the pyramidal fibres, being concerned with muscle posture and tone. *See* Nervous System.

Extrasystole: normally the heartbeat follows a regular pattern; the pacemaker, called the sinuatrial node, which is in the right atrium, sets up an impulse which starts a wave of contraction passing through the atria. When this contraction reaches the atrioventricular node, another group of specialized cells near the tricuspid valve (which guards the opening between the right atrium and the right ventricle), the atrioventricular node sets up an impulse in a bundle of specialized muscle fibres (the bundle of His) which passes into the interventricular septum, the partition between the right and left ventricles, and sets up a wave of contraction in the ventricular muscle. A contraction of the heart arising as the result of an impulse set up anywhere outside the sinuatrial node is called an extrasystole.

Extravasation: an escape or a discharge of fluid from a vessel into the tissues. For example, an extravasation of blood occurs when a blood vessel has been injured, and if large forms a haematoma, if small a bruise. Injuries of the urethra and bladder lead to extravasation of urine.

Eye: the eyes are the organs of vision. They are just under an inch in diameter, and are contained in bony sockets (orbits) in the skull. The eyes are moved in their sockets by muscles called external ocular muscles – four straight muscles (rectus muscles) running from the back of the orbit to cover the top, bottom and sides of the eyeball, and two oblique muscles. The inferior oblique muscle runs from the inner forward part of the floor of the orbit obliquely backwards and is inserted into the upper outer back part of the eyeball, but the superior oblique muscle is more complicated. It starts at the back of the orbit from the inner part of the roof, runs forwards, and then hooks round a fibrous pulley called the trochlea and changes direction completely, running obliquely backwards and outwards to be inserted into the upper outer part of the back of the eye near the inferior oblique. It is important for the doctor to know how these muscles run, because when they are paralysed the eyeballs do not move properly and the patient develops double vision. From a consideration of the character of the double vision the muscles or nerves that are paralysed càn be named. In grosser degrees of paralysis the eyeballs can be seen to move unequally; the paralysis is best seen when the eyes are moved in the direction in which the muscle normally works. Eye movements are co-ordinated in the brain.

Structure of the eyeballs. The outer coat of the eyeball is called the sclera, an opaque strong layer of fibrous tissue which is continuous in front with the translucent cornea. The curve of the cornea is greater than the curve of the sclera so that the cornea protrudes a little. Inside the sclerotic layer is a middle pigmented layer forming the choroid at the back and the ciliary body and iris in front. In this pigmented layer run many blood vessels. The next layer is the retina, which is the expanded end of the optic nerve. It has a complicated structure, but essentially it is made up of nerve fibres, a plexus of their connections with the nerve cells of the retina and the rods and cones, and blood vessels. The rods and cones are receptors sensitive to light, but in order to reach them the light has to pass through the other retinal structures. Filling the main part of the eyeball is the vitreous humour, a transparent jelly. In front of the vitreous humour, shutting it off from the front part of the eye, is the lens, supported by its suspensory ligament which fastens it to the ciliary body, a part of the pigmented layer of the eyeball which contains muscle fibres. In front of the lens is the iris, again pigmented and containing muscle fibres. In front of the iris, forming a translucent window through which the light reaches the inside of the eye, is the cornea, continuous with the fibrous opaque outer coat of the eye, the sclera. The part of the eyeball in front of the lens is filled with aqueous humour, which is like water.

Function: the rods and cones of the retina are specialized cells sensitive to light. The rods contain a pigment called rhodopsin, or visual purple, which is bleached by light. It is made from a protein and Vitamin A, which is therefore essential for vision in dim light. Rods are for monochrome vision; cones are concerned with colour vision (*see* Colour Blindness). The lens focuses images on to the retina; it is transparent, and the back is more curved than the front surface. It is normally held out by the suspensory ligament, so that when the muscle of the ciliary body contracts and the ligament slackens the lens becomes rounder – the distance between the front and back surfaces is greater – and near objects are brought to a focus on the retina. As we get older the elasticity of the lens becomes less so that there is greater difficulty in focusing on near objects. There are two places in the retina where the structure differs from the rest: the fovea, where the retina is thinnest so that the light passes directly on to the sensitive cones (there are no rods at the fovea); and the optic disc, where the fibres of the optic nerve leave the eye and there are no rods or cones at all. The centre of the image formed by the lens normally comes to a focus on the fovea, and the optic disc forms the 'blind spot'. The shape of the lens and of the eyeball itself can produce errors of refraction. If the surfaces of the lens are not spherical, astigmatism (q.v.) follows; if the lens brings the image to a focus in front of the retina, either because it refracts too sharply or because the eyeball is too long from front to back, the result is short sight or myopia; if the opposite is true, and the lens cannot refract sharply enough or the eye is too short, the result is long sight or hypermetropia. These faults are corrected by spectacles. The amount of light reaching the inside of the eye is controlled by the iris, which by contracting makes the pupil – the aperture in the centre of the iris – smaller. The muscle of the iris is supplied by the autonomic nervous system (see Nervous System) and is not under voluntary control. It works reflexly; the sympathetic dilates the pupil where the parasympathetic constricts it. When a strong light falls on the retina the pupil at once contracts to cut down the illumination, but if the eye is in the dark the pupil expands. The movements of the pupil are easily seen; if you stand in front of a mirror and shine a torch in your eye you will see both pupils contract. The response of the pupil to light depends on the central connections of the optic nerve in the brain stem and the integrity of the oculomotor nerve and the ciliary ganglion. The fibres of the optic nerve carry impulses arising in the retina back through the optic chiasm, where half the fibres cross sides so that all the fibres 'seeing' the outer world on the right-hand side (those from the nasal side of the right eye and the outer, or temporal, side of the left eye) now lie on the left side of the brain and all the fibres sensitive to images on the left lie on the right side of the brain. The fibres relay in the mid-brain and the impulses end in the visual cortex, which is at the back of the brain. The impulses from the rods and cones are to some extent correlated by the ganglion cells of the retina which connect the rods and cones to the fibres of the optic nerve. Further analysis of information takes place in the cerebral hemispheres, but the processes by which we recognize objects are by no means understood (*see also* Perimetry, Stereoscopic Vision, Colour Blindness, Blindness). Diseases of the eye are described under their own headings, for example Glaucoma, Cataract, Conjunctivitis, Trachoma.

Injuries: injuries and foreign bodies in the eye should always be treated with the greatest caution. Ordinary dust or grit may be dislodged by blinking. If this fails, then the upper eyelid should be lifted outwards and downwards over the lower lid; when the lid is released the edge of the lower lid may carry away the particle. Sometimes foreign bodies are moved if the patient blows his nose hard, and sometimes they can be picked off the eye with the corner of a clean handkerchief. If the particle does not come away easily then the patient must see a doctor, for it is necessary to be very careful when the foreign body adheres to the surface of the eye or has become embedded in the cornea. Wounds of the eye should always be referred to a doctor, but a black eye, which is a bruise in the eyelids and the loose tissues surrounding the eye, may be treated by the application of cold compresses directly after it has been sustained. Discoloration of the skin round the eye after a blow elsewhere on the head is of more serious significance and needs the doctor's attention.

Eyelids: the eyelids are composed of skin stretched by a thin layer of dense fibrous tissue at the margins; they are closed by the action of the orbicularis oculi muscles surrounding the eye, and the upper lid is raised by the action of the levator palpebrae. At the margins of the eyelids the Meibomian glands secrete sebum or grease and sometimes become blocked to form small Meibomian cysts which may need to be opened on the inner surface of the eyelid. Near the outer canthus or angle of the eyelid lie the lacrimal glands whose function is to secrete the liquid which keeps the surface of the eye clean and moist; normally the tears pass across the surface of the eye, being constantly distributed by the action of blinking, and leave it by the lacrimal puncti which can be seen as two tiny openings above and below at the inner angle of the eye. Ducts lead from the lacrimal puncti into the lacrimal sacs at the inner angle of the orbit and from this a duct passes down into the nose. Strong emotions or irritant vapours and foreign bodies cause an excess flow of tears which is more than can be carried away by the duct so that they overflow on to the cheek, and a similar result occurs when for some reason the duct is blocked, for example by a cold which causes the lining of the nose to swell – hence the watery eyes of coryza or hay fever. When the duct is blocked for any length of time the lacrimal sac swells and the condition known as dacryocystitis (q.v.) results in which a swelling near the inner angle of the eyelids can clearly be seen.

F

Facial Nerve: the seventh cranial nerve. It supplies the muscles of expression of the face (but has nothing to do with the sensation of the face, which is the concern of the fifth or trigeminal nerve); it is sometimes affected by palsy, which shows itself by immobility of one side of the face. *See* Bell's Palsy.

Facies: the face, or in clinical medicine the expression. Various diseases produce characteristic expressions, for example the adenoid facies seen in children – a stupid open-mouthed appearance, or the Parkinson's facies in Parkinson's disease where the appearance is expressionless and stolid. The Hippocratic facies is the face of approaching death – 'drawn, pinched and livid'.

Faeces: *see* Feces.

Fainting: or syncope, a transient loss of consciousness caused by temporary lack of blood supply to the brain. It is therefore brought about by conditions which produce a low blood pressure in the cerebral circulation, such as very hot baths, long standing in one position as on military parades, getting up for the first time after a long period of being confined to bed, an overdose of tobacco or alcohol, blows on the head or in the solar plexus region of the abdomen (when fainting really begins to shade into shock), and from strong emotions in nervous people. Rarely, fainting occurs in heart disease (for example in heart-block and auricular flutter), and it may also occur in severe anaemia, low blood pressure and vaso-vagal attacks, but when it happens in otherwise normal adults by far the commonest causes are emotional and postural. The fainting of a postural type which occurs in soldiers on parade results from prolonged standing with inactivity of the leg muscles which ordinarily aid blood to return to the heart by the massaging effect of movement; the blood collects in the veins of the leg and the lower parts of the body and is therefore not available to supply the brain adequately. Such fainting may be prevented by contracting and relaxing the muscles of the calves while standing for any length of time but, when the premonitory signs of pallor, rapid and weak pulse, a 'sinking feeling', and cold sweat or dimming of vision and hearing occur, the individual should lie down or sit with the head bent forward between the knees which, even on parade, is better than falling down unconscious. Once a faint has occurred, much the best thing to do is to let the patient lie flat with any tight clothing loosened. Other procedures are more for the benefit of the onlookers than of the individual, who will recover without their help. When fainting attacks are at all frequent the doctor should be consulted to find whether some physical or emotional cause requires treatment. As in other types of unconsciousness, no attempt must be made to force an unconscious or partly unconscious person to drink; the brandy is best saved for the period of recovery or for the attending doctor.

Fallopian Tubes: also called uterine tubes, these are two tubes 10 cm long which run from a position close to the ovaries on each side of the pelvis to the upper corners of the womb. The cavity of the tubes is open into the womb, but at the outer end the tube opens directly into the peritoneal cavity. This end is free, but formed from a number of processes shaped like fingers which are applied to the surface of the ovary. The epithelium lining the tubes is ciliated (*see* Epithelium), and the cilia help the passage of ova from the ovaries into the ends of the tubes and so down to the uterus. The ovum is normally fertilized in the tube, and sometimes it starts developing there and embeds itself in the wall of the tube (ectopic gestation). Eventually the tube gives way as the ovum grows. Severe bleeding into the peritoneal cavity follows. If the bleeding is fast the patient, who has missed one or two periods, feels acute abdominal pain and collapses. If the bleeding is relatively slow, the patient has recurrent attacks of lower abdominal pain which may be accompanied by vaginal bleeding. Treatment is surgical: the abdomen is opened, the ectopic pregnancy removed, and the bleeding stopped. The occurrence of a tubal pregnancy does not mean that the patient cannot subsequently become normally pregnant.

Fallot's Tetralogy: a congenital abnormality of the heart. There is a defect in the interventricular septum, that is the dividing wall between the right and the left ventricles, and a stenosis, or narrowing, of the pulmonary artery. This means that the resistance is less in the left side of the heart, from which blood flows into the general circulation, than in the right side from which blood normally flows into the lungs. More blood, therefore, flows from the right side of the heart through the septal defect and out into the body than flows into the lungs to pick up fresh oxygen. Associated with the defect in the septum and the narrowing of the pulmonary artery are over-development of the right ventricle and a shift of the aorta towards the right side of the heart.

SYMPTOMS: the baby is blue – either all the time, or when it exerts itself. The tips of the fingers become 'clubbed'. As it grows, it becomes more obvious that the baby is liable to become breathless and tired, perhaps on the slightest exertion. Breathlessness is relieved by squatting, and this is the position the child takes up of choice. Growth may be retarded.

TREATMENT: the only treatment possible is surgery. Heart surgery has made enormous progress in the last 25 years, a great deal of it in the field of congenital heart defects, particularly in the relief of Fallot's Tetralogy. Each case must be considered on its merits, and it is not sensible to generalize; but every child with cyanosis due to a congenital heart defect should have the benefit of a surgeon's opinion.

Farcy: another name for glanders (q.v.).

Farmer's Lung: a disease of the lungs found mainly in agricultural workers.

CAUSE: inhalation of the dust derived from funguses in mouldy hay, or other mouldy vegetable produce, containing antigens which set up a reaction in the lungs.

SYMPTOMS: a fever, with cough, difficulty in breathing, and feeling of ill health.

TREATMENT: corticosteroids during an attack, and avoidance of the precipitating substances afterwards. Farmer's Lung is recognized as an industrial disease. *See* Bagassosis, Bird Breeder's Lung.

Fascia: fibrous tissue organized to form sheets which lie just under the skin (superficial fascia) and round the muscles (deep fascia). The superficial fascia contains fat and the nerves and vessels running to the skin, while the deep fascia is densely fibrous; its strength varies from place to place, e.g. it is very strong over the outside of the thigh but very thin in the face. It forms sheaths for the muscles and compartments in which groups of muscles lie together.

Fasting: the length of time it is possible to exist without food varies with the circumstances. Thus without water most people would die within a week or ten days, but if water is given and the surroundings are warm it is possible to last for about two and a half months. Terence McSwiney, the Mayor of Cork, died on hunger strike in prison in 1920 after a fast of 74 days, and others have survived after fasting for 50 days or more. Professional fasters rarely subsist on water alone and the fluids they drink usually contain fruit juice or glucose which naturally prolongs the period for which they can go 'without food' considerably. Fasting as a health measure is recommended by many people and it is probably quite a good idea for stomachs which are usually overfull to rest for a while, to pass through a period of low living and high thinking, relieved perhaps by the occasional orange juice. Nevertheless it must always be remembered that it is inadvisable for older people to change their way of life suddenly. If the overfed and sedentary suddenly indulge in violent exercise or fasting all they are likely to get is a coronary thrombosis or stomach ulcer.

Fat Embolus: a complication of broken bones. Fat is released from the bone marrow in severe bone injuries, and globules enter the bloodstream where they act as emboli (q.v.).

Fatigue: fatigue is of two types: (1) physical fatigue due to heavy muscular exercise in which recognizable waste-products appear in the blood, such as lactic acid resulting from the metabolism of muscular tissues; (2) psychological fatigue in which no such waste-products appear since nerve tissue does not become exhausted in the ordinary sense and the effects are really the result of boredom, for example in

273

doing monotonous work against which the mind revolts or in doing work unwillingly with a feeling of resentment. The first type of fatigue is not at all common in our basically sedentary society, and psychological fatigue plays a large part in all tiredness; it is, for example, at the root of most of what used to be called industrial fatigue. Therefore, someone who feels fatigue for psychological reasons when doing a particular form of work is usually quite capable of doing something he or she likes immediately the work is changed; the man who is tired on sentry duty and cannot see in the dark is quite able to meet his girl friend on the darkest night. Thus interest has a potent influence on the subjective feeling of tiredness and we are always likely to become tired when doing something unwillingly. There is no treatment for tiredness along the lines usually advertised in the Press as nerves do not need to be 'fed' nor are they soothed by nerve tonics or milk drinks, although there are many stimulants which cover up the feeling of fatigue such as amphetamine and even alcohol. The advertisements recommending glucose are another piece of humbug, because although it is quite true that glucose supplies energy in the completely academic sense that it is the main fuel of the body, it is not true (a) that glucose is in any way superior to a cup of sweet tea with ordinary cane sugar, (b) that the average person lacks glucose, or (c) that people suffering from fatigue are usually suffering from the sort of tiredness that glucose could relieve – they are lacking not energy but inclination. Most fatigue is a form of boredom mixed with resentment and results from doing something when all one's natural impulses are revolting against it. This sort of fatigue due to warring impulses is quite a common occurrence in neurosis (q.v.).

Fat Necrosis: occasionally a hard lump appears in the breast, sometimes after a blow, fixed to the skin and resembling a cancer but in fact composed of dead fat cells. The diagnosis from a cancer is made by biopsy. Very rarely in the abdomen pancreatic enzymes escape after injury or in the course of a severe inflammation into the abdominal cavity and kill fatty cells in the omentum or the mesentery.

Fatty Degeneration: occurs as the result of anaemia of

certain types, interference with the blood or nervous supply, or from some poisons such as chloroform, carbon tetra-chloride or phosphorus. The organs most frequently affected are the heart, liver and kidneys. The cells degenerate and lose their normal function, and fat globules appear in them.

Fauces: the opening between the mouth and throat bounded above by the soft palate, below by the tongue, and on either side by the tonsils. The two ridges of mucous membrane before and behind the tonsils are called the pillars of the fauces. They both contain muscle fibres.

Favus: a ringworm of the scalp found in countries of the Middle East; it responds to griseofulvin.

Febrifuge: an old name for antipyretic drugs.

Feces: the waste products from the small and large in-testines; the motions.

Feeble-mindedness: *see* Mental Defect.

Feeding: the details of the kind of foods necessary to health are described under the heading of Diet; here we are con-cerned only with other factors such as timing and quantity. There is no evidence that regular meals are of any importance except in cases of peptic ulcer where the rule is a stomach 'never full, never empty'; otherwise the hours of adult feeding are simply a matter of social convenience as are the rules of infant feeding which are, like their bedtimes, arranged for the convenience of grown-ups. Time has dealt harshly with the belief that one should take 'eighteen chews to each bite', for, although it is advisable to chew food thoroughly before swallowing it, the fact is that some people are prone to peptic ulcer no matter how carefully they eat while others swallow all their food in large lumps without suffering in the least. Indeed many people who are wholly without teeth have never had indigestion in their lives, although there is no doubt that in their presence digestion would take place much more rapidly. Because of the in-fantile association between food and love many people in adult life unconsciously associate the two with the result that they may, when anxious or unhappy, overeat (anxiety is an important cause of obesity), or they may attach undue importance to food and accept peculiar ideas about its potency to cure all ills. Thus, apart from vegetarianism, we have in recent years had two curious diets or forms of treatment: one based on the belief, for which there is no medical evidence whatever, that proteins and carbohydrates should not be eaten together in the same meal, and the other on the equally absurd belief that meals are improved by the addition of something called black-strap molasses. Another individual described as an old-fashioned American country doctor advocates the use of sour cider and honey as a cure for nearly every disease under the sun, although why sugar and vinegar should have this remarkable effect is not known – in any case it enabled him to become a best-seller.

It can be said categorically (a) that how one takes one's food does not matter from the medical point of view so long as enough of the essential food materials are available from either animal or vegetable sources; (b) that when one takes one's food does not matter in normal people; (c) that most people eat too much and their food tends to be too rich, too soft, not bulky enough and not fresh enough. There would be healthier teeth and no need to worry about constipation if people would eat hard foods which require biting and chewing with enough roughage to give bulk to the motions and stimulate the bowels. Most of us would be much the better for a period of fasting, and yet one finds that anyone who has the temerity to miss a meal or even chooses to fast for a few days is immediately put under strong social pressure to eat whether he wants to or not. An improved appetite is a sign of better health in the invalid, not the cause of it; nobody should eat (except in some nervous illnesses) if he does not want to.

Vegetarianism (q.v.) is an example of a belief which can be perfectly well justified on the grounds of humanitarianism, personal taste or even health, but is all too often held in the form of an absurd obsession amounting almost to a religion. There is no reason at all why people should not be vegetarians, but neither is there any reason why they should read magazines about it, preach it, and try to convert others. A man who was obsessed with a desire for inch-thick steaks or caviare would rightly be judged a little odd, but so, too, is the vegetarian who allows himself to think that his practice is more than a matter of preference and in effect centres his life around food which, in ordinary civilized life, does not justify more attention than that due to any other cultural commodity. It is worth while pointing out that at a time when vegetarians and other food faddists are ever more vehemently insisting on the importance of diet in curing disease, orthodox medicine tends to pay rather less attention to it than in the past; there are very few detailed diets in medical treatment today and even in the treatment of peptic ulcer it is sufficient in most cases to require the patient to leave out fried foods, spicy or rich foods and to eat little and often. Obesity, diabetes, gastric and some intestinal diseases, and kidney diseases in some instances, require what might be described as special diets, but in fact are only slight modifications of ordinary ones. Dietetic prohibitions form part of certain religious creeds as in Islam and Judaism. One is usually told that the prohibition of pork in both these religions had its origin as a hygienic precaution in areas and at times when 'measly pork' could cause tapeworm infestation. This may be doubted, for prohibition of pork is only one of many food prohibitions in Judaism (for example all the blood must be removed from meat after killing, milk must not be taken with meat, etc.) and the real reasons are probably to be sought in the unconscious mind. Psychoanalytic theory, for example, sees vegetarianism and the eating of kosher meat as reactions against latent aggression or 'bloodthirstiness' and the prohibition against 'seething a kid in its mother's milk' as a primitive incest taboo. A great many food peculiarities are probably better explained in primitive emotional terms rather than in terms of the rationalizations given to account for or justify them. At a time when some of us are worrying about overeating it is worth while remembering that 500 million people in the world are suffering from acute malnutrition and 1,000 million from varying degrees of hunger.

Felon: a suppurating infection of the pulp of the finger. *See* Pulp Infection.

Femur: the thigh-bone, the largest and strongest bone in the body. At its upper end it fits into the acetabulum of the pelvis to form a ball and socket joint. The lower end forms a joint with the tibia, the great bone of the lower leg (the shin-bone) at the knee. The front of the knee joint is covered by the knee-cap. The knee is a hinge joint, and rotation of the trunk on the foot takes place at the hip. The neck and head of the femur are at an angle of 125° to the shaft, and rotation takes place round an axis joining the head of the bone to its lower end; it is along this axis that weight is borne. The part of the femur most liable to fracture, as one would expect, is the neck below the head or as it joins the shaft. This fracture is not as common as it might be among adults in the prime of life, for the inside of the neck and shaft of the femur is buttressed by lines of dense bone formed along the lines of force; but when in old age all the bones lose their elasticity and become brittle, then a fracture of the neck of the femur is always a possibility after a relatively trivial fall. The method of treatment is internal fixation – a special nail is used to fasten the head of the bone in place, and weight-bearing can begin again almost at once, which avoids the fatal necessity for confining an old person to bed for any length of time: A fracture of the shaft of the femur is a serious injury, usually the result of considerable violence. The legs should be bound together and the patient taken to hospital as soon as possible, for there will be a degree of shock associated with the fracture. Treatment is by traction and takes a considerable time – up to three months in bed, then about six months in walking plaster, so that it may be nine months before a man is fit to resume work. During the whole time of treatment the patient must persevere with exercises which are designed to keep the muscles working and the joints moving; otherwise the leg will become weak and stiff.

Fenestration: an operation on the ear which was when first introduced a great advance in surgery, for it enabled many people to hear who would otherwise have been reduced to lip-reading or the use of deaf-aids. Newer operations have been introduced to improve what the first fenestration operation began, but they cannot improve every kind of deafness; impairment of hearing due to damage or disease of the auditory nerve cannot be set right by operation. *See* Ear, Otosclerosis.

Ferments: another name for enzymes (q.v.).

Fern Root: male fern extract is used to treat infestation with tapeworms. The patient fasts for 48 hours before he is given the drug, and 2 hours after the drug has been taken in an emulsion or in a capsule he takes a saline aperient, so that the worm and the remains of the drug are expelled.

Fersolate: trade name for tablets of ferrous sulphate, used in iron-deficiency anaemias.

Fetishism: a sexual abnormality in which sexual excitement is associated with certain objects, such as a woman's shoe, or underclothes.

Fetus: the unborn child, particularly from the stage when it becomes recognizable as belonging to the species of its parents; prior to this it is usually called the embryo. The ovum or egg is fertilized in the Fallopian tube (q.v.) and in the first week of fertilization passes into the cavity of the womb where within a further 2 weeks it grows to about $\frac{1}{2}$ in (12.7 mm) in length. By the fourth week the embryo becomes curved like a comma, and buds appear which will become the ears and the limbs; in the following week the eyes appear and the segments of the limbs are defined. At the end of 2 months the embryo has a definitely human appearance with a nose and separate fingers, and the tail which has hitherto been prominent is reduced to a rudiment; its length is then just over an inch. In the third month the limbs are clearly human, the finger- and toe-nails appear and sex can be distinguished. In the fourth month the foetus is from 4 to 6 in (101–152 mm) long, hair has appeared, and the legs have become proportionately longer. In the sixth month the foetus is about 12 in (305 mm) long, eyelashes and eyebrows appear and a month later the eyes open and the foetus is capable of being born alive. The following 2 months see the child becoming plumper and the skin develops its final colour. At birth it should weigh from $6\frac{1}{2}$ to $7\frac{1}{2}$ lb (2.9–3.4 kg) and be about 20 in (508 mm) long.
Before birth the foetus is dependent upon the mother's blood for its food and oxygen; exchange takes place through

the placenta, a fleshy pad attached to the wall of the womb where interchange of products between mother and foetus is possible, although there is in fact no direct connection.

The foetus is connected to the placenta by the umbilical cord, which after birth becomes atrophied.

Fever: a condition of the body characterized by a temperature above normal, with disturbances of normal function. The normal temperature is usually given as 98.4 °F. (36.9 °C.), but as the body temperature varies throughout the day, anything between 98.4 °F. (or lower) and 99.5 °F. (37.5 °C.), may be taken as, for all practical purposes, normal. Thus the temperature rises after a large meal, during hot weather when it is less easy for the body to get rid of heat, after prolonged or violent exercise, is at its highest level between the hours of 4–9 p.m., and at its lowest between the hours of 1.30–7 a.m. In women, the temperature varies with the menstrual cycle, notably just prior to ovulation (the fertile period), and the method of taking daily temperature readings is used in contraceptive practice to calculate the 'safe period', or, in those who suffer from sterility, to calculate the time when fertilization is most likely to occur. A raised temperature is usually, but by no means always, a sign of bacterial or virus infection; it may be raised very considerably in heatstroke, in certain types of brain injury or disease, and, especially in children, in nervous shock. The body temperature is controlled by a centre in the brain which ensures that there will exist a balance between heat production and heat loss, but in bacterial invasion both these processes are affected. A fever is usually ushered in by a *rigor* which may vary from sensations of chilliness to violent shivering in which the whole body trembles uncontrollably and the teeth chatter. Although this is often termed the cold stage of a fever because the skin feels cold and clammy, it is in fact accompanied by raised temperature within the body, and it is during this stage that convulsions frequently occur in young children. When the fever becomes established the hot stage has arrived, in which the skin is hot and dry and there is a feeling of lassitude, aching muscles, headache and thirst; the urine is scanty, there may be constipation, nausea and vomiting, and the pulse and respirations are speeded up.

This stage is finally succeeded by profuse sweating, a copious flow of concentrated urine, and general relief of symptoms, a process which, if it takes place rapidly, is known as the crisis (for example in lobar pneumonia), or if it occurs more gradually is called lysis.

A high temperature is often accompanied by delirium and even when this is not apparent the patient's mental state is likely to be somewhat confused with a loss of awareness of the passage of time, nightmares, etc. Death during a fever may occur suddenly on slight exertion which the weakened heart is unable to bear, or it may terminate the so-called typhoid state in which the patient gradually sinks into a weakened condition, becomes delirious, and finally comatose. Numerous patterns of temperature curve are seen when regular readings are marked on a chart and these often give valuable information about the nature of the infection. The degree of fever is not always a reliable guide to the severity of a disease, for the temperature in diphtheria, miliary tuberculosis and typhoid fever is sometimes only slightly raised, whereas children with quite mild infections may have a high fever with convulsions and delirium. The commonest type of temperature curve is the *continuous type* in which the temperature rises more or less rapidly, remains at about the same level for some days or even a couple of weeks, and then comes down to normal either by crisis or lysis; to this type belong most of the common fevers that occur in childhood.

In *relapsing fever* the same curve is seen, but after the temperature has been normal for about a week a further bout of fever follows which, after another latent period, may recur two or three times. *Remittent fever* occurs in typhoid when the temperature, although never coming down to normal, shows morning and evening variations, with a higher evening temperature and a lower morning one. This type of chart is typical of many tropical diseases. *Intermittent fevers* such as malaria show attacks of fever recurring at specific intervals with periods of normal temperature in between; quotidian fever occurs every 24 hours, tertian fever every 48 hours, and quartan every 72.

It will be seen from the above that the usefulness of the clinical thermometer at home is strictly limited, because there is little value in a single reading which the user is rarely able to interpret. The degree of fever within wide limits gives no indication of the severity of the disease, as a high temperature may mean quite a trivial disease and a low temperature or no fever at all does not mean that all is well. A patient may be very ill without any fever. Furthermore, the habit of constantly bringing out the thermometer whenever a child complains of feeling unwell is to be deprecated as its sole result may be that the child becomes neurotic about his health. If someone who 'feels a cold coming on' takes his temperature – what information has he gained from the observation that his temperature is 100 °F.? Very little; half an hour before it might have been 102 °F. If it is normal, it still tells him nothing since it does not stop him from feeling ill nor guarantee that he will not feel worse in an hour or so. A doctor using a clinical thermometer is not basing his diagnosis on its readings but merely using it to confirm what he has learned from other sources; thus if a generalized rash is present then a raised temperature makes a diagnosis of scarlet fever more probable while a normal temperature (taken together with other indications) might suggest an allergic rash. True, a child who has been irritable and moody will be treated with more respect if it can be shown he has a fever which may reasonably be supposed to be the cause of his irritability, but the absence of a fever does not justify us in treating him as if nothing were wrong except bad temper. The presence of a fever is always significant, but its absence does not imply the opposite. Fever is a symptom and its treatment is that of its cause.

Fibrescope: an endoscope through which the light is carried by a bundle of flexible fibres. This replaces the more rigid telescopic systems used in older endoscopes. *See* Endoscopy.

Fibrillation: *see* Defibrillation.

Fibrin: a substance which forms the framework of blood clots. *See* Coagulation of the Blood.

Fibrin foam: a preparation, which is subsequently absorbed, for arresting bleeding. It is soaked in a solution of thrombin before it is used. Gelatin foam and surgical alginates (prepared. from seaweed) are other substances used to speed clotting of the blood, for they provide a large surface on which clotting can take place and are absorbed afterwards by the body.

Fibrinogen: a substance circulating in the blood. In certain circumstances it is changed into fibrin in the formation of blood clots. *See* Coagulation of the Blood.

Fibrocystic Disease: a process involving the formation of cystic spaces with overgrowth of fibrous tissues between them. Fibrocystic disease of the pancreas is a complicated hereditary condition in which the abnormal state of the pancreas is only one of a number of disease processes present in the patient. The liver is also involved, but the most serious aspect of the disease is that the patients suffer from staphylococcal infection of the lungs, which has to be treated incessantly with antibiotics to which the staphylococci often develop immunity. In many cases children affected by the disease succumb to lung infection in infancy, and if they survive are liable to die at the time of puberty from heart failure, secondary to the lung condition. Fibrocystic disease of bone occurs in two main forms, one localized and one general. The localized form is not associated with any other abnormality, but the generalized disease is a consequence of overaction of the parathyroid glands (q.v.). As one might expect, the bones in this condition are liable to fracture; not so obvious is the fact that the disturbance of calcium balance results in the formation of kidney stones.

Fibroid: a non-malignant tumour consisting of muscular and fibrous tissue enclosed within a capsule which occurs in the womb, most usually in the main part or body but in about 8% of cases in the cervix or neck. It is commonest in childless women and rarely becomes malignant; most fibroids of the body of the womb are multiple while those of the cervix are often single.

CAUSE: the cause of fibroids is not known, but it is not improbable that some imbalance of the sex hormones is responsible.

SYMPTOMS: are due to the mechanical effect of the swellings which cause congestion of the womb or pressure on

283

surrounding areas. Those due to congestion include flooding during the periods (menorrhagia), or bleeding in between the periods (metrorrhagia). Pressure may cause pain, or more commonly attacks of retention of urine, varicose veins, swelling of the ankles, and piles, all of which are caused by pressure on the abdominal veins. There may be some discharge if sloughing has occurred and sterility or miscarriage is common.

TREATMENT: the treatment for fibroids is removal by operation or, in some cases, especially if the patient has passed the childbearing age and there are many fibroids, removal of the whole womb (hysterectomy).

Fibroma: a simple benign tumour composed of fibrous tissue, usually quite small. Fibroid tumours of the uterus are made up of muscle as well as fibrous tissue; they are called 'fibromyomata' and may grow to a considerable size. *See* above.

Fibrosarcoma: this is a malignant tumour of fibrous tissue which grows relatively slowly, often in muscles near the surface of the body. It invades neighbouring tissue but does not at first spread to other parts of the body; in its later stages it may metastasize to the lung. Treatment is surgical, but the tumour may recur after removal. Fibrosarcomata are not affected by radiotherapy.

Fibrosis: the formation of fibrous or scar tissue in place of normal tissue which has been destroyed by injury, infection or deficient blood supply (*see* below).

Fibrous Tissue: fibrous tissue makes up a great deal of the body. There are two main sorts of fibrous tissue, white and yellow, the former being unyielding when put upon the stretch, the latter highly elastic, less plentiful, but equally strong. White fibrous tissue is composed of thin stringy fibres of a substance called 'collagen' produced by star-shaped cells (fibroblasts) lying between the fibres. It is found forming loose networks called loose connective tissue, or areolar connective tissue, filling spaces underneath the skin, round joints and round organs and muscles, and it also forms the dense sheets of connective tissue that make up tendons, sheathe the muscles, and bind the muscle bundles together in compartments (*see* Fascia). There are a certain number of elastic fibres in loose connective tissue, but elastic fibrous tissue occurs mostly in the elastic walls of arteries and in ligaments where some degree of elasticity is desirable (the ligaments joining the laminae of adjacent vertebrae, etc.).

Fibula: the splint-bone of the lower leg which is situated behind and to the outer side of the tibia or shin-bone. Its upper end forms a joint with the tibia – it does not enter into the formation of the knee joint – and the lower end articulates with the astragalus (talus) at the ankle. The outer projection of the ankle, called the external malleolus, is the lower end of the fibula. *See* Pott's Fracture.

Filariasis: an infection with worms named filariae – they are very thin, about the size of a heavy thread, and vary in length from about 1–2 cm up to 40–50 cm. The adult female worm produces a number of larvae called microfilariae, which are distributed in the blood. When an insect bites an infected man it becomes infected with microfilariae, which turn into filariae proper in the insect. When another man is bitten by the infected insect he in turn becomes infected with filariae.

Varieties of filarial worms: the worms that infect man are Wuchereria bancrofti, Brugia malayi, Onchocerca volvulus and Loa loa. They are found in tropical and subtropical countries. W. bancrofti and B. malayi are responsible for the disease elephantiasis, in which worms block the lymphatic channels and the legs and genital organs become grossly enlarged. The intermediate host is a mosquito.

Onchocerca volvulus produces the disease onchocerciasis, in which the skin itches and is thickened. About the lower waist and in other parts of the body swellings are liable to come up which contain adult worms. These swellings have to be removed surgically, otherwise they are a continuing source of reinfection. Onchocerciasis is sometimes called African river blindness from the effects of the damage the worm can cause to the eyes. The infection is common in Central Africa, West Africa, and South and Central America. The intermediate host is the buffalo gnat, Simulium, and the microfilariae are found in the skin rather than the blood. Loa loa occurs in West Africa, where the intermediate host, the mango fly, bites during the daytime, unlike the mosquitoes which are more likely to bite at night. In Loa loa swellings appear in the skin, called Calabar swellings, and from time to time the worms wriggle across the conjunctiva of the eye, where they can be seen.

TREATMENT: diethylcarbamazine, marketed under the proprietary names Banocide, Hetrazan and Ethodryl, kills microfilariae in the blood and skin, but has less effect on adult worms, especially the Onchocerca. Patients taking diethylcarbamazine are liable to suffer fever, headache and general malaise as a result of allergic reaction to dead microfilariae, and in infections with Onchocerca the eye may be affected and the skin itches severely. The swellings containing adult worms in onchocerciasis are removed surgically, and if the reaction to diethylcarbamazine is marked the patient is given corticosteroids. A drug sometimes used in intractable infection with Onchocerca is suramin (Antrypol), administered intravenously, but it is liable to cause damage to the kidneys.

Fingers: consist of three bones or phalanges joined together by hinge joints and strong ligaments; the thumb has only two phalanges. The movements of flexion (bending) and extension (straightening) are carried out by powerful muscles in the forearm whose tendons pass, two in front and two behind, to each finger. These tendons are covered by synovial sheaths which contain fluid to enable the muscles to work without friction and they are inserted in the base of the middle and end phalanges back and front. At the side of each finger are two small arteries and two small nerves which are of particular importance in view of the great sensitivity of the finger-tips; these are branches of the radial and ulnar arteries and the nerves of the forearm. On the front of the hand the ulnar nerve supplies only the little finger and the adjoining half of the next finger, all the rest being supplied by the median nerve. On the back of the hand, the ulnar nerve supplies the last two and a half fingers; the median nerve supplies the finger-tips, and the radial nerve supplies the rest of the back of the hand and the fingers as far as the tips. At the tip of each finger is the nail, and at the base the finger is joined to the metacarpal bones of the hand, one to each finger. The diseases most commonly affecting the fingers, apart from injuries and infections, are those connected with their blood supply (Raynaud's disease or chilblains), arthritis (usually rheumatoid arthritis), neuritis, skin diseases and, in the nail, ringworm.

Fissure: a crack or small ulcer occurring most commonly at the corner of the mouth or on the mucous membrane of the anus.

CAUSE: in the mouth, various conditions give rise to small fissures which are kept in constant movement and are in contact with saliva containing bacteria, so that they take a long time to heal. They are particularly common in cold weather. Fissures in the anus are often the result of the passage of hard motions which tear the mucous membrane; once this has been done, the fissure is reopened at the passage of subsequent motions and infected by the faeces.

SYMPTOMS: fissure-in-ano is very painful. The patient feels a sharp pain on passing motions, which is severe enough to produce constipation because the patient avoids going to the lavatory. There may be slight bleeding, and very often itching round the anus. Fissures at the corner of the mouth may be both uncomfortable and unsightly.

TREATMENT: if the fissure is at the corner of the mouth, the mouth and face must be kept clean and the patient must avoid licking the fissure with the end of his tongue. Obvious dental sepsis is best cleared up, and sometimes the fissure may heal after application of a caustic stick. A fissure-in-ano is best treated by keeping the motions soft and regular and in the case of mild fissures using an anaesthetic ointment. The anus and the skin round about must be kept clean, and it is best to wash after passing a motion. In more severe cases the surgeon may try the effect of dilating the anus under general anaesthetic, but sometimes the only effective treatment is surgical removal of the fissure and the surrounding skin; the resulting raw area heals in a few weeks.

Fistula: an abnormal channel between a natural cavity and the surface of the body or between two natural cavities, for example between the intestines and the skin surface or

287

between the bladder and the intestines. This may arise from errors of development as when a child is born with a channel running from the region of the tonsil to the surface of the neck; from an obstructed duct as when, a salivary duct being blocked, a fistula develops which discharges saliva on to the cheek; from injury, as when a torn urethra causes a fistula which discharges urine through the tissues and the skin; from disease, as when a fistula arises between the bowel and bladder from an abscess or tumour in the pelvis. One of the commonest types is fistula-in-ano, i.e. a fistula between the lower part of the rectum and the skin surrounding the anus caused by an abscess in the region, sometimes tuberculous but more usually of the ordinary type. In most cases a fistula heals when continuity of the normal channels is restored, but fistula-in-ano is more difficult to deal with as it is kept constantly infected by the faeces which pass through. In this case a minor operation is necessary and care is taken afterwards to ensure that closure takes place in the deepest part of the wound first, and that the scar is solid.

Fits: *see* Epilepsy.

Flat-foot: (Pes planus). A condition normal in infants and many children, and in people who have never worn shoes. The foot in people who wear shoes has two arches – one from side to side, and the other longitudinal. In a wet foot-print on a flat surface there is an empty space between the areas marked out by the base of the toes and the heel bounded only by the imprint of the outer edge of the foot. In flat-foot this space does not exist, and the whole print looks broader.

CAUSE: loss of tone of the muscles which support the arches of the foot, commonly following an illness and being confined to bed; acute strain of the feet; fracture of the bones of the feet, particularly the heel-bone or os calcis; general debility or overweight; long hours of standing; inflammation; arthritis of the foot.

SYMPTOMS: pain, either acute or chronic.

TREATMENT: the treatment includes building up the general health, exercises (walking on tiptoe, raising and lowering the body on tiptoe, walking on the outer edge of the foot, balancing on the outer edge of the foot), supports of the type sold in shops dealing in such appliances which may take the form either of a steel arch or a sponge rubber pad, manipulation, and operation. Supports relieve the symptoms almost immediately, but are not usually to be recommended as they not only prevent the arch from becoming stronger by taking away its normal function, but stretch even further the already lax tendons and ligaments of the sole, thus increasing the degree of flat-foot. Manipulation endeavours to set the foot in the correct position which is maintained for a month or so in plaster; in operative treatment part of the bone may be removed from the inner side of the foot to shorten the instep and make a new arch. The results of operation and manipulation are sometimes disappointing and there is no doubt that, in the early stages, the best treatment is improvement of the general health and exercise. It is worth while noting (*a*) that many people have flat-foot without any symptoms; (*b*) that others become obsessed with the condition and use it, in effect, as a neurotic symptom to evade unpleasant duties (for example the 'excused boots' character well known to the army of former days); (*c*) that flat-foot can be a very considerable disability to those whose work involving standing may be imperilled by the condition.

Flatulence: gas in the stomach or intestines which may become evident in distension of the abdomen, unpleasant rumblings inside, a feeling of fullness and discomfort, or the passage of wind by belching or from the anus. The vast majority of cases of flatulence, i.e. all cases of flatus in the stomach and many cases of flatus in the bowels, are self-inflicted, being caused by the habit of swallowing air which is ingested in increasing quantities as the patient tries to bring up the air he has already swallowed. Although dyspepsia is the predisposing cause of this annoying habit (annoying not only to the patient but to those around him, as many sufferers from flatulence seem to dramatize their disability), it is obvious that unless the patient makes a determined effort not to swallow air his condition will remain. Dyspepsia should, therefore, be treated, but the main emphasis placed on breaking the habit. Flatus in the intestines may come from the stomach, but sometimes results from decomposition of foods within the bowel; this is particularly the case in diseases of the liver or gall-bladder when the flow of bile is impeded. This type of flatulence should be investigated medically.

Flavine: *see* Acriflavine.

Fleas: (Siphonaptera). These annoying insects are of medical importance for they are concerned with the transmission of various diseases – murine typhus, for example, and bubonic plague. Tunga penetrans, the jigger flea, burrows its way into the skin and causes ulceration, but the most peculiar method of passing on disease is that forced upon the rat flea, Xenopsylla cheopis, by the organism of bubonic plague, Pasteurella pestis. The flea bites an infected rat, and the bacteria multiply in its fore-gut until the gut is blocked by a mass of bacteria. The 'blocked' flea bites another creature, but the blood it draws will not pass into its mid-gut. It is, however, contaminated by the mass of bacteria, and when the unfortunate flea regurgitates its meal the bacteria pass into the new victim's circulation. The flea, which cannot keep anything down, tries to feed as often as it can; and when the rats which are normally the fleas' host die of plague, as they may, the flea in its search for a warm-blooded host may light on a man and infect him.

Fleming, Sir Alexander (1881–1955). Nobel Prize-winner with Sir Howard Florey and Sir Ernest Chain for the discovery of penicillin.

Flexibilitas Cerea: an abnormal condition found in advanced catatonic schizophrenia in which the patient's limbs remain in whatever position they are placed by the observer.

Flooding: the common name for excessive bleeding in women whether during the menstrual period, when it is described as menorrhagia, or between periods, when it is called metrorrhagia. It may be a sign of various different conditions and should be reported to the doctor.

Fluid Balance: it is essential for all living things to keep in fluid balance – too little fluid, and the cells dry up; too much and they drown. Bound up with the question of fluid balance is the balance of the electrolytes carried in the fluid without which the cells cannot function. The commonest way for sick people to lose fluid is by vomiting or diarrhoea. The average daily output of fluid as urine is between 1,200 and 1,500 ml, and the usual loss from perspiration and in the breath up to 1,000 ml, so that the average man needs 2 to 3 litres of fluid a day. He also needs 4.5 g of salt and a little potassium. If the patient cannot take fluids by mouth, they must be given intravenously, with appropriate amounts of salt and potassium. It is sensible to keep some check on what a patient drinks and how much water he loses even at home, for some sick people, especially the elderly, drink too little if left to themselves. One of the signs of this is a concentrated urine, but in some cases the kidneys are unable to concentrate the urine and the specific gravity of the urine is no help. In hospital charts are kept of the amounts of fluid lost and taken by a patient. On the whole patients have to be encouraged to drink enough rather than restrained from drinking too much.

Flukes: (Trematodes). Leaf-shaped parasitic worms with suckers which can infest the intestine, the blood, the lungs and the liver. They have at least two hosts in their life-cycle, living as adults in vertebrates and spending their youth in invertebrates, usually some sort of snail. When the adult fluke lives in the intestine the eggs are passed in the faeces. They can only survive in the wet, and if they are fortunate enough to fall into water they develop as free-swimming miracidia. The miracidia then have to find a suitable snail within a short time, for they die in a matter of hours. In the snail the worm goes through a number of stages on the way to becoming a fluke. The eggs of flukes which live in the lungs reach the outer world via the sputum, and the eggs of flukes in the blood are discharged in the urine (*see* Bilharzia). The lung fluke is called Paragonimus, and it is found in the Far East; the liver flukes are Clonorchis sinensis, found in China, and the sheep liver fluke Fasciola hepatica; but the most important fluke of all, Schistosoma, lives in the blood, and gives rise to the widely spread schistosomiasis (bilharzia). *See* Worms.

Fluorescein: an orange-coloured powder used in watery

solution to detect ulcers and abrasions on the cornea of the eye.

Fluorine: one of the halogen series of elements (i.e. belonging to the same group as chlorine, bromide and iodine), which is one of the normal constituents of bones and teeth. Its main interest today is in connection with the controversy about adding fluorine to public water supplies in order to prevent dental caries. It has been shown that those who habitually use water with a concentration of 1 part per million of fluorine are less prone to dental decay than those whose water supply is fluorine-free. Opponents of fluoridation contend: (1) that as a matter of public morality no one has a right to add materials to the water supply which all have to use whether they approve or not; (2) that fluorine has not been proved to have the stated effect beyond all doubt, that it may stain the teeth, and that in larger amounts it is known to be poisonous. Those who support it point out: (1) that in fact many chemicals are already added to the drinking supply in order to purify it and kill any organisms present, and adding fluorine is no different in principle from this; (2) that there is little or no doubt that fluorine prevents decay, and in the amounts used it is neither likely to stain the teeth nor to harm the general health. Reports show that in those drinking fluoridated water all their lives the incidence of caries is 66% less than elsewhere.

Fluoroacetic Acid Poisoning: fluoroacetate is used as a rat poison, and occurs in South Africa in a plant which poisons cattle. The substance is not itself lethal, but is changed in the body to fluorocitrate, one of the most dangerous poisons known, which interferes with metabolic processes.
SYMPTOMS: nausea, twitching, apprehension, convulsions.
TREATMENT: intramuscular injection of acetamide.

Foetus: *see* Fetus.

Folic Acid: (Pteroylglutamic acid). A substance originally found in spinach, and present in the leaves of other plants, yeast and liver. It is part of the Vitamin B complex, and is used in the treatment of the type of anaemia which shows large abnormal red cells (megaloblastic anaemia). Folic acid is sometimes found to be deficient in pregnancy, and is often given with iron compounds as a routine to expectant mothers. It is also used in the treatment of nutritional disorders accompanied by megaloblastic anaemia in which the diet is deficient or there is a defect of absorption from the gut. Alcoholism in particular may lead to a folic acid deficiency.

Follicle: a very small secreting gland or cyst. In the ovary, the ovum develops in a small cystic space called an ovarian follicle.

Follicle Stimulating Hormone: a hormone secreted by the pituitary gland which causes ripening of the ovarian follicle.

Fomentation: generally applied to hot, wet, medicated or non-medicated substances applied to the body to bring blood to the area and absorb discharge. In all cases a kaolin poultice is best because it does not turn the skin into a sodden mess ripe for reinfection. Turpentine, laudanum and other types of fomentation have long been discarded with a more rational approach to medicine. A kaolin poultice should be either heated in the tin in a pan of boiling water and then spread on lint, or spread on the lint cold and toasted under the grill. Unless there is much discharge there is no need to change the dressing every time and it can be toasted again when it grows cold.

Fomites: a term describing all articles which have been in contact with an infected person, for example clothes, bedding, toys, books, etc., which may therefore, at least in theory, spread the disease. Briefly, the risk from such articles is in most cases much less than used to be thought, and it is not necessarily believed to be a bad thing to contract the ordinary childhood fevers early in life as they are likely to be caught anyhow and are much more dangerous in adult life. Whereas formerly all bed-clothing, etc., was sterilized by boiling and books and toys were burned, the ordinary case of measles or scarlet fever today is treated little differently so far as fomites are concerned from any other illness. This, however, does not apply to serious infectious diseases

293

like smallpox or to lice or flea-spread diseases where clothing, etc., may need to be destroyed.

Fontanelle: when it is born the baby's skull has not completely closed, and there are still present gaps in the bone filled by membrane. The largest is in the front of the head where, at the meeting-point of the frontal bone and the two parietal bones that form the side walls of the skull, there is at birth a gap about one square inch in size. This is the anterior fontanelle, and through it can be felt the pulsation of the brain. It is normally closed by the eighteenth month, and delay signifies some arrest in development. In fevers and other states it may bulge, and it will sink in when the infant is dehydrated. There are six fontanelles in all at birth.

Food Poisoning: a very general term formerly applied to diarrhoea caused by almost anything, but more usefully applied to intestinal disorders caused by bacterial contamination of food.

CAUSE: contamination of food with (1) Staphylococci, which multiply and form colonies in the contaminated food. The bacteria themselves are not poisonous, but they produce a toxin which is. Staphylococci are found most frequently in twice-cooked meat or food requiring much handling, for example pies, minced meat and so on. Septic sores on the hands, tonsillitis or a discharging ear are sources of infection. (2) Bacteria of the Salmonella group; S. typhimurium, the cause of mouse typhoid, is often involved. Many other organisms of this group cause infections which originate from cattle, pigs and animal products such as eggs and milk. (3) Contamination of food with the organism Clostridium welchii, which flourishes in meat allowed to cool and then warmed again, for its spores resist heat and so do some of the toxins it produces. It lives without oxygen.

SYMPTOMS: staphylococcal poisoning is acute, produces vomiting and diarrhoea, and is over quickly although it is very unpleasant while it lasts. Salmonella poisoning has a much longer incubation period – perhaps two days instead of two hours. The patient again develops vomiting and diarrhoea, and becomes feverish. Cl. welchii produces symptoms in about a day, and patients recover in about two days.

TREATMENT: symptomatic – antibiotics are not used, efforts being concentrated on stopping the vomiting and diarrhoea and counteracting the loss of water. The simple remedies are best. *See* Diarrhoea, Botulism, Dysentery.

PREVENTION: in tropical and subtropical countries it is sensible to assume that all food, particularly vegetable, is contaminated, and to wash it carefully before use. If possible it should be bought from a source known to be clean. Food must be stored in a cool place free from flies and well ventilated, and all who handle the food and plates and containers used in cooking and serving must be subject to inspection and well educated in the rules of personal cleanliness. No rubbish can be allowed to remain in or near the kitchen, which must always be clean. If anyone in a household develops food poisoning everyone living in the house must be doubly careful about their own personal hygiene, for the infection can spread quickly. It is sensible to avoid eating twice-cooked food in the summer if you do not know the circumstances in which it has been prepared. All frozen meat and poultry should be properly cooked.

Foot: the foot is very similar in structure to the hand, the toes being composed of three phalanges. (There are only two in the big toe.) The toes join the five metatarsal bones which correspond to the metacarpal bones of the hand and, in turn, articulate with the tarsal bones, seven in number, which correspond to the carpal bones of the wrist. The arrangement of the blood vessels and nerves is similar to that in the hand and fingers. The weight of the foot is borne on three distinct points: the heel, the point where the big toe joins the first metatarsal bone, and the same point at the base of the little toe. The elasticity of the foot is greatest in the longitudinal arch, and the transverse arch is so arranged that only the heads of the first and fifth metatarsals bear much weight. This is altered in flat-foot (q.v.). The main tarsal bones are the astragalus which supports the leg-bones and the calcaneus which forms the heel; the others, smaller in size, are the scaphoid, three cuneiform or wedge-shaped bones and the cuboid bone. *See* Corns; Bunions; Chilblains; Gout; Nails; Drop-foot; Club-foot.

Foramen: a natural opening especially into or through

bone for the passage of blood vessels or nerves. The largest foramen is the foramen magnum at the base of the skull through which passes the spinal cord.

Forceps: instruments for taking hold of objects, from tissues in the course of an operation to the head of the baby in a difficult labour. Some have notched handles and two fine blades so that they can be used to hold and compress blood vessels to stop bleeding, some, called bone forceps, are made with blades and handles strong enough to cut through bone. Forceps exist in all shapes and sizes and have many names; perhaps the most famous are Spencer Wells, named after the English surgeon who invented them to stop arterial bleeding, and Chamberlen's obstetric forceps, invented by the man midwife Peter Chamberlen (1560–1631), the original obstetric forceps.

Foreign Bodies: anything found in a part which is not naturally there; foreign bodies are, for example, found in the intestines, ears and noses of children in consequence of swallowing things which cannot be digested or poking small objects into the ear and nose. Foreign bodies often get into the eyes where they cause pain and irritation and can be dangerous. They are of prime importance in military surgery, for if they are not removed they can cause chronic infection and prevent wounds healing. Foreign bodies which have been swallowed may stick in the gullet, or may be dangerous – sharp fragments, open safety-pins – and have to be taken out by the surgeon. Few objects can have been so thoroughly foreign as that encountered by a British surgeon who is alleged to have removed from a patient's rectum a bust of Napoleon.

Formalin: a gas prepared by the oxydation of methyl alcohol. It is used as a solution in water (40%) for fixing and preserving specimens.

Formic Acid: a substance found in the stings of certain insects such as ants, bees and wasps. It has been used in the treatment of arthritis on the assumption that 'natural' products have some virtue not possessed by synthetic ones and that, since it occurs in creatures which are noted for their activity, formic acid will produce a similar freedom of movement in those who take it.

Fractures: in theory fractures of bone may occur in any part of the skeleton, but in practice they are most commonly found in certain well-defined areas; for example the most common fracture of the forearm is a Colles' fracture of the wrist, and the most common fracture of the leg is a Pott's fracture of the ankle. This is partly due to the varying strength or weakness of bones in different areas, partly due to the very similar ways in which people tend to have accidents, for example falling on the outstretched hand in the former instance, 'going over on the ankle' in the latter. Numerous different types of fracture are described: (1) *simple fracture* – the bones are broken cleanly with little laceration of surrounding tissue and no communication with the skin surface; (2) *greenstick fracture* – characteristic of injuries in children when the bones, being soft and not fully calcified, bend rather than break right through; (3) *open or compound fracture* – the fracture communicates with the skin and is obviously in danger of infection; (4) *complete and incomplete fractures* – these are distinguished by the degree of separation of the broken ends – a mere crack needs no further interference whereas a complete fracture with separation of the ends may need to be 'reduced' under an anaesthetic; (5) *comminuted fractures* – much splintering occurs, and part of the bone is broken into small pieces; (6) *impacted fractures* – in these one part of the bone is telescoped into the other.

In early life bones contain a good deal of fibrous tissue and hence are resilient and more likely to bend than break, but with increasing age they come to contain increasing amounts of calcium and therefore become brittle and heal less easily once a fracture occurs. Bones are broken most frequently by indirect violence; the force is applied at some point other than that where the break occurs, and is transmitted from the point of impact as in the Colles' fracture of the wrist already mentioned. Direct violence is usually associated with crushing injuries. The bone is broken at the point of impact and the fracture is likely from the nature of the cause to be complicated or compound. In a few instances a fracture is caused by muscular action (i.e. by the violent and sudden pull of muscles); this is a common cause of fracture of the knee-cap and sometimes happens in throwing at ball games. Finally, those who are suffering from certain diseases associated with decalcification of the bones, cysts, or tumours in bone, may sustain fractures which occur spontaneously with little or no violence; these cases will obviously need further investigation and are to be suspected when a fracture occurs without violence or when a series of fractures occurs with only slight violence. Following a fracture there is a certain amount of bleeding from blood vessels which have been torn both within the substance of the bone and in its surrounding membrane or periosteum. The blood forms a clot which surrounds the broken bone ends, and gradually the clot becomes organized with the formation of small arteries, veins and a certain amount of fibrous tissue. This is known as a soft callus. With the deposition of calcium salts the fibrous tissue soon begins to harden and it forms a hard callus which initially extends in a ring around the fracture, giving it a bulging appearance. Finally, excess bone is absorbed unless the bone ends are not completely in apposition when a bulge may remain to strengthen the area.

SYMPTOMS: certain signs present in most fractures enable them to be recognized. These signs include uselessness of the part (particularly when a limb is affected), pain on movement, and deformity, which usually occurs when the bone ends are displaced, for example the limb is shortened or seems to be in an unnatural position. There is swelling, movement occurs where it should not, and the ends of the broken bone may be heard or felt grating against each other (crepitus).

TREATMENT: obviously, when medical help is expected soon, all that is necessary is to splint the bone with something rigid such as a piece of wood in the position which gives least pain. The patient should be kept comfortable (but not too hot) and given a warm drink. Many types of splint are described, but special splints should only be applied by those who have some experience. 'Reduction' of a fracture is accomplished by exerting a gentle pull on the end of the limb below the break until the ends come into apposition, but this is usually done under an anaesthetic and should not be attempted unless skilled help is not going to be available. Displaced fractures of the flat bones, for example the skull, cannot usefully be dealt with except by a surgeon. The general first-aid rule in fractures of the limbs is that, provided they are not open, the clothes should not be removed, movement should be reduced to a minimum, and splints should be applied to keep the arm or leg still. If splints are not available, the broken leg can be tied to the good one, or the arm tied to the side. In the case of a broken collar bone the arm should be slung just under the neck by the wrist. Fractures of other parts, being nearly always the result of direct violence, are likely to be compound and splinting is either unnecessary or impossible as a first-aid measure. When in doubt the best first-aid rule is 'splint them where they lie'; keep fractures of the leg in an extended position, put the arm in a sling, and for suspected fractures of the spine keep the patient lying flat on his stomach.

Fragilitas Ossium: a condition in which, as the name implies, the bones are fragile. No cause is known to account for the disease; it is sometimes hereditary, and the baby may be born with fractured bones. The ear is affected, patients often being found to be deaf, and sometimes the whites of the eyes – the sclera – are blue. The condition improves after puberty. Deformities may occur because of repeated fractures sustained in childhood.

Framboesia: *see* Yaws.

Freckles: small pigmented spots in the skin caused by exposure to the sun. They are rather like localized areas of sunburn, being collections of the pigment melanin, and occur mainly in blond or red-headed people. They are found attractive by most men and unattractive by women, who waste much time trying to remove them. Once they have formed they cannot be removed – they must be left to fade – but to some extent they can be avoided by the use of sunburn creams and keeping out of the sun. Obviously it is possible to cover freckles with cosmetics or disguise them by attaining a deep degree of sunburn.

Freud: *see* Psychoanalysis.

Friar's Balsam: balsams are substances exuded from the trunks of certain trees which contain resins and oils. They are, or were, mainly used in the preparation of cough medicines; Friar's Balsam, or Compound Tincture of Benzoin, is given as a soothing inhalation for colds in a dose of one teaspoonful of balsam to one pint of boiling water.

Fringe Medicine: a common term used for the methods of people who, sometimes rudely described as quacks, practise medicine usually without orthodox medical qualifications. The word quack is best reserved for uneducated individuals who peddle remedies on their own, often, or generally, knowing them to be worthless. Those we are concerned with here are not like that at all, and there is no reason to doubt that practitioners of fringe medicine are as sincere as practitioners of orthodox medicine. Most of them belong to 'professional' bodies which tend to have the following characteristics: (1) they are usually founded by one man (Hahnemann for homoeopathy, Andrew Still for osteopathy, D. D. Palmer for chiropractic which, more recent in origin than osteopathy, claims to 'adjust the back' and 'correct faulty nutrition'); (2) they are nearly all committed to a 'system', i.e. most of their theories can be framed in the form 'all disease is caused by . . .' with its corollary 'all diseases can be cured by . . .'; (3) unlike scientific medicine, they do not submit their results to scientific criteria of cure. Yet many of these bodies flourish, and we must ask ourselves why. The cynical answers would be (a) that the public is almost infinitely gullible, and (b) that the vast majority of diseases have a large psychological element, and that in any case, although time may not heal all wounds, it helps an awful lot. Most diseases are self-limiting. But the more fundamental answer to the popularity of fringe medicine is, paradoxically, the success of orthodox medicine, which has changed the pattern of disease.

The great plagues, the specific fevers of childhood, the nutritional diseases, are largely wiped out in technically advanced countries. People live longer and suffer more often from the irreversible conditions which sometimes accompany old age, such as inoperable cancer, osteoarthritis, atherosclerosis. In younger people, the infectious diseases have given way to neuroses and stress diseases, the diseases of malnutrition such as rickets to the diseases caused by eating too much. All these are much more difficult to treat, and the clients of unorthodox medicine are the disgruntled, the neurotic, the incurable who although not necessarily seriously ill want to try something else, the overfed, and the sedentary whose faulty posture leads to vague or positively severe aches and pains. These patients, who frankly sometimes bore the family doctor because they are always in his surgery but reject his advice, can often be helped by someone who listens, takes their diet and exercise in hand, and gives them the faith to accept a psychological kick in the pants. Tell a business executive that he must diet while staying at home, and he is unlikely to do so on the free advice of his N.H.S. doctor; but tell him of a place in the country where, for the small sum of 40 or 50 guineas a week, he can be starved, rubbed, and take unwonted exercises, and he will think it not only money well spent but is quite likely to be the better for his stay. There are, after all, plenty of people in the world who think the treatment they get is worth as much as they pay for it. Moreover, it must be remembered that with the exception of a few outstanding figures, scientific medicine hardly existed until about the middle of the nineteenth century, when anaesthetics and antiseptics and drugs which really worked were first discovered. Even at the beginning of the present century the number of drugs which had a specific effect on disease, such as quinine in malaria, Ehrlich's Salvarsan in syphilis, or iron in anaemia, could be numbered on the fingers of one hand and there were probably only about a score of drugs in the whole pharmacopoeia which had any significant effect in alleviating the symptoms of disease. In fact, until about a hundred years ago there was little difference between varying theories of medicine. Now, however, orthodox medicine can reasonably put forward the following objections to fringe medicine. (1) It is simply not true that all disease has a single basic cause and a single basic cure. Thus, although D. D. Palmer's son was prepared to state that diphtheria was caused by a dislocation of the sixth dorsal vertebra, it is only those who sit comfortably at home with complaints largely brought on by their own selfish worrying or inertia who are capable of the idiocy of supposing that the millions who die yearly of infectious diseases in the less well developed lands are really suffering from dislocation of the spine, wrong diet, or would respond to homoeopathic remedies. (2) Although it sometimes happens (as in the case of electroconvulsant therapy in psychiatry) that the orthodox physician does not always know why a particular treatment works, he is always trying to find out why it does. As far as possible, he bases what he does and the results he obtains on scientific criteria of pathology, treatment and cure. But no homoeopath, no osteopath, no chiropractor, has ever even attempted to demonstrate that his theory is true or how his methods work by techniques which would satisfy any scientist. (3) While believing that some cures are produced by manipulation, diet or the 'miracles' of Lourdes, the writer does not accept the official explanation for these cures; every doctor has seen, or at least heard of, cases of 'incurable' cancer which simply disappeared without any treatment, of 'agonizing' pains cured by an injection of plain water, and most doctors remember the notorious example of cortisone which initially caused hundreds of rheumatoid arthritis sufferers who had not walked for years to leap from their wheelchairs, although we now know that, except in selected cases, cortisone in this condition is not more useful than aspirin. (4) Although no risk is involved in numerous cases who go to naturopaths and the rest for treatment, there is very grave danger for those who have some disease which, diagnosed in time, can be cured by ordinary medicine or surgery. Accurate diagnosis may demand complicated and expensive techniques only available to the qualified man in touch with a hospital. Practitioners of fringe medicine may sometimes cure, often alleviate, but either way they are frequently guilty of what T. S. Eliot described as 'the worst treason – they do the right thing for the wrong reason'. *See* Acupuncture, Homoeopathy, Osteopathy, Diet, Naturopathy.

Frohlich's Syndrome: a group of symptoms occurring in pituitary disease which leads to the development of characteristics immortalized by the 'fat boy' in Dickens's *Pickwick Papers*, i.e. a grossly fat child given to overeating, slothful, prone to sleepiness, and sexually and emotionally immature. Treatment depends on the cause, which requires expert diagnosis. *See* Pituitary Gland.

Frostbite: exposure to cold interferes with the vitality of the tissues largely but not entirely by affecting the circulation, and produces frostbite. In response to severe cold the arteries contract so that the limb 'goes dead', and this, if prolonged, leads to gangrene. Removal from the cold in the earlier stages brings about a reaction with flushing and redness which, in minor degrees, is a welcome sign that circulation is returning but in excess may mean inflammation and death of the part. The circulation must be restored gently by warming the affected part against the body of the patient or another person. The treatment which used to be described in accounts of polar exploration which involves rubbing with snow is generally inadvisable, and extremes of heat or cold are likely to cause tissue breakdown. The general circulation of the body should be maintained by walking about if possible and hot drinks. Alcohol is usually forbidden, but although frostbite is more likely to attack those who drink a good deal the action of alcohol in dilating the arteries and stimulating the heart may be helpful as a first-aid measure. The rule is to keep the part warm and dry, avoid extremes of heat or cold, and do not rub.

Frozen Section: when operating for a growth the surgeon may not be able to tell for sure whether the tumour is malignant or not. Because it makes a great deal of difference to the extent of the operation, a specimen of the tissue in question, particularly in the case of tumours of the breast, may be frozen and then cut into sections sufficiently thin for the pathologist to examine under the microscope. The examination can be made in a quarter of an hour while the patient is kept anaesthetized, ready for the operation to be continued according to what the 'frozen section' reveals.

Fructose: fruit sugar, also called laevulose.

Fruit: most fruit contains at least 80% of water, the amount being less in starchy fruit such as bananas and greatest in melons, pumpkins, etc. The pulp consists mostly of starch and sugar, the other main constituents being acids such as citric, tartaric and malic and essential oils or volatile substances which give the characteristic taste. Most fruit contains varying amounts of Vitamin C, which is high in citrus fruit (with the exception of limes), blackcurrants, guavas and rosehips. Dried fruit from which the water has been largely removed, such as prunes, raisins and sultanas, dates, figs, dried apples, pears and apricots, contains large amounts of sugar and starch, but correspondingly little Vitamin C. Minerals in fruit include iron and calcium and most fruit has a slightly laxative action. Rhubarb and strawberries contain oxalic acid and in susceptible people can cause crystals to form in the urine.

Fugue: a patient may suffer from a change of consciousness in which he carries out acts apparently with a purpose, but has no recollection of them afterwards. This is a state of fugue; such a state of altered consciousness may occur in epilepsy.

Fulguration: the use of electricity to destroy tissue, applied usually to the use of diathermy to burn bladder tumours through an operating cystoscope. It is properly used to mean destroying tissue by means of sparks, but fulguration in the bladder is carried out under water.

Fumigation: the process of burning or volatizing substances in order to produce vapours which kill disease germs and vermin. Originally one of the procedures which added a sinister aspect to the infectious fevers when it was used to disinfect the sick-room, it is now rarely employed. Camphor and other resins have no effect whatever on germs and the only justification for their former use was the innate human belief that strong or nasty smells and tastes are more potent in driving out illness, germs, bad things and evil spirits, than odourless and tasteless substances (hence the faith of a large part of the public in 'strong' medicines, i.e. those with a foul taste or smell).

Functional Disease: in the past this was used as a term to describe those diseases in which the main element was believed to be neurotic, no organic disease having been found. Thus functional dyspepsia was dyspepsia in which no damage to the stomach could be demonstrated in a patient who suffered from nervous tension. The diagnosis was often an excuse for doing nothing, but the realization that 'functional' malfunctioning is just as troublesome to the patient as organic disease, is not synonymous with 'imaginary', can lead to structural changes and is susceptible to treatment, has led to the term being discontinued save among those who are entirely mechanically minded.

Fungus: some diseases are caused by fungi and many antibiotics (q.v.) are derived from them. For diseases caused by fungi *see* Athlete's Foot, Ringworm, Candida albicans, Blastomyces, Histoplasmosis, Madura Foot, Farmer's Lung. For poisonous fungi sometimes mistaken for edible ones, *see* Poisonous Plants.

Funny Bone: *see* Humerus.

Furuncle: a boil (q.v.).

G

Gait: the way in which a person walks often gives important information about the medical or surgical conditions from which he may suffer. Typical are the Chaplinesque gait of severe flatfoot with the toes turned out and the feet placed flat on the ground, the dragging leg following a hemiplegia or stroke, the gait of alcoholic and other forms of neuritis in which foot-drop causes the knees to be raised higher than usual as if walking through mud, and the 'festinant' gait of paralysis agitans in which short quick steps are taken so that the legs seem to be trying to keep up with the top part of the body. In damage to the knee joint (for example arthritis) the leg is held stiff, and in hip-joint disease the diseased leg is swung round upon the healthy one, the whole pelvis entering into the movement. When, as in locomotor ataxia, the sensory nerves supplying information from the legs are damaged, the heels are placed on the ground with a stamping motion and the eyes kept fixed to the ground; when they are closed or the patient tries to turn he is liable to fall down. Needless to say, gaits only give suggestions about what might be wrong and an accurate diagnosis is made on other grounds.

Galactagogue: an agent designed to increase the flow of milk.

Galactocoele: a cyst in the breast containing milk; it is caused by obstruction of a milk duct.

Galenical: originally a preparation made from a formula ascribed to Galen, the medical adviser to Marcus Aurelius, the term is now applied to preparations which contain organic as opposed to pure chemical substances.

Gall-bladder: the gall-bladder is part of the biliary system, which is concerned with draining the bile from the liver, storing it and concentrating it, and conveying it ultimately to the intestines. The bile is collected in the liver by small ducts which coalesce until two large ducts are formed; these leave the liver in a deep fissure named the porta hepatis, which also admits to the liver the portal artery and vein with nerve plexuses and small lymphatic vessels.

The right and left hepatic ducts unite to form the common hepatic duct after they leave the porta hepatis, and this duct is continuous with the bile duct which runs down to the duodenum. The name of the common hepatic duct changes during its course because the cystic duct – the duct leading from the gall-bladder – runs into it, and it is at this point that the bile duct is formed, which receives another duct running from the pancreas before it empties into the duodenum. The gall-bladder is a cul-de-sac, and the only way in or out is through the cystic duct. It lies on the undersurface of the liver, and the rounded end may project a little from under cover of the free edge of the liver. It is just under the lower margin of the ribs on the right-hand side, about half-way out from the middle line. The function of the gall-bladder is to store and concentrate bile, discharging it as necessary at intervals. After it has emptied, more bile trickles down the common hepatic duct from the liver, but it cannot escape into the duodenum because a muscle called the biliary sphincter closes the bile duct. The bile therefore finds its way up the cystic duct, through a spiral valve formed by a fold of mucosa inside the duct, into the gall-bladder. Here the mucosal lining withdraws fluid from the bile and concentrates it, and the muscle of the wall of the gall-bladder relaxes to accommodate the increasing volume until the signal comes for it to contract and expel the concentrated bile into the bile duct. This signal is given about half an hour after the beginning of a meal, and comes both from the brain via the vagus nerve and from the intestine, for a hormone called cholecystokinin is released from the mucosa of the duodenum in response to the presence of food. The function of the gall-bladder can be observed by X-rays, for organic iodine compounds are excreted by the liver in the bile and concentrated in the gall-bladder; if the compounds are radio-opaque, they show up the outline of the gall-bladder. It is found that the substances which cause the most complete contraction of the gall-bladder are egg yolk, meat and fat. *See* Cholangiogram, Cholangitis, Cholecystitis, Cholelithiasis.

Galls: are excrescences produced in plants and trees by puncture and laying of eggs within by parasitic insects; they are better known as 'oak apples' or 'witches' brooms' and the commonly used one is the oak apple produced on *Quercus infectoria* by the insect *Cynips gallae tinctoriae*. Containing tannic and gallic acids, galls were used as astringents, particularly in the form of an ointment with or without opium, for applying to bleeding piles, although one may doubt their ability to do more than provide temporary relief.

Galvanism: named after Luigi Galvani (1737–98), who spent much of his life in research on the effects of electricity on animal muscle. Galvanism was a method of treatment and alleviation of pain by the application of electrical currents. Its scope is much limited today, and it is mainly used for muscular stimulation of tissues which, due to disease of the nerves, might otherwise waste, or for the relief of rheumatic pains. Nobody now believes that the passage of electricity through the tissues in itself produces any specific effect, and the decreasing category of diseases of unknown origin for which (as in the neuroses) Galvanism was once used has decreased its interest to the physician, although it is still popular among quacks and in the less scientifically advanced parts of the world.

Gamma Globulin: most antibodies are proteins which fall into the class of gamma globulins. Globulins are proteins which are soluble in salt solutions but not in plain water, and they can be divided into three groups by their electrophoretic mobility – alpha globulins have the greatest, beta intermediate, and gamma the least. It follows that if gamma globulins are separated from the other blood proteins the resulting fraction is very rich in antibodies (*see* Allergy for a discussion of antibodies), and can be used to provide passive immunity. It is used in two forms: one is gamma globulin derived from the serum of ordinary adults who can be expected to have formed an immunity to the common diseases of the communities in which they live, and the second is gamma globulin derived from patients convalescent from the illnesses against which it is desired to protect. Diseases in which gamma globulin is used include measles, infectious hepatitis, yellow fever, occasionally mumps, vaccinia, smallpox, tetanus, and haemolytic disease of the newborn where mothers found to have Rh positive cells from the foetus in their circulation can (if it is available) be treated by gamma globulin with a high content of incomplete anti-D rhesus antibody. *See* Hemolytic Disease of the Newborn.

Gammexane: proprietary name for an insecticide (benzene hexachloride) active against a large range of insect pests.

Ganglion: a word referring to two different entities: (1) a collection of nerve cells in the course of a nerve or a network of nerve fibres; (2) a swelling found in relation to tendon sheaths and joint capsules. The latter is a minor but sometimes annoying complaint. The swelling is formed of a material like jelly contained in fibrous tissue, often as a number of cysts closely bound together; these swellings are found in relation to the wrist, particularly on the back, and less often on the fingers or the palm of the hand. They are not painful, but may be inconvenient. The traditional treatment is a sharp blow with the family Bible, but it is sensible to show the ganglion to the doctor before treating it in such a way for some are due to tuberculosis. In any case the best treatment may be surgical removal, for ganglia tend to recur after they have been burst by a blow or by steady pressure with the thumbs.

Gangrene: a condition in which a part dies while it is still attached to the rest of the body. It is classified as wet and dry gangrene; dry gangrene is the result of blockage of the arteries, and wet gangrene follows arterial and venous insufficiency and bacterial infection. In dry gangrene the part, possibly a toe or a finger, becomes shrivelled and black; a zone of demarcation develops where the living tissue meets the dead, and in time the dead tissue separates and falls off. Gangrene is associated with diabetes; it may follow wounds, burns, long exposure to cold, the action of drugs such as adrenaline and ergot which may cause spasm of the arteries, and exposure to strong acids, alkalies or carbolic acid. (For this reason phenol must not be used on dressings.) Gas gangrene is due to the infection of dead muscle with the organisms Clostridium welchii and Cl. oedematiens, which live on dead tissue without oxygen and produce exotoxins which kill muscle fibres round about, so producing more dead muscle for the organisms to invade. The organisms set up a fermentation in the tissues which leads to the formation of bubbles of gas.

TREATMENT: is surgical. In hospital attempts may be made to improve the blood supply to the part, and to keep dry gangrene sterile and cool until the gangrenous portion separates. In some cases the surgeon may decide to amputate, but he has to do so at a level well above the actual site of the gangrene because the blood supply in a part which has become gangrenous will be insufficient to allow satisfactory healing to take place. Gas gangrene has to be treated by drastic surgery, but with antibiotics the outlook is no longer as uniformly hopeless as it once was.

Gargles: various substances which are brought into contact with the back of the throat without swallowing; they are usually employed for such conditions as tonsillitis, pharyngitis and 'sore throats' in general. Their action is to clean the mouth and throat of mucus and discharge, to increase the blood supply to the throat by reason of their warmth or the chemicals they contain, and, if antiseptics are used, to kill some of the infecting organisms. Gargles are of strictly limited value since the solution is in actual contact with the membranes for too short a period to produce much effect, and the germs, by the time gargling is thought necessary, are too deeply embedded in the tissues to be reached. However, the local anaesthetic effect of aspirin makes soluble aspirin a useful gargle to relieve discomfort (2 tablets in a glass of warm water which can subsequently be swallowed), and a strong salt solution will cleanse the throat of clinging mucus. Neither as gargles nor mouthwashes are strong antiseptics generally advisable, but potassium chlorate (12 grains in a glass of warm water), potassium permanganate (a few crystals similarly used are sufficient to make a pink solution which can be seen through), glycerine with borax and boric acid or with thymol, and most of the reputable proprietary gargles are helpful. As already indicated their main function is to add to the patient's comfort by cleaning the throat and relieving irritation.

Gas Gangrene: *see* Gangrene.

Gastrectomy: surgical operation for the removal of part or the whole of the stomach. The extent of the operation depends upon the condition for which it is being carried out; it is indicated in cases of chronic peptic ulceration, severe bleeding from ulcers, scarring of the duodenum after ulceration leading to obstruction, and perforation of an ulcer. Except in cases of emergency the stomach should not be removed until adequate medical treatment has been tried, but in cases properly selected the results are very good. Gastrectomy is necessary in cases of cancer of the stomach. *See* Stomach Diseases.

Gastric: the word means 'relating to the stomach'. The phrase 'a gastric stomach' is therefore a tautology.

Gastritis: inflammation of the stomach.

Gastro-enteritis: inflammation of the stomach and the intestine, usually due to infection. *See* Dysentery, Diarrhoea.

Gastro-enterostomy: an opening made surgically between the stomach and the intestine in order to bypass the pylorus and the duodenum, and to allow the alkaline juices of the small bowel (the jejunum) to flow directly into the stomach and neutralize excessive acidity. The results of this operation in cases of peptic ulceration are not very good, and about a third of all the patients so treated develop ulceration at the artificial opening within ten years. It is therefore reserved for use in cases which are not suitable because of age or infirmity to undergo the more severe, but more satisfactory, operation of gastrectomy.

Gastroscope: an instrument with an interior telescopic system and light which is passed down the gullet into the stomach so that the inside of the stomach may be examined. The observer may be able to tell whether an ulcer is simple or cancerous, and in cases of doubt may be able to see an ulcer which has not been shown up by X-rays. It is not possible to inspect the whole of the stomach in this way, and a negative gastroscopic examination does not rule out the presence of an ulcer. No anaesthetic is necessary for the examination, which is perhaps uncomfortable but safe.

Gastrostomy: an operation on the stomach whereby an opening is made between the stomach and the exterior through the abdominal wall. It is done in cases where the oesophagus is blocked by a tumour or otherwise obstructed; in the days when such dangerous corrosive poisons as lye or caustic soda and the mineral acids were used widely in the home it was not uncommon for them to be swallowed by mistake or by way of committing suicide, and then a gastrostomy would be necessary so that the patient could be fed. The operation is less performed now than once it was owing to the reduced frequency of this type of accident and the improved surgical techniques which have made the operation of oesophagectomy possible. (In this operation the damaged or diseased part of the oesophagus is removed and the continuity restored.) Gastrostomy may still be valuable in the treatment of growths, for if it is carried out temporarily to short-circuit the area of growth it may make intensive irradiation possible. The tumour is later removed, and the gastrostomy closed.

Gel: a colloid (q.v.) which contains a good deal of liquid but has the consistency of gelatin.

Gelatin: a colourless transparent substance used in making jellies; in medicine it is used as a base for suppositories, etc. It is made from the collagen of connective tissue – from the skin, tendons, fascia and bones of animals. Although it is a protein, it has relatively little nutritive value, so that clear soups and stock made from it, including calves' foot jelly, are less nourishing than is often thought. In the manufacture of jellies, gums and pastilles, vegetable materials such as agar (q.v.) are increasingly used.

Gelsemium: the root of the yellow jasmine, containing gelsemine, a very poisonous alkaloid. It is rarely used except perhaps in the treatment of migraine and neuralgia, because it is unreliable in its effects and toxic except in very small doses.

Gene: geneticists use the word to mean a factor which controls the inheritance of a specific characteristic. It has now been established that deoxyribonucleic acid is the chemical substance through which the patterns of composition of protein and the structure of cells in an organism are passed from parents to offspring, and the gene can be regarded as a region of the very long spiral deoxyribonucleic acid (D.N.A.) molecule responsible for the duplication of a specific inherited molecule.

General Paralysis of the Insane: also known as G.P.I. and dementia paralytica, this disease is a manifestation of the third stage of syphilis (q.v.).

CAUSE: infection of the brain and nervous system with the organisms of syphilis; the brain becomes shrunken and the membranes thick.

SYMPTOMS: the earliest symptom is often mental deterioration. This begins ten or even twenty years after the primary infection, and is found generally in men. The patient becomes forgetful, complains of headaches, may be obviously inefficient at his job, and while he may drink more freely is more susceptible to the action of alcohol. There may be tremor of the tongue and of the muscles of the face, and slurring or stammering speech, while actions are unrestrained and the emotions unstable. Mental changes lead the patient to laugh or weep too readily, or to adopt a general attitude which is over-confident and over-optimistic. Grandiose delusions of wealth may involve him in heavy debt, or in absurd actions such as buying a number of expensive motor cars or getting mixed up in foolish financial schemes which betray his lack of judgment. Some patients become depressed and self-condemning, confessing early sins of a relatively trivial sort. Fits and confusion may mark the early stages of the illness, and as it progresses the patient becomes more paralysed until he is bedridden and incontinent. In the absence of treatment the end is death within about four years.

TREATMENT: a course of penicillin; after preliminary smaller doses, for the destruction of great quantities of spirochaetes may set up a severe reaction (the Herxheimer reaction), 600,000 units of procaine penicillin are given every day by intramuscular injection until a total of 10 million units has

313

been given. This treatment is sometimes combined with intramuscular injections of bismuth 200 mg weekly for 10 weeks, and in the rare cases where penicillin does not improve the disease the patient can be treated in a heat cabinet. Formerly a high temperature was induced by infecting the patient artificially with malaria, but this somewhat erratic and uncontrollable therapy has been replaced by the fever cabinet. The outlook is reasonable if treatment is started early, and in favourable cases a good recovery is possible. If the disease has been in progress for some time partial recovery may be all that is achieved, and in some cases only arrest of the disease can be hoped for; in a very few cases the disease does not respond to treatment. Patients are usually admitted to hospital when the disease is diagnosed, for they can become unmanageable at home – indeed, they may have to go into a mental hospital. Follow-up at stated intervals after treatment is absolutely essential, for there may be a relapse or incomplete long-term response to treatment and the course of penicillin may have to be repeated.

Gentian: the root of the yellow gentian is used as a bitter to stimulate appetite, and is incorporated in various Continental alcoholic aperitifs.

Gentian Violet: an aniline dye used by bacteriologists to stain bacteria and so make them visible under the microscope. It has been used as a skin antiseptic, for example in impetigo, but it stains the skin and clothes a deep violet which is difficult to remove. It has therefore been replaced by less inconvenient remedies.

Genu Valgum: knock-knee.

Genu Varum: bow-legs.

Geriatrics: the branch of medicine that deals with the diseases of old age and studies its problems. The term originates with Dr I. L. Nascher of New York who in 1909 was the first to employ it and to emphasize that something constructive could be done about such problems instead of merely accepting them as inevitable. However, little was done by medicine until after World War 2 when, with an increasing number of old people in the population, the social issues arising therefrom meant that geriatrics had to be taken more seriously. The problem of the old is essentially one of industrial society in which families tend to become small and the old, being unproductive, are regarded as financial liabilities.

The physical and mental changes associated with age come on gradually and at times which depend upon the individual, some being hale and hearty in their nineties while others are already old in the fifties. Broadly, the mental effects of age are due to changes in the brain tissues associated with narrowing and hardening of the arteries which lead to an inadequate blood supply. The memory for recent events becomes poor, whereas that for long-past events is retained; the emotions are superficial and easily aroused so that the individual tends to be sentimental and tearful; and traits which have always been present such as suspiciousness become exaggerated. In more severe cases there is a lack of attention to social conventions and the patient may be dirty, untidy, and incontinent in the control of bowels and bladder. These qualities are exaggerated in those who live alone and take inadequate nourishment. Although there are basic physical changes in the body, it is important to emphasize that much of the disability of old age is socially conditioned, as those who live solitary lives lose interest in themselves and their general attitude changes for the worse. Much can be done in the way of clubs and other communal activities to restore an interest in life to such cases (*see* comments on 'institutional neurosis' under Iatrogenic Disease).

Germ: popular word for the micro-organisms of disease.

German Measles: (Rubella). An infectious disease associated with a skin rash.

CAUSE: rubella is a virus infection spread by direct contact. The incubation period is two to three weeks, and the disease is infective during the time when it is developing and while it is acute.

SYMPTOMS: the obvious sign is a rash, usually starting on the face but spreading quickly to the trunk. The spots are small

– between 1 and 3 mm across – and pink, and they last for about two days. The day before the rash appears the patient may feel ill, and complain of a stiff neck and headache. The eyes become pink, and a very characteristic sign of rubella is enlargement of the lymph glands, particularly those behind and below the ear. Complications are extremely uncommon, although adults with the infection may develop pain in the joints of the hands and feet. As far as children are concerned, the disease is virtually harmless, but there is one condition in which the consequences of rubella may be grave – and that is pregnancy. If a woman in the first three months of pregnancy is infected with rubella, the foetus may show microcephaly, deafness, heart defects or cataract, and may be stunted. The risk to the foetus is great, for it is particularly susceptible to the virus. As rubella is innocuous in childhood, it is logical and sensible to recommend that every effort should be made to encourage the spread of the infection among young girls.

TREATMENT: none is necessary in the vast majority of cases. If a woman in the first three months of pregnancy thinks she has run the risk of infection she must seek medical advice. In some cases gamma globulin (q.v.) has been found effective in preventing the development of the disease, but it is not entirely reliable. *See* Immunization.

Gestation: pregnancy.

Giardiasis: Giardia lamblia are single-celled organisms with four flagellae (i.e. appendages shaped like whips which they use to propel themselves along). The organisms are found in the duodenum and the bile duct, and to a certain extent along the small intestine; they may produce diarrhoea, especially in children, which is treated with mepacrine.

Giddiness: *see* Vertigo.

Gigantism: a tumour of the acidophil cells of the pituitary gland (q.v.) occurring before growth is complete produces gigantism, for the tumour secretes abnormal quantities of the growth hormone. Those afflicted may grow until they are 7 or 8 feet tall, and go blind because of the pressure of the tumour on the optic nerves as they cross over above the pituitary body. Pituitary giants are not as strong as their appearance suggests. *See* Acromegaly.

Gin: an alcoholic drink made from rye or barley with the addition of juniper berries and hops and formerly used medically as a diuretic (q.v.). Its alcoholic content is the same as that of whisky or brandy and the idea once held that it is more likely than other alcoholic drinks to cause cirrhosis of the liver is quite unfounded. *See,* Alcohol, Cirrhosis.

Ginger: is prepared from the roots of Zingiber officinale, which comes from East India and the Caribbean, and is used as a condiment or medically as a carminative to stimulate the digestive juices and relieve flatulence. White ginger is the root after scraping; if it has only been scalded it is black.

Gingivitis: inflammation of the gums. *See* Teeth.

Glanders: a contagious disease of horses, donkeys, mules, and also cats, guinea-pigs and dogs, which is (very rarely) communicated to man through abrasions on the skin or through the eye, mouth or nose.
CAUSE: the micro-organism Loefflerella mallei present in the saliva and nasal discharge of infected animals.
SYMPTOMS: a small boil appears on the spot first infected and if this is on the hand the lymph vessels running up the arm soon appear as angry red lines. The germ enters the general circulation and two or three weeks after contact the temperature rises and the patient starts vomiting and coughing, and develops pustules and ulcers over the surface of the body, pains in the joints and growing weakness. The acute form of the disease is likely to be fatal within two weeks but chronic infections may last for months, sometimes abating, sometimes becoming more acute, but usually ending in death.
DIAGNOSIS: this is effected with mallein prepared from the glanders bacilli and used in the same way as tuberculin to detect tuberculosis. In stables it is extremely difficult to diagnose and many animals are likely to die and new arrivals be infected before the disease is even suspected. Affected animals must be destroyed and their stables disinfected. The term glanders is sometimes used specifically for the nasal

form of the infection, the term 'farcy' being used of the skin eruptions and the underlying nodules.

TREATMENT: the infecting organisms are tested for sensitivity to antibiotics and the appropriate preparations are given. In some infections the use of vaccines has proved helpful.

Glands: a word used to describe several different types of structure within the body: (1) the large organs such as the liver, kidney and pancreas which produce a secretion (i.e. some substance to be used by the organism, for example bile from the liver, the pancreatic enzymes from the pancreas) and discharge it through a duct to the area where it is needed; or an excretion (for example urine, the waste excreted by the kidney); (2) the small glands which secrete digestive ferments (for example the salivary glands and the glands lining the gastro-intestinal tract) or those which protect and lubricate the skin (the sebaceous glands); (3) the endocrine glands, which secrete substances directly into the bloodstream, upon which the whole functioning of the body and mind depend. They are often described as the ductless glands (for example the pituitary, thyroid, suprarenal and sex glands); (4) the lymph glands. It is with the last-named we are concerned here, the others being dealt with under their respective headings.

Lymph glands are found throughout the body but particularly at junctions, so that there are glands behind the knee and in front of the elbow, under the arm-pit and at the angle of the jaw, in the groin and behind the ears; deep glands lie in the region where the mesentery or cellophane-like membrane supporting the intestines is attached to the back of the abdominal cavity, at the junction of the right and left bronchi, and in many other areas. Together they form the lymphatic system, and between them run lymphatic vessels which finally join to form the thoracic duct which pours lymph into the bloodstream at the point where the internal jugular vein meets the subclavian at the root of the neck on the left side; a smaller duct collecting lymph from the right arm and the right side of the chest and neck enters the venous system on the right side of the same point.

Lymphatic vessels and glands have four main functions: (1) the lacteals in the intestinal walls collect certain food-stuffs during digestion which, passing through the mesenteric glands, are poured into the bloodstream via the thoracic duct; (2) the glands are the site where the lymphocytes, one type of white blood corpuscle, are formed; (3) they produce antibodies in response to the local presence of antigens; (4) they act as a filter preventing infection from entering the bloodstream. The last is the most obvious function of the lymph glands as they become swollen in the presence of infection in the region and if overwhelmed may break down and suppurate. In a serious infection of the hand the red lines of the lymphatics can be seen running up the arm and the glands in the arm-pit become swollen and tender; in foot or leg infections a similar change occurs in the groin; in lung infections the glands where the bronchi leave the lung to join and form the windpipe are affected, and swellings in the neck in cases of sore throat or ear disease are familiar to most people. Enlarged glands of this sort anywhere in the body are described as adenitis, a condition which can only be dealt with by seeking and dealing with the source of infection. The glands themselves are best left alone unless they break down and suppurate. Generalized enlargement of the lymph glands may occur in various systemic as opposed to local infections, and local enlargement is found in cases of malignant disease where the glands hold up cancerous cells breaking away from the primary growth.

Glandular Fever: (Infective mononucleosis). An acute fever, usually occurring in isolated cases but sometimes seen in epidemic form. It is commonest between the ages of 15 and 25.

CAUSE: infection by one or more varieties of virus, some cases apparently being infected with the Epstein-Barr, or E.B., virus, others with the cytomegalovirus.

SYMPTOMS: sore throat, with difficulty in swallowing and sometimes severe inflammation of the tonsils, coming on between four days and three weeks after exposure to infection. The lymph glands in the neck are enlarged and tender, and often there is general enlargement of the glands. There is a fever, which may be considerable; after a week a rash may develop which looks like the rash of German measles, and in severe cases there may be jaundice. The disease may recur after an apparently complete recovery, and it often drags on for weeks while the patient feels 'run

319

down' for months afterwards. The diagnosis is made by examining the blood, which shows an increase of lymphocytes and sometimes special glandular fever cells. An antibody can be demonstrated in the serum of many patients which is capable of agglutinating the red cells of a sheep (the Paul-Bunnel reaction).

TREATMENT: no special treatment is possible. Secondary infection of the throat may have to be cleared up by penicillin or tetracycline.

Glauber's Salts: sodium sulphate, used as an aperient. It works by drawing fluid into the intestine and not by irritating the wall of the gut, and is therefore useful on the rare occasions when aperients are necessary.

Glaucoma: a disease of the eye usually occurring after middle age.
CAUSE: the pressure of the fluid inside the eye rises and the optic disc and retina are damaged so that in time the eye becomes blind. The aqueous humour (*see* Eye) in normal circumstances drains away at the angle between the surface of the iris and the margin of the cornea, where there are a number of fine channels which lead into the canal of Schlemm and so into the veins. If the channels are blocked, or the secretion of fluid is too great to be drained, the pressure inside the eyeball rises.
SYMPTOMS: acute headache, severe pain on the affected side with perhaps nausea and vomiting, and change in vision. Coloured haloes are seen round lights, acuity is lost and vision dimmed, the eyelids are swollen and the eye is red. A light shone into the eye shows up greenish grey, and the eyeball feels hard when touched through the eyelids. The disease starts in one eye and if untreated may affect the other.
TREATMENT: this is a matter for the specialist, and should be undertaken as soon as the eye becomes affected. The longer the interval between the onset of the disease and a visit to the doctor the less likely treatment is to be successful. The doctor may treat acute glaucoma by using eyedrops of eserine or pilocarpine which contract the pupil and widen the angle where the canal of Schlemm runs between the iris and the margin of the cornea, so that fluid has a greater chance of escaping from the eye, but it may be necessary to

operate on the eye in order to provide a wide path through which the fluid can escape. Such operations are not severe and if undertaken in time are usually successful.

Gleet: the slight watery discharge characteristic of chronic gonorrhoea.

Glioma: a tumour of the brain and spinal cord which arises from the tissue of the nervous system as opposed to tumours which arise from the membranes covering the brain (meningiomas) and those which arise from the blood vessels (haemangiomas). Gliomas are regarded as malignant tumours because they invade and infiltrate the nervous tissue in which they lie, so that there is no clear line between normal and tumour-bearing tissue. They do not spread by metastasis (q.v.), but it is not often possible for the surgeon to remove them without doing such damage to the brain as to leave the patient gravely crippled – with no guarantee that the tumour will not recur. Treatment is rarely undertaken by the surgeon except when the tumour is cystic, in which case the tumour tissue may be confined to a small area in the wall of the cyst, or when the glioma is confined to an area of the brain which can be amputated without entirely crippling effect. X-ray therapy may be effective on some sorts of glioma. Symptoms caused by gliomas depend on which part of the brain they destroy, and upon whether they cause a major rise in pressure inside the skull. The course of the illness depends on the speed of growth of the tumour; gliomas are classified broadly into four groups, grade 1 being the least malignant and grade 4 the most malignant. Death may ensue from a grade 4 glioma within a few months, but a patient may survive for years with a grade 1 tumour.

Globulin: a class of proteins found in the blood, insoluble in water but soluble in weak salt solutions. Divided into alpha, beta and gamma globulins according to their electrophoretic activity. *See* Gamma Globulin.

Globus Hystericus: the feeling that there is a 'lump in the throat' preventing swallowing or producing choking, characteristic of certain neuroses and caused by anxiety.

Glomerulonephritis: a disease of the kidneys affecting the glomeruli (*see* Kidney).

CAUSE: the disease follows infections usually with haemolytic streptococci of the throat, skin or burns. It used to occur in association with scarlet fever. It is brought about by an antigen-antibody reaction in the glomerulus which interferes with function and leads to the retention of salt, water and nitrogenous substances, with overloading of the circulation and oedema or swelling of the limbs.

SYMPTOMS: blood in the urine, pain in the small of the back, headache, and swelling of the legs or the face. In the majority of cases there is a history of a sore throat, and the patient may have a slight fever. He may become nauseated and start to vomit, and as the condition progresses the urine becomes more concentrated, the oedema more obvious, and the patient may develop headaches and a cough caused by oedema of the lungs and may become breathless. The acute phase of the disease is usually over within two weeks.

TREATMENT: rest in bed, and the use of penicillin to clear up any residual infection of the throat and prevent infection reaching the waterlogged lungs. The intake of water must be cut down, and the diet must be free from salt. The intake of fluid is regulated by the output, about half a litre being added to the amount of water passed the previous day. Complications such as rise of blood pressure, heart failure or oedema of the lungs or brain are treated as they arise; they are among the only conditions still logically treated by blood-letting. Patients are allowed out of bed about two weeks after the urinary output has returned to normal, but they must take things easily for another few weeks and be followed up carefully, for although the majority of cases make a complete recovery, some continue to pass red blood cells in the urine and show positive tests for protein, and among this small group of patients will be some who progress to kidney failure unless they are treated properly and promptly.

Glomus Tumour: there are normally in the finger tips and in other parts of the body such as the ears and the face communications between small arteries and veins which when open allow blood to bypass the capillary vessels. These short-circuits are called glomus bodies and are concerned with the regulation of skin temperature. Occasionally they form tiny pink tumours which are extremely painful and tender; they may occur under the nail, and the only treatment is surgical removal of nail and tumour.

Glossina: the tsetse fly, a biting fly which transmits the trypanosomes of sleeping sickness.

Glossitis: inflammation of the tongue.

Glossopharyngeal Nerve: the ninth cranial nerve. It contains both motor and sensory fibres, supplying motor impulses to the stylopharyngeus muscle in the throat, the secretory nerve to the parotid gland, and sensory fibres to the posterior third of the tongue and the throat and tonsil. These fibres include some conveying the sensation of taste from the posterior third of the tongue.

Glottis: the part of the larynx in which the voice is produced, i.e. the vocal folds or cords and the opening between them, the rima glottidis.

Glucagon: a hormone found in the pancreas which causes a rise in circulating blood sugar by increasing the release of glucose from the liver. It is used in the treatment of low blood sugar occurring in the diabetic patient, for it can safely be given by a layman and can be left with a member of the family of a diabetic in case he fails to balance his dose of insulin with an adequate intake of food and goes into coma.

Glucose: or grape-sugar; this is found in most fruit and in honey, and is the main form into which all other sugars and starches are reduced by digestion in the body. With the exception of alcohol it is the only natural food immediately absorbed by the stomach without being digested. It is therefore useful as an energy-producing substance in those who are too weak to digest heavier meals and is sometimes given in such cases intravenously. Since proportionately more energy is used up during fevers and the appetite may at the same time be lost, mildly effervescent lemon-flavoured glucose drinks are very useful in such conditions, being clean to the taste and acceptable when others are not. But it is sheer rubbish to suggest as is often done that normal people when tired require glucose, as most fatigue is a psychological state allied to boredom which has nothing to do with energy lack but rather with the lack of will to apply it.

Gluteal: the region of the buttocks, applied as an adjective to the muscles, nerves and blood vessels therein.

Gluten: the protein part of wheat flour which becomes sticky (cf. the word 'glutinous') on the addition of water. Since it can be separated from the starchy carbohydrate part of flour gluten is used in making diabetic bread and rolls which can be included in reducing diets. In some children intolerance of gluten gives rise to a condition in which fat cannot be absorbed from the intestine. *See* Coeliac Disease.

Glycerin: (Glycerine, Glycerol). An alcohol used in medicine occasionally as a purgative in doses of 1–2 teaspoonfuls but more often because of its pleasantly sweet taste added to various medicines. With gelatin, it forms the base of many pastilles, and it is used in suppositories to soften the motions if the passage of hard stools is painful.

Glycerophosphates: formerly much used as 'nerve tonics' because of the (false) assumption that since glycerophosphoric acid is a constituent of nerve tissue, glycerophosphates would feed the nerves. In fact the condition commonly named 'nerves' has nothing to do with the state of nourishment of the nerve cells, and glycerophosphates are excreted unchanged.

Glyceryl Trinitrate: the nitrites and organic nitrates relax smooth muscle fibres in the body and therefore lower the resistance of blood vessels to the passage of blood, for the vessel walls contain smooth muscle which narrows the aperture of the vessel when contracted. They are accordingly used in the treatment of angina pectoris (q.v.) for two reasons: they increase the flow of blood in the coronary arteries of the heart, and they reduce the pressure against which the labouring heart has to pump the blood into the arterial circulation and so reduce the work it has to do. Glyceryl trinitrate is taken in tablets containing 0.5 mg, and the amount required varies from one to four tablets. They should be chewed and sucked in the mouth, for the drug is best absorbed through the mucous membranes. It is useless to swallow the tablets. The effect is felt in a few minutes, and lasts for half an hour; this knowledge enables a patient suffering from angina to take glyceryl trinitrate before he has to make an effort which normally would bring on the pain.

Glycogen: the liver normally stores about 100 gm of glycogen, from which glucose can be derived as needed by the body. Glycogen is broken down into glucose by enzyme action under the influence of the hormones adrenalin and glucagon when increased amounts of glucose are needed, and is formed from glucose under the action of other hormones, notably thyroxine and cortisol. The uptake of blood glucose by the cells is influenced by the hormone insulin, which may also increase the formation of glycogen in the liver. The muscles contain glycogen in substantial amounts.

Glycosuria: the presence of sugar in the urine. *See* Diabetes.

Goitre: a swelling of the thyroid gland in the neck which may be (1) simple, that is, not associated with under- or over-activity of the gland, nor with malignancy; (2) malignant; (3) associated with under-action of the thyroid gland or hypothyroidism; (4) associated with over-action of the gland or hyperthyroidism.

1. *Simple goitre*
CAUSE: deficiency of iodine in the diet is the commonest cause, and as one would expect leads to a greater incidence of goitre among people who live in certain geographical areas such as the Himalayas, the Andes, and the Alps in Europe where the supplies of iodine in the water are low or absent. In such cases the over-growth of the thyroid is in response to the increased activity which is needed to try to keep up the supplies of the hormone thyroxine to the body.
SYMPTOMS: are caused by the size of the tumour, which can vary from the scarcely perceptible to enormous swellings like a grotesque collar which press upon the windpipe and gullet hard enough to make breathing and eating rather difficult.

325

TREATMENT: the administration of iodine in the diet as iodized salt or sodium iodide will prevent the formation of such goitres. If they have reached a size large enough to cause obstruction they must be removed surgically; when there are nodules in the thyroid they can be removed separately. In some cases haemorrhage occurs into these nodules and blows the gland up suddenly, so that a sudden worsening of symptoms occurs. Goitres in adults can sometimes be reduced by treatment with thyroid hormones, but this does not diminish the nodules.

2. *Malignant goitre.* A rare disease, if anything most common in areas where simple goitres are found.

SYMPTOMS: in younger patients a solitary nodule may be found, which is hard. In patients above 40 a different type of malignant growth develops, again showing itself in the thyroid by the presence of a growing nodule, but often making itself felt for the first time by the effect of secondary deposits particularly in the bones and the lungs. In patients over 60 malignancy of the thyroid takes the form of a diffuse enlargement of the gland with the development of obstruction of the gullet and the windpipe. The patient may be hoarse because of involvement of the nerves (recurrent laryngeal) which supply the larynx.

TREATMENT: in younger patients the thyroid gland is removed surgically with any lymph nodes that are obviously affected. The results are good. In the second type of tumour described above, the thyroid gland is removed and the secondary deposits are irradiated by giving the patient radioactive iodine. In some cases iodine is not taken up by the tumour tissue and external radiotherapy must be used. In all cases where the thyroid gland is removed the patients must be given thyroid hormone by mouth for the rest of their life. The last type of malignancy is best treated by radiotherapy.

3. *Hypothyroidism,* or *under-action of the thyroid gland.* In areas where the supply of iodine is deficient, or in cases where the thyroid gland is absent or unable to make its hormone satisfactorily, lack of the hormone (thyroxine) produces in children the cretin, and in adults the disease myxoedema. The condition may or may not be associated with a goitre.

SYMPTOMS: the cretinous baby looks normal at birth, but by the third month it may be seen that it is not feeding properly, and tends to fall asleep too much. In time it develops a coarse appearance, with a dry skin, large tongue which sticks out, and mental deficiency. In myxoedema the patient, who is commonly a woman of middle age, develops amenorrhoea, deafness, anaemia, a certain coarseness of the hair which becomes sparse, and increasing mental and physical slowness with aversion to the cold.

TREATMENT: in the case of an infant treatment must be started within six months of birth if it is to be fully effective; the administration of thyroxine must continue for life. The treatment of adult myxoedema is very satisfactory providing that the dose of thyroxine is not discontinued as soon as the patient has returned to normal. Again, the drug must be taken for life.

4. *Hyperthyroidism*, or *over-action of the thyroid* (Graves' disease, thyrotoxicosis). A disease found mostly in young female adults.

SYMPTOMS: the goitre is smooth but not as large as the simple goitre. The patient is excessively nervous, has a fine tremor of the hands, which are moist, loses weight although the appetite is increased, and has an increased pulse rate which may be felt as palpitations. She often becomes breathless on exertion, and dislikes hot weather. The condition is sometimes called exophthalmic goitre, because one of the common symptoms is protrusion of the eyes so that they appear to be staring. The lids are drawn back, and the white sclera can be seen all round the iris of the eye. An early symptom of hyperthyroidism may be diarrhoea.

TREATMENT: surgical removal of part of the gland is advisable if the goitre is large, or if the patient is between 30 and 45 years old, or if treatment with antithyroid drugs has proved ineffective. Antithyroid drugs act by interfering with the formation of thyroxine by the thyroid gland. The most commonly used drug is carbimazole. Methyl thiouracil and propyl thiouracil are also used, but in larger doses. Indications for the use of these drugs are the age of the patient – they should be used when the disease is present in children and in young adults – and pregnancy, but there is a considerable relapse rate when they are used on older patients. Once the disease has been controlled by the use of antithyroid drugs, a process which may take about eight weeks, it is necessary to continue taking a maintenance dose administered under medical supervision, for the drugs may have toxic effects which include enlargement of the lymph glands, fever, vomiting, abnormality of the formation of blood cells, rashes on the skin and swelling of the legs. Any patient taking antithyroid drugs who develops a sore throat must at once stop taking the drug and go to the doctor. The third method of treatment is the administration of radioactive iodine, which is very satisfactory but requires access to properly equipped departments concerned with the medical aspects of radiation. It is therefore not always available now, but should become more widely used in the future. In most cases a combination of antithyroid drugs and surgery offers the best chance of successful treatment, and in general it is true to say that few branches of surgery produce such gratifying results as that concerned with the thyroid gland.

Gold: gold salts were formerly used in the treatment of tuberculosis, but this has been abandoned. Gold is still sometimes used in cases of rheumatoid arthritis, but its mode of action is not understood. It should not be used when the patient suffers from disease of the liver or the kidneys or has anything wrong with his skin, for gold is liable to give rise to toxic effects which include generalized skin reactions, damage to the kidneys leading to the passage of blood and albumin in the urine, and diminution in the number of white cells in the blood. Gold may prove poisonous to the liver, and it may produce vomiting, diarrhoea and jaundice.

Golden Eye Ointment: yellow mercuric oxide ointment commonly used to relieve inflammation of the eyelids.

Gonad: the male or female sex gland.

Gonadotrophic Hormone: there are at least two distinct gonadotrophic hormones secreted by the pituitary gland which control the activity of the ovaries and the testicles. The first, called F.S.H. (follicle stimulating hormone), causes growth of the follicle which contains the ovum in the female and formation and development of spermatozoa in the male, and the second, L.H. (luteinizing hormone), brings about the release of the ovum from the ovary, the formation of the corpus luteum (q.v.) and the secretion of oestrogens and progestogens. In the male L.H. is concerned with the secretion of testicular androgens. Secretion of the gonadotrophic hormones by the pituitary body is controlled by the brain via the hypothalamus, upon which many varied stimuli act, not all of which are unconscious.

Gonorrhoea: a venereal disease usually spread by sexual intercourse with an infected person. Eye disease may reach the infant from an infected mother, and the young female child may catch vaginitis from infected towels or clothes.
CAUSE: the infecting agent is the diplococcus Neisseria gonorrhoeae.
SYMPTOMS: in men, a thick yellow discharge from the urethra at the end of the penis after an incubation period of 2–10 days, and pain on passing water. Later, if the disease is untreated, the discharge becomes clear and sticky, and the associated organs (testicles, bladder, prostate gland at the base of the bladder) may become inflamed and painful. Still later complications are scarring of the urethra so that urination becomes difficult or impossible (stricture), arthritis of the knee, ankle, wrist or elbow, usually supposed by the patient to be 'rheumatism', septicaemia with inflammation of the heart-valves (endocarditis), or abscesses in various parts of the body. In women, there is yellow vaginal discharge, pain on passing water and inflammation of the glands at the entry to the vagina; chronic infection may pass to the womb, Fallopian tubes and ovaries leading to frequent miscarriages, sterility, and, less frequently, peritonitis which may be fatal. The eye disease of infants (ophthalmia neonatorum) is much less frequent since the use of silver nitrate eyedrops on all newborn babies became general, but, neglected, is one of the commonest causes of blindness. The treatment of early gonorrhoea has been revolutionized by the discovery of penicillin, which cures (very often in a single injection) most cases of this ancient affliction of the human race. It need hardly be pointed out that early treatment is absolutely essential and no false modesty should prevent those who fear they may have become infected from seeking advice, although a great many people who report with urethral discharge are suffering

from a non-specific urethritis. The discharge from acute gonorrhoea is thick, creamy and plentiful, that from non-specific urethritis thin, colourless and scanty; nevertheless, *all* abnormal discharges should be investigated and the specialist's conclusions accepted as it is quite common for those who are not naturally promiscuous to become neurotic about a non-venereal discharge although, in fact, there is no dubiety whatever about the results of diagnosis in the hands of a venereologist. *See* Venereal Disease.

Gout: a disease characterized by pain and swelling in certain joints, notably the great toe, the fingers, thumbs, knees, wrists and elbows, occurring mainly in men, and in women only after the menopause.

CAUSE: a predisposition to gout is hereditary, but the development of the disease is thought to be bound up with hearty eating and drinking although it is possible for very abstemious people to suffer from gout. Crystals of uric acid are deposited in the affected joints; people liable to gout show a raised level of uric acid in the blood, and as uric acid is derived from the breakdown of cell nuclei it can be expected that eating well will increase the formation of uric acid because a high protein diet must include many cells. The mechanism by which alcohol influences the blood level of uric acid is not understood. It is notable that gout does not occur in women of childbearing age, and it might be expected that this has something to do with the presence of sex hormones in the blood, but nothing precise is known.

SYMPTOMS: acute gout starts with a pain which comes on suddenly, generally in the great toe, which becomes red and shiny and very tender. Usually it is almost impossible to put any weight on the affected foot in the acute stage, but even without treatment the really painful period only lasts for a few days, during which the patient may run a slight fever and feel disinclined to eat. Sometimes he feels actively unwell, but he may not be at all upset in general health. After a number of attacks of acute gout the symptoms may never completely resolve, so that the disease becomes chronic; the joints are deformed, and 'gouty tophi' form – deposits of urates which are found round about the affected joints and also in the ear cartilages.

TREATMENT: the acute attack is controlled by the use of the

drugs colchicine or phenylbutazone, and the chronic state by increasing the excretion of uric acid through the kidneys by the use of probenecid (Benemid) or sulphinpyrazone (Anturan) combined with the intake of a great deal of fluid. It is recommended that sufferers from gout who wish to keep entirely free of the disease should not eat kidneys, brain, liver, fish roes or sardines, and should not drink beer, wines or spirits. Spinach, strawberries and rhubarb are also forbidden. The formation of uric acid in the body can be reduced by the drug allopurinol (Zyloric), but when it is first given it may precipitate an acute attack of gout, and it should not be taken during the course of an existing attack. It is important to realize that the deposition of crystals in the joints is characteristic of gout alone, and that manufacturers of proprietary medicines who seem to imply that 'rheumatics' in general have something to do with 'crystals in the blood' which have to be 'dissolved away' are talking nonsense. *See* Colchicum, Rheumatism.

Graft: the term applied to a piece of tissue removed from a person, animal or plant and implanted in another or the same organism in order to make good some defect or (in the case of plants) to build a composite individual plant. In modern surgery the commonest types of graft are skin, bone, and blood vessel. Skin grafts are used to cover areas which have been denuded of skin by burns, accidents or surgical operation; since grafts from one person to another are generally unsuccessful for reasons to be mentioned later, and the only successful ones of this type take place between identical twins, they have been largely abandoned and the skin used is taken from another part of the patient's own body in one of four ways: (1) *pinch grafts*, used for covering small areas, are round pieces of the superficial layer of the skin about a quarter of an inch in diameter often taken from the thigh and placed on the affected part where they take root and grow together to cover it; (2) *split-thickness grafts* are sheets of skin removed by hand or by a special instrument known as a dermatome consisting of a sharp knife attached to a drum which can measure accurately and slice a graft of about 4 by 8 inches containing both the superficial and part of the deep layer of skin of the thigh, abdomen or back – this type of graft is employed usually on large burned areas where the skin is completely destroyed; (3) *full-thickness grafts* contain all the layers of the skin except the basal fatty one, are used in parts subject to friction or pulling where (2) would not be suitable, and are cut exactly to size and stitched into place (the donor area is also closed by stitches); (4) *pedicle grafts*, in which one end of a piece of skin is attached to the area to be covered while its other end remains attached by a pedicle containing the necessary blood vessels and nerves to its original site until the graft has taken, when the connection can be severed. In this way pieces of skin can be 'leap-frogged' from one part of the body to another, for example a piece of skin from the abdomen is attached at one end to the arm or hand and, when it becomes firmly attached there, is cut free from the abdomen and attached to the face while retaining its connection with the arm. When it takes on the face it is disconnected from the arm. In *blood-vessel grafts* portions of a vein from the superficial tissues of the arm or a segment of an artery from a blood-vessel bank are used to replace a segment of a vital artery which has been destroyed, or affected by such conditions as severe arteriosclerosis. *Bone grafts* are usually taken from the patient himself (autogenous graft). They are removed from the crest of the ilium above the hip, or from the fractured bone above the affected part; occasionally they are obtained from a bone bank (homogenous graft), and may be a piece of rib removed at a chest operation or a piece of bone taken from an amputated leg or a dead body at post-mortem examination. They are used in cases where the healing of a fracture refuses to take place normally or where some loss of bone has occurred between the fractured ends. The grafting of whole organs from one organism to another is now called transplant surgery, and is discussed under that heading.

Gram's Stain: a method of differential staining of bacteria devised in 1884 by J. H. C. Gram, a Danish physician, who showed that staining with a parafuchsin dye such as methyl violet for 5 minutes, then with iodine for 2 minutes, and then treating the slide with acetone for 5 seconds and washing with water resulted in some bacteria taking up the dye and some being decolorized. The bacteria which stain purple are called Gram positive, and those which are decolorized and can subsequently be stained with other contrasting dyes are called Gram negative. This technique separates bacteria into two large groups, but the exact nature of the underlying reaction is obscure.

Grand Mal: *see* Epilepsy.

Granulation Tissue: the tissue formed by fibroblasts and endothelial cells which grows over any raw surface as a prelude to healing. It looks like red velvet and is very resistant to infection. As healing proceeds it is covered by epithelial cells which eventually form skin; the endothelial cells form small blood vessels and lymphatic vessels, and the fibroblasts lay down fibrous tissue which, as the process of healing continues, contracts to form a scar. Formation and contraction of fibrous tissue is increased by the presence of infection, so that scarring is always at its worst after a wound has been infected. The process of the formation and development of granulation tissue into a scar is called organization. Tumours (in the strictly medical sense in which the word means a swelling) of granulation tissue are formed in tuberculosis and syphilis, and are called granulomata.

Granuloma Inguinale: a contagious disease usually contracted by sexual intercourse and more common in tropical countries. The infecting organism is Donovania granulomatis, and the distinguishing lesion is a granulomatous (*see above*) ulcer usually on the genital organs. The ulceration may spread, but it is not painful. Treatment is by antibiotics, in particular tetracycline, and if there is a relapse the drug should be repeated.

Gravel: a popular term for small kidney stones.

Graves' Disease: *see* Hyperthyroidism *under* Goitre.

Gravid: pregnant.

Greenstick Fracture: a type of fracture found in the long bones of children, usually due to indirect violence, where the bone does not break completely but rather bends owing to the preponderance of connective tissue over calcium apatite in its structure, which makes it flexible. *See* Bones, Fractures.

Gregory's Mixture: or powder is pulvis rhei compositus, a mixture of rhubarb, heavy and light magnesium carbonates, and ginger once used as an antacid and purgative for digestive upsets. It is now known as rhubarb compound mixture but remains just as disagreeable.

Grey Powder: a powder containing mercury and chalk once used in cases of diarrhoea in infants, but now abandoned because it is liable to cause mercurial poisoning. Not for nearly half a century after the first description of a new disease called 'pink disease' in infants was it recognized as being due to mercury poisoning contracted from 'teething' powders.

Grinder's Disease: a disease of the lungs, once common among knife-grinders, caused by inhaling particles of steel.

Gripes: the colic of infants.

Grippe: a popular name for influenza.

Griseofulvin: an antibiotic which is active against fungus infections. It is used in ringworm of the scalp and body, and if used for long enough is effective in cases of ringworm of the nails, but it is disappointing when used against tinea pedis (athlete's foot).

Groin: an area which includes the upper part of the thigh and the lower part of the abdomen; the groove running across it covers the inguinal (Poupart's) ligament and its main abnormalities are hernia and enlarged inguinal lymph glands or 'buboes'. It is also a non-medical euphemism for the genitalia, as in 'a kick in the groin'.

Growing Pains: pains occurring in children during the course of their development, usually felt in the legs and back. They are due to a variety of causes none of which are to do with growing, and although such pains are unlikely to be serious skilled advice should always be sought.

Growth: a popular term for all sorts of swellings, especially those that are due to malignant tumours.

Gubernaculum: a cord of tissue formed during the development of the testis which connects the testis with the scrotum while it is still inside the abdominal cavity. When the testis descends into the scrotum during the seventh and eighth months of intra-uterine life the gubernaculum guides the way and keeps the channels open.

Guinea Worm: *see* Dracunculus.

Gullet: the oesophagus (q.v.), a muscular tube 10 inches long which connects the throat with the stomach.

Gumboil: an abscess at the root of a decayed tooth which produces pain and swelling on the outside of the face. In its early stages pain may be relieved by hot mouth-washes, packing the cavity in the tooth with cotton wool soaked in oil of cloves, aspirin, and hot applications to the cheek. Penicillin and a visit to the dentist are the remedies usually prescribed by the doctor.

Gumma: a hard granulomatous swelling (*see* Granulation tissue) caused by the third stage of syphilis, commonly affecting the skin, liver, bones, testicles and the central nervous system. *See* Syphilis.

Gums: hard fibrous tissue which is closely related to the bone of the upper and lower jaws and is applied to the necks of the teeth. The gums are covered by mucous membrane which is continuous with the membrane covering the alveoli, the sockets of the teeth. The gums are subject to various diseases including Vincent's angina (q.v.).

Gynaecology: that branch of medicine dealing with the diseases of women.

Gynaecomastia: abnormal enlargement of the male breast which may occur in diseases of the pituitary gland or the sex glands, cirrhosis of the liver, and deliberate or accidental administration of female sex-hormones.

Gyrus: one of the convolutions of the surface of the brain.

Haema-, haemato-, haemo-: for words beginning with these elements, *see* under Hema-, Hemato-, Hemo-.

Hair: there are many misconceptions about hair, perhaps because it falls into the no-man's-land between medicine and cosmetics. Only a few can be noted here, but it must be realized that hair is a dead structure which is kept glossy by the secretion of the sebaceous glands of the scalp. It is therefore untrue that cut hair loses some property which can be prevented from escaping by singeing, and, so far as one knows, hair cannot be fed externally, for such nourishment as the scalp requires must come to it from the bloodstream. There is no 'correct' number of times to wash the hair during the week as this depends on aesthetic considerations and individual variations in the natural oiliness of the scalp; women may shampoo their hair once weekly or once every two weeks, and some men wash it daily, but this would be a mistake if the scalp is naturally dry unless oil is added afterwards. Washing the hair has nothing to do with physiological functions although many women believe that it should not be done during the menstrual periods, a totally fallacious belief. Nor are there any hair tonics which prevent hair falling although it is not impossible that stimulant lotions which act by improving the blood supply to the scalp may delay loss of hair which, by and large, is controlled by heredity and the endocrine glands. Where baldness (q.v.) is due to disease it is obviously possible to do something about it, but most men will become as bald and as grey (or otherwise) as their fathers and at the same age no matter what they do. The fact that men often become bald whereas women rarely do has been attributed by the lunatic fringe to numerous factors, for example that women keep their hair long, or brush it more frequently, but the fact most probably is that large amounts of male sex hormone in the blood tend to cause baldness while the female sex hormone prevents it; both types of hormone are found in either sex and there is some foundation for the belief that baldness is in some measure associated with virility and preponderance of the male hormone. Eunuchs do not go bald. The main point to be made, however, is that most forms of 'scalp treatment' are a waste of money as they do nothing whatever for normal hair, and diseased hair requires proper medical diagnosis and treatment by a skin specialist. *See* Baldness, Superfluous Hair.

Hair-ball: if hair is swallowed over a period of years, it may collect in the stomach and form a hair-ball or trichobezoar. Hair-balls may be associated with gastric ulcers.

Halibut Liver Oil: a particularly rich source of Vitamin A and Vitamin D. It can be put up in capsules, and it is a more convenient means of giving the vitamins than cod liver oil, which is less concentrated.

Halitosis: *see* Breath, bad.

Hallucinations: these are not to be confused with *illusions* or *delusions*. An *illusion* is an error of sense perception in which a person misinterprets something that he actually experiences (for example mistaking a piece of clothing hanging on a door for a ghost), whereas a *delusion* is a faulty belief peculiar to the individual himself and not shared by others of the same social group (thus a man who believes himself to be Napoleon shares his belief with no one, whereas one who believes that the British people are descended from the lost ten tribes may be wrong, but his belief is shared by others of the British Israelite sect; a similar belief is held by the Mormons who believe that the Red Indians are the missing tribes). It is the social acceptability of a belief not its truth which is the criterion of its normality, and a delusion is a false belief private to the individual. Hallucinations are false sense perceptions in which the individual experiences something which others agree is simply not 'there' and, unlike an illusion, is not simply a misinterpretation of what really is there; hallucinations are often backed by delusions and, in fact, it might well be said that a delusion is father to an hallucination in that the person frequently experiences what he expects to experience. Hallucinations may be visual, auditory or related to the senses of smell or touch, those connected with hearing or smell being usually purely psychological in nature while those of sight, touch, and sometimes smell may have an organic basis. Ordinarily hallucinations have been regarded as symptomatic of insanity, but there can be no doubt that trance states in hysteria may bring them about as can drugs, alcohol (especially the visual hallucinations of delirium tremens), brain disease, the trances of mediums and witch-doctors, and religious ecstasy. Schizophrenia is the classical cause of auditory hallucinations, but it is certain that simple or deeply religious people experience similar phenomena without any mental or physical illness being present, although these are disapproved of in our predominantly materialistic and rationalistic culture which does not accept the metaphysical views upon which they are based. The significance of hallucinations must be judged (*a*) in the context of the individual's ordinary beliefs and cultural level, and (*b*) in relation to the rest of his behaviour. *See* Mental Illness.

Hallux: the great toe.

Halothane: (Fluothane). The 'modern chloroform'. A colourless volatile liquid, the vapour of which is used as an anaesthetic. It is not irritating, and it acts quickly, but it is not to be used by the inexperienced for it lowers the blood pressure and slows the breathing. It has a direct relaxing effect upon muscles, and although it tends to slow the heart rate, an action which is reduced by the administration of atropine, unlike chloroform it does not stop the heart's action, nor does it poison the liver. It is expensive, but widely used because of its flexibility and the ease with which breathing can be controlled.

Hammer Toe: the toe in this deformity is drawn up and bent like an inverted V, and it is liable to be painful because of the corns that form on it. The condition is probably caused by badly fitting shoes, and is treated by straightening the toe surgically and fixing the first joint so that it cannot afterwards move.

Hamstrings: the tendons behind the knee; there are inner and outer hamstrings. To hamstring is to cut these tendons, so that the knee becomes unstable and cannot be flexed.

Hand: the ability of man to oppose the thumb to the other fingers so that small objects can be grasped is one of the distinguishing features of the human race and is related to the hand's extreme delicacy and intricacy as an instrument. When the brain, in which the hand is represented over a much larger area in man than in other animals, becomes diseased, loss of the finer movements of the hand is one of the first signs that all is not well. The hand possesses 27 bones: 8 carpals in the wrist roughly arranged in two rows of four each; 5 metacarpals in the palm; and 14 phalanges in the fingers, the thumb containing only two and the rest three. From the muscles of the forearm 12 tendons run in front of the wrist passing under a ligament and enclosed in a complex synovial sheath to be attached to the fingers where they bring about flexion; at the back of the wrist a similar number of tendons cause extension. The turning of the palm downwards is termed pronation, and supination, which again is most highly developed in man, is the turning of the palm upwards, and these movements are brought about by the pronator and supinator muscles assisted by the biceps. Because supination is the more powerful movement this has determined the thread direction in such instruments as corkscrews and woodscrews. Forming the ball of the thumb and little finger and filling in the spaces between the meta-carpal bones are the short muscles whose function is to separate and bring the fingers together and to bend the hand at the knuckles. The blood supply comes from the ulnar and radial arteries, the former passing down the inner side of the arm, the latter down the same side as the thumb; they form two arches, deep and superficial, in the tissues of the palm, from which branches run down both sides of each finger. The ulnar nerve supplies the skin with sensation over the little finger and the inner half of the next one on the front of the hand, and the little, fourth and half the middle finger on the back of the hand. The median nerve supplies the other fingers on the front of the hand and the back of the tips of the fingers, while the radial nerve supplies the remainder of the back of the hand.
Few parts of the body tell so much about the individual as

his hand; ignoring as superstition the theories of the palmist and treating with reserve beliefs that the shape of the hand is related to the personality, so that long sensitive fingers are associated with artistic tendencies (as in the chimpanzee?) or short stubby ones with practical virtues, it is nevertheless true that we can infer a great deal about a man from his hands, for example his care, or lack of care, his work (especially in the case of craftsmen), his general sensitivity or lack of it, etc. From the medical point of view the doctor will note the shape and size, sometimes finding the large hand of acromegaly (q.v.), the claw-hand of ulnar paralysis, the 'main d'accoucheur' (midwives' hand) with the thumb and fingers held in a cone as with tetany, paralysis agitans, and other nervous diseases, the clubbed fingers of chronic heart and lung disease, the nodules of gout, the swollen joints of rheumatoid arthritis, and so on. Then there is the tremor of the alcoholic (sometimes accompanied by wrist-drop) and the different types of tremor associated with organic disease or mere nervousness, the purplish discoloration of the palm in cirrhosis of the liver, the white or blue fingers of Raynaud's disease and other circulatory conditions, the loss of the sense of pain in syringomyelia, often indicated by old scars from unheeded cigarette-burns or cuts, and many other signs too numerous to mention. But it need hardly be said that no diagnosis would be made on the basis of any one of these signs or symptoms taken in isolation. They are suggestive rather than conclusive.

Hanging: in general, apart from judicial hanging, this activity is carried out with suicidal intent (although cases are not unknown where murder has been committed by suspension). Death in such cases is ordinarily due to strangulation, and since this is a relatively slow means of dying an individual found hanging should be cut down immediately, his body being supported while this is being done, the noose loosened and removed, and artificial respiration applied at once. Steps to stimulate the heartbeat must be taken (*see* Cardiac Massage) and efforts at resuscitation carried on for some time until it is certain that life is extinct or recovery begins. In judicial hanging the cause of death has been different since the late Mr Hangman Berry devised his scientific formula for calculating a drop which would neither cause death by slow strangulation nor, as all too frequently happened, pull the condemned man's head completely off – an unaesthetic sight at the best of times. Functioning in England at the turn of the century, Mr Berry, who took his profession so seriously that he used to hand the condemned evangelical tracts suitable to their condition, showed that the best results were obtained by a drop of six feet on an average varying inversely with the weight of the body. Such a drop would dislocate the neck without undue mutilation or, medically speaking, cause the odontoid process at the base of the skull to break through its ligament and crush the vital centres in the medulla. But accidents will happen and it was necessary for Sir Bernard Spilsbury to amend the formula and recommend an increase of three inches in the drop. Since those who accept capital punishment in spite of the fact that it has been abolished in most civilized countries are hardly likely to listen to reasoned argument, nor is this the place for it, we may leave further discussion to moralists and politicians.

Hangover: most of the symptoms of hangover (excluding those caused by the consumption of impure alcoholic drinks of dubious ancestry) are brought about by two main factors: (1) alcohol is a diuretic, so that one is bound to get rid of more fluid than is drunk; (2) alcohol irritates the stomach so that in excessive amounts it produces gastritis. It is instructive in this context to pour a little whisky or gin on to a cut. The remedy for both these conditions – dehydration and gastritis – is the same: two pints of water drunk before retiring for the night. Two pints is a lot of water, and it may take some determination to drink down four tumblers, but the results are worth the effort. Remaining gastritis or oesophagitis may be relieved by alkalies, for example sodium bicarbonate, taken the next day.

Haptene: a chemical group which determines the antigenic specificity of a molecule. A molecule may also act as a specific antigen on account of its 'foreignness' to an organism, thus horse serum may set up an antigenic reaction in a human being. If a substance is to be able to set up this reaction it must have a large molecule, i.e. have a molecular weight over 5,000. The size of a haptene, however, is not

341

significant, but it must be attached to a substance of high molecular weight.

Hare-lip: *see* Cleft Palate.

Harvey, William (1578–1657): an English physician who discovered the circulation of the blood (q.v.).

Hashimoto's Disease: a disease characterized by a diffuse enlargement of the thyroid gland resulting from an increase of fibrous tissue and infiltration of lymphocytes rather than an increase of colloid material as in the commoner type of goitre. The patient, usually a middle-aged woman, has a general enlargement of the gland. Initially there are no symptoms elsewhere and no signs of thyrotoxicosis, but the condition usually ends in myxoedema caused by lack of thyroid hormone. The disease is now considered to be due to a disorder of the immune reaction, whereby the patient produces antibodies against her own thyroid cells.
TREATMENT: this is by the administration of thyroid hormone, and if the gland obstructs the windpipe it may (rarely) be necessary to remove part of it.

Hashish: *see* Cannabis Indica.

Hay-fever: an allergic disease characterized by irritation of the mucous membranes of the eyes, nose and air passages brought about by the pollen of various grasses and plants and therefore seasonal in incidence, coming on regularly at the same time each year.
CAUSE: as explained elsewhere (*see* Allergy) all foreign proteins when they get into the body unchanged act as antigens, i.e. they stimulate the formation of antibodies against them. In allergic subjects, a reaction takes place in the cells of the body with the formation of various poisonous substances including histamine. Hay-fever is the allergic disease affecting predominantly the eyes and nose, just as asthma affects the bronchial tubes and certain types of allergic dermatitis the skin. Most cases of hay-fever occur in summer and spring when the antigen is grass-pollen, but some occur in autumn when the pollen of ragweeds is the usual cause.

A tendency to allergy seems to be inherited but the specific form taken by the disease is not, so that it is quite common in a family to find one member suffering from hay-fever and another from asthma or occasional skin rashes. Such subjects are more often men than women and tend to be sensitive and highly strung; structural defects are sometimes found in the nose by enthusiastic ear, nose and throat specialists, but the same defects often exist in the absence of hay-fever. Not unnaturally, the condition usually improves following a period of rain or at the seaside.

TREATMENT: this may take the form of a course of vaccine prepared from pollen which must be given throughout the preceding winter each year, or the use of drugs which must be taken throughout the season. A change of environment to escape the pollen is not open to everyone and is rarely necessary; the nose is best left severely alone so far as operative measures are concerned. Drugs have different effects on different individuals and if one does not help or has unpleasant side effects another should be tried.

Hazeline: or witch-hazel is prepared from the leaves and bark of Hamamelis virginiana and used as an astringent extract or ointment for the skin and anus. It is soothing and stops minor irritation, bleeding and discharge; it is sometimes used as a rubbing lotion for strained muscles and sprained joints.

Headache: this is one of the commonest symptoms in medicine and it is a fair estimate that at least 90% of all headaches have no basis so far as structural defects are concerned. This does not, of course, mean that nothing at all is happening in the body but rather that what does happen is temporary and often of emotional origin, the most frequent emotions being anxiety or suppressed anger and resentment. In such cases the immediate cause of pain is in all probability a spasm of the sheet of muscle passing over the scalp from the eyebrows to the back of the neck or of other muscles in the neck region; this is possibly an evolutionary relic of a type of reaction seen in the lower animals (cf. the angry or suspicious dog or ape whose hair stands on end over the back of the neck as the muscles tense for action). Some kinds of headache appear to be caused by dilatation of the arteries

343

in the brain or tension in the membranes covering it; for the brain itself has no capacity to feel pain and can, in fact, be operated on or touched with impunity while the patient is fully conscious. In migraine (q.v.) the headache may be of this type, as may also be the very severe headaches in brain tumour or other space-occupying diseases within the skull. Congestion inside the spaces of the skull such as the sinuses causes severe pain, and even mild congestion within the nose makes most people feel 'headachy'. Possibly eye defects can produce headaches by congestion, but it is unlikely that all the many people with headaches who seem to think that this is an immediate indication for having their eyes tested are right – even if they rarely leave their oculist without a new pair of glasses. It is true, of course, that some of the more serious eye diseases such as glaucoma (q.v.) cause very severe pain.

Other causes frequently given for headaches are dental sepsis, constipation, indigestion, kidney disease, 'rheumatism' and high blood pressure, but there is not the slightest reason to believe that any of these directly lead to headaches, although worry about them very well may. The idea that high blood pressure and headaches are inevitably associated dies hard, but the fact is that the vast majority of cases of hypertension have no symptoms at all and the condition is found accidentally; people who know that their blood pressure is raised often develop headaches but this is largely due to anxiety. For practical purposes it is important to note how the patient describes his pain: the nervous headache is often described as 'terrible' and likened to 'red-hot needles' and so on because it is really a dramatization of the individual's quite real problems. Furthermore it is 'all over' the head and in this way quite unlike the physically caused headache which is sharply localized to a particular part, keeps the patient still rather than restless and talkative, and is usually associated with other symptoms. Severe localized headache accompanied by vomiting attacks always requires immediate attention as these are signs of raised pressure inside the skull. In migraine the headache is frequently preceded by vomiting and there are eye symptoms which are described elsewhere. The headaches of sinusitis may be anywhere in the forehead or face depending upon which sinuses are affected; they may be just above the eyes, at the base of the nose, in the corner of the eyes, over the cheeks, and so on, and there is usually a history of nasal discharge and 'catarrh'. The treatment of headache is the treatment of its cause. *See* Hypertension, Neurosis, Migraine, Sinusitis.

Head Injury: head injuries are not uncommon, and are often sustained in motor-car accidents; they may be open or closed, and may involve any degree of interference with consciousness from a momentary dizziness to coma and death.

Types of injury. The scalp, skull, the membranes covering the brain and the blood vessels associated with them, and the brain itself can all be injured. *The scalp* is commonly bruised or lacerated, and because the blood supply is so free any laceration of the scalp bleeds profusely and looks far worse than it is. Bleeding is controlled by pressing the scalp against the bone round the bleeding area so that the vessels are obliterated; a pressure dressing can be applied when the worst of the bleeding has stopped. Hair quickly becomes matted with blood; and this makes many injuries look worse than they are. There should be no hesitation in cutting hair off if it makes it easier to see the extent of the wound and to control bleeding, for damage to the hair is the least of possible injuries. Open injuries that involve the bone and the underlying brain should be covered with a clean dressing or freshly washed cloth; no attempt must be made to apply disinfectants or other medication. *The skull* itself is often fractured by a serious blow on the head, although the scalp may look undamaged, but a fracture of the skull is not important (except that it gives an indication of the force encountered) unless it runs across the region of the temple, the ear or the nose, or the bone is depressed. It is not usually possible to tell that the skull has been fractured in a closed head injury without X-rays, and it is more important to attend to the problems of an unconscious patient than to wonder if his skull is fractured. Apart from direct violence and open fractures, where the damage is obvious, *the brain* may be severely injured in closed injuries because the head is accelerated or decelerated at the moment of the accident and the brain moves after the skull, so that there is first a moment when the brain stays still and the skull moves sharply enough to bruise it, and a second moment when the

345

skull has stopped moving but the brain continues, to strike against the stationary or rebounding skull on the side opposite to the site of injury and produce 'contre-coup' injury. Rotating forces cause shearing strains in the brain which are also of great importance in the mechanism of brain injury. Sometimes, particularly when the skull is fractured, *blood vessels* running in the membranes that line the skull are torn and bleed. In the case of arteries, the middle meningeal is most often injured in the temple, and the escaping arterial blood forms a haematoma or swelling between the dura mater and the skull (*see* Extradural Hemorrhage). When a vein is torn, the bleeding is inside the dura mater and may form a swelling over a period of hours, days or even months (*see* Subdural Hematoma). These collections of blood press on the brain and lead to increasing headache, to epileptiform fits, and to loss of consciousness and coma which, if the condition is not relieved by surgery, ends in death.

TREATMENT: this will vary according to the degree of injury, but after the obvious wounds have been dealt with it is imperative to keep the patient under observation, for if he has suffered a degree of violence sufficient to cause him to lose consciousness even for a little while it is possible that he is developing a collection of blood inside the skull or a swelling of the brain in response to the injury that will take time to develop. The usual period of observation is 24 hours. If the patient has suffered a very severe injury it is possible that he may have to be treated by an artificial breathing machine, and in the worst cases he may only be 'alive' while the machine is working (*see* Death). Collections of blood within the skull are let out by the surgeon, and such cases often have a good result; but it is always possible for epileptic attacks to follow head injury, and for post-traumatic headaches to develop (but *see* Compensation Syndrome). The really important thing to remember about the immediate treatment of an unconscious patient with a head injury is that the airway (q.v.) must be kept clear so that he can breathe easily. *See* Concussion.

Healing: *see* Granulation Tissue.

Health: the basic principles of a healthy life are well-known: care of the teeth; a well-balanced diet with adequate supplies of vitamins and minerals in addition to suitable amounts of carbohydrates, proteins and fats; adequate exercise; cleanliness and fresh air; freedom from undue anxiety and nervous tension, and the rest. However, a look at these requirements in the light of modern knowledge must result in their being somewhat modified. It is true that a well-balanced and well-digested diet is important but this is obtained in different parts of the world in widely differing ways: examples are the vegetarians with their relatively low protein diet, the Eskimos with their high fat diet, hunting tribes with their almost wholly meat diet, and Latins with a diet high in carbohydrate and vegetable oils. All seem to be equally suitable although it has recently been suggested that diets rich in cholesterol, i.e. animal fats, eggs, liver, kidneys, etc., make one prone to coronary thrombosis. What seems much more likely is that overeating is harmful. The correlation between coronary disease and lack of exercise leads one to believe that a moderate amount of exercise is important to the ordinary individual although many invalids who are totally immobilized live long lives; violent exercise as in athletes correlates in no way at all either with subsequent health or with long life.

Apart from keeping free from infection it would seem that the main function of bathing is cosmetic and, indeed, very few infections enter the body through the skin, most of those in temperate climates being airborne or ingested in the food or in water. Some diseases (for example poliomyelitis) in fact are more prone to attack the healthy than the weakling, but there can be no doubt of the connection between bad housing and insanitary surroundings and such diseases as bronchitis, rheumatism, tonsillitis and adenoids, and upper respiratory tract infections. Climate has been discussed under that heading and when climate is separated from the conditions associated with specific climatic states it will be seen that climate in itself plays a relatively small part in the maintenance of health or the production of disease. Thus malaria used to be common in England and its presence in tropical climates is in a sense incidental, for when the disease is wiped out the climates will have remained virtually unchanged. There are few doctors today who believe that cold and damp in themselves produce illness but there can be little doubt that the incidence of colds and sinus diseases is closely related to sudden changes of temperature when we leave our overheated rooms to go into the cold air outside or vice versa. Addiction to alcohol is an important factor in causing disease both directly and indirectly (*see* Alcoholism), yet the moderate drinker lives longer than the total abstainer and there is not the slightest evidence that puritanical attitudes in life lead to longevity and a healthy life. Constipation is dealt with elsewhere and, except as a symptom of other diseases, is of little significance. Even the presence of serious disease does not necessarily shorten life and most doctors know of patients with chronic bronchitis or bronchial asthma and enlarged hearts who live to a ripe old age in spite of their troubles; indeed, one of the most striking experiences of medical practice is how these cases live on while apparently healthy patients are carried away in their prime. We must reconcile ourselves to the fact that a great part of longevity and health is, in a technically advanced society such as ours, based on constitution and inheritance and is not to be wooed by taking thought, diet, or care – except that necessary to keep out of the way of accidents.

Hearing Aids: essentially small electronic devices designed to amplify sound waves, hearing aids should always be obtained from specialists in the matter because they can be supplied to fit in with the characteristics of the loss of hearing of each patient. It is sometimes the case that people will not wear hearing aids; this is all very well if they do not mind being thought stupid, but uncorrected deafness may unjustly get a child a reputation for backwardness which could be avoided.

Heart: *Function.* The heart is essentially two pumps lying side by side, one pumping the blood from the lungs out into the body, and the other pumping the blood from the body into the lungs. Each pump has two chambers; in the first, the atrium, the blood collects from the veins which bring blood either from the lungs or the body. When the atrium is full it contracts, a non-return valve at its inlet from the veins closes, and the blood passes into the second chamber, the ventricle. When the ventricle contracts the non-return valve between the ventricle and the atrium closes, and the blood is pumped out into the arteries, to go into the lungs or round the body. When the ventricle relaxes another non-return valve prevents blood running back into it from the arteries. The pump which circulates blood from the body into the lungs is named the right side of the heart, and that which pumps blood returning from the lungs out into the body is the left side of the heart.

Anatomy. It is not strictly true to say that the two pumps, which in function are quite separate, lie side by side, for the anatomy is such that the right side spirals and partially encircles the left. The heart is an entirely muscular organ, which lies in the centre of the chest in between the two lungs behind the breastbone. It lies obliquely so that the apex, which is in fact part of the right ventricle in front and the left ventricle behind, is behind the fifth space between the ribs on the left side of the chest about in a line with the left nipple or inside this line. The left ventricle has a thicker wall than the right, and when the ventricles contract the heart turns and the apex can be felt beating against the chest wall.

Connections with large vessels. The heart is fed by the venae cavae, superior and inferior, on the right side. These two large veins form part of the wall of the right atrium. The right ventricle pumps into the pulmonary artery – this artery therefore contains venous or de-oxygenated blood, for it has been returned from the veins of the body. When the blood has passed through the lungs and is full of oxygen it returns to the left atrium through the four pulmonary veins, which contain arterial or oxygenated blood. This blood is pumped through the mitral valve into the left ventricle, whence it is pumped into the aorta, the great artery of the body, and so round the arterial tree, through the capillaries and into the veins again to be returned in the two venae cavae to the right side of the heart.

Valves. The non-return valve between the right atrium and the right ventricle is named the tricuspid valve because it has three flaps, like all the other valves of the heart; it is only the mitral valve between the left atrium and left ventricle which has two flaps, rather like a bishop's mitre. A considerable pressure is set up when the ventricles contract – up to 150 mm Hg on the left, and about 30 mm Hg on the right – and the mitral and tricuspid valves are supplied with cords and muscles like guy-ropes which run between the cusps of the valves and the inner surface of the ventricles to prevent the cusps being blown inside out. The other inlet non-return valves and the outlet valves, the pulmonary valve on the right and the aortic valve on the left, have no such support. All the valves are set in fibrous rings in the heart muscle.

Heart sounds. The valves open silently, but when they close they set up vibrations in the bloodstream which can be heard through the chest wall as sounds. The heart sounds are traditionally represented by the words 'lubb-dup'; the first sound is made by the mitral and tricuspid valves closing, the second sound by the aortic and pulmonary valves. If the valves are diseased and cannot open or shut properly, eddies are formed in the bloodstream and 'murmurs' are heard through the stethoscope.

Contraction of the heart. When the heart relaxes the blood flows in, and contraction in the atria is set off by a pace-maker, an island of specialized tissue called the sinuatrial node, or S.A. node, which lies in the right atrium. The wave of contraction spreads very quickly throughout the atrial muscle on the right and left sides, and reaches another island of specialized tissue on the right near the tricuspid valve called the atrioventricular, or A.V. node. From the A.V. node there runs the atrioventricular bundle of very fast conducting fibres which descend into the partition or septum between the right and left ventricles and then branch out into the ventricular muscle on each side. When the wave of atrial contraction reaches the A.V. node impulses run into the right and left ventricles and the ventricular muscle contracts.

Electrocardiogram. The electrical changes in the heart muscle can be picked up from the chest and amplified so that a trace representing the changes of potential can be recorded and studied. *See* Electrocardiogram.

Pericardium. The heart is enclosed in a bag of fibrous tissue named the pericardium, which has two layers, one inside the other, separated by a thin film of fluid. This enables the heart to move in relation to the structures round about.

Blood supply of the heart. Although the heart is always full of blood, it has to have its own blood supply which comes from the coronary arteries. *See* Coronary Disease.

Diseases of the heart. These are described under their own headings. *See* Heart Failure, Valvar Disease of the Heart,

Endocarditis, Myocarditis, Pericarditis, Coronary Disease, Angina Pectoris, etc. The *symptoms* of heart disease, curiously enough, are not very frequently such as one would directly relate to the heart. Thus pain over the heart, palpitations, and discomfort in this region in the vast majority of cases are caused by gastric upsets, flatulence and nervous tension, which is by far the commonest cause of palpitations. The exceptions to this rule are the pains caused by pericarditis in the early stages – although in this case the patient is usually incapacitated by some other disease – coronary thrombosis and angina pectoris. In the latter two diseases the pain is severe and tends to pass down the left arm or shoulder; coronary thrombosis often occurs while the individual is resting or asleep, but in angina the pain is brought on by exertion. Although it is often claimed that palpitations can be caused by local sepsis, excessive smoking, etc. (*see* Tachycardia), there can be little doubt that the most important factor is nervous tension. The worried patient holding his hand over his heart and thinking that he is going to drop dead at any moment prompts questions directed to his home and business worries rather than to his heart; whereas *as a generalization* the patient who really has heart disease is often unworried and unaware of the connection between his symptoms and his heart. The symptoms are likely to be: breathlessness, tiredness, swelling of the ankles which is worse at night-time, headache and giddiness, sometimes fainting attacks, 'bronchitis' and spitting of blood, and 'sleep-starts' when the patient wakes up suddenly at night unable to get his breath. All of these are caused by inadequate oxygenation of the blood due to impaired circulation or to congestion in particular areas. *Surgery of the heart.* Surgical treatment of heart disease (both congenital and acquired) is described with the diseases in which it is used. *See* Patent Ductus Arteriosus, Septal Defect, Fallot's Tetralogy, Valvar Disease of the Heart, etc. Transplantation of the heart is discussed under the heading Transplant Surgery.

Heartburn: a burning pain in the region of the heart and up the back of the throat. It is particularly common in hiatus hernia (*see under* Hernia). It is relieved by alkalies, for example sodium bicarbonate, as advertisements for many

patent medicines point out. Excess of alcohol may cause
inflammation of the oesophagus and consequent heartburn.
See Hangover.

Heart Failure: the heart may fail to carry out its function
because of congenital or acquired disease, and the failure
may be mainly of the right or left side of the heart (*see* Heart).
The commonest type of failure is left heart failure following
disease of the mitral or aortic valves, coronary insufficiency,
or high blood pressure. Congenital heart disease leads more
often to failure of the right side, as does chronic disease of the
lungs. One of the end consequences of left heart failure is a
congestion of the lungs, which leads to right heart failure
because of back pressure.

SYMPTOMS: *Left heart failure*. The first symptom is loss of
breath; the patient becomes breathless on exertion, and as
the condition progresses the amount of exercise he can carry
out diminishes. In time it becomes difficult to take breath,
and patients often find that they breathe much more easily
sitting up than lying down. Attacks of breathlessness may
occur especially at night, when the patient wakes up fighting
for breath. Sitting up relieves a number of cases, but if the
breathlessness is due to waterlogging of the lungs the patient
may go blue, and may slip into unconsciousness. The patient
apart from developing breathlessness on exertion feels tired
and unwilling to make much effort to do anything.

Right heart failure. As in left heart failure the blood fails to
return from the lungs, and the pressure of the blood in the
lungs rises, so in right heart failure the return of blood from
the rest of the body is diminished and the pressure rises in
the veins. The consequence is swelling of the liver and waterlogging (oedema) of the ankles and legs under the influence
of gravity; if the patient takes to his bed swelling develops in
his back. There is pain and tenderness on the right side of
the abdomen in its upper part, and congestion of the intestines and stomach which produces loss of appetite, nausea
and even vomiting.

TREATMENT: the most important single factor in the treatment of heart failure is rest; in severe cases the rest must be
absolute, but in milder cases it should be in proportion to
the degree of failure. In some instances it is enough to lie
down during the afternoon, or to go to bed early. Holidays

HEATSTROKE

although valuable should not be energetic. Movement of
the legs even in those who have to go to bed is important,
for muscular action helps to return the blood to the heart and
cuts down the retention of water in the tissues. Unless the
patient is being treated for heart failure which is part of a
coronary infarction he can get out of bed to go to the bathroom, and sit out of bed for part of the day. It is dangerous
to let old people become completely bedridden, for they
develop infection of the lungs which may be fatal, or bedsores which can reach dreadful proportions in spite of careful
attention. The second factor in the treatment of heart failure
is the drug digitalis (q.v.), which has a strengthening action
on the heart muscle, and is beneficial in all cases of heart
failure. The third factor is the possibility of increasing the
flow of water from the kidneys by using diuretics, that is to
say drugs which act on the kidneys to make them secrete
more urine. Waterlogging of the lungs and the collection of
water in the dependent parts can be diminished by the use of
these drugs, which are often given to the patient every other
day rather than daily because they are very powerful.
Acute heart failure and attacks of breathlessness caused by
water in the lungs secondary to left-sided heart failure are
best treated by injections of morphia, which quieten the
patient and enable him to rest and so give his heart the best
chance of recovery.

Heart-lung Machine: these machines, of which there are
now several designs, take in venous blood and mix it with
oxygen by letting it come into contact with the gas in a thin
film. The oxygenated blood is then pumped back into the
arterial system. This essentially simple conception is of course
complicated by a number of factors – for one thing, the blood
has to be prevented from clotting, and for another, it must
be kept absolutely sterile. It must also be kept at the right
temperature. The machines are used in heart surgery to keep
the blood circulating and oxygenated while the heart is
bypassed so that it can be opened and manipulated.

Heatstroke: sunstroke. Until fairly recently it was usual to
distinguish between heatstroke and sunstroke, the former
being said to be produced by excessive heat whether in the
tropics or in a steel foundry in northern Europe, the latter

353

being produced by the rays of the sun beating down on the head or spine. In fact, no such state as sunstroke exists if by this it is implied that the rays of the sun in themselves and apart from a hot climate can cause any damage other than sunburn of the skin. The only useful function of solar topees is to keep a bald scalp from being burned by the sun, or to keep bright sunlight out of the eyes; any other broad-brimmed hat would do just as well.

SYMPTOMS: sunstroke and heatstroke are the same entity and result from a hot atmosphere, particularly one which is also damp, in which excess heat cannot escape from the body. In the early stages there is excessive sweating leading to salt loss and therefore to painful cramps and concentration of the blood which disturbs the circulation; in the later stages the whole heat-regulating system breaks down, sweat is inhibited, and delirium and coma herald a fatal end in serious cases. In the mild case there is only slight or severe headache, sweating, cramps, irritability and fatigue.

TREATMENT: this consists in removal to a cool place and giving large amounts of normal salt solution (1 teaspoonful of salt to a pint of water) either by mouth or intravenously. In severe cases the naked body should be wrapped in a wet sheet and kept fanned until the temperature falls to about 102 °F. (38.9 °C.). Delirium, cessation of sweating, and a temperature above 105–7 °F. (40.6–41.7 °C.) are bad signs. Some people seem more liable to heatstroke than others, but beyond ordinary sensible precautions experience has shown that much of the traditional rigmarole about midday suns, special clothing other than that which commonsense suggests, and the rest is unnecessary as, indeed, a glance at the local inhabitants might have suggested, or even a glimpse at the past. The 'light morning diet' formerly advised looks rather silly in face of the hot bulky curries of India and the 'light airy clothes' in face of the clothes of our forebears like the explorer Mungo Park, who at the end of the eighteenth century sought the source of the Niger dressed in his every-day Scottish suit and top hat.

Hebephrenia: a state of rapid deterioration of the mind with lack of social interest, self-centred delusions, hallucinations and absurd behaviour. It forms one of the subdivisions of schizophrenia.

Heberden's Nodes: small hard lumps that appear at the joints of the fingers in some cases of arthritis.

Heliotherapy: treatment by the sun's rays or ultraviolet rays produced by a special lamp. Formerly much used for medical purposes the method has fallen into relative disuse and its only common function is now cosmetic.

Helminths: a name for parasitic worms. *See* Worms.

Hemachromatosis: (Bronzed diabetes). An hereditary disease due to an abnormality of iron metabolism, resulting in the deposition of iron pigment, haemosiderin, in the skin and other parts of the body, so that skin becomes dark. It is a disease of men.
CAUSE: there is an increased quantity of iron in the blood which in the form of brownish granules of haemosiderin is taken up by the liver, pancreas, spleen, the heart and the testicles as well as by the skin. The presence of the pigment leads to fibrosis in the organs affected.
SYMPTOMS: the obvious change is the darkening of the skin, but the patient also feels tired and lacking in energy. The testicles may shrivel and the breasts enlarge, and as the disease progresses damage to the pancreas causes the development of diabetes mellitus, or 'sugar diabetes' (q.v.). The heart muscle may be damaged so that the symptoms of heart failure appear.
TREATMENT: the diabetes and heart failure, if present, are treated as usual; the abnormal level of iron in the blood which is a feature of the disease is best treated by bleeding the patient of about half a litre of blood at regular intervals.

Hemangioma: a tumour of blood vessels. *See* Angioma.

Hematemesis: the vomiting of blood, a symptom which should always be brought to the attention of the doctor as soon as possible. Small amounts of blood often come from the back of the throat and nose and may be swallowed and vomited later; such blood is likely to be dark in colour due to partial digestion. Gastritis following the intake of irritating foods or strong alcohol sometimes results in similar amounts of blood being vomited, but larger amounts come from

355

gastric or duodenal ulcers, in which case the vomit may look like coffee-grounds. A considerable haematemesis is almost always the result of an ulcer breaking into a blood vessel, or the rupture of portal varices – varicose veins which arise in cases of cirrhosis of the liver at the end of the oesophagus and in the upper part of the stomach due to congestion of the portal circulation. Such haemorrhages are severe and often fatal, and have to be treated with the greatest urgency. Less commonly haematemesis accompanies certain fevers and blood diseases.

Hematocoele: a cavity containing blood, formed for example when an injury or the rupture of an aneurysm (q.v.) causes blood to flow into a natural cavity or into loose connective tissue.

Hematocolpos: the retention of menstrual blood in the vagina by an imperforate hymen which completely closes the entrance. A small and painless incision immediately frees the accumulation.

Hematology: that branch of medicine which deals with the blood in health and disease.

Hematoma: a collection of blood in the tissues resulting from injury or operation.

Hematuria: the presence of blood cells in the urine which may come from any part of the urinary tract and be of serious or relatively trivial significance. Some indication of the site of the bleeding may be obtained from the appearance of the urine, which is dull brown or smoky rather than red when the blood comes from the kidneys. Blood from the bladder is more red and may come from inflammation as in cystitis or from a stone, in both of which cases it is likely to be mixed with pus, but bright red blood in fair amounts is nearly always the result of a papilloma or wart on the wall of the bladder. A fractured pelvis, inflammation of the urethra, bilharzia in the tropics, prostatic enlargement, scurvy, purpura and other blood diseases are other causes of haematuria. Rarely, haematuria occurs periodically without any discoverable disease being present. All cases require speedy investigation in order to discover the site of bleeding; this may often necessitate a cystoscopic examination and special X-rays. *See* Cystoscope, Pyelography.

Hemeralopia: a state of day-blindness in which the individual can see better in the half-light than in full daylight.

Hemianaesthesia: loss of sensation down one side of the body.

Hemianopia: (Hemianopsia, hemiopia). Loss of one half of the field of vision. It may be congruous (homonymous), when the loss in each eye is symmetrical and in the same position, or incongruous (heteronymous), when the loss is asymmetrical and in different positions in each eye. By a careful consideration of the character and size of the defects, the physician can draw conclusions about the site of the disease process within the skull which is causing them by pressing on or destroying some part of the nervous pathways through which impulses are carried from the retina to the parts of the brain concerned with sight.

Hemiatrophy: wasting of one side of the body, or half of a part of the body such as the face, resulting either from defects in the course of development or from some disease process.

Hemicrania: headache limited to one side, or pain on one side of the head.

Hemiparesis: weakness of the muscles on one side of the body.

Hemiplegia: paralysis of one side of the body. Both hemiparesis and hemiplegia may follow a stroke, the left side being affected if the vascular accident is on the right side of the brain, and the right side of the body (and the power of speech in right-handed people) if the blood vessels of the left cerebral hemisphere are at fault.

Hemisphere: half of any round structure or part of the

357

body, usually used of the cerebral and cerebellar parts of the brain. *See* Nervous System.

Hemlock: the name given to a group of plants which contain the poison coniine, the common hemlock Conium maculatum being the plant from whose juice Socrates died, for this was the official method of execution in the Athens of his day. Its effects are well exemplified in the account given by Plato. Socrates after drinking was told to walk about until his legs felt heavy (motor paralysis) and later, when his foot was pressed, he could not feel (sensory paralysis). Death finally occurred from paralysis of the respiratory system. The effect of coniine in diminishing muscular contractions was once valued by doctors and the drug was used to treat chorea, whooping-cough and epilepsy. Its use is now extinct.

Hemocytometer: a special microscope slide marked in squares for counting the number of white or red cells in the blood.

Hemoglobin: about one-third of the substance of the red cells of the blood is haemoglobin, a pigment containing iron in four 'haem' groups and protein in the globin portion. It is made by the developing red blood cells. The function of haemoglobin is the transport of oxygen to the tissues, and it is also concerned with the removal of CO_2 after the tissues have used up the oxygen. Oxyhaemoglobin is bright red but the colour of reduced haemoglobin is much darker; it has the same chemical formula as chlorophyll, the green colouring matter of plants, save that the latter contains magnesium instead of iron.

Hemoglobinuria: free haemoglobin will pass through the kidneys into the urine and colour it a dark red. The presence of blood pigment free in the bloodstream is due to the breakdown of red blood cells (haemolysis), and is caused by a number of agents, some chemical such as arsine, potassium chlorate or quinine, some infectious such as yellow fever and malaria (blackwater fever), and some traumatic such as extensive burning or crushing. Attacks of haemoglobinuria may occur in otherwise normal people after exposure to cold or violent muscular exercise, and there is a condition called 'paroxysmal nocturnal haemoglobinuria' in which paroxysms of haemolysis during the night result in the passage of darkly stained urine in the morning. The mechanism of the disease is based on a defect in the circulating red blood cells, and patients with this rare disease develop anaemia.

Hemolysis: the breakdown of red blood cells and the liberation of blood pigment into the bloodstream. It may be caused by a number of conditions, including haemolytic disease of the newborn and the bites of those venomous snakes whose venom contains a haemolytic factor.

Hemolytic Disease of the Newborn: this is due to incompatibility between the blood cells of the foetus and the blood of the mother, whose antibodies may pass through the placenta and destroy the cells of the foetus. The incompatibility nearly always involves the Rh factor (*see* Blood Groups), and depends on the sensitization of an Rh-negative mother by an Rh-positive foetus, some of whose red cells may from time to time escape into the mother's circulation across the placenta. It is fortunately possible for the disease to be recognized from the time when a pregnant woman's blood is found to be Rh-negative; tests during the pregnancy will detect a rising amount of antibody, and the baby can be born in hospital with all possible resources for treatment at hand. Various methods of treatment are used, varying from early induction of labour and even intra-uterine transfusion of the foetus to the replacement of all the blood of a baby born at full term. It may in the future be possible to prevent the disease developing by injecting mothers found to have Rh-positive foetal cells in their circulation with an appropriate gamma globulin (q.v.). The disease may be fatal to the baby if it develops generalized oedema (hydrops foetalis), but jaundice does not mean that the child will not recover.

Hemophilia: a disease of the blood in which there is a deficiency in the blood clotting mechanism. The disease is hereditary, and is passed down in the female line although only the males suffer from haemophilia. It is sometimes known as the royal disease, for it has in the past run in royal

359

families. Queen Victoria carried haemophilia, passing it to her daughter, the Czarina of Russia; her son had the disease, with consequences that went beyond the confines of Russia. The Hapsburgs are also said to have suffered from haemophilia.

CAUSE: one of the factors concerned in the formation of plasma thromboplastin (*see* Coagulation of Blood) is missing, so that conversion of prothrombin to thrombin is delayed and the production of fibrin insufficient.

SYMPTOMS: a large number of haemophiliacs are only slightly affected, and they may only be recognized when they have a tooth taken out or have to undergo a surgical operation, when it is found that the blood clots slowly and bleeding is excessive. In severe cases the patient bleeds spontaneously especially into his large joints, so that in time the joint becomes disorganized and useless with wasting of the muscles that act upon it and even deformity. Bleeding may occur into soft tissues, for example the kidney, where it gives rise to passage of clots in the urine and consequent colic. Bleeding tends to be less as age advances; it usually starts when the child begins to crawl and walk, and it occurs in attacks between which the patient may be free of symptoms.

TREATMENT: in milder cases little treatment is needed beyond a general caution against running unnecessary risks of injury, and careful preparation if any surgery has to be carried out or if a tooth has to be extracted. In severe cases the child and his parents are faced with a number of difficult problems, for the recurrent bleeding can interfere with education, social life and work. Once the diagnosis is made, patients are best referred to special centres where haemophilia is studied and treated by experienced physicians. With care a haemophiliac can lead a reasonable life, but a case of any severity has to exist as it were padded with cotton wool. In Great Britain special identity cards are carried by sufferers from haemophilia and related diseases so that there should be no delay in instituting special treatment if they fall victim to an accident away from home.

Hemoptysis: the spitting up of blood from the respiratory system (i.e. from the larynx, trachea, bronchi or lungs). True haemoptysis may be due to pulmonary tuberculosis, valvular disease of the heart or heart failure (especially mitral stenosis and left ventricular failure), bronchiectasis, pulmonary infarction (i.e. a clot of blood in the lungs), pneumonia, tumours of the bronchi or lungs, abscess or gangrene, wounds, and some of the less common infections. It may also occur in blood diseases (for example purpura, pernicious anaemia, leukaemia), in severe deficiency of Vitamins C and K, measles, high blood pressure and emphysema. False haemoptysis is caused by blood coming from the throat, gums or nose and this is on the whole more frequent than the genuine type, although all suspected bleeding must be investigated by the doctor.

Hemorrhage: bleeding. Haemorrhage may be external or internal, arterial, venous, or capillary. If an artery is cut the blood is bright red and jets out with the beat of the heart; venous blood is dark and flows in a constant steady stream, whereas oozing from the capillaries is intermediate in colour. The main points to observe in controlling severe bleeding are to make the patient rest, to keep him moderately warm but not hot, and to avoid all stimulants, as anything which stimulates the heart will also increase bleeding. Movement should be avoided. In internal bleeding no food or drink may be given but the patient may suck pieces of ice. External bleeding from wounds or other injuries can be dealt with by a tourniquet when the limbs are affected, but the tourniquet must be loosened frequently otherwise the part of the limb from which the blood is cut off will be seriously damaged. A tourniquet must always be visible and the patient must not be given into other hands without its being pointed out that a tourniquet has been applied. Pressure should be put on the bleeding area and in venous bleeding this should be greatest on the side away from the heart, the limb being raised; in arterial bleeding pressure should be greatest on the side nearest the heart. (The pressure-points familiar to the first-aider are better derived from some knowledge of anatomy and physiology than learned by rote.) Various types of internal haemorrhage dealt with elsewhere are epistaxis or bleeding from the nose, haematemesis or vomiting blood, haemoptysis or spitting blood, haematuria or blood in the urine, and melaena or blood in the motions. *See also* Coagulation of the Blood, Hemophilia.

361

Hemorrhoids: *see* Piles.

Hemostatics: substances which control the flow of blood in haemorrhage, and also (although the word is infrequently used in this sense) instruments used to control haemorrhage. The most commonly available haemostatic agents are heat and cold and on the whole heat is more efficient than cold. Both the heat and the cold must be severe enough to be uncomfortable to the hand if they are to work. Haemostatics include adrenaline, perchloride of iron, cobwebs and witch-hazel but they are only effective in slight or capillary bleeding. Haemorrhage from larger vessels is best controlled by pressure.

Hemothorax: blood in the pleural cavity, the space between the chest wall and the lung.

CAUSE: penetrating wounds or injuries, the presence of malignant tumours, occasionally leukaemia; it may occur spontaneously as the result of the tearing of an adhesion between the pleural membrane covering the chest wall and that covering the lung.

SYMPTOMS: if the haemothorax is the result of injury the pain, shock and shortness of breath associated with the haemothorax will be greater than that expected from the size and severity of the injury to the chest wall. The onset of symptoms is slow or quick according to the severity of the bleeding, and in the development of a slow haemothorax the patient may begin to run a fever as well as experience increasing pain and breathlessness, with an increase of pulse rate. He may suffer from pain in the upper abdomen if the blood irritates the diaphragm.

TREATMENT: blood lost, if the haemothorax is of any size, must be replaced by transfusion, and the blood in the chest must be drawn off through a large-bore needle under local anaesthetic. If it becomes clear that the haemorrhage is not stopping it may be necessary for a thoracic surgeon to open the chest to identify and deal with the bleeding points.

Heparin: a substance first isolated in the U.S.A. in 1916 which prevents the clotting of blood. It is found in the liver, lungs, muscles and intestines, where it is concentrated in the mucosal lining. It prevents the formation of fibrin by interfering with the action of thrombin on fibrinogen, and is used in medicine when clotting of the blood must be avoided, for example in blockage of the vessels of a limb by blood clot or in cardiac surgery when the blood is being circulated outside the body (*see* Heart-lung Machine, above). Heparin can be administered intravenously in single doses or as a continuous drip. *See* Coagulation of Blood.

Hepatitis: generally used to refer to infective hepatitis, an infection of the liver accompanied by jaundice.

CAUSE: infection by a virus which is transmitted in food contaminated by the excreta of a person suffering from the disease. A very similar condition named homologous serum jaundice is transmitted by blood and serum used for transfusions, and by needles and syringes used on an infected person; the use of disposable needles and syringes should cut down the incidence a great deal. In both conditions the liver swells and the cells are damaged, sometimes beyond recovery.

SYMPTOMS: the incubation period of infective hepatitis is about three weeks, but that of homologous serum jaundice much longer – between two and six months. Before the jaundice shows itself, the patient feels miserable and ill with nausea, loss of appetite and possibly discomfort in the upper abdomen. The diagnosis does not become clear until the second week of the infection, when jaundice appears and the skin and whites of the eyes turn yellow. The urine is dark and the motions light. The patient commonly feels better once the jaundice has appeared, but is often depressed throughout the illness and for a time afterwards. The duration of the illness varies, but recovery is shown by the gradual return to their normal appearance of the urine and the motions and the disappearance of the yellow discoloration of the skin. It usually takes about a month and a half to two months for the patient to feel fit again. Relapses may occur, and on the whole homologous serum jaundice is more severe than infectious hepatitis.

TREATMENT: the patient need not be strictly isolated, but it is imperative that the excreta should be carefully dealt with so that there is no chance of the infection spreading. The patient is kept in bed, and should be at rest. Alcohol is forbidden and the diet is light – generally there is no desire for anything much to eat. Gamma globulin (q.v.) will protect against the disease, and one attack confers immunity.

Heredity: this vast subject which forms the theme of the science of genetics can only be dealt with summarily here. The scientific study of heredity was initiated by the Austrian monk Gregor Mendel (1822–84) who, although one of the greatest of scientific geniuses, died virtually unknown, his work being published only after his death. Mendel's most important experiments were carried out on the common garden pea in which it is a relatively simple matter to distinguish several inherited characters and to cross-fertilize one plant with another. Thus some seeds are round, others wrinkled; some are green, others yellow; some plants are tall, others dwarf. By deliberately fertilizing one plant with another, Mendel was able to show how such character-istics are handed on. It might be supposed that traits of this type mingle to produce others which are a compromise between the two, for example that the offspring of a tall and a dwarf parent would be medium-sized, and so it sometimes turns out in a state of nature where few characteristics occur in the pure form. But Mendel was able to show that when the two pure lines are crossed the offspring are hybrid talls because the characteristic of tallness is dominant and when these are interbred the third generation are in the proportion of one pure tall to one pure dwarf and two hybrid talls. The pure lines when mated with each other breed true, only producing talls or dwarfs; but when the hybrids (who all *appear* tall) breed, the above proportions appear.

The reason for these proportions, although not known to Mendel, is apparent when we consider the processes of cell-division and reproduction. Every living cell (with rare exceptions such as the human red blood cell) contains a central nucleus which controls cell metabolism and carries the material which is the agent of heredity in the form of the chromosomes; ordinarily these are in a confused network which resembles a roughly crumpled skein of wool, but when cell division is about to occur this breaks up into numbers of separate chromosomes. These are rod, comma or globular-shaped bodies along which are strung the genes which are the actual carriers of the units of heredity. The cell narrows at the middle and the chromosomes divide equally down the centre of each so that when the narrowing becomes a distinct 'waist' and then a dumb-bell shape just before the two new cells separate, each part will contain exactly the same genes as the other. This process is known as mitosis and obviously there is little possibility of variation, for the two cells which have separated in this way contain identical hereditary material. But the mechanism of evolution and progress is divergence and it is this factor which is introduced by sexual reproduction when two cells unite each with a different hereditary content. Before this can happen, however, the number of chromosomes must be halved in the sex cells – otherwise the chromosome number would be doubling each time mating occurred. So in the development of the sex cells or gametes the chromosomes, instead of dividing down the middle, go half to one cell and half to another, thus the human body cells each contain 46 chromosomes but the germ cells only 23, the rest coming at fertilization from another individual of the opposite sex.

Now let us consider once more Mendel's tall and short pea plants. It will be seen that each pure-bred tall pea and each pure-bred dwarf carries in every body cell two units (or genes) for tallness or dwarfness so that when they divide to form the sex cells all will contain only factors for tallness or dwarfness. The hybrid types, on the other hand, have body cells which contain one gene for tallness and one dwarf gene and when they divide to form sex cells some will carry only tall characteristics and others only dwarf ones. When the two hybrids are crossed the possibilities for the offspring are: tall unites with tall, tall unites with dwarf, dwarf unites with tall, dwarf unites with dwarf. So there will be a proportion of two hybrids which appear tall but are not pure-bred, and one each of pure tall and dwarf stock; in short, three will appear tall and one dwarf. Most characters have a variation which is, in a sense, its opposite like tallness and shortness, blue eyes and brown eyes, and the one which imposes its appearance on the hybrids is known as the dominant gene, the other being the recessive one. According to commonly accepted theory the genes are totally unaffected by any events in the life of the individual who carries them and changes in the genetic constitution of a species are brought about by natural selection, which weeds out the useless traits by causing those who carry them to die out

365

earlier than those with useful variations. To take an example, in a wood near London a certain kind of moth had a wing coloration which perfectly fitted in with the light grey bark of the trees on which it usually rested and so it was invisible to prowling birds. But gradually the smoke of the growing city blackened the trunks of the trees and the light-coloured moths were easily seen and picked off by their enemies; some, however, had chance variations of wing-colour which were nearer in tint to the blackened trunks and these not only survived but increased since they naturally produced a higher proportion of dark-winged offspring. Today no light-winged moths survive. This is natural selection, which only involves the carrying on of useful variations already present and their multiplication in a favourable environment. The other main mechanism of evolution is mutation, in which the genes are radically changed by factors which, on the whole, are not fully understood. X-rays and atomic radiation can produce them, but such mutations are in the majority of instances harmful, only a minority being useful and progressive. From this it follows that the parents' way of life has little bearing on the inherited traits of their offspring. Lamarck's theory which, roughly speaking, implies that giraffes acquired long necks by constant stretching to reach the more tender leaves at the tree-tops and handed this acquired trait on to their offspring is thoroughly discredited, although the Soviet geneticist Lysenko made himself notorious by maintaining something of the sort. Acquired traits are not inherited.

What implications have these discoveries for general medicine? The answer must be at this time extraordinarily little. A number of diseases are inherited (for example certain forms of idiocy, haemophilia, Huntingdon's chorea) in a fairly definite way, but with most the issue is far less clear. For instance, the fact that obsessional neurosis is more frequent in the children of obsessional parents is more suggestive of training than heredity, and many other diseases in which there is a familial incidence are extremely complex problems. Epilepsy, for instance, seems commoner in the families of epileptic parents but it would be an overconfident physician who would recommend a man not to marry a woman whose aunt had suffered from epilepsy or even a woman who had a history of epilepsy herself. In general there is only a tiny minority of cases where the question of heredity is so clear-cut that those with the defect would be well-advised not to have children. *See* Eugenics, Hemophilia.

Hermaphrodite: everybody is born either male or female, because this characteristic is handed down with the sex chromosomes which determine sex rigidly at the moment of conception. There are, however, some children in whom the sexual organs are abnormal so that it is difficult to tell which sex they are. This is caused by failure of the gonadal tissue to differentiate properly in the embryonic stage, with the result that some children have both male and female sex organs present – gonads as well as external organs. There are three categories of hermaphrodites: (1) the sex of the predominant gonads (testicle or ovary) agrees with the sexual characteristics inherited in the cells; (2) the sex of the predominant gonads is not the same as the sexual characteristics of the cell; (3) the sex of the gonads cannot be identified. It is not in fact possible for anyone to change their sex, but it is possible for the male or female characteristics of the other sex to be removed by plastic surgery or sometimes supplemented by hormonal treatment. If gonads of both sorts are present, the incongruous tissue can also be removed. Nothing, however, can change the inherited sexual characteristics of the cell nucleus.

Hernia: the protrusion of any organ in whole or part from the compartment of the body normally containing it. The human body has a number of distinct compartments, for example the head, chest and abdomen; out of these compartments important structures run, such as the blood vessels which run out of the abdomen into the legs, the spermatic cord which runs from the abdomen into the scrotum, and the oesophagus which runs through the chest and into the upper part of the abdomen. It is at such points where the continuity of the wall of the compartment is normally incomplete that hernias are prone to develop. There are many sorts of hernia, and they are best described under separate headings.

1. *Inguinal hernia.* This is the most common type of hernia; it may be congenital or acquired, direct or indirect. In the congenital type there is a pre-existing weakness of the

abdominal wall which may give way under the strain of increased pressure inside the abdomen such as comes with chronic coughing, straining to pass motions, unaccustomed lifting of heavy weights, etc. In the acquired type the muscles of the abdominal wall become weak, with age for example, and therefore give way under strain. Inguinal hernia is commonest in men.

Indirect congenital hernia: the commonest type. In this hernia there is a congenital weakness where the testis once descended from the abdomen into the scrotum during early development – the path taken persists into adult life as the inguinal canal, which normally contains the spermatic cord, its coverings and blood vessels. In an indirect congenital hernia a sac of peritoneum, continuous with the abdominal cavity, is found associated with the cord inside which lie the contents of the hernia, which may be intestine or omentum (the fatty 'apron' which hangs down in front of the intestines).

SYMPTOMS: an aching pain associated with a swelling in the groin. The swelling may only come when the patient strains or coughs, or it may always be seen, especially on standing upright.

Direct inguinal hernia: this type is usually acquired and is caused by a weakness in the muscles of the region round the inguinal canal. This weakness allows the intestines or omentum to bulge out, and the swelling weakens the muscles still more.

SYMPTOMS: swelling and discomfort in the groin. The difference between a direct and indirect hernia is academic as far as the patient is concerned, for the treatment is the same for both.

TREATMENT: operation for reduction and repair of the hernia is always best. If the patient for one reason or another is not fit for operation a truss may be used, which must be put on while the hernia is reduced. This means that trusses must always be put on while the patient is lying down, and only removed if the hernia slips out or the patient has gone to bed. In general it is true to say that if a truss is comfortable it is not doing its job properly. It should consist of a firm pad attached to a belt round the waist, which is often reinforced by a steel spring.

2. *Femoral hernia.* This type of hernia is commoner in women

than in men. In it the protrusion is below the inguinal ligament instead of above it, as in inguinal hernia, and the hernia is directed downwards into the top of the thigh.

SYMPTOMS: again, the hernia presents as a swelling in the groin, but it is a little lower than the inguinal hernia and does not extend downwards towards the genital organs.

TREATMENT: this should be surgical, because it is virtually impossible to control a femoral hernia by means of a truss and because this type of hernia is very prone to strangulation (*see below*).

3. *Umbilical hernia*. The true umbilical hernia is commonest in infants. Almost indistinguishable from the true umbilical hernia, which comes through the umbilicus, is the para-umbilical hernia which comes through a gap in the mid-line of the abdomen just above the umbilicus. This, too, is found in children; the difference is that the true umbilical hernia can confidently be expected to close by itself, while the para-umbilical hernia may have to be repaired by operation. Para-umbilical hernia also occurs in the elderly, usually in women.

TREATMENT: true umbilical hernia found in infants may be left until it closes by itself. Some believe that strapping a coin over it helps by keeping the hernia reduced, but no convincing evidence has been offered that this is indeed so. In children an operation may be necessary to repair para-umbilical hernias, and it is usually advised that it should be done after the child is 4 years old because this type of hernia does not become strangulated (*see below*). Surgical repair of a para-umbilical hernia in the elderly may tax the ingenuity of the most skilful.

4. *Incisional hernia*. This is a hernia which comes through a part of the abdominal wall weakened by a surgical incision. It is a hernia of middle and old age, and although surgical treatment is advised it may not be practical. In such cases the patient ought to wear a tight belt to keep the abdominal contents in place.

5. *Epigastric hernia*. This is a hernia of fat through the mid-line of the abdominal wall between the umbilicus and the lower end of the breastbone. It is on occasion painful and tender, and in big hernias intestine or omentum may eventually be contained. The discomfort arising from an

369

epigastric hernia is sometimes mistaken for the pain of a gastric ulcer.

6. *Diaphragmatic or hiatus hernia.* This is a hernia involving the upper part of the stomach (cardia) more often seen in late middle or old age than in youth, except for cases that are found in infants where it is thought to be associated with an abnormally short oesophagus.

SYMPTOMS: the commonest symptom is heartburn; discomfort on swallowing, regurgitation of food and 'wind' are often present. In the infant there may be vomiting which may be bloodstained.

TREATMENT: in the infant, every effort is made to keep the child upright day and night – it is sat up in bed, and fluid feeds are given up as soon as possible in favour of thicker food. If, exceptionally, the stomach does not descend to its proper position in the upper abdomen, an operation can be carried out through the chest wall to reduce the hernia. In adults, those who are overweight are advised to reduce, tight clothes are never worn, and the patient is propped up in bed at night. The worst position for the hernia is lying down – exactly the opposite case to the hernias described above. The 'wind' is caused by swallowing air, and a treatment for this condition is described under Aerophagy. Cases that do not respond to medical treatment, which should include treatment of oesophageal irritation by alkalies such as magnesium trisilicate and a reasonable period of rest, are often operated upon with success.

Reduction of hernias. Hernias that can be replaced in the abdominal cavity are said to be reducible. Reduction, if difficult, is helped if the patient lies down.

Hernias which cannot be reduced are said to be irreducible, and fall into one of the two classes described below.

Incarcerated hernia: a hernia which cannot be reduced because the contents, which may be intestine or omentum, will no longer pass through the opening through which they came. This can happen when the empty bowel in a hernial sac becomes full.

It is important to note that the bowel in an incarcerated hernia is alive, and that its blood supply is intact.

Strangulated hernia: in strangulation, as the name implies, the contents of the hernial sac are strangled at the opening into the hernia, and their blood supply is cut off. This sets up a vicious circle, for as the effects of the stoppage of blood develop, the dying and dead contents of the hernia swell and increase the constriction at the neck of the hernial sac. Gangrene sets in and immediate operation with removal of the dead part of the bowel or omentum is imperative. As the hernia becomes strangulated it becomes painful and swollen and the skin over it may redden. Femoral hernias are prone to develop a particular type of strangulation in which only a part of the wall of the gut is caught in the hernial sac and cut off. This is called Richter's hernia, and the diagnosis may be difficult because obstruction of the intestine is not complete, and the contents of the gut may still pass the site of the partial strangulation.

Heroin: (Diamorphine). A drug of addiction formed from morphine by a slight alteration of its chemical formula. It is more potent than morphine weight for weight – that is, a smaller amount of heroin is needed to produce an effect – but otherwise it has no real advantages. It is probably the fact that a little goes a long way that has made it so popular with drug takers; indeed, the World Health Organization wishes the manufacture of heroin to be banned entirely. It is illegal to use the drug medically in the U.S.A., and it is not usual to use it to treat pain in Great Britain. *See* Drug Addiction.

Herpes: 1. *Herpes zoster, Shingles.* A painful disease of the sensory nerves with inflammation of the skin supplied by the nerve affected.
CAUSE: infection with the same virus that causes chickenpox. The relation is not quite straightforward, for although children can catch chickenpox from an adult with herpes zoster, adults do not seem to catch herpes from children with chickenpox or from another adult with herpes. It may be that the virus causing herpes zoster in adults has survived in the body in a dormant form from an infection in childhood.
SYMPTOMS: there is first a period of slight fever with pain in the part of the body supplied by the affected nerves. The disease usually extends round the side of the body like one half of a belt (the effect of herpes is in most cases on one side

371

only). After a few days the skin becomes red and then small blisters form over the affected area. They break down and dry scabs take their place; when the scabs eventually fall off a white scar is left. Herpes may occur in one of the divisions of the fifth cranial nerve, the nerve which supplies the sensation of the face and head. If it affects the first or ophthalmic division of the nerve the eye may suffer badly and may even become blind. After herpes has resolved, the patient may continue to suffer from persistent and crippling neuralgia or pain in the area supplied by the affected nerve, although the scars left are insensitive.

TREATMENT: there is no specific treatment. Pain is controlled by the use of drugs as powerful as are required, and the blisters are covered with collodion (q.v.) and kept dusted with sterile powder. They must not be allowed to become infected. Pain which persists after an attack of herpes zoster is one of the most difficult problems the physician has to face, and it may be almost impossible to treat the condition successfully.

2. *Herpes simplex*, or '*Cold Sore*'. At the corners of the mouth, sometimes near the genital organs, and occasionally on a finger occur small blisters often in association with a cold or other infection.

CAUSE: a virus, different from that which causes herpes zoster, which remains in the cells and is activated from time to time.

TREATMENT: corticosteroid ointment combined with neomycin. Whereas one attack of herpes zoster confers an immunity from further attacks of the disease, herpes simplex recurs.

Hetacillin: a penicillin derivative which can be given by mouth. It is a broad-spectrum antibiotic similar to ampicillin, but administration by mouth produces higher levels in the blood; undesirable side effects are much the same, and include diarrhoea, heartburn, nausea and skin rashes.

Hexamine: a substance made by the action of ammonia on formalin; in acid fluids it liberates the antiseptic formaldehyde. It was until recently used as a urinary antiseptic, the urine being kept acid by the administration of acid phosphate of sodium.

Hexoestrol: a synthetic ovarian hormone related to stilboestrol and with similar but weaker action. It is not often used.

Hexylresorcinol: a drug, usually given in capsules, active against roundworms, threadworms and hookworms (*see* Worms). It is useful in treating mixed infections, the dose being 1 g. The drug is also used as a surface antiseptic.

Hiatus Hernia: *see* Hernia.

Hibitane: (Chlorhexidine). A substance which is active against bacteria, particularly Grampositive bacteria, used widely as an antiseptic. In hospitals it is used to prepare the skin before operations, often in combination with cetrimide. Hibitane cream 1% is used a great deal by surgeons and midwives, and can be used with advantage in the home on minor wounds and abrasions.

Hiccup: a spasmodic inspiration which ends suddenly as the vocal cords close. It is caused by involuntary contractions of the diaphragm, and although it usually stops fairly quickly there are conditions in which it persists and exhausts the patient.

CAUSE: irritation of the diaphragm or of the nerves supplying the diaphragm, or rarely disease of the brain (encephalitis) or disorder of blood chemistry (uraemia).

TREATMENT: various 'cures' are recommended which include drinking cold water out of the wrong side of a glass, holding the breath, and the administration of a stiff fright. More scientific remedies are the inhalation of carbon dioxide (which can be achieved by breathing in and out of a paper bag), pulling the tongue forwards with reasonable force, or the inhalation of a capsule of amyl nitrite. The doctor should be called to cases of persistent hiccups.

Higginson's Syringe: a type of rubber syringe which consists of an elliptical bulb with a tube at each end. Non-return valves are incorporated in the junctions of the tubing with the bulb in such a way that pressure on the bulb forces fluid out through one tube and expansion of the bulb draws fluid in through the other. Higginson was a nineteenth-

373

century surgeon who practised in Liverpool, and his syringe is usually employed to administer enemas.

High Blood Pressure: *see* Hypertension.

Hip Joint: a ball and socket joint formed by the ball-shaped head of the femur (thigh-bone) and the acetabulum, a cup-shaped hollow in the side of the pelvis. Because it has a very strong fibrous capsule with powerful ligaments it is rarely dislocated in the adult, but some children are born with an ill-formed hip joint which is easily dislocated. This condition is called congenital dislocation of the hip, and is most common in northern Italy and some parts of central Europe. If it is diagnosed early in life it can be cured, but if it is left the individual walks with a waddling limp for the rest of his life and is prone to develop osteoarthritis. Another disease liable to affect the hip joint in early life is osteochondritis of the head of the femur (Perthes' disease), a disease in which the head of the femur becomes flattened and shaped like a mushroom. The joint is painful and in later life tends to become the site of osteoarthritis. Perthes' disease is more often found in boys than girls. Tuberculosis of the hip may occur in either sex and at any age; treatment takes a long time and often involves orthopaedic surgery. Because the hip joint transmits a considerable weight and is in constant movement it is in later life very inclined to become the site of osteoarthritis even in the absence of any predisposing disease, and various operations have been devised to reduce pain and restore movement. The most effective operation to reduce pain, however, is an arthrodesis, in which the articular surfaces of the joint are fused together so that movement is no longer possible. This is a state of affairs which is unacceptable to many people, and today newer operations to replace the diseased joint surfaces by artificial structures are proving increasingly successful.

Hippocrates: a Greek physician who flourished in Cos from about 460 to 370 B.C. and left many writings. He is universally recognized in the West as the Father of Medicine; he left a famous oath for the guidance of the profession which has been accepted as the foundation for codes of medical conduct ever since:

I swear by Apollo Physician, by Asclepius, by Health, by Heal-all, and by all the gods and goddesses, making them witnesses, that I will carry out, according to my ability and judgment, this oath and this indenture: To regard my teacher in this art as equal to my parents; to make him partner in my livelihood, and when he is in need of money to share mine with him; to consider his offspring equal to my brothers; to teach them this art, if they require to learn it, without fee or indenture; and to impart precept, oral instruction, and all the other learning, to my sons, to the sons of my teacher, and to pupils who have signed the indenture and sworn obedience to the physicians' Law, but to none other. I will use treatment to help the sick according to my ability and judgment, but I will never use it to injure or wrong them. I will not give poison to anyone though asked to do so, nor will I suggest such a plan. Similarly I will not give a pessary to a woman to cause abortion. But in purity and in holiness I will guard my life and my art. I will not use the knife either on sufferers from stone, but I will give place to such as are craftsmen therein. Into whatsoever houses I enter, I will do so to help the sick, keeping myself free from all intentional wrong-doing and harm, especially from fornication with woman or man, bond or free. Whatsoever in the course of practice I see or hear (or even outside my practice in social intercourse) that ought never to be published abroad, I will not divulge, but consider such things to be holy secrets. Now if I keep this oath and break it not, may I enjoy honour, in my life and art, among all men for all time; but if I transgress and forswear myself, may the opposite befall me. (*The Doctor's Oath*, by W. H. S. Jones, Cambridge University Press.)

Hippus: normally the pupil of the eye contracts and dilates rhythmically but imperceptibly – hippus is a condition in which the movement is exaggerated and obvious. It continues all the time and is not stopped by changes in the level of illumination or by accommodation.

Hirschsprung's Disease: (Aganglionic Megacolon). A condition in which there is malfunction of the large intestine, which becomes loaded with faeces and grossly distended. CAUSE: absence of the nervous fibres which normally form a plexus in the wall of the intestine and control muscular activity. A segment of the colon is affected, usually just above the rectum, and in this segment there is no peristalsis, the rhythmic movement by which the intestine moves its contents along. The bowel at the level of the abnormality and below it is narrow and empty, but the bowel above is distended and full because the area without peristaltic movement acts as an obstruction.

SYMPTOMS: the newborn baby passes no motions; the abdomen may become blown up. The child is always severely constipated and may show signs of intestinal obstruction.

TREATMENT: the segment of abnormal bowel is removed surgically and functional continuity of the intestine restored.

Hirsuties: (Hypertrichosis). The growth of superfluous hair especially in women with distribution of the male type both on the face and body, It is sometimes associated with disorders of the suprarenal glands.

Histamine: a very important substance present in the bodies of many animals including man, and found in various plants, for example the stinging nettle. It has many pharmacological actions, which are by no means fully understood, but perhaps the action of greatest practical importance in the present state of knowledge concerns allergy (q.v.) and similar states. At the beginning of this century it was noticed that the effect of injecting histamine into guinea pigs and rabbits was very like anaphylactic shock (q.v.), and later it was seen that 'pricking' histamine into the skin produced a reaction very like the response to running a blunt point firmly in a line along the skin – a red line surrounded by a reddened area, followed by swelling of the line which forms a distinct wheal (the triple response of Lewis). Moreover, a large injection of histamine and a severe tissue injury both lead to a state of surgical shock. It was therefore thought that histamine, which is known to be in the tissues, is liberated or formed when cells are damaged. Later work has shown that cellular injury produces an increase in the formation of histamine, particularly in the lungs and skin, and that the disintegration of cells in an antibody-antigen reaction liberates granules of histamine.

It follows that substances which antagonize the action of histamine ought to relieve the symptoms of allergic reaction and anaphylactic shock; such substances are adrenaline, which acts very quickly, and a number of drugs called antihistamines (which can themselves cause sensitivity reactions if applied unwisely to the skin). Antihistamines are better at preventing reactions than treating them; when a reaction has developed, it is best treated in the first instance by the injection of adrenaline or hydrocortisone and the subsequent regular use of chlorpheniramine (Piriton or Chlor-Trimeton) or promethazine (Phenergan). Some diseases, notably asthma, react disappointingly to antihistamines, and this is thought to be due to the release of substances other than histamine as part of the allergic process. Antihistamine drugs have other actions beside counteracting the effects of histamines; they produce drowsiness and are used as sedatives, they prevent motion sickness, and they alleviate giddiness caused by disease of the balancing organ in the ear (Menière's disease). The production of drowsiness may be very important if a patient taking antihistamines tries to drive a motor car or operate machinery.

Histology: the study of the microscopic structure of tissues.

Histoplasmosis: a disease more common in the U.S.A. than in the United Kingdom. The organism that causes it is the fungus Histoplasma capsulatum, which lives in dust and in the soil. If it is inhaled it infects the lungs and sets up chronic foci of irritation which result in the formation of small granulomata, or even pneumonia. Histoplasmosis may be confused with tuberculosis.

Hives: nettle-rash or urticaria (q.v.).

Hoarseness: commonly due to infectious conditions of the throat and larynx. The treatment of hoarseness is the treatment of the condition causing it. Chronic or continuing hoarseness may be due to irritation of the vocal cords by misuse; they become oedematous and thickened, and may even grow polypi – small warty excrescences. The treatment is to give up shouting. Those whose voices become hoarse in the absence of infection or misuse are advised to seek medical advice, for such a change of voice may be a sign that a tumour is present in the larynx. A change of voice can also be produced by disease affecting the recurrent laryngeal nerve which supplies the larynx, which in its course through the neck may be damaged by disease in such different places as the thyroid gland, the apex of the lung, or the aorta. Removal of the thyroid gland may result in damage to the recurrent laryngeal nerve and weakening and hoarseness of the voice.

Hobnail Liver: *see* Cirrhosis.

Hodgkin's Disease: (Lymphadenoma). A disease of the reticular and lymphatic tissues of the body, commonest in young men.

CAUSE: unknown.

SYMPTOMS: the glands in the neck slowly become enlarged, but do not hurt. They are not tender but feel rubbery, are separate, and move about easily. As the disease progresses other groups of glands enlarge and the patient may have intermittent fever, the bouts lasting for about ten days at a time. Groups of enlarging glands begin to interfere with the function of structures nearby, for example the glands round the bronchi may compress the air passages so that the patient becomes breathless and parts of the lung collapse. The liver and spleen enlarge, and cause abdominal discomfort, and pressure on nerves may produce pain or paralysis. In rare cases pain is felt in the enlarged glands if the patient drinks alcohol.

TREATMENT: radiotherapy is effective against isolated groups of glands, and cytotoxic drugs are used in cases where enlargement is widespread. Agents often used are nitrogen mustards, which are related to mustard gas. Other cytotoxic drugs such as Vinblastine sulphate, derived from the periwinkle, and Chlorambucil may be tried. The disease is accompanied by anaemia which is sometimes so marked that it has to be treated by transfusions.

Localized pressure causing pain or interference with function can in some cases be relieved by surgery.

Homatropine: an alkaloid derived from atropine used to dilate the pupil of the eye. The effect of a 1% solution wears off in a few hours, but may cause considerable blurring of vision while it lasts. The drug is sometimes used in order to make examination of the back of the eye by ophthalmoscopy possible.

Homoeopathy: a system of medicine founded by C. F. S. Hahnemann (1755–1843) at the end of the eighteenth century. Born at Meissen in Saxony he studied medicine at Leipzig and Vienna, finally graduating at Erlangen and settling down as a physician in Leipzig. Dissatisfied (quite justifiably) with the state of medicine at that time Hahnemann put forward in 1796 his new principle of 'the law of similars' to the effect that diseases should be treated by drugs which produce symptoms similar to them in healthy people (*similia similibus curantur*).

This concept, if not of universal application, was considerably in advance of contemporary medicine as it is true that many symptoms can be regarded as resulting from the body's attempt to throw off the disease, for example diarrhoea is clearly an attempt to get rid of irritant matter or disease-causing germs, and before the discovery of antibiotics and sulpha drugs it was more appropriate in many cases to give a purgative such as castor oil to aid the process rather than opium to slow it down. But this does not apply to all symptoms and even when it does diarrhoea, for example, may be so severe that its original function is lost in the harm it is doing to the patient by loss of fluids and damage to the intestine; in such cases it must be stopped regardless of the lesser harm done by the temporary retention of poisonous or irritant products. Four years later Hahnemann produced his other principle, that drugs should be given in almost infinitesimal doses and, with all respect due to a great man, this has been accepted by no one save homoeopathists even when based on the pseudo-scientific theory of dynamization, or increase of force with diminution of matter, such dynamization being allegedly produced by trituration or grinding to a fine powder and extreme dilution. Although many eminent physicians have given their approval to homoeopathy it is remarkable that this theory which could be quite easily put to the test in animal experiments has never in fact been so tested and one can only conclude that its practitioners are aware of the fallacies involved. Tests on the human being are rarely valid if we are to rely solely on subjective feelings of improvement, since it is entirely obvious that these are more likely to depend upon faith and suggestibility than objective results; the fact that 90% of patients feel better after a certain line of treatment tells us nothing whatever except that that is how 90% of patients felt. How they objectively are is quite another matter. Hahnemann's system caused great antagonism and he had to leave Leipzig, finally ending up in Paris, where he ran a successful practice based on his principles (which, as has already been admitted, were infinitely superior to the bulk of orthodox medicine at that time). Homoeopathy is practised by a decreasing number of orthodox physicians and there are a number of excellent homoeopathic hospitals in England which, so far as one is aware, pay comparatively little attention to Hahnemann's original principles and certainly do not use specific drugs such as sulphonamides and antibiotics in diluted doses. There are no homoeopathic hospitals left in the United States. In contrast with homoeopathy orthodox medicine is described as allopathy or heteropathy, meaning that it treats diseases by giving remedies which produce opposite results from the symptoms. This, however, is a misnomer because modern medicine is based on scientific research unsupported by any one overall theory. The trouble with homoeopathy is that it is a system, and nature cannot be confined to any such rigid schemes. It may be taken almost as an axiom that any system which begins with the assumptions: *every* disease is caused by . . .' or *every* disease can be cured by . . .' as do osteopathy, Christian Science, homoeopathy, and the rest is bound to be wrong.

Homograft: a graft taken from another individual of the same species.

Homosexuality: *see* Sex.

Hookworm: Ankylostoma duodenale and Necator americanus are the hookworms which infect man. Both of them are small – about ten millimetres long – and they live in the intestines where they suck blood.
CAUSE: the hookworms lay eggs which pass out of the gut,

but can only develop into larvae in moist or damp places where it never freezes. The larvae are able to burrow through human skin, so that anyone coming into contact with water or mud where larval worms are present runs a risk of becoming infected. The same risk is present if drinking water becomes infected, but simple sanitation will prevent this. When the hookworm has entered the skin it makes its way into a small blood vessel, and is carried into the lungs. There it escapes from the bloodstream, and crawls up the air passages into the trachea. When the worm reaches the top of the larynx it crosses into the oesophagus and drops down into the stomach through which it creeps into the first part of the small intestine, the duodenum, where it commonly lives.

SYMPTOMS: the places where the larvae enter the body break out into a dermatitis, with small infected pustules. This is often referred to as 'ground itch', and lasts a number of days. When the larvae reach the lungs, irritation leads to over-secretion of mucus, which is coughed up; but the main symptoms are caused by worms sucking blood from the walls of the intestine. In a heavy infestation there is anaemia, pain, discomfort in the upper abdomen which may be confused with the symptoms of peptic ulceration, and obvious malnutrition. There may be diarrhoea with blood in the motions.

TREATMENT: the disease only occurs where sanitation is defective and there is water or mud. The first objective is of course to destroy the worms in the patient, which may be done by doses of bephenium hydroxynaphthoate (Alcopar), but the disease can never be controlled until the conditions which make it possible are altered; if this is not done the patient will become infected again, for an attack confers no immunity on the sufferer. *See* Worms.

Hordoleum: (Stye). Inflammation of a sebaceous gland in the eyelid.

Horehound: a group of perennial herbs found throughout Europe, although not very common in Britain where the white or common horehound is infrequently found and black horehound only occurs south of the Forth and Clyde. The dried leaves of the former (Marrubium vulgare) are used to

relieve coughs; they are either mixed with sugar or prescribed in a fluid extract (1–2 teaspoonfuls) although more
often nowadays by herbalists than physicians. Horehound
candies are used in the United States for cough.

Hormones: substances which, secreted by the ductless or
endocrine glands, influence tissues and organs in other parts
of the body, being carried thither in the bloodstream.

Horner's Syndrome: a group of signs and symptoms
resulting from paralysis of the sympathetic nerves in the
neck. They are: drooping of the upper eyelid; sinking in of
the eyeball; pupillary constriction; and loss of the power of
sweating on the affected side.

Hospital: a place for the reception and treatment of the
sick. The word, derived from the Latin 'hospitalis', and
meaning pertaining to a host or guest, has also given rise to
the words hotel and hostel which now have a different
significance. There were hospitals of a sort attached to the
temples of ancient Egypt from about 4000 B.C. where patients
slept in the hope that the gods would cure them, but the
temple of Asclepius (Aesculapius) at Cos associated with
Hippocrates (q.v.) 'the Father of Medicine' who died *c.*
370 B.C., although originally based on the same principles,
became much more scientific as under his influence diseases
came to be better understood. In the East the Indian emperor
Asoka founded a hospital at Surat and the famous sultan
Harun al-Rashid who died in A.D. 809 built numerous
hospitals in Baghdad. Constantinople under the Byzantine
empire had the Pantocrator which was far in advance of
anything in medieval Europe, with specialists in various
branches of medicine, women doctors for childbirth, a
pharmacy and an almoner's department, disinfection of the
patients' clothes on admission and issue of clean clothing and
bedding while under treatment, and so on. But until the
eighteenth century there was comparatively little provision for the institutional treatment of the sick in Britain
where, by 1710, the only general hospitals in London were
St Thomas's and St Bartholomew's. Subsequently the
number of hospitals slowly increased and during the nineteenth century numerous dispensaries, some of them founded

by religious bodies, were set up to provide some form of out-patient treatment. The important events which made hospitals as we now know them possible were (*a*) the discovery of anaesthetics (q.v.), which put an end to the bloody, agonizing, and necessarily brief surgical operations carried out only as a last resort, and opened the way to modern surgery; (*b*) Lister's introduction of the antiseptic technique in surgery (1865), which reduced the dangers of sepsis; (*c*) the improvements in the standard of nursing carried out by Florence Nightingale as the result of her experience during the Crimean War and later introduced by her to St Thomas's nursing school in London.

Hourglass Stomach: the appearance seen in an X-ray of a stomach which is constricted in the middle either because of spasm or more commonly old ulceration. *See* Stomach Disease.

Housemaid's Knee: a swelling of the bursa which lies in front of the knee-cap due, as the name suggests, to excessive kneeling.

Humerus: the bone of the upper arm, articulating with the shoulderblade at the upper end in a ball and socket joint and with the radius and ulna, the two bones of the forearm, at the lower end in a hinge joint. The inner prominence of the humerus at the elbow is called the funny bone; the ulnar nerve runs behind it directly under the skin, and a blow upon it is extremely painful.

Humour: a term now used only for the aqueous and vitreous humours of the eyeball, but formerly associated with a theory of the nature of disease originating with the Pythagorean philosophers in the sixth century B.C., but accepted by Hippocrates (400 B.C.), Aristotle (300 B.C.), Galen (A.D. 200), and in one form or another by most other physicians up to the end of the eighteenth century. The theory ascribed temperaments and diseases to excess or deficiency of humours, which were classified as sanguine (full-blooded), phlegmatic (dull-watery), choleric (fiery, due to yellow bile), and melancholy (depressed, due to black bile). Although as a theory of disease this view is long outdated, some still use the terms to classify inherited temperaments; for clearly there is some ground for supposing the types of optimist and pessimist, the quick to anger and slow to be moved, to be basic psychological categories of personality.

Hunterian Chancre: the primary sore of syphilis, which has an ulcerated hard base. The discharge is thin and watery; it derives its name from the eighteenth-century surgeon John Hunter, who inoculated himself with syphilitic matter in order to demonstrate how the disease was passed on and how it developed.

Huntington's Chorea: a disease inherited as a Mendelian dominant. It shows itself between the ages of 30 and 40, and is characterized by the sort of involuntary movements seen in chorea and progressive mental deterioration. Finally the movements become gross and the patient completely paralysed and demented. The condition is slowly progressive and there is no known treatment. Institutional care is usually necessary in the later stages.

Hutchinson's Teeth: the narrowed and notched incisor teeth typical of congenital syphilis, named after the physician Sir Jonathan Hutchinson (d. 1913) who first described them.

Hyaluronidase: a naturally occurring enzyme which has the property of breaking down the cement substance, or ground substance, of the tissues so that the tissue planes are opened up. Hyaluronidase is sometimes used to speed up the absorption of injected drugs and fluids.

Hyatid Cyst: a disease in which parasitic cysts are formed in the liver, lung, brain or other organs.
CAUSE: the tapeworm Taenia echinococcus lives in the intestines of the domestic dog, the wolf and the fox, and gravid segments are passed in the creature's faeces. Some of these segments may stick to the animal's fur, and he may by scratching shift them to any part of his body. In one way or another, usually by eating food or drinking water contaminated by an infected dog, the segment of worm containing eggs is passed to the intermediate host, which is

usually a sheep, but may be a man. In the intermediate host embryo worms are liberated in the upper part of the small intestine where they burrow into the wall of the gut and by way of the portal circulation make their way to the liver. The embryos either stay in the liver or travel onwards to the lungs and so into the systemic circulation and into other organs, notably the brain. They then form cysts, called hydatid cysts, which contain fluid and many daughter cysts, each one of which is capable of starting further cyst formation if it is liberated in the tissues. The cycle is complete when a dog eats infected sheep offal.

SYMPTOMS: the cysts cause symptoms according to their site; for example in the brain they can cause epilepsy and paralysis. Occasionally they rupture spontaneously and the fluid escaping from the cyst may precipitate anaphylactic shock, as well as seeding many daughter cysts in the surrounding tissues.

TREATMENT: if the cysts become very large they can be removed surgically, but the surgeon has to be careful not to break them and let the fluid escape. It is dangerous to aspirate the cysts; they must always be removed completely. Prevention of the disease depends on strict hygiene, and attention to worming dogs. In sheep-rearing areas where the disease is known to occur children should be prevented from coming into very close contact with dogs, and the dogs must be prevented from eating sheep offal. *See* Worms.

Hydatidiform Mole: a disease of the superficial layer of the chorion, the outer of the two membranes covering the foetus, in which the uterus becomes full of vesicles like grapes; no embryo is found, for it is destroyed by the mole.

SYMPTOMS: the patient progresses as she would in the first months of pregnancy. After about four months' amenorrhoea there is a certain amount of bleeding, sometimes a watery discharge and occasionally the escape of vesicles from the mole. There may be pain in the back and the loins, and the uterus is generally bigger than expected for the date.

TREATMENT: the mole must be removed as soon as possible, or in one in ten cases it undergoes malignant change. If the patient is satisfied to have no more children the uterus is removed with the mole, to make sure that there is no risk of malignant growth. If the mole alone is removed, the patient

385

must attend the clinic to be examined at regular intervals for a time to make sure that there is no recurrence.

Hydrargyrum: mercury.

Hydrocele: a common condition of men in which there is a collection of fluid in the tunica vaginalis, the sac which surrounds the testicle. It may occur at any age, but old men are perhaps more prone to the condition.

CAUSE: in most cases unknown, but in some cases the collection of fluid is caused by an underlying disease which is discovered by analysis of the fluid or by examination of the testicle after the fluid has been drawn off.

SYMPTOMS: painless, smooth, and elastic enlargement of the scrotum. The hydrocele is translucent; that is, if a bright light is placed upon it in the dark the whole swelling lights up. If it is painful it usually means that it has become infected, or has been the site of a haemorrhage.

TREATMENT: the best treatment is by operation, when the sac containing the fluid is removed. The testicle itself can be inspected at operation to verify that there is no underlying disease. If the patient is not fit to have an operation, the fluid in the hydrocele can be drawn off through a wide-bore needle without difficulty or discomfort, but the swelling always recurs and aspirations have to be performed at regular intervals. Hydrocele in infants needs no surgical treatment because it usually disappears by itself.

Hydrocephalus: the brain contains cavities called ventricles which are normally full of cerebrospinal fluid. There are two lateral ventricles, right and left, one central ventricle into which the lateral ventricles drain, called the third ventricle, and a fourth ventricle into which fluid from the third passes and which communicates with the outside surface at the base of the brain. At the exit of the fourth ventricle the cerebro-spinal fluid passes into the subarachnoid space between the pia and arachnoid membranes surrounding the brain and the spinal cord, and runs upwards over the outer surface of the brain. It is absorbed through special valves in the arachnoid membrane, called arachnoid villi, into the blood contained in the venous sinuses of the outer membrane covering the brain, the dura mater. The cerebro-spinal fluid is formed in the ventricles by plexuses of blood vessels called the choroid plexuses. Interference with the passage of cerebro-spinal fluid through the ventricles to the outside of the brain, or with its passage to that part of the arachnoid membrane where arachnoid villi pass it back into the bloodstream, or excessive production of the fluid, results in hydrocephalus – abnormal amounts of water, or fluid, in the head. The condition may be congenital, in which case investigation may show that it is possible for an artificial valve or communication to be established to restore the circulation of the fluid, or acquired; commonly acquired hydrocephalus is the result of blockage by a tumour, but sometimes it occurs as the result of inflammation or rarely of injury, In both types of hydrocephalus, congenital or acquired, the only treatment is surgical. In congenital cases the head itself may be obviously swollen and deformed. If the condition is not relieved the patient suffers from severe headaches and interference with vision, hearing and eventually mental functions.

Hydrochloric Acid: a gas which when dissolved in water forms a strong corrosive acid. It is found in normal gastric juice in a much diluted form; it may be present to excess in cases of peptic ulceration, but in other conditions it may be absent. An excess of acid of itself does not cause symptoms, nor does a deficiency.

Hydrochlorothiazide: a substance which promotes the secretion of urine and the excretion of sodium. It is used to increase loss of fluids from the body in conditions where the tissues are in danger of becoming waterlogged, for example in congestive heart failure or oedema associated with kidney disease. There are numerous proprietary preparations in use. *See* Diuretics.

Hydrocortisone: *see* Corticosteroids. Hydrocortisone is used for injections and for local applications to the skin.

Hydrocyanic Acid: (Prussic acid). A poisonous substance which produces its effect by depriving the cells of oxygen. Recommended antidotes are: amyl nitrite capsules inhaled at once, injection of sodium nitrite into the veins (10 ml of

3% solution) given slowly, intravenous injection of 25 ml 50% solution of sodium thiosulphate, again given slowly, and if there is reason to believe that the poison is in the stomach, a washout of 25% sodium thiosulphate. These injections, and capsules of amyl nitrite, should always be available in places where there is a risk of cyanide poisoning; cyanide poisoning first-aid kits are commercially available.

Hydrogen Peroxide: being decomposed into water and oxygen when brought into contact with the tissues, especially in the presence of dead cells and pus, hydrogen peroxide exercises its effect as an antiseptic by virtue of its freed oxygen. It is mild, safe, ordinarily non-irritant, and is most useful in removing dressings that stick, in disinfecting small amounts of drinking water, in cleansing suppurating wounds where the bubbles formed help to remove discharge and destroy anaerobic organisms, as a mouth-wash and in the treatment of inflammations of the gums, in removing wax from the ears, and in stopping bleeding from capillary oozing.

Hydronephrosis: distention of the pelvis of the kidney with greater or lesser destruction of the kidney tissue and loss of renal function.

CAUSE: the cause of primary hydronephrosis is not known. Some postulate an intermittent obstruction to the outflow of urine by defective neuromuscular control of the ureter, in the same way that in Hirschsprung's disease (q.v.) absence of co-ordination of neuromuscular action results in obstruction of the large bowel. Secondary hydronephrosis, as its name suggests, is secondary to some other pathological process which causes obstruction or damage to the ureter. Such conditions are stones in the ureter which block the outflow of urine on one side or the other, tumours of the pelvis of the kidney, and stones, tumours, obstructions and strictures of the bladder or the urethra including those caused by enlargement of the prostate gland. Obstructions higher than the bladder will affect the kidney on the diseased side; obstructions of the bladder or the urethra will affect both kidneys.

SYMPTOMS: pain in the loin, usually colicky as well as dull and aching. There may be blood in the urine, or signs of infection such as pain on passing water and frequency. The patient may suffer from nausea, and may actually vomit from time to time. In secondary hydronephrosis added symptoms are due to the primary condition.

TREATMENT: the treatment of secondary hydronephrosis is the treatment of the primary condition. If the kidney is completely disorganized and lacks all function it is removed, but efforts are always directed towards saving all the functioning kidney tissue possible.

Hydropathy: the use of water in treatment whether internally or externally, once extremely popular – so popular that the fortunes of whole towns were founded upon their waters. Although nobody would deny that baths and the rest are both useful and pleasant, few today would be prepared to allow hydropathy to occupy the grandiose position it once held, and very few doctors recommend their patients to 'take the waters'. Perhaps hydropathy was at its best in treating afflictions which were vague and ill-defined – or even non-existent; nevertheless, certain natural waters contain salts which taken internally are purgative or diuretic, and may today be bought in bottles.

Hydrophobia: *see* Rabies.

Hydrotherapy: *see* Hydropathy.

Hygiene: the science of the preservation of health.

Hyoid Bone: a small U-shaped bone at the base of the tongue which can be felt in the front of the neck about an inch above the Adam's apple. It is usually broken during strangulation, a fact which may prove to be very important in the investigation of death.

Hyoscyamus: from this plant is prepared hyoscine, or scopolamine, a drug used to counteract the action of the parasympathetic nervous system. It has a potent effect in relieving pain caused by muscular spasm of the involuntary muscles, for example in the bladder, ureter or urethra. Hyoscine is also a cerebral depressant used in states of mental excitement such as mania, delirium tremens or the delirium of fever. It is used to prevent seasickness, is useful in the treatment of Parkinson's disease and is combined with morphia or its derivatives for use before surgical operations as a 'premedication'. It is not without its dangers, and unwise administration can cause hallucinations, a fact which has to be borne in mind if the drug is used to relieve the pangs of duodenal ulcer by reducing muscular spasm and lessening the secretion of hydrochloric acid in the stomach, for patients are liable to take too much of the mixture as a routine.

Hyperacusis: abnormal sensitivity to sounds, or an abnormally acute sense of hearing.

Hyperaemia: congestion of a part with blood.

Hyperaesthesia: increased sensitivity to touch, or to pain in the skin, or abnormally increased sensitivity in one of the organs of special sense.

Hyperbaric Oxygenation: the exposure of patients to oxygen at high pressure in a special chamber has been used to render cancer cells more sensitive to X-ray therapy, to treat gas gangrene – a disease where the causative organism flourishes only in the absence of oxygen – and to treat carbon monoxide poisoning. The technique has also been used to treat accident victims in whom arteries have been damaged so badly that the survival of limbs is in doubt. The treatment is not without complications, for a patient breathing oxygen is liable to oxygen poisoning, which may produce fits but is transitory; after long exposure to oxygen he may develop a form of broncho-pneumonia. The attendants in a high-pressure chamber, who breathe air, may develop caisson disease, and the risk of fire is considerable.

Hyperchlorhydria: excess of hydrochloric acid in the stomach.

Hyperemesis: excessive vomiting, which when it occurs in pregnancy is named hyperemesis gravidarum. This is commonest with the first child and begins before the fourth month, usually from psychological causes. The vomiting responds to removal of the patient from her home to hospital in most cases, but careful consideration of the problems of the expectant mother and efforts to ease them, combined with firm reassurance, are often enough to cure the condition without hospital treatment.

Hyperglycaemia: excess sugar in the blood. *See* Diabetes.

Hyperhidrosis: (Hyperidrosis). Excessive sweating. This may be caused by interference with the normal action of the heat-regulating system, for example in thyrotoxicosis or by drugs such as alcohol, by an exaggeration of the normal response to emotional stress (particularly in young people), or it may be an inherited tendency.

Hypermetropia: long sight, caused by the eye being too short from lens to retina or having a lens without sufficient refractive power. The ability to focus on objects near at hand is restored by a convex spectacle lens. *See* Spectacles.

Hypernephroma: a malignant tumour of the kidney, which affects men more than women and is commonest in those over the age of 50.
SYMPTOMS: blood in the urine, sometimes occurring painlessly but sometimes associated with colic caused by the passage of clots down the ureter. There may be discomfort in the loin, or even a swelling. The tumour may announce itself by signs of secondary invasion of the lungs or of bone.
TREATMENT: investigation of the whole of the urinary tract must be carried out in cases of unexplained blood in the urine, and the discovery of a tumour of the kidney will be followed by a search to see if there has been any secondary spread. If none is found the kidney is removed, surgical treatment often being combined with radiotherapy. Sometimes a secondary deposit is found months or even years after the primary tumour has been removed, usually in the lung but also in bone; if the deposit is solitary removal is often worth while.

Hyperpiesis: another word for high blood pressure or hypertension.

Hyperplasia: abnormal increase in the number of cells

391

in a tissue, and consequent increase in size of an organ or structure.

Hyperpyrexia: a high temperature.

Hypertension: high blood pressure.

CAUSE: hypertension may be primary or secondary. In primary hypertension, no underlying cause can be found; secondary hypertension follows disease of the kidneys, pregnancy in which the mother develops toxaemia, and sometimes malfunction of endocrine glands. The majority of cases are primary, and in some there is a family history.

SYMPTOMS: it is not easy to unravel the complicated state into which patients can get once they have been told they have a high blood pressure, for to symptoms caused by hypertension they add a number of complaints which are in fact to be explained on psychological grounds, and arise largely because of anxiety. The true headache of hypertension is very severe, is felt towards the back of the head and is associated with vomiting; but many patients complain of other types of headache which resemble those found in states of anxiety and nervous tension. Most physicians estimate the progress of the disease by its effect on the arteries of the eye, which can be seen by ophthalmoscopy, the state of the heart, and the examination of the urine, rather than by the symptoms of which the patient complains.

TREATMENT: it must first be realized that people can live normal lives with a high blood pressure, and the fact of hypertension does not automatically mean that a person is going to develop crippling or fatal complications. If the high blood pressure is secondary, then the underlying cause must be dealt with. If it is primary, or 'essential', the patient must be calmed and advised to come to terms with his hypertension. He must avoid excessive anxiety, and in some cases sedative drugs are useful. A regular routine is beneficial, the weight should be watched, and excessive smoking discouraged if the patient finds it too much of a strain to give up smoking entirely. There is no reason why he should not enjoy alcohol, but every reason why he should not indulge too freely. He should avoid the use of salt at table, and give up food which obviously contains large quantities of salt. In cases which do not respond to simple measures the physician may use one of the modern drugs which lower the blood pressure. There are now a number of these drugs, which act in a number of different ways, but a primary requirement in all is very close co-operation between the patient and the doctor. The use of drugs merely to lower the blood pressure is not sensible, for it is not the number of millimetres of mercury which the blood pressure will support which is important but the effect of the rise in pressure upon the brain, heart and kidneys, and the level of pressure found to be damaging varies from case to case. Patients are naturally prone to ask for the figures as an index of their progress, but the figures mean very little compared to the examination of the whole man. The only cases in which the actual figures are an indication to start drug therapy are those rare ones in which the blood pressure is so excessively raised that the doctor knows complications are likely to develop.

COMPLICATIONS: the complications of hypertension include heart failure, coronary disease and angina pectoris. There may be bleeding from the nose, or bleeding into the gut. The brain is often affected by associated arterial disease which may cause thrombosis or haemorrhage, and there is a condition peculiar to hypertension known as hypertensive encephalopathy in which the patient may suffer from attacks of epilepsy, loss of consciousness, blinding headache and vomiting, paralysis, loss of vision or the power of speech, and subsequently recover in response to treatment or spontaneously. The kidneys are affected in advanced disease.

Hyperthermia: the treatment of certain diseases by the artificial induction of a high fever. The method has largely fallen into disuse. The word also means a high body temperature.

Hyperthyroidism: over-action of the thyroid gland. *See* Goitre.

Hypertrophy: increase in size of an organ, usually as a result of increased work or stress imposed upon it for which it has to compensate. Examples are the enlarged heart of the athlete, or the increased size and strength of the arms in people who have lost the use of their legs.

Hypno-analysis: the use of hypnosis or drugs with a hypnotic action such as thiopentone (Pentothal) to abbreviate the process of analysis in psychological illness. Such methods are sometimes used to allow the patient to get rid of repressed emotions by abreaction (q.v.), or to give positive suggestions of health, but hypno-analysis properly speaking refers only to *analysis*, i.e. the recovery of repressed material and its neutralizing by explanation and understanding rather than by suggestion or the release of emotion.

Hypnosis: a state of artificially induced trance which causes the individual to be more open to suggestion. It has also been termed mesmerism, animal magnetism, odylic force, and induced somnambulism. Induced trances of one sort or another have been part of the stock-in-trade of the medicine man, witch-doctor, religious devotee, the reputable and not so reputable physician, and many other would-be influencers of mankind from the dawn of human history. Indeed, it is difficult to say where suggestion begins and rational attempts to convince end – what the politician says by way of logical argument is not independent of his personality nor is the physician's bed-side manner irrelevant to the effectiveness of the remedy he prescribes. But for practical purposes hypnosis is a deliberately induced trance in which there is an emotional rapport between the operator and his subject such that he is enabled to produce the desired results with greater facility than otherwise and demonstrate certain phenomena characteristic of the hypnotic state, for example anaesthesia of parts of the body, the recovery of forgotten memories, etc. This definition is admittedly inadequate, for it must be remembered that some animals can be hypnotized (in which case emotional rapport is presumably absent, the main feature being inhibition of some fields of behaviour); and that there are various degrees of hypnosis in the sense of increased suggestibility without the production of trance. In this respect the vast majority of people can be hypnotized, although only a minority of individuals can be deeply hypnotized to such a level that complete anaesthesia of a limb or other part is capable of being induced. It should be unnecessary to add that there is nothing mysterious about hypnosis, which in its simplest form is simply the inhibition or 'putting to sleep' by monotonous stimuli of a part of the brain (much as a clock, no matter how noisy, ceases to be heard after a few minutes), added to a maintenance of contact by the hypnotist with the uninhibited part.

Anybody can induce hypnosis when shown how to do so and although many highly intelligent people use the method, undue confidence, a feeling of superiority, and a measure of stupidity are undoubtedly a help. Hypnotism has always appealed to the charlatan and humbug; historically its first significant appearance in European society dates from the sensational work of Anton Mesmer, who from 1774 onwards was the rage first of Vienna and then of Paris. The physicians who made hypnosis respectable were Braid of Manchester, who suggested that hypnosis was merely a form of sleep which could be produced by gazing at a bright light, Professor Elliotson of University College, London, and Esdaile, an army surgeon in India who was able to perform surgical operations under hypnosis. Nobody can be hypnotized against his will and allegedly bad effects produced by performers on the stage or over the radio are cases of unconscious self-deception by hysterics looking for some excuse on which to hang their symptoms. Results brought about by deep hypnosis or hysteria (which for the present purpose can be regarded as a state of self-hypnosis) include: anaesthesia of a part which, however, does not correspond to the anatomical distribution of its nerves; apparent symptoms of organic illnesses which similarly do not bear expert examination; the recall of long-forgotten events and even their enacting; apparent double personality; the disappearance of symptoms, at least temporarily; hypersensitivity of the senses which may enable the subject to appear capable of telepathy; and less frequently physical phenomena such as bleeding and stigmata, and pseudo-religious or mystical mental states.

In medicine hypnosis is used in inducing anaesthesia, for example in childbirth, in hypno-analysis (q.v.) where information about the causation of symptoms may be obtained and used for cure, and occasionally for making positive suggestions of health. The latter process is poorly regarded by psychiatrists in general since, on the reasonable assumption that every symptom has a cause, the removal of symptoms without dealing with their cause is likely to lead to nothing more dramatic than another symptom taking its place. Drawbacks to hypnosis are: its unreliability, since not everyone can be deeply hypnotized; its tendency to produce an emotional attachment (transference) between operator and subject which is precisely what most doctors want to avoid lest it should get out of control; and the suggestion (often not entirely unjustified) of hocus-pocus and mystery which is likely to exist in the mind of the subject if not of the operator. Basically any method which is not uniformly reliable is unsatisfactory to the physician.

Hypnotics: drugs which induce sleep.

Hypocalcaemia: a low level of calcium in the bloodstream, that is, less than 7.5 mg/100 ml in the plasma. The condition may follow damage to the parathyroid glands or their accidental removal in operations on the thyroid gland, and it may be found in rickets if the diet is very deficient in calcium. Low plasma calcium values are associated with tetany, a condition in which the nerves are abnormally excitable; there are tingling sensations in the face and the hands, and muscles of the legs and feet, forearms and hands, may go into spasm so that the hands and feet are stiff and distorted. Spasm of the muscles of the face may produce a caricature of a grin called the risus sardonicus. Tetany can be produced by overbreathing, which temporarily lowers the blood calcium level; it is not to be confused with tetanus.

Hypochlorhydria: deficiency of hydrochloric acid in the stomach. Complete absence of the acid is called achlorhydria. Neither of these conditions by themselves cause symptoms, but they may be found in association with cancer of the stomach, pernicious anaemia and sometimes chronic gastritis.

Hypochlorous Acid: the main active ingredient in such antiseptics as Eusol, which is prepared from bleaching powder and boric acid.

Hypochondriasis: a fixed belief in the existence of physical disease although there is no evidence of it. The hypochondriac may be suffering from a specific mental illness such as a depressive state, a neurosis, or even schizophrenia, but a large number of cases fit into none of these categories, being middle-aged people, usually men, often with a family history of preoccupation with bodily functions. Complaints usually centre around the abdominal organs, for example vague pains in the bowels, or peculiar feelings described in a bizarre way, and nothing said by the physician or demonstrated by special examination will convince the patient more than briefly that nothing is wrong. In these cases there is often a considerable risk of suicide.

Hypochondrium: the outer upper parts of the abdomen, under the ribs; the right and left hypochondria lie to each side of the epigastrium.

Hypodermic: this word means 'under the skin'; a hypodermic, or subcutaneous, injection is one which is given under the skin. Injections in general are used as a way of introducing into the body drugs which would be destroyed by the processes of digestion if they were swallowed. Injections also ensure that drugs will be absorbed fairly quickly; hypodermic injections are absorbed least quickly, intramuscular injections more quickly and intravenous injections very rapidly.

Hypogastric: the hypogastric region is the middle lower part of the abdomen between the umbilicus and the pubic area.

Hypoglossal Nerve: the twelfth cranial nerve, which supplies the muscles of the tongue. *See* Cranial Nerves.

Hypoglycaemia: a low level of sugar in the blood.
CAUSE: during the treatment of diabetes mellitus administration of insulin or similar drugs without adequate carbohydrate coverage may precipitate an attack of hypoglycaemia. It can also occur in Addison's disease, myxoedema and pituitary disorders, in tumours of the islet cells of the pancreas which secrete insulin, and in patients who are sensitive to insulin.
SYMPTOMS: palpitations, excessive sweating, tremor of the hands and excitability with a sensation of hunger. The onset is sudden and the patient may quickly become confused and clumsy; if the condition is not treated he may become unconscious or very sleepy.

TREATMENT: the patient must be given sugar, at least four lumps or teaspoonfuls, if he can take food. If he cannot, then an injection of glucagon will increase the blood sugar level and may bring him round so that he can take sugar by mouth. An injection of adrenaline will have the same effect but it is not as safe; the dose is 0.6 ml of adrenaline 1/1,000, and it is given subcutaneously. *See* Diabetes, Glucagon.

Hypomania: a state of mental excitement less in degree than that of mania.

Hypophosphites: the hypophosphites of calcium, iron, etc., like the glycerophosphates, are sometimes given in 'tonics'. They have no effect.

Hypophysectomy: removal of the hypophysis or pituitary gland.

Hypopiesis: low blood pressure. *See* Hypotension.

Hypopituitarism: deficiency of the secretions of the pituitary gland. If the anterior part of the pituitary is functionless, as it may be in a condition which sometimes follows the delivery of a baby complicated by a severe haemorrhage, or as the result of a tumour or other local disease, the patient develops amenorrhoea, intolerance to cold, hypoglycaemia, water retention, loss of hair, atrophy of the genital organs, and a peculiar yellowish pallor. Loss of only one of the pituitary hormones may lead to atrophy or lack of development of the sex organs, or dwarfism. The condition is treated not by an attempt to replace the missing pituitary hormones, but by giving cortisone, thyroid hormone, androgens and oestrogens, for loss of the pituitary hormones produces failure of the secretory functions of the thyroid, the adrenals and the gonads. Damage to the posterior part of the pituitary gland leads to diabetes insipidus, a condition in which the patient passes large quantities of dilute urine and consequently suffers from excessive thirst. This is relieved either by small doses of posterior pituitary extract, or, unexpectedly, by the use of thiazide diuretic drugs, which in the absence of the posterior pituitary hormone have an anti-diuretic effect. *See* Diuretics.

Hypoplasia: underdevelopment of an organ. *See* Hyperplasia.

Hypopyon: an accumulation of pus in the anterior chamber of the eye.

Hypospadias: a congenital malformation of the penis, in which the genital folds fail to unite normally in the midline, and the orifice of the urethra – the external meatus – may lie anywhere along the undersurface of the shaft of the organ. If the deformity is severe the two halves of the scrotum may fail to unite, and the testes fail to descend. It may then be difficult to decide the sex of the child on superficial examination. Treatment is by plastic surgery when the child is 4 years old.

Hypostasis: the pooling of blood in the vessels and of fluid in the tissue spaces of the dependent parts of the body when a poor circulation is unable to overcome the effects of gravity. Hypostatic congestion of the feet and ankles occurs in heart failure, and those who are old, enfeebled and bedridden develop hypostatic congestion of the base of the lungs which may lead to pneumonia.

Hypotension: low blood pressure. Apart from the obvious causes (excessive blood loss, or pain) there is a condition called postural hypotension in which the blood pressure falls when the patient stands upright or sits up suddenly from the lying position. The effects vary from a momentary giddiness to outright fainting. Postural hypotension may be secondary to heart disease, or may be brought on by various drugs, especially those used for the relief of high blood pressure; there is also a condition rarely found which occurs in men, often in middle age, in which giddiness or fainting on standing up is associated with impotence and an absence of sweating.

Hypothalamus: a very important part of the forebrain which lies below the thalamus and forms the lower part of the wall of the third ventricle and its floor. Its integrity is essential for life, for it is concerned with the 'vegetative' functions. It plays a major part in regulating the temperature of the body, the body weight and appetite, sexual behaviour, blood pressure and fluid balance, and it can be said to be the physical basis of the emotions. *See* Nervous System.

Hypothermia: low body temperature. There are certain techniques by which the temperature of the body may be artificially lowered to enable the surgeon to take advantage of the fact that tissues which are colder than normal need less oxygen, so that the time he has to operate on the heart or the brain in a bloodless field is increased. This type of therapeutic hypothermia is under control, but it is possible for a loss of temperature to occur spontaneously, particularly in the aged, which is dangerous to life. This type of heat loss is found among the elderly and poor, the lonely and mentally confused, who are unable to afford adequate heating, bedding or clothing. In the case of younger people heat loss would be made up by the production of heat by the body but the mechanism does not work adequately in older people, especially in winter in northern countries. This emergency has largely been overlooked in the past because those affected do not ordinarily complain of cold in spite of the fact that their temperature may have fallen to 90 °F. (32.2 °C.) or less. Besides age, weakness and inadequate protection against cold, other factors influence hypothermia, such as heart disease, pneumonia, certain drugs and alcohol. The signs and symptoms are a semiconscious state, mental confusion, slow breathing and pulse rate, and low blood pressure. Although even those parts of the body which have been covered feel cold to the physician, they do not feel cold to the patient.

TREATMENT: this is urgent. The important thing is *not* to apply heat to the body as, in the poor state of the circulation, any warming of the skin will carry the blood away from the essential organs. The patient should simply be covered to prevent further loss of heat and the temperature allowed to rise of itself. More specific treatment has to be applied by the doctor. Hypothermia can also affect newborn infants. *See* Cold Injury.

Hypothyroidism: deficiency of the hormone secreted by the thyroid gland. *See* Goitre.

Hysterectomy: the surgical operation of removing the womb. Subtotal hysterectomy removes the body but not the cervix (i.e. the portion projecting into the vagina) and is commonly performed for fibroids (q.v.); total hysterectomy may be carried out both for malignant tumours and fibroids, the cervix being removed. When other pelvic structures (the tubes and ovaries, broad ligaments, the upper third of the vagina and associated lymph glands) are removed the operation is described as Wertheim's operation. Still more radical, when nearly all pelvic structures are removed, is the procedure of pelvic exenteration. When the womb is small, the ligaments supporting it lax, and the condition benign, a vaginal hysterectomy may be performed to remove the womb through the vagina instead of through the abdomen as in other types of operation. The question often arises in hysterectomy whether the ovaries should be removed or one or both left, and this ordinarily will depend upon the age of the patient, since removal might be less important to a woman at the change of life than to a young one, and upon the condition of the ovaries and tubes. Removal of both ovaries means not only sterility but loss of the ovarian hormones, a loss which leads to important physical and psychological effects upon the whole body; these do not follow if one ovary is left behind. Contrary to general belief hysterectomy does not lead to loss of sexual desire.

Hysteria: a nervous disorder characterized by dissociation (i.e. the apparent cutting-off of one part of the mind from the other); a high degree of suggestibility both from the self (autosuggestion) and from others; and a great variety of phenomena which may give the impression at first of organic disease, although the condition is wholly psychological in origin. *See* Neuroses.

Hystero-epilepsy: supposedly a state in which fits occur mid-way in type between those of hysteria and true epilepsy. Since the fits in these two disorders are very rarely even remotely alike there is no reason to think that any such condition exists, although epileptics may show hysterical manifestations.

401

I

Iatrogenic Disease: a disease unwittingly produced by the doctor, for example the mere fact of taking the blood pressure, especially if done repeatedly, can lead to anxiety on the part of the patient and an obsession with the subject even when this is objectively unnecessary. Patent medicine advertisements and indeed medical dictionaries can produce the same result if read by susceptible people (i.e. those who have a fund of unattached anxiety waiting for an apparently rational hook on which it may be hung). This is particularly true of matters which stir the individual's guilt feelings such as sex, mental disorder and venereal disease which are frequently and often illogically associated together. Obviously the physician must be careful to avoid the development of such a situation, but it is fair to point out that it is only those already suffering from anxiety or guilt who respond in this way, and the main part played by the doctor is that he may present a more 'rational' excuse for worry than would otherwise have been presented. A much more serious type of iatrogenic illness occurs in those unfortunates who by reason of old age or chronic mental illness are confined to institutions largely because society in the form of their friends and relatives no longer has any use for them. This 'institutional neurosis' takes the form of a progressive dementia or deterioration of conduct which seems to be due to a physical degeneration of the brain or the disease for which they were admitted, but is in fact largely caused by the lack of social contact and the inevitable loss of the personal touch in overcrowded and understaffed hospitals and homes.

Ichthammol: (Ichthyol; Ammonium ichthyolsulphonate). A dark brown viscous fluid of distinctive fishy odour obtained by the distillation of certain bituminous schists and subsequent treatment with water and ammonium sulphate. Ichthyol has some antiseptic action and is mildly irritant to the skin, and is used in some chronic skin diseases. It has been given by mouth for numerous conditions, but there is no reason to believe that it is in any way effective. Large doses cause diarrhoea.

Ichthyosis: a disorder in which the skin becomes coarse and cracked. It may be congenital or acquired; the congenital type shows a dry, scaly skin with a tendency to be worse over the shins and the backs of the elbows. There is very little disability apart from the appearance of scaliness, and the condition does not predispose to other skin troubles. The acquired type is seen in old people, in whom scaly skin is common, and it differs from the congenital type in that it itches.

Icterus: jaundice.

Icterus Gravis Neonatorum: congenital haemolytic anaemia, erythroblastosis foetalis; all terms referring to a condition in which the newborn baby suffers from breakdown of the red blood cells and consequent jaundice. The cause is that the baby carries in its blood the Rhesus factor (*see* Blood Groups) while the mother is Rhesus negative. Cells from the child cross the placenta into the mother's circulation, and she elaborates an antibody to them. An alternative way in which an Rh-negative woman can become sensitized to the Rh factor is by receiving a transfusion of Rh-positive blood. However sensitization may arise, Rh antibodies cross the placenta and destroy the Rh-positive red blood cells of the child. The reaction is worse in the case of the second and subsequent children.

TREATMENT: in a number of cases the baby has to be given an exchange transfusion, in which blood is withdrawn a little at a time from the umbilical vein and replaced by fresh blood. If it is thought that the baby is likely to be severely affected while still in utero, it is possible either to induce a premature birth and institute exchange transfusions at once, or to perform intra-uterine transfusions. To do this the foetus is visualized by X-rays and a needle passed into its peritoneal cavity. Through the needle packed Rh-negative red blood cells are injected.

PREVENTION: it is possible to prevent the disease by the injection of gamma globulin into Rh-negative mothers within 48 hours of the birth of their first Rh-positive baby, for it is at birth that most of the foetal cells gain entrance into the mother's circulation. It is particularly valuable to use this technique if the mother's and the baby's blood are compatible under the ABO classification, for incompatibility prevents to a great extent foetal blood cells exciting the Rh reaction in the mother. The gamma globulin is obtained from the blood of Rh-negative mothers who have been immunized to the Rh factor.

Idiocy: idiocy is legally defined as a form of mental defect in which persons are 'so deeply defective in mind from birth or from an early age as to be unable to guard themselves against common physical dangers'. It is the lowest of the three grades of mental defect – idiocy, imbecility and feeble-mindedness – and the condition is readily recognizable from a very early age. Physical deformities are common in idiots, and paralysis and convulsive attacks are also frequent. In the United States, the term severely retarded is used for this degree of mental deficiency. *See* Mental Defect.

Idioglossia: the continued utterance of meaningless sounds as in some mental defectives or demented schizophrenics. In certain religious sects it is regarded as a sign of peculiar holiness.

Idiogram: a diagram showing the 'chromosome complement' of an organism.

Idiopathic: a term applied to diseases to indicate that their cause is unknown, thus 'idiopathic epilepsy' is true epilepsy not secondary to some other organic disease.

Idiosyncrasy: a response to a certain drug or substance in a given individual which is different from the normal one. Allergy (q.v.) is an idiosyncrasy of some people to protein or other substances which have no effect on normal people.

Ileitis: localized area of inflammation occurring in the ileum (the last two-thirds of the small intestine). It is also called Crohn's disease.
CAUSE: not known, although some are convinced that it is yet another manifestation of the antibody-antigen reaction.

The bowel wall becomes swollen and red, and feels like a thick hose, and the loops of intestine become matted together by adhesions. The disease commonly occurs in the ileum, but it may be found anywhere along the small or large intestines.

SYMPTOMS: abdominal pain and diarrhoea. The appendix is often suspected and an operation carried out, during which the surgeon finds the inflamed area of bowel and makes the correct diagnosis. In some cases, however, the ileitis is not apparent, and later the intestine may adhere to the wound made at operation and in time form a fistula – a communication between the inside of the bowel and the outside of the body. The formation of a fistula is characteristic of ileitis; not only can it happen through an operation wound, but it occurs in the region of the anus, and a fistula about the anus can be the first sign of the disease.

TREATMENT: in the beginning the condition should be treated medically, if it has been diagnosed correctly without being mistaken for a surgical disease, and the patient put to bed and encouraged to eat a high-protein diet. Sometimes atropine relieves the colic associated with the disease, and corticosteroids may be given, but the response may be slow. Antibiotics and sulphonamides are not used as a routine, but are kept for acute attacks of inflammation. Iron is given to treat anaemia, which often results from incomplete absorption of food, and vitamins are given for the same reason. Obstruction, if it occurs, is treated by continual gastric suction through a stomach tube and intravenous fluids and electrolytes, but if, despite energetic treatment, the obstructed intestine will not open, it may become necessary to operate on the abdomen and either remove the diseased section of intestine or make a short-circuit round it. Surgery is not curative; the disease tends to recur even if all the obviously abnormal bowel has been taken away, and surgical and medical treatment must proceed hand-in-hand.

Ileocaecal Valve: (Ileocolic valve). The lower end of the small gut, called the ileum, opens into the large gut at the place where the colon joins the caecum, the blind end that lies in the right lower part of the abdomen and from which the appendix arises. At the junction of the large and small intestines there is a valve which consists of two 'lips' surrounded by a thickening of the circular muscle of the intestine. The function of the ileocaecal valve is not clear, but it may act as a means of preventing the contents of the ileum from running too easily into the large bowel.

Ileostomy: the establishment of an artificial opening between the ileum and the exterior. An ileostomy is usually carried out as part of the surgical treatment for ulcerative colitis, in which the colon and rectum are removed and the intestinal tract ends on the surface of the abdomen in the right iliac fossa – the right lower part of the abdomen. Although the idea of this seems revolting, in fact patients with an ileostomy are a good deal better off than they were with ulcerative colitis, and they can lead a perfectly normal life.

Ileum: the last three-fifths of the small intestine, continuous above with the jejunum and below with the colon. The differences between the jejunum and the ileum develop slowly and progressively so that the separation of the small intestine into two-fifths jejunum and three-fifths ileum is arbitrary. The true length of the small intestine is a matter for mild dispute, for though after death it can be stretched out to 7 or 8 m, in life when the muscles are normally contracted it only measures about 3 m.

Ileus: obstruction of the intestines.
CAUSE: (1) *Mechanical*. Obliteration of the cavity of the intestine by a tumour, strangulation in a hernia, twisting of the intestine round an adhesion or round itself in a loop. (2) *Paralytic*. This results from paralysis of the muscles of the wall of the intestine, often accompanying an 'acute abdomen', peritonitis or abdominal injury.
SYMPTOMS: the abdomen is distended and the patient vomits. No motions or flatus are passed, nor are bowel sounds heard on auscultation of the abdomen. The condition is only painful if it gives rise to colic, as it may do with a mechanical obstruction.
TREATMENT: gastric suction and intravenous administration of fluids and electrolytes until a firm diagnosis is made and the patient's general condition is as good as it can be; then if necessary surgical operation.
In paralytic ileus gastric suction and intravenous fluids are

continued until the bowel begins to move again.

Ilium: the haunch-bone, which forms a firm joint with the sacrum behind and is continuous with the pubic bone in front and the ischium below. The ilium together with the pubis and ischium forms the os coxae or hip-bone; the two hip-bones with the sacrum form the pelvis. The crest of the ilium can be felt just below the lower ribs.

Illusion: a false mental interpretation of a real sensory stimulus.

Imbecility: the second most severe degree of mental defect, legally defined as occurring in 'persons in whose case there exists from birth or from an early age mental defectiveness not amounting to idiocy, yet so pronounced that they are incapable of managing themselves or their affairs, or, in the case of children, of being taught to do so.' In the United States, the term moderately retarded is used for this degree of mental deficiency.

Imhotep: the first physician whose name has come down to us, Imhotep was an Egyptian who lived during the Third Dynasty (*c.* 2600 B.C.). As time went on he became worshipped as a god of healing.

I.M.I.: intramuscular injection.

Imipramine: a drug used in the treatment of depression. It takes three or four weeks to become fully effective, but it is active in a great number of cases. Its action resembles a normal remission, and the attendant symptoms of depression such as impotence, insomnia and agitation respond to it. It has a beneficial action in Parkinson's disease and to a certain extent in trigeminal neuralgia and post-herpetic neuralgia. Side effects include lowering of the blood pressure, especially in elderly people, a dry mouth, sleepiness, interference with accommodation and consequent slight blurring of vision, and in old men retention of urine.

Immersion Foot: a condition seen in people who have spent a long time with their feet in water at a temperature

407

below 50 °F. (15 °C.). The smaller arteries become constricted, and the feet turn blue and then white; they swell up, and the skin may ulcerate. The feeling goes out of them, and the condition is painless until recovery begins. Immersion foot is found in shipwrecked sailors and airmen who descend into the sea and have to spend hours in a partially submerged dinghy or raft.

TREATMENT: is at first directed towards keeping the patient's body warm and his feet cold, for until the blood supply has returned it is beneficial to keep the feet cool in order to cut down their requirements of oxygen. The patient is put to bed and not allowed to walk; the feet are kept clear of the bedclothes and propped up on a pillow without being covered with dressings. A fan is used to keep them cool for several days until the swelling and the pain have begun to go, when the temperature of the feet can be allowed to rise. *See* Frostbite.

Immunity: immunity is of two sorts, active and acquired. Active immunity comes by surviving an infectious disease, although the attack may be so mild as to pass unnoticed. The infecting organisms produce antibody reactions which persist in some cases for as long as a lifetime. Immunity can be acquired by intentional exposure to infectious organisms, usually altered so that they can produce an antibody reaction but cannot produce severe symptoms of disease. Preparations used to produce intentional immunity include living organisms, organisms killed or rendered inactive by chemical treatment or heat, and substances produced by organisms which are thought to play a leading part in disease processes. *See* Allergy, Immunization.

Immunization: the action of making a person immune to a disease; immunization may be passive or active. In the production of passive immunization, an antitoxin already elaborated in another creature is injected; the creature used for example in the case of tetanus is usually a horse, in which an active immunity is induced by the injection of antigen. The serum of the horse may then be used to protect an injured man who has not been actively immunized against tetanus, but there are drawbacks. In the first place, because horse serum is a foreign protein, patients may react violently to it, and may develop urticaria, or even anaphylactic shock; and secondly the immunity conferred lasts only for a short time – a matter of weeks – and has no value against subsequent attacks of the infection. The first drawback will in time be overcome by the use of gamma globulin from human beings who have an immunity against the disease in question, but the drawback of transient value is inherent in the method. In active immunization a substance is injected into the patient which will provoke the formation of antibodies in the patient's own blood. The substances used are generally referred to as vaccines, and although they are intended to imitate the infections which produce various diseases they are designed to do so without producing the symptoms of disease. The immunity conferred lasts a very long time, in some diseases for life. The effectiveness of active immunization is shown by the figures for the incidence of diphtheria in Great Britain since 1940. Up to that time, the yearly cases of this disease were between 70,000 and 80,000. In 1940 active immunization against diphtheria started on a nation-wide scale; in 1967 the number of cases was 6. There have been no deaths from diphtheria in immunized people since 1948. The risk involved in immunization is infinitely less than the risk of serious infection in the unprotected child.

Vaccination (q.v.) or active immunization is now recommended for:

Diphtheria, tetanus and whooping-cough. First injection between third and sixth months, second after 6 weeks, then again after 6 months.

Poliomyelitis. Oral vaccine given at the same intervals.

Measles and smallpox. During the second year.

Tuberculosis in susceptible children. B.C.G. vaccine between 10 and 13.

Injections of diphtheria and tetanus and oral doses of polio vaccine are repeated at 5 years old, or when the child first goes to school, and revaccination against smallpox is carried out at the same time. Tetanus toxoid and polio vaccine are repeated on leaving school, and smallpox revaccination is carried out again.

Impaction: the jamming of two objects together; for example, an impacted tooth is one so firmly lodged in its socket that eruption is impossible, an impacted fracture is one where the two ends of the bone are pushed into each other, and impacted faeces are motions which have become so hard and dry that they cannot be passed out of the rectum without special measures being taken.

Impetigo: a skin disease spread by contagion.

CAUSE: infection of the skin with Staphylococcus pyogenes, followed by streptococci.

SYMPTOMS: at first a fluid-filled vesicle appears on the skin. When this breaks a yellow scab quickly forms, and the infected area spreads. The scab enlarges to keep pace with the infection. The disease is commonest in children, and the areas affected most often are the face, the neck and the scalp. It may follow chickenpox, or be associated with lice or scabies. Impetigo may hide an underlying ringworm infection.

TREATMENT: chlortetracycline ointment, and if necessary an antibiotic by mouth. The child should be prevented from picking the scabs, and because the disease is so contagious great attention has to be paid to keeping towels and linen from being used by other people. Correctly carried out, treatment is always effective.

Impotence: the inability of the male to perform sexually, which may be due either to organic or psychological factors and be temporary or long-lasting.

CAUSE: failure to achieve an erection can result from endocrine disease affecting the testicles, the thyroid gland or pituitary body. Occasionally there may be local defects, such as a tight foreskin, and diseases of the central nervous system such as tabes dorsalis or serious general diseases like untreated diabetes or chronic alcoholism may cause impotence. The vast majority of cases, however, are psychological in origin, and result from feelings of guilt, anxiety, distaste for the sexual act either in general or in a particular case, latent homosexual tendencies and sheer ignorance. The ability in men to have sexual intercourse satisfactorily is dependent upon many factors, among which are self-confidence and self-regard, and it frequently happens that failure on one occasion perpetuates itself owing to the fear on each subsequent occasion that all will not be well.

Since erection is almost impossible in the presence of the conflicting emotions of anxiety and desire, love and fear, impotence results in such circumstances.

TREATMENT: the comparatively rare organic types can often be dealt with by the use of appropriate hormones (for example testosterone propionate), but otherwise treatment must be directed towards removing anxiety. Aphrodisiacs to increase sexual excitement, such as cantharides or 'Spanish fly', are both useless and dangerous because they produce their effect by local irritation of the urethra. Since any such method also irritates the kidneys, often to the point of causing blood to appear in the urine, it should never be used. Sexual desire should not be treated as a mechanical procedure to be stimulated by mechanical means and in the absence of desire or affection for the partner nothing is likely to be successful. Nearly all men are at some time impotent, but if a single occasion is regarded anxiously as indicating the possibility of future failure the condition will be likely to persist. Desire and introspection cannot exist together, and anxiety is the most potent anaphrodisiac.

Inanition: the state of the body in starvation.

Incisions: there are a great number of named surgical incisions, particularly in the abdomen, perhaps the most famous of which is McBurney's incision, made in the right lower part of the abdomen about an inch inwards from the anterior superior spine of the iliac bone. This approach is made mainly by splitting rather than cutting the abdominal muscles, and is used when taking out the appendix. Another named incision is that of Pfannenstiel, which is made transversely just above the pubic bone so that when it heals it is covered by the pubic hair. It is used for pelvic operations in women. The standard surgical incisions in the abdomen are the median, which may be above or below the umbilicus, the paramedian which is to one side of the mid-line, the transverse and the oblique, which may, in the case of operations on the renal tract, run round along the lowest ribs to the front of the abdomen. Combinations of these incisions may be used as necessary, but the surgeon always tries to avoid weakening the abdominal wall.

Incisors: the front four teeth of upper and lower jaws; their function is cutting.

Incompetence: in relation to the valves of the heart incompetence refers to a condition in which the valves will not close completely because of disease. When this occurs the blood pumped out is liable to flow back into the chamber which it has just left.

Incontinence: the inability to control bladder or bowels found in conditions where they are diseased or injured, or, more commonly, where disease or injury of the nervous system has taken away the power of control. Incontinence occurs both in infancy and the second childhood of old age, and is common in attacks of epilepsy.

Inco-ordination: the inability to co-ordinate movements, brought about by damage to the sensory nerves which inform the brain about the position of the body in space, defects in the brain, or disorder in the motor system or the muscles.

Incubation Period: the period elapsing between infection with the germs of a disease and the appearance of the first symptoms. In any given disease it is relatively constant; a person who has been exposed to an infectious disease and may be incubating it is known as a contact. Contacts should be watched carefully, because they may become highly infectious as soon as the first symptoms of disease appear. Roughly speaking incubation periods may be divided into short, intermediate and long, and the incubation periods for the common infectious diseases are:
Short (up to seven days)
Diphtheria; scarlet fever; bacillary dysentery; influenza; plague; cholera; meningitis (meningococcal cerebro-spinal fever, spotted fever).
Intermediate (one to two weeks)
Smallpox; measles; chickenpox (may be up to three weeks); glandular fever; typhoid fever; whooping-cough.
Long (more than two weeks)
German measles (rubella) (up to three weeks); mumps (up to three weeks); virus hepatitis (up to four weeks); serum

412

hepatitis (a matter of months).

The quarantine period is the maximum incubation period with two days added, but for the usual childhood infections quarantine is not practical. Cases should be kept as far as possible in isolation at home as soon as they develop symptoms, except in the case of German measles (rubella), where it is advisable for the disease to be spread as widely as possible among young girls to prevent them contracting the infection in later life when they are pregnant. Contacts of diphtheria and close contacts of typhoid and paratyphoid fever should be swabbed and kept at home until the results of the swabs show them to be clear of infection. Contacts of poliomyelitis should be kept at home, and those who have been in contact with a case of meningococcal meningitis should be given sulphadimidine as a prophylaxis.

The periods of infectivity of common fevers are:

Chickenpox. Until the scabs have all gone. In the United States it is considered non-contagious after a week following the rash.

German measles. One week from the beginning of the rash.

Measles. One to two weeks from the first appearance of the rash.

Whooping-cough. Three weeks from the first symptoms.

Diphtheria. Until swabs from nose and throat are negative.

Mumps. One week after the glands go down.

Indian Hemp: *see* Cannabis Indica.

Indifference, Belle: found in hysteria and schizophrenia, it is a state of complacence about the disease from which the patient is suffering.

Indigestion: *see* Dyspepsia, Stomach Disease.

Indole: one of the compounds which is normally found in faeces and is in part responsible for the characteristic smell.

Indomethacin: (Indocid). A drug which is effective in about a third of all cases of rheumatoid arthritis, and in cases of acute gout. It is valuable in relieving pain in osteo-arthritis. Side effects include headache, nausea and vomiting, dizziness, depression and even confusion. Treatment with the drug is therefore started with small doses which are gradually increased to an upper limit of 200 mg a day. The drug should be taken with food, milk or an antacid preparation, and patients should remember that the drug may make them dizzy; if it does, they must not drive or operate machinery.

Induration: hardening of a tissue or organ.

Industrial Disease: *see* Occupational Disease.

Infantile Paralysis: *see* Poliomyelitis.

Infants and Infant Welfare: it is important to realize that the term 'normal infant' simply means the average; this may be quite misleading in an individual case (for example so far as weight is concerned infants who are quite healthy may fall considerably short of, or greatly exceed, the average weight). The figures given here are only rough guides and no anxiety should be felt if one's own child does not conform unless there are other signs that its condition is not satisfactory.

Weight. At birth the average infant weighs 7–7½ lb (3.2–3.4 kg); the weight is approximately doubled by the fifth month, trebled by the end of the first year, and at the end of the second year the child should weigh about 28 lb (12.7 kg). Apart from the first week when there is a slight initial loss, the weight increases by about 6–8 oz (170–226 g) a week, but minor variations are of little significance and small infants (since infants vary within the normal as much as their parents) may do quite satisfactorily with a weekly gain of 4–6 oz (113–170 g).

Height. This again varies as greatly as does the height of the parents but, broadly speaking, the hereditary factor in height does not make its influence felt until about the fifth year; before that time height is largely dependent upon nutrition. At birth the average infant is about 20 in (508 mm), and at the end of the year about 28 in (701 mm); the height increases about 3½ in (90 mm) a year thereafter until the fifth year when the hereditary factor begins to make itself felt.

Sleep. During the first month an infant sleeps nearly all the time except for feeding and dressing, but by the sixth month this has gradually altered to about 12 hours at night, 2 hours in the morning, and 2 or 3 hours in the afternoon. At 1 year the period of sleep is 12 hours at night, 2 in the morning and 1 in the afternoon, and at 18 months the afternoon hour is omitted since too much sleep during the day may result in loss of sleep at night. Bedclothes should be warm but light, the room darkened and well ventilated, but without draughts.

The Cot. For the first two or three months the most convenient type is the Moses basket. When the baby grows bigger, it needs a cot which has a solid head to keep off draughts, and bars closely set to prevent the head passing through and becoming stuck.

Movements and walking. Newly born babies can grasp objects, suck, and swallow, but movements of the arms and legs are not at first co-ordinated although by the end of the third month the child can usually lift up its head. By 6 months it begins to sit up, by the ninth month to crawl and by 10 months to stand up. Walking begins about the twelfth or fourteenth month.

Speech. Single words may be spoken by the end of the first year, but what can reasonably be described as speech does not make its appearance until the end of the second.

General management. The mother should be free from anxiety, relaxed and not given to fussing. Many feeding difficulties arise from the infant's awareness of the mother's tension and in later life there is no surer way to make a child neurotic than to fuss over it, thus giving the impression that the world is a dangerous place. Neurosis is one of the most infectious diseases known.

Feeding. Feeding should be under the direction of the home nurse, health visitor, Welfare Centre or the paediatrician himself, but it is worth while pointing out that, no matter what advances have been made in our knowledge of breast-milk substitutes, infant morbidity in breast-fed infants is still much below that of the artificially fed. This is partly because breast-milk contains antibodies (or is believed to do so), and because the risk of infection is obviously much greater in artificial feeding. The idea that a fixed schedule of feeding should be ruthlessly adhered to regardless of the child's cries of hunger is no longer popular and it will be found that if the child is at first fed on demand it will gradually develop a regularity suited to its own needs.

Clothes. Should be light and loose and preferably made of wool, silk and wool, or cotton material, and must be non-inflammable. The body should be able to get a reasonable amount of fresh air and sunshine and be free to move. All cotton clothes should be washed before they are worn for the first time because they are often dressed with starch which may irritate the baby's skin.

Bathing. After birth the baby is thoroughly washed in water a little above blood heat (100 °F.; 37.8 °C.): this can best be tested by the attendant's elbow. The stump of the umbilical cord is dried by swabbing, dusted with antiseptic powder and covered with lint. Daily sponging is carried out thereafter while keeping the cord quite dry until it separates on or about the tenth day. In a month or so the temperature of the bath should be lowered to tepid and after the daily bath the child should be allowed to lie naked in front of the fire to kick freely.

Dentition. The lower central incisors appear from the fifth to the eighth month and the other incisors follow first in the upper jaw and then in the lower. The 20 milk teeth should all be present by the end of the second year and the permanent teeth begin to erupt from about the fourth.

Weaning. Weaning should be a natural process, and from the fourth month, or as directed, the feed should be supplemented by broth and egg-yolk, minced meat being used by the ninth month. Fruit juice and cod-liver oil supplements or vitamin concentrates must always be given and the child should have something hard to exercise its teeth on. Weaning proper usually begins by the ninth month; the midday feed is omitted and replaced by cereal milk foods, broth and hard crusts. A week later milk, hard crusts and butter, lightly boiled egg and bread-crumbs or porridge with milk, may replace the breakfast feed. In the third week, crisp toast with milk should replace the teatime feed and finally the other feeds should be stopped and replaced by milk or fruit-juice.

General health. Symptoms and signs of ill health include fever, restlessness and irritability, lethargy and persistent crying (crying itself is not necessarily anything to worry about and the mother will soon learn to distinguish the cry of pain or discomfort). Colds, which block the nose, are

416

extremely distressing to babies and coughs should always be referred to the doctor or welfare clinic. Vomiting small amounts is not necessarily serious; the normal child brings up small amounts of food especially if it is overfed, but violent vomiting with or without diarrhoea should receive medical attention. Diarrhoea is an indication for asking for professional help, but constipation is rarely a cause for worry and many babies who are perfectly healthy tend to be constipated. It is only worth considering when it is prolonged or accompanied by other signs of ill health. Here it should be pointed out that the habit of 'potting' regularly at a time when the child is quite unable for anatomical reasons to control its bowels is a bad thing and to be avoided; most bowel troubles and neuroses in later life are caused by the parent's obsession with the child's bowel functions, which should be allowed to develop control in their own good time.

Infarction: when an artery is suddenly blocked by thrombosis or by an embolus and there is no collateral (alternative) circulation to keep the tissue nourished, then a wedge-shaped area will die, the apex of the dead tissue being where the blocked vessel begins to be solely responsible for the supply of nourishment and oxygen. The area of dead tissue is called an infarct, and the process whereby the blood supply is cut off and necrosis ensues is called infarction.

Infection: infectious diseases are those caused by invasion of the body by organisms from outside; they are characterized by the fact that the disease can be passed on from one person to another or from an animal to a person. Once organisms have gained entrance to the body they provoke a total reaction, even though the area directly affected may be quite small. Vermin which live on the surface of the body are said to infest rather than infect the individual. The bacteria causing disease are classified according to shape as bacilli (rods), staphylococci (bunches), streptococci (chains), diplococci (pairs), vibrio (comma-shaped), etc., and other pathogenic or disease-producing organisms can be classified as spirochaetes (these are corkscrew-shaped, move about by wriggling, and cause the two important diseases syphilis and spirochaetal jaundice), viruses, fungi and protozoa. Viruses are usually too small to be seen under an ordinary micro-scope; they can, however, be photographed under the electron microscope, which uses a magnetic field in place of a lens and a stream of electrons in place of a beam of light. Viruses cause such diseases as influenza, measles, mumps, poliomyelitis, smallpox, encephalitis, yellow fever, in-fective jaundice and chickenpox, and also such plant and animal infections as tobacco mosaic disease and foot and mouth disease. Other virus diseases are swine fever in pigs, and myxomatosis in rabbits. Viruses are responsible, so far as research has been able to show, for the common cold.

The main characteristics of viruses may be briefly sum-marized: (1) They can only grow in living cells and must be cultured in the laboratory on living tissue, unlike bacteria which grow readily on plates containing jelly made from meat broth, gelatin, milk and other delicacies; (2) they are so small that they can usually pass through the pores of the finest bacteriological filter; (3) one attack of a virus disease often produces immunity for life, second attacks of the diseases mentioned above being very rare save in the cases of influenza and the common cold; (4) viruses reproduce themselves and show other characteristics of living things yet in some respects act as non-living objects, for example some can be reduced to crystalline form without losing their ability to produce disease; (5) numerous viruses have shown themselves to be little affected by the antibiotics and other drugs. Some infections are caused by fungi, i.e. organisms belonging to the same group as moulds, mushrooms and toadstools. Perhaps the most serious fungal infection is actinomycosis; however, most are relatively trivial and restricted to the surface of the skin as in the case of ringworm and athlete's foot.

Protozoa are the lowest division of the animal kingdom; they are one-celled organisms. The main human diseases caused by protozoa are: amoebic dysentery (not to be confused with bacillary dysentery), sleeping sickness (trypanosomiasis) which is caused by an organism known as a trypanosome, and malaria, caused by the plasmodium. Other organisms which it would be more correct to describe as infesting the human body are animal parasites and worms. The former live on the skin and, if uncomfortable, are not in themselves dangerous; nevertheless, some can carry the germs of dangerous diseases, for example the flea, plague, and the louse, typhus. Worms live in the human intestine – the tiny threadworm, the roundworm somewhat resembling an ordinary garden earthworm, and tapeworms which are flat and segmented and may reach a length of 10 ft (3 m) or even 20 ft (6 m). Many parasitic worms lead a kind of double life, spending part of their existence in the human intestine and part in the muscles of some animal which is used for food. For example, in the case of Taenia solium, the common pork tapeworm, eggs are laid in the intestine of the human host which pass out with the faeces and are then swallowed by pigs (especially in those parts of the world where human excreta are used as manure). In the pig the eggs form cysts in the muscles and produce 'measly pork' which, being eaten by human beings, starts the cycle all over again. The life-cycle of the worm Taenia saginata, the common beef tapeworm, is much the same. The Russian tapeworm grows to nearly 30 ft (9 m) and is spread by raw or undercooked infected fish. Dog worms are responsible for serious larval infestation in children. In Egypt and other warm countries, including a large part of Africa and some parts of South America, live small leaf-shaped flatworms called schistosomes which lay eggs that are passed into canals and pools in the urine of infected people, hatch out as miracidia, enter a water-snail, leave it in the form of small parasites called cercariae, pierce the skin of bathers, pass to the liver, and subsequently reach the bladder or rectum. Bilharzia, as this disease is called, is a serious infestation described more fully elsewhere. Ankylostomiasis, filariasis (which causes elephantiasis), the disease dracontiasis caused by the Guinea-worm, cysticercosis and hydatid disease, are all worm or helminthic diseases.

The spread of infection. One of the commonest means of spread of bacterial and virus diseases is by droplet infection. Minute drops carrying germs are coughed or sneezed into the air by someone already suffering from the disease. Such droplets can be projected at least 10–15 ft (3–4.5 m). Next commonest mode of spread is perhaps by way of infected food, water and infected hands in the kitchen; cholera, dysentery, food-poisoning and typhoid fever are passed on in this way. Spread by direct contact is less common than might be supposed since the skin unless broken forms a formidable barrier, but parasites are generally spread this way and when the mucous membranes of the mouth or genitals are involved protection is slight. Hence sexual contact is a common cause of infection which is then called venereal. Spread through an intermediary host has already been mentioned; the carrier may be an insect or parasite such as the rat-flea which carries plague from the rat to man. Lastly infection may sometimes come from within one's own body, for some bacteria are harmless in one part but not in another; for example the bacillus coli does no harm in the human intestine but can cause pyelitis or cystitis (inflammation of the pelvis of the kidney or bladder) when it gets into the urinary tract.

How the body deals with infection. The body has numerous methods of defence but the main ones are, firstly, the substances known as antibodies and antitoxins produced in response to an infection, the former rendering the invaders helpless and the latter neutralizing their poisons; and secondly, special white cells in the blood (phagocytes), which engulf and destroy the germs after they have been attacked by the antibodies. Antibodies and antitoxins can be transferred from one individual to another, or from an animal such as a horse to man. The process is known as passive immunization and is used in medicine both to prevent infection and to cure it. Obviously it is much better if the body can be stimulated to produce its own antitoxins and antibodies and this is done by active immunization – the injection of a solution of killed bacteria (for example T.A.B. for typhoid) or one of live but weakened organisms (vaccination). Active immunity may last a long time, but passive immunity is always short-lived. The manner in which the body deals with local infections is discussed under the heading of Inflammation. *See* Immunity, Immunization.

Infectious Mononucleosis: *see* Glandular Fever.

Infestation: the invasion of the body by parasites, which may be found in the hair, the clothes, on the skin, or in the intestines.

Inflammation: the reaction of the defences of the body to injury caused by: (1) bacteria, viruses, fungi, protozoa and worms; (2) mechanical objects and physical agents such as heat, cold and radiation; (3) the immune reaction, which is the reaction of antibody against antigen (*see* Allergy); (4) cancer. Inflammation may be acute or chronic, and may end in one of several ways: resolution, which is a return to normal; fibrosis, or scarring, which replaces tissue destroyed; suppuration, which is the formation of pus; ulceration; gangrene or death of the tissues.

The characteristics of inflammation were described by Celsus, a physician who flourished in Rome in the first century A.D., as Rubor (redness), Calor (heat), Tumor (swelling) and Dolor (pain). This basic conception was last modified in the second century A.D. by Galen, who added Functio laesa, impairment of function. Acute local inflammation starts at the point of damage by dilatation of the blood vessels, so that the blood circulates more quickly, and the skin appears red and feels hot. Soon the circulation at the centre of the inflamed areas slows down, white blood cells stick to the walls of the smallest vessels and begin to make their way through the vessel walls into the damaged tissues, and fluid passes from the blood into the tissue spaces causing swelling. The white blood cells have several functions: they destroy and remove invading organisms, remove dead tissue, and then aid in the processes of repair.

Antibodies pass through the vessel walls with the fluid, or serum, as well as fibrin, which helps to contain the infection. A thick cellular barrier is formed as a fence round the infected area, but some bacteria may escape. If they do they often pass into the lymphatic vessels, and in a bad infection of the hand or foot red streaks (lymphangitis) are seen spreading up the limb to the lymphatic glands at the knee and elbow, and thence to the glands in the arm-pit or groin which become swollen and painful and themselves inflamed. In the worst cases the inflammatory reaction is not successful, and bacteria and infected matter enter the bloodstream to cause bacteraemia or septicaemia. *See* Blood Poisoning.

Influenza: (Grippe). An infection of the upper respiratory tract.

CAUSE: infection with the myxoviruses, influenza A, B, or C.

SYMPTOMS: a sudden onset characterized by a high

temperature, shivering, headache, aching pain in the bones and muscles and a cough, dry at first and then productive. If secondary bacterial infection supervenes the condition may progress to broncho-pneumonia or pneumonia. Depression often accompanies influenza.

TREATMENT: in the uncomplicated case, bed and aspirin. If the cough is troublesome a linctus may help, and there is little doubt of the medicinal value of whisky. Influenza may have a toxic effect upon the heart muscle, which means that middle-aged patients ought to rest for a few days after the infection has passed. Elderly patients should stay in bed longer than they may like, and must take life easily when they get up. If broncho-pneumonia or pneumonia develop, treatment is by antibiotics (penicillin, tetracycline, erythromycin, ampicillin) and must be energetic, for post-influenzal pneumonia is sometimes resistant and slow to resolve.

PREVENTION: there are three types of influenza virus, A, B and C. The A viruses are further divided into A_0, A_1 and A_2. General immunity to a particular strain of virus develops over about ten years, and the type ceases to spread. A new variant then emerges and epidemics break out again. The great pandemics of 1917–19 and 1957 were caused by A strains. The 1917 outbreak killed more people than the fighting in World War 1; the A_2 strain responsible for the 1957 outbreak was first identified in China, then spread to Hong Kong, and thence round the world. The mortality was reduced by the use of antibiotics. The importance of this is that infection with a particular strain of influenza virus gives only partial protection against infection with other related types, so that general inoculation to produce active immunity and control of the disease is not possible. The best control is secured by isolation of influenza victims, but the disease is not one which traditionally keeps the patient away from work if he can walk; curiously, there is thought to be some kind of virtue in 'refusing to give in' to colds and influenza, and in spreading infection freely. It is possible to protect some people from current epidemics by active immunization, but protection does not last long nor is it invariably effective; nor is it possible to forecast the incidence of epidemics or the type of virus likely to spread.

Infra-red: radiations below the red end of the spectrum, used both to heat the tissues in physiotherapy and in photographing areas of the body in which the pattern of blood vessels may be abnormal – infra-red photography for example may show up greatly increased vascular patterns in the skin over the breast in cases of malignant growth. *See* Thermography, Ultraviolet.

Infusions: watery preparations of vegetable drugs made by steeping the appropriate part of the plant in water and straining. Following this they must be suitably standardized, one of the weaknesses of herbal preparations being the variability of the amount of drug in different samples. Senna, digitalis, quassia, gentian, cinchona, tea and coffee are made this way.

Inguinal Region: the groin.

Inhalation: a means of introducing drugs into the air passages and lungs in the form of gas, vapour or finely divided particles. Some anaesthetics are given by inhalation – nitrous oxide, the vapours of ether, halothane, etc. – and other drugs are conveniently given by this method in cases of asthma and diseases of the bronchi and lungs. In particular the drugs isoprenaline (isuprel) and disodium cromoglycate are used by inhalation in asthma; isoprenaline has a powerful dilating effect on the air passages, and disodium cromoglycate (Intal) has the unique action of interfering in some way with the antibody-antigen reaction which underlies asthma.

Inhibition: the process whereby one nervous process by its strength overwhelms another. At the physiological level this can refer, for example, to the slowing-down of the heart's beat by the action of the vagus nerves; at a 'psychosomatic' level one may speak of the inhibition of gastric secretion by worry, or at the highest psychological level one finds inhibition of anti-social drives by the action of self-regarding sentiment, superego, or conscience, i.e. by other dominant aspects of the mind which realize them to be inappropriate. In the popular (which is not the scientific) sense a person is said to be inhibited or to have 'inhibitions' when he is shy, unsociable, or afraid of expressing his emotions. Inhibition may be a conscious or unconscious process; repression is always automatic and unconscious. Both are used as equivalent to each other in everyday speech if not in psychology.

Injection: may be intradermal (into the skin), hypodermic or subcutaneous (under the skin), intramuscular (into a muscle), or intravenous (into a vein). The most rapid way of getting a drug into the general circulation and so into the organs upon which it is intended to act is by intravenous injection. Intramuscular injection is the method to use in an emergency if you don't know how to make an injection. Wash the skin with soap and water if possible, or swab it with an antiseptic, and enter the needle for about $\frac{1}{2}$–1 in straight through the skin into the upper outer part of the arm about 3 in below the point of the shoulder or into the upper outer part of the backside, where the needle can be allowed to travel farther into the muscles. An injection made into the upper arm is more quickly absorbed by a shocked patient than one made into the rump. Empty the syringe slowly but firmly, having first pulled the plunger back a little to make sure the point of the needle is not in a blood vessel. If you are using soft ampules with a needle attached for emergency injections you will not be able to do this, but if you make the injection in the places mentioned above no harm is likely to be done. Enemas are correctly, but not frequently, spoken of as injections.

Innocent: sometimes used of benign tumours as opposed to malignant growths.

Innominate: literally, nameless; applied (1) to the hipbones which form the two sides of the pelvis (innominate bones); (2) to the largest branch of the aorta, the great artery which arises from the arch of the aorta behind the breastbone, passes upwards, backwards and towards the right side of the root of the neck, and divides there into the right subclavian and common carotid arteries (innominate artery); (3) to the two great veins formed on the right and left sides by the junction of the subclavian and the internal jugular veins which unite to form the superior vena cava (innominate veins).

Inoculation: the accidental or intentional introduction into an organism of bacteria or other agents causing disease. *See* Immunization.

Inquest: an inquiry into the circumstances and cause of a death, held before a Coroner (q.v.).

Insanity: *see* Mental Illness.

Insecticides: any substance that is lethal to insects is called an insecticide. These substances are of the utmost importance in preventive medicine as well as being essential for efficient agriculture, and their numbers are continually growing. Insecticides in common use include (1) the chlorinated hydrocarbon substances and (2) the organo-phosphorus compounds.

1. *Chlorinated hydrocarbons.* (a) D.D.T. This compound is also called Dicophane, and it is poisonous to arthropods but only slightly toxic to vertebrates, unless it is injected intravenously. It kills mosquitoes, houseflies, lice and fleas; since 1944 when a typhus epidemic was successfully controlled by the use of D.D.T. in Naples, it has proved invaluable in the prevention of malaria, plague, yellow fever, and all the diseases spread by flies. Lately D.D.T. has become a villain rather than a hero, but the matter must be seen in proportion; the unsuspected presence of D.D.T. in human beings as the result of its widespread use is a small price to pay for the number of lives it has saved and the amount of suffering it has prevented. Its successes and dangers spring from the same property – its physical inertness and stability, which give it extraordinary residual properties. (b) Lindane (gamma B.H.C.). This is more toxic than D.D.T. to flies, mosquitoes, lice and bedbugs, but has less residual activity. (c) Chlordane, Dieldrin. Dieldrin is very toxic to insects but unfortunately toxic to human beings as well, so that although it acts very quickly and has a very persistent action its use is limited.

2. *Organo-phosphorus compounds.* These compounds are very poisonous both to insects and to human beings, and their

use is limited to places in which the chlorinated hydrocarbons have failed.

Insecticides are not by themselves capable of controlling the spread of disease, but form part of a much larger programme which includes adequate sanitation and the clearance of places where insects can flourish. Their use must not be indiscriminate, not only because they may be poisonous to man but also because insects become resistant to insecticides. Continual vigilance is necessary to ensure that any change is noted and that the right insecticides are being used.

Insomnia: inability to sleep may take numerous forms – inability to get to sleep on going to bed, waking up too early, disturbed sleep following which the individual does not feel sufficiently rested in the morning, or sleep accompanied by frightening dreams and nightmares. Its cause in the vast majority of cases is psychological. Sometimes it is due to the sleeper's fear of relaxing control over his mind; in other cases the individual is unable to get to sleep because anxiety or worry makes him unable to relax; sometimes, particularly in the case of a brainworker, the mind has been so active all day that it cannot be turned off at bedtime, even though the thoughts are not necessarily unpleasant. The state of mind may well be (and in children often is) one of pleasurable expectation for the following day. Worry, however, is the chief killer of sleep, and other factors are either obvious or uncommon. Thus it is hardly necessary to point out that pain can prevent sleep, that drugs which are mental stimulants can have the same effect, that there are some organic nervous conditions which interfere with sleep, and that there are some people who sleep so lightly that they are easily distressed by a full stomach, cold feet, noises, and so on.

The cure of insomnia depends first of all upon realizing that no harm can come from it; the body is a self-regulating system (on the whole a very effective one), and it ensures that everyone always in ordinary circumstances gets enough sleep. Of course, as in the case of constipation, if one believes that a particular process is harmful then harmful it will be even if this is only manifested in the way the person feels; one is hardly likely to feel well when living in the belief that mysterious 'toxins' are slowly poisoning the system or that lack of sleep is about to lead to insanity. The latter belief is based on the argument that because those who have subsequently become mentally ill previously could not sleep, the lack of sleep caused the mental breakdown. This is to put the cart before the horse since the inability to sleep was caused by the approaching illness rather than the other way round. Insomnia is a sign of anxiety, not a cause of it, and many great men have slept very little. There have even been claims from some saying they never slept at all, for example, one Dr Pavoni in northern Italy who died in his eighties. He did not sleep to any significant degree for over 60 years, but instead amassed a comfortable fortune by doing other doctors' night calls. The treatment of insomnia is the treatment of its cause. In mild cases, a hot soothing drink at night, warm but not too heavy bedclothes, the avoidance of intellectually stimulating activity late at night, and the avoidance of late tea or coffee, may be sufficient especially when combined with a state of mind which looks forward to sleeping but allows a healthy indifference towards the possibility of failing to do so; nobody can sleep if his mind is filled with the thought that he will have a breakdown if he does not. A good way of wooing somnolence is to read in bed, choosing a book which is pleasing but not enthralling. Pain and other strictly medical conditions which interfere with sleep must be dealt with by the doctor, as should the question of sleeping tablets. In general unless one is ill or old it is thoroughly bad to get into the habit of using sedatives (although it is unnecessary to be puritanical about this). Natural hypnotics such as hot whisky can do no harm, nor can the beverages advertised as suitable for 'night starvation', even if no such state is known to medical science. In severe insomnia, however, such measures are unlikely to succeed, and if psychological problems seem to be at the root of the trouble it is best to ask the doctor's advice about a psychiatric opinion.

Insufflation: the blowing of a suitable powder into a cavity in order to treat local disease, for example in the ear.

Insulin: the pancreas has two sorts of cell. One type of cell elaborates a digestive juice which is carried into the duodenum through the pancreatic duct, and other cells, which form isolated groups called the Islets of Langerhans, secrete the hormones insulin and glucagon. The existence of insulin was postulated in 1909, but the hormone was not isolated until 1922 when Macleod, Banting and Best working in Toronto finally succeeded where many others had failed. They shared a Nobel Prize, for their discovery meant that diabetes mellitus (q.v.) could be treated.

Action of Insulin. Insulin, roughly speaking, enables the body to use sugar. When the level of sugar in the blood rises, insulin is secreted into the blood. It has two main actions: it increases the rate at which the sugar is withdrawn from the blood and passed into the tissues, and it decreases the rate at which sugar is added to the blood by the liver. Insulin brings about an increase in the rate of muscular storage of glycogen, the forerunner of glucose, increases the rate at which glucose is used in the tissues, and prevents the formation of glucose in the liver. It stimulates the formation of protein in muscle, stimulates the formation of fat, and prevents its breakdown.

Intal: (Disodium cromoglyconate). A substance which has the property of preventing the antibody-antigen reaction in the lungs which is the basic cause of asthma. It is administered by inhalation. *See* Allergy.

Intercostal: word used to describe the blood vessels, nerves and muscles lying between the ribs.

Intercurrent: applied to a pathological condition occurring during the course of another disease.

Interferon: although many of the infectious diseases have been brought under control and in some cases almost eliminated, one large group stands out as resistant to most methods of treatment. This is the group of the virus diseases; the list for which there is no specific cure runs all the way from mild conditions such as the common cold, chickenpox, rubella and mumps, to such fatal conditions as encephalitis and yellow fever. The importance of interferon is that it may possibly one day prove to be active against virus diseases. Interferon was first described in 1957 as the result of a study of the effect on live influenza virus in a chick embryo of killed virus introduced after the infection had taken. It was found that the fluid surrounding the cells that had been treated with killed virus contained a substance which protected them against the live one. This substance was called interferon. It is now known that many types of tissue exposed to live or dead viruses produce this substance, which is apparently non-poisonous and effective against most viruses within the same species (i.e. rabbits would not be helped by chick interferon). Although nearly all the work so far has been carried out on animals, it has been shown that a great number of virus diseases infecting chickens can be prevented or halted by this substance; perhaps one of the most significant findings is its ability to halt the development of a cancer in chickens known as Rous sarcoma which is caused by a virus. Opinions vary about the use of interferon in controlling virus infections in man, and certainly a great deal of further research has to be done. Nevertheless, this discovery, like the initial discovery of penicillin, opens a new window on another approach to controlling infectious disease and possibly, in the long term, even cancer.

Intermittent Claudication: a pain or cramp which comes on in the muscles of the legs as a result of exercise. The pain is relieved by rest. It is caused by inadequate blood supply to the muscles, with consequent ischaemia or lack of oxygen and accumulation of the products of muscular activity which should have been removed. The underlying disease of the arteries is usually atherosclerosis, and medical treatment is by drugs designed to produce dilatation of the arteries; as most of them are diseased and their walls are fixed, the effects of the drug may be disappointing. *See* Arterial Disease.

Interstitial: interstitial tissue is 'background' tissue, which supports the active cells of an organ. It is usually fibrous.

Intertrigo: chafing between two skin surfaces that rub together, for example beneath the breasts, or at the groin in the obese.

Intestine: the alimentary canal after it leaves the stomach.

It is divided into small and large intestine; the small intestine is the longer, and it starts at the lower end of the stomach where it is called the duodenum. This is a short section of gut divided for descriptive purposes into four parts which form a C with the concavity to the left, filled by the pancreas. The bile duct and main duct of the pancreas enter the second part of the duodenum; duodenal ulcers form in the first part. The duodenum gets its name from the fact that its length is about equal to the breadth of twelve fingers, being usually given as 25 cm. The rest of the small intestine is divided into jejunum and ileum; the jejunum and ileum together are in life about 3 m long, but in death, when the muscles have lost their tone, the small intestine can be stretched to a length of 8 m. The jejunum (the first two-fifths of the small intestine) and the ileum (the remaining three-fifths) are attached to the back wall of the abdominal cavity by the mesentery, a membrane which is only about 15 cm long at its base but as long as the small intestine at its intestinal edge. It fans out into many convolutions, and carries the arteries which supply the small intestine with blood. The duodenum has no mesentery, but is applied to the back wall of the abdominal cavity, and the same is true of the ascending colon, the first part of the large intestine. The terminal part of the ileum joins the large intestine in the right lower region of the abdominal cavity just above the caecum and the appendix.

The difference between the ileum and the colon is not only in size but also in appearance, for whereas the small intestine has a continuous muscular coat the colon has three longitudinal bands of muscle starting at the appendix and running the whole length of the large gut to the rectum. These longitudinal bands are called the taenia coli, and they pucker the gut lengthways; it is divided into sacculations by circular muscles. Another difference from the small intestine is that there are small bags of fat scattered on the surface of the large intestine called appendices epiploicae. The ascending colon runs up the right side of the abdominal cavity to the hepatic flexure near the liver, and then turns to run across the upper part of the abdomen as the transverse colon. This part of the large intestine has a mesentery by which it is suspended, and from its lower border hangs the back fold of the omentum (q.v.). The transverse colon turns downwards on the left side of the abdomen near the spleen at the splenic flexure, where it loses its mesentery and is again adherent to the back wall of the abdominal cavity. At the brim of the pelvis, the descending colon becomes the sigmoid colon, which has a mesentery until it joins the rectum. The rectum passes downwards out of the peritoneal cavity and is continuous with the anal canal 3 cm above the anus.

The functions of the intestine are described under the heading Digestive System, and its diseases under separate headings. *See* Abdomen, Peritoneum.

Intoxication: the state produced by poison; in particular, it refers to the state of being poisoned by alcohol.

Intracranial: inside the skull.

Intradermal: in the skin.

Intramedullary: within the spinal cord or the cavity inside a bone.

Intramuscular: inside a muscle.

Intrathecal: within the sheath – the membranes covering the spinal cord. An intrathecal injection is made between the arachnoid membrane, which is the middle layer, and the pia, which is the inner covering, for it is in between these two membranes that there is a space normally filled with cerebro-spinal fluid.

Intravenous: a term meaning within a vein.

Intussusception: a condition in which the small intestine telescopes into the large intestine, or less commonly part of the small or large intestine telescopes into the next segment of intestine lower down.

CAUSE: most cases occur in male infants between the fourth and ninth months, and although it can occur in adults, it is very rarely seen after the age of 2 years. In adults there is almost always an obvious cause, usually a benign tumour such as a polyp, sometimes a cancer. In infants there is no

431

obvious cause, but it is thought that in some cases patches of lymphatic tissue in the wall of the intestine in the region of the intussusception are swollen as the result of local infection. If the patches of lymphatic tissue are very swollen it is possible that they could act in the same way as tumours in the adult, and irritate the intestine so that it tries to expel them; in doing so it must telescope itself.

SYMPTOMS: a sudden onset, with colic and pain, causes the child to scream and draw its knees up, and it may vomit. The attack passes and the child seems perfectly normal until the next bout of pain. A sign of the condition is the passage of motions which contain mucus stained with blood; this is called a 'red currant jelly stool'. Careful examination of the abdomen will in many cases disclose the presence of a swelling which may be felt, often in the right upper part of the abdomen under the ribs. The doctor must be called without delay.

TREATMENT: there are two possible courses to follow in a case which is seen by the surgeon within 12 hours of onset. The first, which is not entirely satisfactory but is simple, is to administer a barium enema under X-ray control. The intussusception may be reduced by the pressure of the enema. The second course of action is to open the abdomen under general anaesthetic and reduce the intussusception by hand. At the same time the intestine can be inspected to detect any sign of gangrene which may require removal of the damaged section of gut, and explored for the presence of a tumour or other abnormality which might have caused the intussusception.

Treatment in adults is always by surgical operation.

Inunction: a method of treating disease by rubbing into the skin a mixture of drugs and oil or fat.
This unpleasant and unsatisfactory procedure was once used for administering mercury in the treatment of syphilis.

In Vitro: term applied to a biological reaction which takes place under experimental conditions, literally 'in glass', as opposed to in vivo, which means 'in life' and is applied to reactions occurring in the living animal or human body. The fact that a particular drug has a certain action in vitro does not mean that it has the same action in vivo.

Involution: (1) a return to normal size, used particularly of the uterus after pregnancy; (2) the shrinking in old age of various organs.

Iodine: this is now mainly used in medicine in the radio-active form, usually as I^{131}, which has a half-life of 8 days, and is valuable in the investigation and treatment of thyroid disease. Tincture of iodine was formerly used to clean wounds or to apply to the skin before surgical operations, and has also been used as a means of applying counter-irritation to chronically inflamed joints and glands. A mixture of iodine and potassium iodide (Lugol's iodine) is often given to patients before an operation for thyrotoxicosis, and a similar mixture in glycerine is used to paint the throat in inflammatory disorders. Potassium iodide is used in cough mixtures, where it acts as an expectorant. In excess, iodine causes 'iodism', which is a state very much like the common cold with an associated skin rash. Deficiency of iodine causes goitre. Sensitivity to iodine is present in some people and can be a nuisance, for iodine on the skin then produces a severe reaction, and iodine preparations used in radiography to outline various structures, for example iodized oil sprayed into the bronchial tree for bronchography, may cause trouble.

Iodoform: a substance obtained by the action of iodine on alcohol in the presence of potassium carbonate. Although it has been used a great deal on wounds, especially in the Latin countries, its antiseptic action is slight. It has, however, a pleasant if penetrating smell, diminishes pain, and forms a protective covering over damaged tissues.

Iodophthalein: a compound excreted quickly by the liver into the bile ducts and gall-bladder. It is radio-opaque, and is therefore used to show up the outine of the gall-bladder on X-ray plates and to give an indication of the efficiency of the secretion and concentration of bile by the biliary apparatus. *See* Cholangiogram.

Ionizing Radiation: the atomic nucleus is composed of protons, which have a positive charge, and neutrons which have no charge. The nucleus is surrounded by electrons

433

which have a negative charge. If a piece of metal is bombarded by electrons travelling at a great pace, X-rays, which are electromagnetic radiations, are given off. Gamma rays are also electromagnetic radiations, which have no mass or charge, but they arise from nuclear reactions which may be the result of the decay of unstable elements or may be induced. Both X-rays and gamma rays are of high energy, and when they encounter the human body they produce pairs of oppositely charged ions by displacing electrons and protons from atoms in the deep tissues. In general gamma rays are of higher energy than X-rays, but the energy of X-rays depends upon the voltage used to accelerate electrons towards the metal target. X-rays are used a great deal for medical purposes and they are responsible for most human exposures to ionizing radiation, although the use of radioactive isotopes is increasing. The effects of radiation on the tissues are not fully understood, but it seems clear that the reaction of water in the cell, which results in the production of hydrogen atoms and highly reactive OH radicals, is basic. It is also clear that the amount of oxygen in the tissues influences sensitivity to radiation, and a number of substances are known which reduce the sensitivity of the tissues to radiation by reducing the amount of oxygen. Other actions of ionizing radiations on animal organisms include a reduction of the numbers of dividing cells, and damage to chromosomes which may produce mutations. *See* Atomic Radiation.

Iproniazid: *see* Isoniazid.

Iridectomy: a surgical operation performed under general or local anaesthetic, usually for glaucoma, in which a segment of the iris is removed.

Iris: the iris is that part of the pigmented coat of the eyeball which lies behind the cornea. It has a central aperture called the pupil through which light enters the eyeball and falls on the retina. The amount of light admitted is controlled by the size of the pupil, which varies with contractions or relaxations of the muscle fibres in the iris.

Iritis: inflammation of the iris, the ciliary body or the choroid, which together make up the middle coat of the eyeball, is called iritis, iridocyclitis or iridocyclochoroiditis, according to which structures are involved; in the last condition the whole of the pigmented part of the eye is affected.

CAUSE: the disease is commonest in young adults and in many cases the cause is syphilis. Other cases are caused by corneal ulcers, diabetes, rheumatic conditions, dental abscesses or infections of the nose. The iris, ciliary body and choroid are all involved in sympathetic ophthalmia, a condition which develops in an intact eye after a penetrating wound of the other eye. The disease is probably due to formation of antibodies to the tissues of the eye which do not normally have any connection with the blood or lymphatic systems, but which are put into communication with them as a result of injury.

SYMPTOMS: iritis causes considerable pain in or just above the eye, which waters copiously and looks red and congested. There is discomfort on looking at bright lights, the cornea becomes hazy, the pupil is small and often irregular, and the light reflexes are lost. The iris itself is discoloured, and vision is greatly impaired. An attack may last several weeks.

TREATMENT: is that of the original cause together with rest dark glasses, cessation of reading, warm bathing, aspirin for the pain, and the use of atropine drops or 1% atropine ointment.

Iron: this is used primarily in the treatment of iron-deficiency anaemias, for which it is specific. There are three misapprehensions concerning the use of iron, which is a perfectly straightforward means of cure in the appropriate type of case, and these are worth mentioning here:

1. It is untrue that iron must be given in some special form or that there is a substitute for iron. The belief used to be common that 'organic iron' is more readily absorbed than inorganic, and it is often contended that iron pills containing additional substances such as copper, vitamins of the B and C groups, stomach extract etc., are better than the ordinary ones of the pharmacopoeia. This is not so; iron is best given as the official preparations, which are ferrous sulphate, ferrous carbonate (Blaud's pills), iron and ammonium citrate mixture, or such simple proprietary preparations of these as Fersolate. Complicated proprietary preparations with 'blunderbuss' formulae of the type mentioned above

are not only no better than the official preparations – they are positively harmful, as those containing stomach extract will conceal the existence of pernicious anaemia if it happens to be present so that it remains undiagnosed. There is no place for the use of liver or stomach extract in the treatment of simple anaemia. Injections of iron may impress the rich, but they are not necessary save in those isolated cases where the oral route causes gastric upset. Iron-containing (chalybeate) natural waters are, by and large, useless since they do not contain iron in sufficient concentration to treat anaemia, and those who are not anaemic do not require iron beyond that supplied in their diet.

2. Iron is not a tonic and it is unscientific to give it in the absence of anaemia. All talk of 'tired blood' or 'weak blood' as a cause of fatigue which requires an 'iron tonic' is nonsense. Anaemia is either present in a measurable degree or it is not and it is so easy to carry out tests for anaemia that iron should never be given unless they have been done.

The conception of iron as a non-specific tonic is very old, and dates from the time of Hippocrates, who knew that in many cases iron salts improved a patient but did not know why. In the Middle Ages, when diets were not nearly as adequate as they are today and for various reasons anaemia was not uncommon, some patients improved after drinking water in which a sword had stood. A natural confusion between the clinical effects of iron in cases of unrecognized anaemia and the semi-magical properties of a warlike metal has persisted to this day.

3. Iron, if given during meals, need not upset the stomach; if it does, it is usually possible to find another preparation which does not. It is extremely doubtful whether there are really many people who have a 'tendency to anaemia' requiring frequent courses of iron, and it is certain that if they do there is something else wrong with them. *See* Anaemia.

Irradiation: treatment by ionizing radiations.

Irrigation: the washing out of a cavity or wound by large amounts of water with or without added substances.

Ischaemia: inadequate blood supply to a particular part of the body caused by spasm or disease of the blood vessels.

It may also follow general failure of the circulation, which results in widespread ischaemia and death.

Different tissues resist ischaemia for varying times – for example, the brain is very sensitive to the effects of oxygen lack and cannot survive intact for more than five minutes' ischaemia, whereas the skin survives for many hours. If it did not, it would be impossible to sit still for very long. Muscle survives for over an hour, but it is not advisable to keep a tourniquet on a limb for such a long time. The kidney can survive for an hour, and in some cases up to two hours, facts which are very important in transplant surgery; the heart survives intact for only a short time, as does the liver, and if they are to be used for transplantation they have to be removed or at least helped by an artificial circulation as soon as the circulation of the original owner is unable to keep them supplied with oxygen. The susceptibility of all tissues to ischaemia is reduced by lowering the temperature, but too low a temperature will itself prove dangerous. Kidneys perfused with chilled solutions immediately after removal have survived for up to eight hours. Partial ischaemia of muscle is painful, and lack of oxygen consequent upon an inadequate circulation with accompanying abnormal concentration of waste products of metabolism is the cause of the pain of angina pectoris, intermittent claudication, and various sorts of cramp.

Ischiorectal Abscess: an abscess between the rectum and the ischium, a part of the hip-bone (*see* below). This type of abscess is very often associated with a fistula between the rectum and the skin, a *fistula in ano*. Treatment is surgical.

Ischium: the lower posterior part of the hip-bone upon which one sits. The actual part that bears the weight of the sitting body is called the tuberosity, and it can be felt under the skin as a large bony prominence. The ischium is a separate bone in early life, but like the pubic bone fuses with the ilium to form the os coxae or hip-bone before adult life. The lines of fusion run through the acetabulum, the socket of the hip-joint.

Ishihara Test: a Japanese test for colour-blindness which consists of several plates illustrated with a large number of spots in different colours. These spots are arranged in patterns some of which cannot be seen by the colour-blind, while others only appear to the colour-blind and not to those with normal vision.

Iso-immunization: the immunization of an individual by an antigen lacking in himself but present in other normal individuals of the same species. An example is the immunization of an Rh-negative mother by an Rh-positive foetus, so that the mother produces anti-Rh agglutinins which harm the child by coagulating its red blood cells. *See* Icterus Gravis Neonatorum.

Isolation: *see* Incubation period.

Isoniazid: (Isonicotinic acid hydrazine; I.N.H.). The most powerful drug known in the treatment of tuberculosis. It is given by mouth and is relatively non-toxic but, like streptomycin, it tends to produce resistant strains of organism. It is therefore given in combination with streptomycin and P.A.S. (para-amino-salicylic acid) so that each drug destroys the organisms that have become resistant to the others. Two interesting facts about isoniazid are: (1) that unlike many chemotherapeutic agents it is a simple chemical substance easily manufactured in the laboratory; (2) that the effect of its derivative iproniazid (Marsilid) in improving the mood of tuberculous patients out of proportion to their clinical improvement led to the discovery of the monoamine oxidase inhibitors which have a remarkable effect on psychiatric cases suffering from severe depression.

Isoprenaline: a drug that has at least twelve proprietary names, isoprenaline is most effective in treating asthma. It can be given as tablets, in which case although it acts quickly it may produce palpitations, or it can be given as a spray or aerosol. Isoprenaline is useful in the treatment of Stokes-Adams attacks occurring in cases of heart block.

Isotonic: solutions which have the same osmotic pressure, i.e. which will not bring about diffusion one into the other through an intervening membrane. A 'normal' salt solution, which contains 0.9 g in 100 ml, will not draw fluid from human tissues nor be absorbed into them, for it is isotonic. On the other hand, hypertonic solutions will withdraw fluid from the tissues and hypotonic solutions will be drawn into them.

Isotope: a chemical element which has the same atomic number as another, but a different atomic mass. It has the same number of protons in the nucleus, but has a different number of neutrons. Radioactive isotopes change into another element over the course of time, the change being accompanied by the emission of electromagnetic radiations, and they are used in medicine both because they can be traced and because some of them become concentrated in one place in the body and can then influence the surrounding tissues by their radiation. Examples are the use of I^{132}, which has a half-life of $2\frac{1}{2}$ hours, for testing the function of the thyroid gland, and the use of I^{131}, which has a half-life of 8 days, for local irradiation of the thyroid gland. Other isotopes are used to irradiate tissues from the exterior, or are implanted by surgery into the part which is to be irradiated. *See* Atomic Radiation.

Itch: popular name for scabies (q.v.).

Itching: *see* Pruritus.

I.V.P.: (Intravenous pyelogram). A radiological technique for demonstrating the kidneys, ureters and bladder on an X-ray plate by giving a patient an intravenous injection of a substance which is selectively excreted by the kidneys and is opaque to X-rays. The substances used contain a great deal of iodine, and as some people are sensitive to iodine the procedure has its risks. An I.V.P. shows the concentrating power of the kidney as well as its anatomical outline, for if the pelvis of the kidney fails to show up clearly the probable cause is that the dye is not concentrated properly. The ureter is seen throughout its course in a successful I.V.P., and the bladder is outlined so that any abnormalities can be recognized. Pictures are taken after the patient has emptied his bladder, for incomplete emptying of the bladder is a feature of some conditions, notably enlargement of the prostate.

J

Jaborandi: the leaves of a South American plant which contains the alkaloid pilocarpine.

Jacksonian Epilepsy: otherwise known as focal epilepsy, is usually the result of a localized area of disease or damage in the brain, but may occur in idiopathic epilepsy. Consciousness may or may not be lost, and the fit may affect motor or sensory parts of the brain. If it is a motor fit, it tends to start in the thumb, the angle of the mouth, or the great toe. Jerking of the muscles spreads to a greater or lesser extent and is usually finished in a few seconds. Sensory attacks may start in the same places, and consist of sensations of tingling, or sometimes more complicated sensations. The essentials of a Jacksonian fit are that it should start in a definite place and spread from there in a definite progression, usually without loss of consciousness. (Hughlings Jackson, 1835–1911, was a London neurologist.)

Jalap: a powerful purgative obtained from the dried root of the Mexican plant Exogonium purga. It is now rarely used. (Sometimes mis-spelt jolip.)

Jaundice: yellow discoloration of the skin and the tissues as the result of the deposition in them of the pigment bilirubin. Bilirubin is a product of the breakdown of haemoglobin derived from spent red blood cells which is normally separated by the reticulo-endothelial system into iron, which is stored, and bilirubin, which is excreted by the liver in the bile.

CAUSES: there are classically three main causes of jaundice: haemolytic, obstructive, hepatic.

1. *Haemolytic jaundice.* If many red blood cells are destroyed in the bloodstream, as in acholuric jaundice and icterus gravis neonatorum, the liver may have to deal with an abnormal amount of bilirubin and may fail to do so. The excess bilirubin circulates in the plasma and stains the skin and tissues. In this type of jaundice the motions are dark and

the urine of normal colour, although it may darken to orange on standing.

2. *Obstructive jaundice.* If the bile passages (i.e. the hepatic ducts from the liver, or the bile duct below the cystic duct) are blocked, the bile cannot be excreted and is re-absorbed into the bloodstream. A common cause of blockage is a stone from the gall-bladder. Because the bile cannot reach the intestine the motions are as light as clay, and because the bilirubin, unlike that circulating in haemolytic jaundice, is not associated with protein it can be excreted by the kidneys and the colour of the urine becomes very dark.

3. *Hepatic jaundice.* This includes jaundice caused by disease of the liver cells themselves and that caused by obstruction of the very small bile channels within the liver by swelling of the liver cells in the course of liver disease. Yellow fever and poisoning with phosphorus, chloroform, carbon tetrachloride, etc. destroy the liver cells, and cause liberation of the bilirubin they contain into the bloodstream; as the disease progresses the jaundice deepens because bilirubin cannot be excreted by the damaged liver. In other infectious diseases, e.g. virus hepatitis, damage to the liver cells at first causes the jaundice and then the cells by their swelling obstruct the minute bile passages inside the liver. In the first stages of the disease the motions will therefore still be coloured and the urine will be dark; in the later stages the motions will become paler and the urine darker.

TREATMENT: the treatment of jaundice is the treatment of the underlying condition. Most cases of jaundice are due to obstruction, and gallstones may have to be removed surgically. There is no specific treatment for hepatitis nor for yellow fever, and the only measures that can be taken are general, such as attention to the nutritive value of the diet. The emphasis should be on proteins; if the jaundice is of long duration, Vitamins A and D with calcium gluconate should be given. Obstructive jaundice may be associated with intense itching, and in such cases local application of calamine lotion with 1% phenol may help. Sedatives, which should be used with caution in cases in which there is liver damage, and antihistamine preparations are disappointing in their action.

Jaundice, epidemic: *see* Hepatitis.

Jaw: the upper jaw is formed by the two maxillary or cheek bones and the lower jaw by the mandible. There are 16 permanent teeth in each jaw, and the upper teeth, those in the maxillae, slightly overlap the teeth of the lower jaw, those set in the mandible. The upper jaw is fixed, but the mandible articulates with the temporal bone just in front of the ear. If you put your finger into your ear and move your jaw you will feel the head of the mandible moving to and fro. In addition to a simple hinge movement, the head of the mandible can slide forwards and backwards, so that the point of the chin can be moved from side to side and a grinding motion imparted to the teeth. The muscles that act on the lower jaw are the two temporal muscles, which can be felt to harden in the temples when the teeth are clenched, and the pterygoid and masseter muscles which aid in closing the jaws and moving the lower jaw from side to side. A number of weaker muscles aided by gravity drop the lower jaw. In the joint between the head of the mandible and the temporal bone there is a disc of cartilage, which should facilitate movement but sometimes clicks and occasionally gets out of place and locks the jaw. Dislocation of the jaw can only take place forwards, and the remedy is to stand in front of the patient and place the thumbs on the back teeth, while the fingers are put under the point of the jaw. Press the thumbs down and the fingers up, and the muscles will pull the head of the mandible into its socket. First-aid treatment of a fractured mandible consists of supporting it by a bandage passing under the jaw and up over the top of the head. A fractured mandible has to be splinted by wiring the teeth of the upper and lower jaws together.

Jejunum: *see* Intestine.

Jerks: the 'jerks' elicited by the doctor when he strikes the patellar or other tendons are the response of the muscles to sudden stretching. If a normal response is present it shows that the muscle stretch receptors are working, and that the nerves which carry the impulses from the stretch receptors to the spinal cord and carry the motor impulses back again are in order; above all it shows that the segment of the spinal cord in which the reflex path lies is healthy. A successful response also shows that the muscle itself is in working order. Abnormal responses involve absent or exaggerated jerks.

Jigger: (Tunga penetrans). A flea which burrows into the skin of the feet and gives rise to acute irritation. In the course of infestation ulcers are produced.

Joint Diseases: joints are classified into movable and immovable, the latter being those such as connect the bones of the skull or join the teeth to their sockets, while the former are further subdivided into perfect and imperfect. The best example of a movable perfect joint is the knee where the articular surfaces fit together closely but comfortably. In this case the cartilaginous surfaces are separated by interarticular plates of cartilage (the semilunar cartilages). Movable joints are enclosed in a synovial membrane, a sac containing a sticky lubricating material called synovial fluid. Outside this is a covering of fibrous tissue known as the capsular ligament, in which thickenings form ligaments.

An imperfect joint is one in which bones are connected by cartilages or ligaments the flexibility of which alone permits any movement, for example the vertebrae of the spinal column, which are separated by thick plates of fibro-cartilage. Other types of movable joint defined in terms of the movement they permit are ball and socket, gliding, hinge, saddle, and pivot.

In general the joints most commonly affected by disease are the knee, the hip, the ankle and elbow since these are most frequently exposed to injury. Apparently severe injuries of a joint may not be serious provided the skin and the joint cavity are not penetrated or broken, but penetrating wounds of joints are among the most serious injuries that a man can suffer. Synovitis is the name given to inflammation of the membrane lining the joint cavity; it may be caused by infection, rheumatic diseases or gout, which are dealt with separately. 'Sprain' is a loose term implying any sort of twisting injury to a joint. If of moderately severe degree, a sprain probably results in a slight outpouring of synovial fluid into the joint cavity with or without stretching or tearing of the ligaments. Stiffness may follow a sprain because of the effusion of fluid in and around the joint.

TREATMENT: the treatment in such conditions is usually

443

aspirin, rest, and heat applied to the joint. Sprains are sometimes treated with injections of local anaesthetic which relieve the pain; although the duration of anaesthesia is only about $\frac{1}{2}$–1 hour, sometimes the pain does not return after the injection.

Jugular: the anterior, external and internal jugular veins convey blood from the head and neck to the chest. The Latin for neck is 'iugulum'.

Jurisprudence, medical: the application of the principles of the law to the practice of medicine. The term is also applied to that branch of medical knowledge and activity which is concerned with the criminal and civil courts, but for this the term forensic medicine is better used.

K

Kahn Test: one of the serological tests used in the diagnosis of syphilis. The other commonly used tests are the Wassermann reaction and the V.D.R.L. (Venereal Diseases Research Laboratories) test. This test may give a positive result in non-syphilitic disease, for example yaws.

Kala-azar: a tropical disease also known as 'black' or 'dumdum' fever found throughout the tropics but most common in West Africa, India, China and the Sudan. Sandflies transmit it.

CAUSE: infection with the organism Leishmania donovani, which multiplies in the reticuloendothelial system (q.v.).

SYMPTOMS: incubation period one month to several years. The patient may develop the symptoms suddenly, in which case he has a paroxysmal fever with sweating, or slowly, when the fever comes in waves which eventually reach a considerable height. The spleen and liver become very large, the skin goes brown, and the patient loses a great deal of weight. There is considerable anaemia, and the white cell count falls. Children with the disease become emaciated and look as though they are victims of famine.

TREATMENT: antimony is specific. It is administered in pentavalent compounds, of which there are a number, by intravenous injections which are given every day for from ten to fifteen days, according to the preparation used. On the whole cases encountered in East Africa and the Sudan are more likely to be resistant than cases occurring elsewhere, and more than one course of injections may be needed.

PROPHYLACTIC TREATMENT: dogs are common reservoirs of infection, and it may prove necessary to destroy them where the disease is widespread. Sandflies must be dealt with by clearing up their breeding grounds and using insecticides. In addition to dogs, jackals, rodents and foxes may harbour the disease.

Kanamycin: an antibiotic used to treat Gram-negative

445

infections (*see* Gram's stain). It is given by intramuscular injection in doses of 250 mg every six hours, and is reserved for severely ill cases, for it can be toxic and staphylococci develop resistance to it easily. In its properties kanamycin is very like streptomycin, and it may damage the auditory nerve in the same way. It can also damage the kidneys in cases where function is already impaired.

Kaolin: is aluminium silicate powdered and freed from grit. It is used as a dusting-powder, internally in the treatment of diarrhoea, and in the kaolin poultice, which is a mixture of kaolin, boric acid, methyl salicylate and the oils of peppermint and thymol with glycerine. This is by far the cleanest and most effective form of poultice and although it can be heated in the can and spread hot on lint the easiest method is to spread the kaolin on cold and toast the dressing under a grill. A mixture of kaolin and morphia is very useful in the symptomatic treatment of diarrhoea. Kao-pectate is another preparation used commonly in the United States for diarrhoea.

Keloid: *see* Cheloid.

Keratin: the substance of which horn, hair, the surface layer of the skin, and the nails are composed. It is a fibrous protein.

Keratitis: inflammation of the cornea.
CAUSE: it may accompany certain kinds of conjunctivitis, or result from unremoved foreign bodies, but *interstitial keratitis*, in which the substance rather than the surface of the cornea is affected, is caused by inherited syphilis. Other causes are infection with various micro-organisms, general debility, and possibly local sepsis elsewhere.
SYMPTOMS: the dangers of keratitis are ulceration of the cornea and the formation of opaque patches which interfere with vision; syphilitic keratitis does not lead to ulceration. The symptoms of keratitis in general are pain, light-sensitivity (photophobia), an overflow of tears, spasm of the eyelids, and deterioration of vision.
TREATMENT: no time should be lost in seeking treatment, preferably by an ophthalmologist, once the condition is

suspected. The eyes are ordinarily both affected, the corneas being dull and hazy, and the attack may last for several months. Hot compresses, atropine drops and tetracycline ointment are used in treatment. Residual opacities of the cornea can be dealt with by the use of corneal grafts. Corneal transplants are obtained from an eye bank (they come from eyes with a healthy cornea removed at operation or from dead bodies); they are satisfactory in over 60% of cases but, of course, do not relieve blindness due to other causes – they can only help those whose defect is due to corneal scarring. Cases due to syphilis require intensive treatment for this condition.

Kernicterus: the staining with bile of the basal nuclei of the brain occurring in icterus gravis neonatorum which may lead to toxic degeneration of the nerve cells with resultant disabilities. In 10% of cases the child becomes spastic and mentally defective and develops an accompanying cirrhosis of the liver. This is one of those interesting conditions in which mental defect is due, not to heredity, but to influences operating within the womb during pregnancy. *See* Icterus Gravis Neonatorum.

Kernig's Sign: is characteristic of meningitis. With the patient lying flat, the hip-joint is flexed until the thigh is at right angles to the body; the leg cannot then be extended at the knee and any attempt at straightening the knee produces great pain.

Kerosene Poisoning: the fumes of paraffin oil (kerosene) and petrol are mildly intoxicating, and the effect of drinking these fluids is the same as drinking ethyl alcohol. Poisoning is not necessarily fatal, and there have been cases in which individuals have become addicted to drinking petrol. Paraffin in the lungs causes pneumonia.

Ketones: substances produced in the body by the imperfect oxidation of fats and proteins. The presence of ketones in the urine is typical of severe diabetes mellitus.

Khellin: (Dimethoxymethylfuranochromone). A substance obtained from the fruit of an eastern Mediterranean plant,

Ammi visnaga, which has for centuries had the local reputation of curing renal colic. It is an antispasmodic, and is used in the relief of asthma and angina pectoris, for it dilates the bronchi and the coronary arteries.

Kibe: an alternative word for chilblain (q.v.).

Kidney: *Anatomy.* The kidneys lie one on each side of the spinal column behind the peritoneum on the back wall of the abdomen at the level of the second lumbar vertebra. They move up and down with the movements of breathing. Applied to their upper poles are the suprarenal glands, and leading from their inner borders are the ureters, the tubes through which the urine is conveyed to the bladder. Human kidneys are about four inches long, they weigh about 150 g, and they are covered by a tough layer of fibrous tissue which forms a capsule. The arteries, veins and nerves enter and leave the substance of the kidney at the same point as the ureter; this point on the inner side of the kidney is known as the hilum.

If the kidneys are cut in half lengthways, it can be seen that their substance is divided into cortex, the paler part near the surface, and medulla, much darker tissue which forms pyramids pointing towards the pelvis of the kidney, the cavity in the hilum into which the urine drains and from which run the ureters. The kidney is made up of about a million microscopic structures called nephrons, which are the functioning units of the organ. Each nephron starts as a small bunch of capillary blood vessels called a glomerulus surrounded by a membrane enclosing a space. The combined structure of glomerulus and surrounding membrane is called a Malpighian body, after the Italian who first described it in the seventeenth century. From the Malpighian body runs the tubule, which is about 30–40 mm long. Its first part is twisted, and is therefore called the proximal convoluted tubule. After the convolutions the tubule runs straight down towards the medulla, bends back like a hairpin and becomes twisted again to form the distal convoluted tubule. Eventually the tubules end in a collecting duct which drains about ten nephrons, and joins with other collecting ducts to open into the pelvis of the kidney. The blood supply to the kidneys is from the two renal arteries, which branch directly from the abdominal aorta; venous blood drains through the renal veins into the inferior vena cava. The lymphatic channels follow the course of the blood vessels.

Function. The kidneys are responsible for keeping the acid-base balance of the blood constant, for keeping the water and electrolyte content of the body balanced, and for getting rid of waste matter containing nitrogen. A human being can survive without kidneys for only two or three weeks. In health a large volume of blood passes through the Malpighian body, where fluid is filtered off through the capillary walls into the tubule. In the proximal convoluted tubule a great deal of water is re-absorbed, along with salt and other substances, but waste products are left with a certain amount of water to keep them in solution. The processes of adjusting the amounts of water and electrolytes absorbed, as well as the regulation of the reaction of the blood, are carried further to ever finer limits in the rest of the tubule. Three main factors influence the activity of the kidney: the blood pressure in the capillaries; the rate of circulation of the blood; and the state of the cells lining the tubules. The hormones which regulate the function of the kidney are: aldosterone and corticol, which have a profound effect on the fate of sodium in the kidney; vasopressin, or the antidiuretic hormone, secreted by the pituitary body which as its name suggests regulates the excretion of water; the growth hormone, also secreted by the pituitary, which has an influence on the excretion of sodium; the parathyroid hormones, which influence the excretion of phosphates; and the hormones secreted by the gonads, which have some effect on the regulation of water and sodium balance.

The kidney itself secretes an enzyme called renin, which acts on the substance angiotensinogen formed in the liver to make angiotensin. This is capable of producing intense constriction of blood vessels, particularly renal blood vessels, and also increases the secretion of aldosterone by the suprarenal glands. It is possible that renin, which by constricting blood vessels puts up the blood pressure, is part of the link between kidney disease and high blood pressure. A substance called erythropoietin, which is essential for the production of red blood cells, is also dependent on the kidney for its formation although the kidney does not contain it.

449

The function as well as the outline of the kidneys can be estimated by taking X-ray pictures at intervals after the intravenous injection of a contrast medium excreted in the urine (Uroselectan, Urografin, etc.). Another way of examining the function and shape of the kidneys is to pass a cystoscope into the bladder, and then to introduce ureteric catheters – fine, fairly stiff tubes – into the right and left ureters. Through these the urine from the right and left kidneys drains off separately; the amount of urine secreted by each kidney, its appearance and chemistry can then be determined. Contrast medium can be injected through the ureteric catheters directly into the pelvis of each kidney for X-ray examination if necessary. Another way of outlining the kidney is to inject air round it, for this will show up on X-ray plates (*see* Ventriculography). The blood supply of the kidneys can be examined by inducing a fine catheter made of polyethylene into the aorta through a puncture made in the femoral artery in the groin. Contrast medium is then injected so that it passes into the renal arteries, and a series of X-ray plates are exposed rapidly at short intervals. *Diseases of the kidney.* These are discussed under their own headings. *See* Nephritis, Renal Calculus, Hypernephroma, Polycystic Disease, Pyelitis, etc.

Kinaesthetic Sensation: sensory impulses are generated in the muscles and joints to indicate their position and degree of tension so that the brain can control and correlate the complicated motor signals which must be sent to the muscles to produce smooth motion or to maintain the posture. Kinaesthetic sensations do not appear in consciousness all the time, but the position of the limbs is normally accurately known; this is the end result of a number of different sensory impulses. A breakdown in the system is disabling, for it is not then possible to generate fine movements nor relate the position of the limbs to the body with the eyes shut. Various everyday activities become impossible. One of the ways in which a patient can become aware of a deficiency in kinaesthetic sensation is that he totters when he bends over a wash basin and closes his eyes in order to wash his face.

King's Evil: or scrofula, is tubercular swelling of the glands of the neck, which in former times was believed curable by the touch of the royal hand. The power was claimed by (or imposed upon) the royal houses of England and France, and maintained in England until the time of the Stuarts; it died out under the Hanoverians, although the Stuart claimants practised it during their exile and even during their invasions of the country.

This does not necessarily imply that they believed in the power – Charles II, for one, certainly did not.

Kino: this is obtained from the dried trunk of the Indian tree Pterocarpus marsupium and is an astringent. It is (or was) used internally for diarrhoea, and also as a gargle for oedema of the larynx and vocal cords arising from inflammation or misuse of the voice.

Kleptomania: the pathological urge to steal objects which are not necessarily, or even usually, wanted. Those who steal compulsively in this way are commonly elderly or middle-aged women of impeccable character who have a compulsion to steal objects which are trivial, useless, and which they would be well able to buy. The unconscious motive is usually a symbolic stealing of love or an attack against the virtuous, dull, or uninterested husband who will be most injured by the publicity given to his wife's shocking behaviour. Kleptomania has, of course, no connection whatever with ordinary shoplifting for which excuses are sometimes made along these lines, nor is it a specific disease entity but rather a symptom of general neurosis or unhappiness.

Knee: although the knee is one of the biggest and strongest joints in the body, it transmits so much weight and is liable to so much stress that it often operates at the limit of its strength and in the case of athletes, especially footballers, it not uncommonly becomes a source of real or imaginary disability. It is a hinge joint, formed between the lower expanded end of the thigh-bone and the upper end of the tibia, and it is stabilized by the action of the great muscles of the thigh, aided by ligaments. Neither the patella, or knee-cap, nor the fibula, the subsidiary bone of the lower leg, take part in forming the weight-bearing joint. Two semilunar cartilages divide the joint, lying between the

451

femur and the tibia on the right and the left. The capsular ligament forms the fibrous capsule of the joint; it is indistinguishable in places from tendinous expansions which are closely applied to the joint, and it is lacking above the patella and in the region of the patella itself. There is a well-defined medial ligament, running from the femur to the tibia, which is adherent in its upper part to the edge of the medical semilunar cartilage, but the lateral ligament, which is much more like a cord, is not adherent to the lateral cartilage; it runs from the femur to the top of the fibula.

There are two very important ligaments inside the joint, the anterior and posterior cruciate ligaments. They cross each other, running from the tibia below up to the internal surfaces of the two condyles of the femur. The anterior cruciate ligament runs from the inner side of the tibia at the front end of the internal semilunar cartilage upwards, backwards and outwards to the femur, and the posterior cruciate ligament runs from the outer part of the tibia near the back end of the internal semilunar cartilage upwards, forwards and inwards to the inner condyle of the femur. The cruciate ligaments are very strong and prevent the joint from being dislocated forwards or backwards. They are tightest when the knee is fully extended.

The patellar ligament, which passes across the front of the joint, is the tendon of the quadriceps muscle of the thigh, and the patella or knee-cap is a sesamoid bone in the tendon. The tendon is inserted into the tibia just below the knee-joint, and it covers and strengthens the front of the joint. It is stretched when the knee is flexed. The tendon of the semi-membranous muscle strengthens the joint behind, and sends off an expansion which forms the oblique posterior ligament. The part of the capsule which arches across the popliteus muscle is thickened to form the arcuate ligament.

Injuries of the semilunar cartilages. Of all the structures in the knee, the intra-articular semilunar cartilages are the most likely to be damaged. They are commonly torn, and the thin central part then projects into the joint and locks it so that it cannot be straightened.

CAUSE: the cause is a twist of the leg while the knee is slightly flexed with the weight upon it.

SYMPTOMS: the knee is very painful, locked and impossible to straighten, and an effusion rapidly forms in the joint so that the knee swells up. The internal cartilage is most often injured because it is more firmly fixed to surrounding structures. If the joint is examined, there is tenderness in the line of the joint about three-quarters of the way round towards the front over the cartilage affected.

TREATMENT: rest, manipulation of the knee to straighten it (which may require a general anaesthetic), a pressure bandage and exercises for the quadriceps muscles. If the tear is severe or recurrent, the cartilage must be removed.

Dislocation. This is rare; more commonly the joint is displaced enough to rupture part or the whole of the medial ligament without permanent deformity. If great force is applied the cruciate ligaments can be torn, and the knee becomes unstable, so that the tibia can be moved forwards and backwards on the femur.

SYMPTOMS: pain is felt in the joint, and there is an effusion of fluid.

TREATMENT: rest, a pressure bandage, and careful examination of the joint, including X-rays, to make sure that there is no accompanying injury of the bones. It is likely that there may be because of the force needed to dislocate or displace the bones from each other. Because the knee relies so much on the strength of the surrounding muscles to keep it stable, people with injuries to the knee must always start doing exercises for the quadriceps muscles of the thigh as soon as they can. The muscles waste very quickly if the knee is immobilized, and once their strength has diminished it is very difficult to restore the stability of the joint.

Knock-knee: (Genu valgum). Caused in children by rickets; sometimes occurs with no known cause. The condition is commoner in girls than boys, and unless the deformity is gross it corrects itself with age. It may be associated with other minor deformities, particularly of the backbone.

Koilonychia: spoon-shaped fingernails, commonly found in chronic anaemia. Such nails may be brittle.

Kola: the nut of the African tree Kola acuminata contains caffeine in about double the amount of that in coffee, but about the same as in tea. It is used as a beverage in Africa and in mineral waters elsewhere, but has no medical applications.

Koplik's Spots: small white spots appearing on the inside of the mouth and cheeks in cases of measles. They appear about three days before the skin rash develops.

Korsakow's Syndrome: a mental disorder occurring in toxic states resulting from both organic and inorganic poisons and frequently associated with polyneuritis. Its typical features are: poor memory for recent events, a tendency to invent tales of non-existent happenings, and disorientation for time, place and person, for example the patient does not recognize the doctor nor does he know where he is or the date or what he was doing the day before, but he may make up for this loss by addressing the doctor by another name and giving a long and circumstantial account of a fictitious visit to his home that very morning although he may have been in the hospital for many weeks. The commonest toxin causing Korsakow's syndrome is alcohol, but other poisons such as lead and bacterial toxins in typhoid and malaria may be responsible. The outlook depends on the initial cause but, by and large, a considerable measure of recovery is likely in a few weeks with concentrated vitamin therapy (particularly those of the B group) as this is partly a vitamin deficiency brought about by defective absorption or intake resulting from the poison. However, complete recovery is likely to take a long time and in many cases there remains a varying degree of memory defect and emotional deterioration shown by an easy suggestibility, emotional facility, and lack of efficiency.

Krameria: or rhatany, is the root of a South American plant (Krameria triandra from Peru or K. argentea from Brazil), which has much the same astringent action as kino (q.v.).

Kummell's Disease: results from undiagnosed crush fracture of a vertebra. The patient complains of pain, stiffness and varying degrees of deformity of the spine.

Küntscher's Nail: transverse fractures of long bones,

particularly the femur, may be fixed internally by such a nail which is hammered over a guide wire down the length of the bone inside the medullary cavity.

Kupffer Cells: star-shaped endothelial cells of the blood sinusoids in the liver which are part of the reticulo-endothelial system (q.v.).

Kwashiorkor: malignant malnutrition, found in children from very poor homes all over the world.

CAUSE: extreme deficiency of protein in the diet. It usually develops when the child is weaned from the breast.

SYMPTOMS: diarrhoea, oedema or swelling of the legs which may become general, patches of peeling skin which may leave raw areas, apathy, loss of appetite and failure of growth. The liver is enlarged.

TREATMENT: first-aid treatment is the administration of protein, and it is found that most cases respond well to dried skimmed milk. This can be mixed with bananas, or flour and butter; vitamins, especially Vitamins A and C, should be given with iron. Potassium should also be given if the child has much diarrhoea, as potassium chloride, dissolved in water and added to the feeds – about half to one gramme to each feed. Any accompanying infections or parasitic infestations must be treated, especially infestation with worms, although in these cases energetic treatment should be postponed until the child is convalescent. Parents must be instructed how to use their dietetic resources to the best effect in providing protein for their children.

Kyphosis: pathological curvature of the spine in which the concavity of the curve is directed forwards – hunchback.

L

Labium: part of the vulva (q.v.), or external female genitals.

Labour: in animals and most primitive races labour (parturition) is not a great problem. In animals this is due to anatomical differences but there can be little doubt that, whatever anatomical differences may be present, the relative ease with which primitive peoples bring forth children is in the main due to (*a*) better muscular development which is associated with a more active life, and (*b*) a different psychological attitude to pregnancy and childbirth. Many modern women secretly resent their role or have been adversely affected by tales of the terrors of labour, and the resulting tension may lead to difficulties. That this is so is shown by the good results obtained by hypnosis or relaxation therapy which would hardly be possible if the problem was purely one of structure. When pregnancy has lasted, more or less, for 280 days the contractions of the uterus known as labour pains begin. The pains initiate the act of expelling the child from the womb.

Labour is divided into three stages: (1) the child is lying head downwards in the womb surrounded by the amniotic fluid and enclosed within the cellophane-like membranes; as the contractions proceed the opening of the neck of the womb which projects into the upper part of the vagina begins to dilate, the process being aided by the thrusting forward of a part of the membranes like a finger of a rubber glove into the space. Soon the pressure and the stretching cause the membranes to burst and with a rush of clear fluid mingled with blood to the outside, the first stage ends. (2) The head of the baby now takes the place of the membranous projection and is thrust downwards first through the cervix which stretches even more widely and then through the vagina itself. The uterine contractions become stronger, more frequent and prolonged, and the abdominal muscles begin to help until the child is finally expelled. Sometimes in a so-called breech presentation the buttocks present first and this, if not diagnosed earlier, may lead to difficulties. (3) The third stage of labour consists of the expulsion of the placenta and the membranes. After a resting period of 20–30 minutes, uterine contractions begin again until the after-birth has been expelled. Most pregnancies would terminate normally even in the absence of skilled help, but obviously it is desirable for a trained midwife to assist what is, after all, a normal process.

As soon as the child is born and before the third stage begins the umbilical cord binding it to the placenta in the mother will have to be tied and cut and the usual lusty yells which begin immediately after birth help to establish the unfamiliar process of breathing. Apart from breech presentations (3.5% of all cases), there may be face presentations (0.4% of cases) or the rather rare cross presentation in which the child is lying transversely across the womb and the pelvis. These, like the breech presentation, require skilled attention. The dangers of the puerperium (the period after childbirth) are haemorrhage and sepsis. Post-partum haemorrhage can be dangerous and occasionally fatal but now it is nearly always controllable. Immediate measures to deal with it are compression of the womb through the abdominal wall and injections of ergometrine or pituitrin. Sepsis was formerly a very grave condition and many mothers died of 'child-bed fever' before the Viennese physician Semmelweiss was able to show its connection with faulty hygiene in the early nineteenth century. It is now almost a thing of the past in civilized communities.

Labyrinth: *see* Ear. Labyrinthitis is inflammation of the labyrinth, or otitis interna.

Lacrimal Apparatus: the parts concerned with the secretion, storage and absorption of tears.

Lactation: the period during which the infant is suckled at the breast. During pregnancy the milk-secreting tissue of the breast proliferates, and towards the end of pregnancy the ducts are full of colostrum, a pale yellow fluid. The secretion of milk begins about the third or fourth day after the birth of the child in response to the anterior pituitary gland hormone prolactin. It is thereafter affected by the infant's suckling, which promotes a reflex secretion of oxytocin from the posterior part of the pituitary. Oxytocin causes the muscle cells in the walls of the minute ducts in the breast to contract and expel milk; it also causes the uterus to contract, and this may be noticed by the nursing mother. Lactation is profoundly influenced by the mother's emotional state, so that emotional upset will cause the milk to dry up just as surely as inadequate stimulus from the child. If the child is not to be breast-fed the flow must be stopped by the administration of an oestrogen. A typical dose is 0.1 mg Ethinyloestradiol 3 times a day for 3 days, followed by 0.1 mg once a day for 6 days.

Lactic Acid: made by the fermentation of milk-sugar or lactose by lactobacilli, as in the souring of milk. Lactic acid is also produced in the muscles by the breakdown of glycogen to provide energy for work in the absence of oxygen. If it is allowed to accumulate in the muscles, for example by inadequate circulation of blood, muscular fatigue follows and further contractions are stopped. At one time sour milk in the form of koumiss or yoghourt was thought to prolong life, but unfortunately the figures do not bear out this claim. Lactobacillus odontolyticus is said to rot the teeth by producing acid from the fermentation of sugar in the mouth.

Lactose: milk-sugar.

Laevulose: one of the constituents of grape-sugar or dextrose.

Lamblia Giardia: *see* Giardiasis.

Lamellae: tiny discs made of gelatin and glycerin impregnated with various drugs (atropine, homatropine, cocaine and physostigmine) to be placed behind the lower eyelid, where they dissolve.

Lameness: *see* Gait.

Laminectomy: when operating upon the spinal cord it is first necessary to remove parts of the overlying vertebral arches or laminae. The operation is called laminectomy, and

458

is carried out in cases where there is pressure on the cord or the nerves issuing from the cord from tumours, prolapsed intervertebral discs, fractures or spondylosis, or when tracts of nervous tissue in the cord are to be interrupted as in cordotomy.

Lancet: a small two-edged pointed surgical knife; formerly used for opening abscesses and letting blood.

Lanolin: fat obtained from sheep's wool and used as a base for ointments because it does not go rancid, and can penetrate the skin as mineral substances cannot. Lanolin is capable of absorbing and mixing with water.

Laparotomy: surgical operation to open the abdominal cavity either to make an inspection of the contents or as a preliminary to further surgery. To be quite correct, laparotomy means incision through the flank, but the word is hardly ever used in this sense now.

Laryngectomy: removal of the larynx, an operation carried out for malignant growths. Patients with no larynx can be taught to speak very well by using various techniques.

Laryngitis: inflammation of the larynx.
CAUSES: (1) virus infection, as in the common cold or measles; (2) irritation of the throat by harmful dust or vapour; (3) misuse of the voice; (4) syphilis or tuberculosis.
SYMPTOMS: a tickling dry cough, harsh or hoarse voice, a feeling of rawness in the throat, and a slight fever. The vocal cords are red and swollen.
TREATMENT: the voice must be rested; often inhalations and a simple linctus help. Smoking aggravates the condition, and may in excess itself produce chronic laryngitis.

Laryngoscope: an instrument for looking into the larynx. It may be a mirror on a long handle, to use when the examiner wears a head mirror so that he can reflect light into the throat along his line of sight. Another form of laryngoscope carries its own light, and yet another, for use when the patient is anaesthetized, carries a light on a blade with which the base of the tongue is drawn forwards so that the larynx is seen under direct vision.

Larynx: the larynx is a fairly rigid framework of cartilages held together by ligaments and moved by attached muscles. It is lined with mucous membrane which is continuous above with that of the throat and below with that of the trachea or windpipe. It is the organ which, on the outside of the neck, forms the lump known as the Adam's apple, and its chief function is speech, brought about by the movement of air through its passage while the vocal cords narrow or widen its aperture. Apart from the conditions mentioned elsewhere, the three main categories of disease in the larynx are obstruction, paralysis and tumour.

1. *Obstruction*

CAUSE: the commonest causes of obstruction are abscess of the lining of the laryngeal cartilage (perichondritis), allergic oedema, acute infections of the throat or floor of the mouth, injuries or wounds, foreign bodies, burns from scalding liquids or steam, and irritation from harmful vapours.

SYMPTOMS: these begin suddenly and progress quickly; there is difficulty in breathing, pallor, restlessness, and later cyanosis (blueness).

TREATMENT: this must be immediate and if the cause can be removed this must be done at once. But when life is threatened and the cause cannot be removed, tracheotomy must be performed as quickly as possible. In this operation an incision is made low in the front of the neck cutting the trachea, and a tube is inserted. Relief is almost immediate. Later, when the cause has been dealt with, the opening can be closed and breathing once more takes place in the ordinary way.

2. *Paralysis*

CAUSE: bulbar poliomyelitis (poliomyelitis of the base of the brain), injury to the nerves supplying the larynx (occasionally during surgical operations on the thyroid gland), and cancer of the thyroid, oesophagus, or neck glands involving the laryngeal nerves.

SYMPTOMS: paralysis of one vocal cord causes hoarseness and a change in the voice, but when both are paralysed and relax towards the midline, breathing in, although not breathing out, is severely affected.

TREATMENT: when both cords are paralysed an operation can sometimes be carried out to fix one in an open position and relieve the situation.

3. *Tumours*

Tumours of the larynx are relatively common and it is a general rule that anyone who is hoarse for more than two weeks should forthwith see a doctor. Most laryngeal tumours are benign; nevertheless, these must be removed, and cancerous growths, commonest in men over the age of fifty, will require both operation and X-ray therapy. The latter seem to be associated with the excessive use of tobacco, overuse of the voice, and the habit of drinking hot liquids. Both partial and complete laryngectomy are performed in this type of case and although the complete operation necessitates the removal of the entire sound-producing apparatus, quite a good voice may in fact be achieved without a larynx. *See* Throat.

Lassar's Paste: a paste used in the treatment of dermatitis. It is made of petroleum jelly (Vaseline), zinc oxide, starch and a little salicylic acid. It is soothing, softening and antiseptic. Lassar's Betanaphthol paste is made of precipitated sulphur, soft soap, and betanaphthol in petroleum jelly.

Lathyrism: a disease caused by eating vetch seeds or varieties of chick-pea. There is pain in the loins and spastic paralysis of the legs.

Laudanum: tincture of opium, until modern times a popular preparation for deadening pain and bringing sleep.

Laughing Gas: nitrous oxide gas, used in dental and other short operations by itself; and in combination with volatile anaesthetics in longer procedures.

Lavage: washing-out of the stomach, usually for severe alcoholic intoxication or after the ingestion of poisons.

Laxatives: *see* Constipation.

Lazaretto: a hospital for plague or contagious diseases.

Lead: lead used to be important in medicine because of the relative frequency of poisoning both in industry and in the home from lead water pipes and lead paints, but now few paints contain lead and the composition of water pipes is carefully supervised. Nevertheless, in the United States lead poisoning is recognized as a fairly frequent illness among children living in slum areas. It is caused by the eating of flaking lead-containing paint and loose plaster in old, deteriorating housing or by inhalation of fumes from used car batteries burnt for warmth. These children appear chronically ill and often show signs of liver damage and acute encephalopathy. Treatment does not always succeed in restoring mental function so that the brains of some victims remain damaged throughout life. Except for such cases poisoning now chiefly occurs among workers with lead in industry, particularly from fumes and dust. An intake of about 2 mg a day is usually excreted before it is absorbed, but above this figure lead may be absorbed and is then incorporated in bone. Here it affects the manufacture of red blood cells; the cells become fragile, and they break up in the bloodstream. Lead also interferes with the formation of haemoglobin, and may damage nervous tissue. It is possible that a minor degree of lead poisoning may follow inhalation of automobile exhaust fumes, for petrol commonly contains tetra ethyl lead.

SYMPTOMS: severe anaemia, and in some cases paralysis due to damage to nervous tissues which leads to wrist- and foot-drop, optic neuritis with blindness, and delirium and delusions of a specific type (*see* Korsakow's Syndrome). The intestines are subject to intense attacks of colic, which is felt as a severe pain centred round the umbilicus.

TREATMENT: for acute colic, local heat to the abdomen, a mixture containing belladonna and magnesium trisilicate, and the administration of an enema. Lead is removed from the tissues by the intravenous infusion of calcium disodium edetate, E.D.T.A.

Leaders: popular name for sinews or tendons.

Lecithin: a complex fat found in large amounts in the brain and nerves as well as in the yolk of eggs and in semen.

Leeches: the medical leech, Hirudo medicinalis, was once used to withdraw blood from 'congested areas', for example from the temples in the case of headache – although the presence of leeches on the temples might very well persuade the patient that the headache was not as bad as he had thought, congestion or no. The leech is shaped like a worm and has a mouth like a sucker at one end which contains three teeth to break and grip the skin. Leeches secrete a substance which prevents the blood coagulating, which can be extracted from their heads. Gnathobdellid leeches are found widely in tropical swamps and wet places and they fasten themselves on to the legs without causing pain, so that the victim either finds unsuspected leeches stuck to his legs when he comes out of the water or finds bleeding bites, for the wounds bleed freely for a long time under the in-fluence of the anti-coagulation secretions.

Left-handedness: or mancinism, is a much more deep-rooted and all-pervading problem than is usually thought. Being due to dominance of the right side of the brain rather than the left as is usual in right-handed people, it is not merely a matter of a preference for the left over the right hand; for such people are often 'left-eyed' too and their natural tendency to read from right to left and even to produce mirror-writing (i.e. writing which is wholly reversed and can only be read by its reflection in a mirror) may result in considerable retardation in learning to read and often unhappiness and frustration. In a world of right-handed people the left-handed person may be at a disadvantage in numerous everyday situations. It is difficult to believe that there can be any harm in causing such a child to use his right hand from the earliest days, but it is equally difficult to believe that it does much good and, of course, although the fact of so training him is harmless it is likely to be carried out in a spirit of annoyance on the part of the parent and resentment on the part of the child which is bad for both. Nor is the tendency 'cured' and such a child, no matter how competent he has become with his right hand, will in moments of tiredness be found reading MAT as TAM. Probably the best solution is to allow the child his left-handedness (making it clear that it is not regarded as an abnormality) and in later years to encourage him to become ambidextrous. Left-handedness is occasionally associated with stammering and squint, but it is probably true to say that it is equally often associated with exceptional achievements; Leonardo da Vinci, for example, was left-handed.

Leg: although in common speech the whole of the lower limb is referred to as the leg, in anatomy the leg is that part which lies between the knee and the foot.

BONES: there are two bones in the leg, the tibia and the fibula. The tibia is the larger bone and it articulates with the femur at its upper end to form the knee joint (q.v.) and with the talus at the ankle. The fibula is the smaller bone of the leg, and it lies to the outer side of the tibia; it takes no part in forming the knee joint, but it does form the outer part of the ankle joint. It does not bear any of the weight of the body, which is transmitted from the knee to the ankle through the tibia.

JOINTS: at the knee the two articular cartilages are attached to the upper surface of the tibia, and intervene between it and the articular surfaces of the femur. The upper and lower joints between the tibia and fibula allow very little movement, especially at the lower end, for the stability of the ankle joint depends a great deal upon the two bones remaining bound closely to each other.

MUSCLES: the muscles are divided into anterior, lateral and posterior groups.

Anterior group. These muscles raise the foot at the ankle, and in doing so raise the inner border of the foot. They also extend the toes. One of them, the peroneus tertius – really the muscle that extends the little toe – tends to raise the outer border of the foot.

Lateral group. There are two lateral muscles, peroneus longus and peroneus brevis. They pull the foot down at the ankle, and tend to turn the foot out. The peroneus longus tendon helps to maintain the arch of the foot.

Posterior group. These are in two divisions, superficial and deep. The superficial muscles are the muscles of the calf, and are large and strong. They pull the foot downwards at the ankle, and their names are soleus, gastrocnemius and plantaris.

Deep group. This includes the popliteus, which acts upon the knee joint to flex it, and the flexor muscles of the toes, which join with the tibialis posterior and the superficial muscles of the calf to pull the foot down.

Deformity of these muscles and their tendons results in club-foot (q.v.). The anterior muscles are supplied by the anterior tibial nerve, the superficial posterior muscles by the medical tibial or popliteal nerve, and the deep posterior muscles by the posterior tibial nerve except for the popliteus, which is supplied by the medial popliteal nerve. All are branches of the sciatic nerve. The principal arteries of the leg are the anterior tibial and posterior tibial branches of the popliteal artery, which is itself the continuation of the femoral artery. The deep veins run with the arteries, but there are many superficial veins running just under the skin which drain into the large superficial veins on the back and front of the leg. These are called the long and short saphenous veins, and are often the site of varicosities. *See* Varicose Veins.

Leiomyoma: a tumour of the unstriped or involuntary muscle of the internal organs.

Leishmania: a species of protozoa which causes in man the disease kala-azar (Leishmania donovani), oriental sore (L. tropica), Chiclero's ulcer (L. mexicana), and espundia (L. brasiliensis). It is an intracellular parasite, multiplying within an infected cell until the cell bursts to release a great number of new parasites to infect other cells. *See* Kala-azar.

Leishmaniasis: a group of diseases, notably kala-azar and tropical sore, caused by protozoa of the genus Leishmania. The vector is the sandfly.

Lemon: a source of Vitamin C, its juice containing 60 mg of ascorbic acid per 100 g. Hot lemon drinks are said to promote sweating during a cold, if the patient wants to sweat, but of itself lemon juice is not slimming. A diet of unsweetened lemon juice could conceivably lead to a loss of weight by destroying the appetite.

Lempert's Operation: fenestration, the forerunner of modern operations for deafness.

Lens: the lens of the eye is normally held out at the edge by the suspensory ligament so that it assumes its greatest diameter and has its least thickness. When the ciliary muscle contracts, it slackens the pull of the suspensory ligament so that the lens becomes more globular; its refractive power is increased, and images of near objects are brought to a sharp focus on the retina. The lens is made of a firm central part or nucleus, surrounded by a softer substance. It is contained in a fibrous capsule; in the foetus it is soft, reddish, very elastic and almost round, but in old age it is flatter, less resilient and slightly yellow. In cataract the lens slowly becomes opaque, and eventually the patient can no longer see through it. The opaque lens can be removed by a surgical operation, and the sight restored by the prescription of glasses.

Leontiasis: hypertrophy or overgrowth of the bones of the face and the forehead which eventually produces an appearance resembling that of a lion. A similar process sometimes takes place in leprosy.

Leprosy: occurs all over the world, but especially in India and China, the West Indies, and South Africa. Its highest incidence in Europe is now in Iceland, but the disease was once common in other European countries.
CAUSE: the Mycobacterium leprae, which in many ways resembles the organism of tuberculosis, being 'acid fast' and forming typical nodules of granulomatous tissue.
SYMPTOMS: there are two main types of leprosy: nodular or lepromatous, and neural or tuberculoid. In the former there are repeated attacks of fever and reddish swellings on the face which gradually harden and become painful, spreading until they coalesce in areas which are insensitive to touch. The ears, face, the inside of the nose, the forearms and thighs become involved and in the late stage the face is 'leonine' in appearance – round, puffy, the eyes sunken in the swollen tissues, the nose flattened. There is ulceration of the tongue, larynx and pharynx, and severe scarring occurs on healing. In the neural type the nerve trunks are first

affected and large atrophic patches appear on the buttocks and body which gradually become pale and without feeling. Because of this loss of sensibility ulcers, sores, and finally gangrene of the fingers and toes appear.

TREATMENT: isolation is not usually necessary, for the disease is not very infectious. Much of the horror it aroused in former times must have been due to the fact that leprosy persists for a long time, is readily distinguishable, and very disfiguring. There is little danger of contracting leprosy, even in a leper colony, provided that intimate personal contact is avoided, but it is often better that healthy children should be taken out of a leprous family until the disease has been controlled. The drug of choice is dapsone, which is given twice a week first in doses of 25 mg, then after 2 weeks 50 mg, after 4 weeks 75 mg, and after 6 weeks 100 mg. The treatment may have to be kept up for years, and the dosage raised slowly to as much as 300 mg twice a week.

Leptospira: micro-organisms like very fine corkscrews, which are in constant motion. They are part of the Spirochaete group, and two of the species produce disease in man, Leptospira icterohaemorrhagica, which is the organism of Weil's disease, and L. canicola, which produces canicola fever. Weil's disease is caught from the urine of infected rats, and canicola fever from the urine of dogs and pigs.

Lesbianism: female homosexuality. *See* Sex.

Lesion: a non-specific term meaning damage or disease in any part of the body. (Latin 'laesio', from 'laedere', to hurt.)

Leucocyte: the leucocytes are the white cells of the blood. They are classified as granulocytes or polymorphonuclear leucocytes, lymphocytes and monocytes. Granulocytes are further divided into neutrophils, basophils and eosinophils according to their staining reactions. Leucocytes range in size from 0.005 mm to 0.015 mm, and the proportions in which they are present in the blood in health are:

Neutrophils   2,500 – 7,500 per mm^3 (40–75%)
Lymphocytes 1,000 – 4,500 per mm^3 (20–45%)
Monocytes   200 –   900 per mm^3 (2–10%)

| Eosinophils | 50 – | 400 per mm³ (1–6%) |
| Basophils | 0 – | 200 per mm³ (up to 1%) |

The total number of leucocytes per cubic millimetre ranges between 4,000 and 10,000. It is raised in inflammatory conditions and abnormally low in other conditions – for example, poisoning of the bone marrow by drugs. The state in which the count is increased is called leucocytosis, and that in which it is decreased leukopenia.

Leucoderma: a condition of the skin in which patches of white appear. The sole harm it causes is the social embarrassment of the patient. The disease may occur in Negroes.

Leucopenia: *see* Leucocyte.

Leucotomy: a brain operation in which the fibres connecting the front part of the cerebral cortex to the rest of the brain are severed to a greater or lesser degree. Devised in the 1930s by Moniz of Portugal for the treatment of otherwise incurable mental disease, the operation has taken different forms and varies in the extent of the incision and its locality, but there are those who strongly disapprove of it in any form in spite of an equal or greater number who have made exaggerated claims on its behalf. On the whole the possibility of permanent damage to the mental functions makes it advisable to reserve leucotomy for cases where all other methods have been tried and failed and there is no reasonable hope of spontaneous recovery. A leucotomized patient whose emotions are shallow and behaviour unreliable may be better than a demented one as far as the relatives and attendants are concerned, but he has lost something which cannot be recovered.
Recent tremendous progress in the drug therapy of mental conditions has made surgeons even more cautious about taking irrevocable measures, with the result that the operation is now rarely performed.

Leukaemia: a group of diseases in which the white cells of the blood are greatly increased in number.
CAUSE: unknown. Although it is not possible to assert that radiation causes leukaemia, it is thought that exposure to

468

ionizing radiations increases the likelihood of developing the disease. The leukaemias are divided into three main groups: acute, chronic myeloid or granulocytic, and chronic lymphatic.

1. *Acute*. A disease commoner in men than women, and the commonest form of leukaemia in children.

SYMPTOMS: the patient has a sore throat, pain in the bones and joints, has a fever and feels generally ill. He may develop small haemorrhages into the skin, and is prone to bruising. He becomes anaemic, and begins to bleed into the gut and from the nose; there may also be blood in the urine. The lymph glands are enlarged, and there is some discomfort on pressure over the breastbone. The diagnosis is made on clinical appearances and by the examination of the blood under the microscope. Acute leukaemia is not a common disease, but it is thought to be on the increase.

TREATMENT: this is by corticosteroids such as prednisone and chemical cytotoxic drugs, for example vincristine sulphate, a drug derived from the periwinkle. The course of the disease and the progress of treatment has to be watched carefully by the pathologist, and blood counts are carried out at least every fortnight. Blood transfusions and the use of antibiotics may be necessary in treating accompanying anaemia and infection.

2. *Chronic myeloid*. This disease is not common among children, but is found in middle age in both sexes.

SYMPTOMS: discomfort in the abdomen, continual tiredness, night sweating and fever, and general ill-health develop, and the spleen becomes very large and may be felt in the upper left part of the abdomen; as the disease progresses the spleen may become so big that it can be seen moving under the abdominal wall as the patient breathes. The diagnosis is made certain by examination of the blood under the microscope, which shows about 200,000 to 300,000 neutrophil white cells (*see* Leucocytes) per cubic millimetre.

TREATMENT: irradiation with X-rays, or the use of the cytotoxic drug busulphan (Myleran).

3. *Chronic lymphatic*. Found more often in men than women, and occurring in middle and later life.

SYMPTOMS: gradual enlargement of lymph glands all over the body. The spleen and liver may enlarge, and the patient loses weight, feels generally ill and tired, and suffers from fever and sweating at night. He may complain of indigestion, may develop symptoms indicating interference with the nervous system, and may suffer from herpes zoster. He is prone to fall victim to acute infection in the later stages of the disease. The diagnosis is made on the microscopic appearance of the blood, which shows a great number of lymphocytes, although the total white cell count is only about half that found in myeloid leukaemia.

TREATMENT: radiotherapy, cytotoxic drugs and corticosteroids.

Leukocyte: *see* Leucocyte.

Leukoplakia: a condition in which the patient, usually a man over 40, develops thickened white patches on the tongue, and sometimes on the gums and the inside of the cheeks. The usual cause is chronic irritation due to sepsis in the mouth, excessive smoking of strong tobacco, alcohol, or syphilis (or, as commonly happens, all four).
The condition may progress through the formation of fissures to carcinoma.

Leukorrhoea: abnormal white discharge from the vagina.

Levallorphan: a derivative of the drug levorphanol, which has a powerful action very much the same as morphine. Levallorphan, however, is an antagonist to morphine and other narcotic drugs and relieves the respiratory depression associated with their use, although it has to be given very cautiously to addicts for it provokes acute withdrawal symptoms.
The drug nalorphine, which is derived from morphine, is another antagonist to narcotic drugs, including morphine, but its action is rather less powerful than that of levallorphan.

Lewisite: a war gas containing arsine compounds which acts upon the lungs, skin and eyes.

Libido: the sex impulse.

Librium: (Chlordiazepoxide). A drug which induces a feeling of 'tranquillity' without sending patients to sleep.

Used in cases of minor anxiety, and therefore prescribed in enormous quantities. The drug is safe, but can produce habituation or dependence, and it potentiates the action of alcohol. *See* Tranquillizers.

Lice: parasitic insects. *See* Louse, Parasites.

Lichen Planus: a skin disease, which has been attributed to mental stress, consisting of an eruption of small lilac papules, smooth on the surface and each with a dent at the top. They increase in number and often form a pattern on the skin like lace which leaves marks behind as it fades. Any part of the body may be affected, but most commonly lichen planus develops on the flexor surfaces of the arms and legs (i.e. the upper surface of the forearm and the back of the legs). There is severe itching. The condition can become quite troublesome; there is no specific treatment, but cortisone preparations help as in other itchy skin rashes.

Ligaments: strong bands of fibrous tissues which hold the bones together and stabilize the joints.

Ligature: a piece of thread used to tie off a blood vessel or a hollow tubular structure, for example the base of the appendix before it is removed.

Lightening: not a discharge of electricity in the heavens, as claimed by a certain medical student, but an occurrence in the 36th week of pregnancy when the head of the foetus engages in the brim of the pelvis, and the uterus and its contents descend a little in the abdomen.

Light treatment: the ordinary medical lamps sold for use at home usually produce both ultraviolet and infra-red rays. The former give the effect of sunlight, the latter of deep heat. Ultraviolet treatment was regarded by some about thirty years ago as almost a cure-all, but those days are gone and anybody who believes that ultraviolet rays do anything more than stimulate the skin and produce unnecessary Vitamin D by irradiating the ergosterol of the body must be exceptionally credulous. Sunlight, of course, is good and it makes most people look good (often a great deal better than they are), but its effects as a general stimulant and tonic are largely psychological. Indeed, in an experiment carried out some years ago when sunbathing under ultraviolet lamps was provided for the benefit of industrial workers, it was found that everybody who had this treatment felt better than those who had not been given it – but the workers who had been unknowingly exposed to lamps with an invisible screen cutting out all the 'health-giving' rays felt just as well as those who had been given the real thing. Infra-red rays are those emitted by a hot body of any sort, for example a coal or electric fire; they penetrate the body up to a depth of 1 inch and increase the blood-flow to the part, and are therefore used to treat muscular and rheumatic pains. (Really deep penetration requires diathermy, q.v.) Ultraviolet rays are sometimes used in rheumatic conditions, where they work by a process of counter-irritation; but it must be remembered that such rays can be very dangerous and cause severe burning from overexposure. Most 'sunlight lamps' do not produce the bronzing of the skin and the sunburned appearance that the advertisers promise.

Lignocaine: (Procaine). A local anaesthetic which acts quickly when applied in concentrations of up to 4% to mucous membranes and when injected as a 0.5 to 1% solution into the skin or round sensory nerves. It is also a cardiac depressant, and may be given intravenously in cases where the ventricles develop extra beats, or the pulse rate is abnormally increased.

Linctus: any syrupy medicine, usually a cough mixture.

Linea Alba: a white line running down the middle of the wall of the abdomen formed by the junction of the flat tendons of the external oblique, internal oblique and transverse muscles of the abdomen after they have split to enclose the two longitudinal rectus muscles.

Liniments: or embrocations are oily or spirit (alcohol) applications rubbed into the surface of the body for muscular or joint pains. Older applications contained such substances as aconite, belladonna, camphor (camphorated oil), and methyl salicylate (oil of wintergreen), but with the exception of the last these are little used today, being both messy and poisonous. Most proprietary applications contain salicylates, presumably because of their association with rheumatism when taken internally, but the real function of a liniment is to increase the blood supply to the part and soothe by warmth and counter-irritation. Demands are frequently made of the doctor for a 'strong' liniment but there is no evidence that these are any more effective than the milder ones and they may cause quite a severe rash on the skin. Some proprietary preparations claim to penetrate the skin, bringing derivatives of nicotinic acid and salicylates into contact with the affected area, but there is little proof that they do so and even less that, if they did, the effect would be beneficial. For practical purposes methyl salicylate liniment is probably the best and safest; some of the proprietary preparations are equally good and certainly cleaner, most of them being in the form of creams which have the advantage of not being liable to be swallowed by mistake. The so-called horse oils are best left to horses.

Lip: there are not many disorders to which the lips are subject, but among the commonest are fissures and cracks which, although they often appear in cold weather, are frequently associated with septic conditions of the mouth (this is particularly the case when the corners of the mouth are affected). Ordinary remedies can be tried, but if they prove inadequate it may be necessary to cauterize the fissures with silver nitrate.

Herpes simplex, not to be confused with herpes zoster, is commonly called a cold sore and may be painted with 'new skin' or collodion which protects it until the condition departs spontaneously. Ulcers on the inner surface of the lips are a sign of mouth infection and should be treated accordingly, and any form of septic sore or boil on the outer surface of the lips, especially the upper lip, must be regarded seriously. Occasionally a chancre, the primary sore of syphilis, is seen on the lip. Hare lip is dealt with under Cleft Palate, and cancer, usually of the lower lip in elderly men (since women stopped smoking dirty pipes), is dealt with under Cancer.

Lipaemia: the presence in the blood of abnormally large

473

amounts of fat or fatty substances including cholesterol.

Lipiodol: a radio-opaque oily substance containing iodine, used in contrast radiography.

Lipoma: a benign tumour composed of fat cells. It may reach a considerable size, but removal is nearly always simple.

Liquorice: (Glycyrrhiza). The peeled or unpeeled root and underground stem of Glycyrrhiza glabra. Used in making sweets, or in medicine to cover up the bad taste of other ingredients of a mixture, for example cascara sagrada. Carbonoxolone sodium, a derivative of liquorice, helps to heal peptic ulcers.

Lithiasis: a condition in which stones are formed.

Lithotrity: the operation of crushing a stone in the bladder by an instrument introduced through the urethra so that the fragments can be passed in the urine (also known as litholapaxy). A lithagogue is a drug which supposedly helps stones to pass out and lithotriptics are drugs which allegedly dissolve stones. No such substances exist, although fortunes have been made in selling preparations which purport to do these things. The lithotomy position in an operation is one in which the patient lies on his back with the legs held up in the air and bent at the knee in order that the surgeon may reach the perineum. These names derive from the eighteenth century when 'cutting for the stone' was one of the few operations, apart from amputations, that doctors could do successfully. In fact, there was even a special class of surgeon expert in the operation and described as a lithotomist; from which we may deduce that either stone was much more common then than it is now or that many nonexistent ones must have been 'removed'.

Little's Disease: (Congenital Cerebral Diplegia). A condition which used to be regarded as the result of injury at birth, but is now thought to be due to various defects of development in the central nervous system. The child is backward, and late in sitting up. It walks with difficulty, if at all, for the legs are stiff and cross-legged and 'scissors' gait is common. Fits and increasingly obvious mental deficiency make their appearance, and while some cases improve others progressively deteriorate.

Liver: the liver is the largest gland in the body.

Anatomy. It lies under the right side of the diaphragm under cover of the lower ribs, reaching as high as the sixth rib. It weighs about 1,500 g and is soft, as can be verified in the butcher's shop. It is divided into four lobes for the purposes of description, but to all intents is a single organ shaped like a wedge. It is supplied with blood by the hepatic artery, a branch of the abdominal aorta, and the portal vein, which brings to the liver blood from the intestines. About one-fifth of the blood reaching the liver comes through the hepatic artery, the remaining four-fifths coming through the portal vein. Blood drains from the liver through the hepatic vein into the inferior vena cava. Branches of the portal vein and the hepatic artery run in company to the 'sinusoids' inside the liver, small blood spaces which take the place of capillary vessels. The sinusoids are lined by liver cells across which the blood has to pass before it is collected in the veins which join to form the hepatic vein. Although they are not separated from each other the liver is made up of about twelve functional segments, each one of which has a branch of the portal vein, hepatic artery, hepatic vein and hepatic duct, and it is possible to remove certain segments of the liver surgically while leaving healthy segments undamaged. The hepatic ducts, through which bile drains from the liver, run from the segments to coalesce and emerge from the liver substance. Right and left ducts join to form a common duct which then joins the cystic duct from the gall-bladder (q.v.) and becomes the bile duct.

Function. The liver is responsible for many chemical processes essential for life; it is not possible for an animal to live without a liver. The main functions of the liver are concerned with the formation and breakdown of proteins, fats and carbohydrates, and their storage. Various hormones are broken down, drugs are changed and excreted, urea is formed, and bile is secreted; the Vitamins A, D, E and K are stored. The functions of the liver are so many and so complicated that it is almost impossible to test them all in

475

the clinical laboratory, and a set of representative tests are carried out for the purposes of diagnosis and treatment. The chemical processes occurring in the liver take place in the cells of the hepatic lobules, formed by collections of sinusoids surrounded by hepatocytes. The hepatic venules which drain the blood run in the centres of the lobules, and the branches of the hepatic artery, which brings fresh blood from the rest of the body, and of the portal vein, which brings blood carrying food substances from the intestines, run at the periphery. In company with them run the biliary vessels. The liver has large reserves of functioning tissue, and life can be supported after quite considerable amounts of liver substance have been removed or destroyed by disease, but if the liver's reserves have been cut down it cannot always deal with toxic substances as quickly as it once did. This is the reason for the reduced tolerance to alcohol that follows severe cases of hepatitis. It is worth remembering in connection with alcohol that a starved liver, one containing few of the normal proteins, carbohydrates and fats, is more liable to damage by disease than one properly nourished, for many people who are very fond of their drink are not so fond of their food. However, the regenerative powers of adequately nourished liver cells are quite remarkable.

Liver Disease: the diseases of the liver are described under separate headings (*see* in particular Jaundice and Cholecystitis), but one or two general remarks may be useful.

Since the liver plays such an important part in the economy of the body it is obvious that many troubles may theoretically befall it, but fortunately damage is minimized by the fact that unlike other tissues it is capable of regeneration and the amount of liver tissue available is normally in excess of what is needed. Few diseases are primarily liver conditions, although there are many in which the liver is secondarily affected. Incidentally, there is no reason to think that there is really such a state as being 'liverish' as so many people suppose when an evening of ill-chosen food or too much drink leads to gastritis. Some people are unduly impressed when vomit contains bile and believe this to be an infallible sign that the liver is affected; but anyone who has vomited the contents of his stomach must inevitably if he vomits again produce the contents of his duodenum, which are likely to contain bile – that is, if the liver is working properly. In spite of the vast number of pills sold for liver disorders and in spite of the fact that all drugs pass through it, there are very few which significantly influence liver function or disease. There is nothing that in the liver corresponds to the alkalies so freely and satisfactorily given for stomach affections. The only effective drugs which can be used to stimulate the flow of bile are bile itself, its salts, and magnesium sulphate (Epsom salts), and they are sometimes given in chronic infections of the gall-bladder or in cirrhosis of the liver but, even so, the value of stimulating the flow of bile is doubtful.

Liver Extract: this is used in the treatment of pernicious and other macrocytic anaemias (*see* Anaemia). It is given by injection, and is quite useless in the treatment of any other form of anaemia.

Liver Fluke: Clonorchis, Fasciola and Opisthorcis are flukes (q.v.) which attack the liver and obstruct the bile passages. Clonorchis is found where people eat raw fish, particularly in the Far East. Fasciola is the sheep-liver fluke, and can be acquired by eating infected vegetables.

Liver Pills: *see* Liver Diseases.

Loa Loa: a filarial worm of West Africa which infests the subcutaneous tissues, causes transient swellings (Calabar swellings) and itching, and is sometimes seen crossing the eyeball beneath the conjunctiva. The vector and intermediate host is the mango fly. *See* Filariasis, Worms.

Lobectomy: the operation of cutting out the lobe of a lung for such diseases as lung abscess, cysts, tumours or bronchiectasis. Removal of the whole lung is called pneumonectomy.

Lobelia: the dry flowering herb of Lobelia inflata, the Indian tobacco, which among its alkaloids contains lobeline. This has the same action as nicotine in increasing the ventilation of the lungs and dilating the bronchi. It is used in asthmatic powders for burning in cigarettes, and is incorporated in asthmatic cough mixtures. Injections of

477

lobeline are sometimes given to stimulate respiration in cases of poisoning or asphyxia from coal gas. Recently it has been introduced in tablet form and used by those who wish to stop smoking. *See* Smoking.

Lobotomy: the operation performed in leucotomy (q.v.) which consists of cutting the frontal fibres of the brain for mental disorders.

Lochia: the normal discharge from the womb lasting one or two weeks after childbirth.

Lockjaw: *see* Tetanus.

Locomotor Ataxia: (Tabes Dorsalis). A disorder of the central nervous system which follows old syphilitic infection; one of the manifestations of tertiary syphilis.

CAUSE: inflammation and then degeneration of nerve fibres in the posterior root ganglia and in the posterior columns of the spinal cord in which sensory fibres ascend to the brain. The main damage is probably in the posterior root ganglia, degeneration in the spinal cord being secondary.

SYMPTOMS: tabes dorsalis is a slow disease which usually attacks men past middle age. The patient often complains of lightning pains, which are sharp severe pains commonly felt in the leg, and he may say that he feels as if he is walking on cotton wool. He may also complain of difficulty in passing water, impotence, transitory attacks of double vision, and unsteadiness in the dark. As the disease progresses he becomes ataxic (unco-ordinated) and picks his feet up too far when walking, stamping them down on the ground again because he does not know where they are. There is a defect of the ability to sense where the limbs and body are in space which causes the tabetic to sway and fall if he tries to stand up with his eyes closed. There may also be profound disorder of the nerves supplying the abdominal organs, which produces tabetic crises in which the patient feels acute severe abdominal pain accompanied by vomiting and even rigidity of the abdominal wall, so that the state is easily confused with an 'acute abdomen' until the reflexes are examined. The knee and ankle jerks are lost, and the eye shows the Argyll Robertson pupil (q.v.). The knee joint is sometimes disorganized as the result of repeated un-noticed small injuries (Charcot's joint), and ulceration may develop on the soles of the feet. Blindness may follow atrophy of the optic disc.

TREATMENT: penicillin and bismuth injections, with careful follow-up and a repeat if necessary.

Loop: one of the shapes for an intra-uterine contraceptive device. *See* Contraception.

Lorain Infantilism: named after a Parisian physician of the last century, this condition results from underfunction of the anterior lobe of the pituitary gland. The child does not grow, nor do the secondary sexual characteristics appear; but the mentality may be normal. *See* Pituitary Gland.

Lordosis: forward curvature of the spine in the lumbar region; the natural curve is exaggerated.

Lotion: a liquid used for washing or for application to the skin. Lotions are watery, and cool the skin by evaporation, an action which is often increased by the addition of alcohol to the liquid. Astringent substances may be added to diminish exudate from skin lesions.

Louse: lice qualify for the description of permanent parasites on human beings, but although a couple of hundred species of lice have been described only two affect the human race. These two can only breed on man, and can live only an hour or two away from their natural surroundings, human skin and hair. It follows that infestation with lice can in the ordinary run of events only be acquired from contact with a lousy person. One type of louse, Phthirus pubis, the crab, lives in the pubic hair and is spread by venereal contact; the other type, Pediculus humanus, lives in the underclothes and in the hair of the head. Lice lay their eggs, which are called nits, on the hair or underclothes; they suck blood, and set up an irritation which in chronic cases results in thickening and pigmentation of the skin. Lice carry Rickett-siae, the organisms that cause typhus; Rickettsia prowazeki, the specific organism of epidemic typhus, is carried particularly by the crab louse, Phthirus pubis, and typhus, as one

479

would expect, is a disease of colder climates and places where people are crowded together and cannot wash properly or change their clothes. Above all it is a disease of wars and of refugee camps.

The diagnosis of infestation with lice is made by seeing the lice on the skin, hair or underclothes. They are about 1 to 4 mm long; the nits, which are very small, grey-white and oval, can be seen attached to the hair or clothes. Head lice are a little smaller than body lice and of a lighter colour, and Phthirus pubis is the smallest and is dark. Marks of scratching can usually be seen where lice have been, and the scratch marks become infected and scabbed.

TREATMENT: this is by dusting with D.D.T. or using a D.D.T. emulsion. Gamma benzene hexachloride (Quell) is also effective; but it must be remembered that the lice do not die at once, but may survive for a few days and have to be attacked again. The hair in cases of infestation is best cut short.

L.S.D.: (Lysergic Acid Diethylamide). A drug derived from ergot which has an effect on the brain in minute doses – 1 µg/kg is enough to produce symptoms, which start with a period of vague apprehension and disturbance of the autonomic nervous system (showing itself perhaps as feelings of heat or cold) followed by visual hallucinations and feelings of anxiety, persecution, depression and hostility with considerable confusion. The symptoms of intoxication come on about 30 minutes after the drug has been taken and last for a few hours, but the effect of the drug does not wear off completely for a day. The antidote is chlorpromazine (Largactil or Thorazine) or another phenothiazine tranquillizer, but it may not always be possible to control the effects of L.S.D. easily; it has been known for people under the influence of the drug to become criminally violent. Although an unbiased observer is in no doubt that the effects of L.S.D. are quite disagreeable in many cases, and not an unmixed pleasure in others, the attraction of the drug as a means of titillation of the senses has proved irresistible to some and it has been accepted as part of the modern drug-taker's armamentarium. Although L.S.D. is not a drug of addiction, it is not recommended, for it sometimes provokes long-term damage to the mentality with the formation of a

480

persistent psychosis, particularly when the drug-taker has been a little abnormal to start with.

Lucid Interval: the interval of consciousness which may follow a period of unconsciousness and precede a lapse into coma in cases where a head injury has started an artery (the middle meningeal or one of its branches) bleeding outside the dura mater. *See* Extradural Haemorrhage, Head Injury.

Lues: syphilis.

Lugol's Iodine: *see* Iodine.

Lumbago: a term used to describe a pain in the lower part of the back of considerable severity for which no obvious cause can be found. It is not a diagnosis but a description of a symptom. The treatment is aspirin, rest and heat.

Lumbar Puncture: the introduction of a hollow needle into the spinal canal in order to withdraw a specimen of cerebro-spinal fluid for laboratory examination or to introduce drugs, radio-opaque substances for X-ray examination, spinal anaesthetics, etc. The puncture is made in the lumbar region between the third and fourth or fourth and fifth vertebral bodies, where the point of the needle cannot harm the spinal cord because it ends at the level of the second lumbar vertebra; it is usually carried out under local anaesthetic.

Luminal: proprietary name for phenobarbitone.

Lunar Caustic: silver nitrate.

Lunatic: one who is moonstruck or mentally deranged. *See* Mental Illness.

Lung: the lungs are the organs in which an exchange of gases and vapours takes place between blood and air (or whatever gas is being breathed in). The complete respiratory system consists of lungs, air passages, the muscles which control breathing, and the pleural cavities.
Gross anatomy of the lungs. The right and left lungs are divided

481

into lobes – the right lung has three, upper, lower and middle, and the left lung two – and each lung has an apex which reaches up to the level of the collar bone, and a base which rests on the diaphragm, which is roughly at the level of the tenth rib, although it reaches the level of the twelfth rib behind and is as high as the eighth rib in front. The bronchi and the blood vessels enter the lungs at the root or hilum on the inner surface. The lungs are fibrous and elastic, and are covered by the pleural membrane. They are separated by the structures of the mediastinum – the heart and great vessels, the oesophagus and, in the upper part, the trachea. Although it is not apparent from superficial inspection, each lobe of the lungs is separated by fibrous tissue sheets into two to six segments, each of which has its own segmental bronchus and blood supply.

Inspired air enters the mouth and nose, passes into the pharynx, and enters the trachea through the larynx. The trachea is a tube prevented from collapsing by rings of cartilage; it is about 25 cm long and at the lower end it branches into the left and right bronchi. The right bronchus divides into branches for the upper and lower lobes of the right lung, branches for the middle lobe coming from the lower main bronchus. The lobar bronchi in turn branch into smaller air passages and so division continues until the smallest air passages of all, the bronchioles, are only 0.2 mm in diameter. The left main bronchus divides in the same way into upper and lower lobar branches, and so eventually into bronchioles. Branches of the pulmonary artery and vein accompany the bronchi. When the bronchioles reach their terminal branches small air-sacs protrude from them, and these are the respiratory as opposed to the conducting parts of the lung. Into the air-sacs open many smaller air spaces called alveoli which have walls only one cell thick. On the other side of the alveolar wall runs a capillary vessel containing blood, and the distance between the blood and the air in the alveolar sac is extremely small, less than 1 μm. The total area of surface available for the exchange of respiratory gases is over 50 square metres. It is a matter of common knowledge that the main function of the lungs is to bring oxygen to the blood and to take the waste product of metabolism, carbon dioxide, away; the only confusing fact about the function and anatomy of the lungs is that the pulmonary artery brings blue, or venous, blood to the lungs and the pulmonary vein carries bright red oxygenated arterial blood back to the heart.

Respiratory movements. Because the inner surface of the chest wall and the outer surface of the lungs are covered by the pleural membranes, they can slide over each other. The lungs themselves have very little muscle in them, and that only to control the size of the bronchi and bronchioles; they cannot move themselves but respond to changes of pressure inside the chest because they are elastic. The movements of breathing are carried out by the muscles which move the wall of the chest and by the diaphragm. When the chest·wall is raised and the diaphragm held still or lowered by contraction of the diaphragmatic muscle, the capacity of the thorax is increased and air is drawn into the lungs. When the ribs are lowered and the dome of the diaphragm rises, air comes out of the lungs. The process depends on the chest being airtight and air only being able to enter through the mouth and nose (*see* Pneumothorax). The nervous control of breathing is automatic, so that we do not have to remember to breathe, but the automatic control can to a certain extent be overridden. There comes a time, however, when the breath can voluntarily be held no longer and automatic control comes into action again. This is because there is a rising concentration of carbon dioxide in the blood, and the respiratory centre in the brain is extremely sensitive to the presence of carbon dioxide.

Lung Diseases: most are dealt with under their own headings (*see* Bronchitis, Bronchiectasis, Emphysema, Pleurisy, Pneumonia, Tuberculosis, etc.), but some will be dealt with here.

Abscess. This is not common, but may follow pneumonia, the inhalation of a foreign body, a wound, or the breakdown of a malignant growth.

SYMPTOMS: cough, pain in the chest, purulent sputum, fever and general ill-health.

TREATMENT: antibiotics, postural drainage of the lungs and physiotherapy, and if necessary surgery.

Collapse of the lung. This is caused by obstruction of the air passages; in the case of obstruction of a large bronchus the collapse is massive, but if only a small bronchiole is blocked the area of collapse is confined to a tiny part of the lung tissue. Obstruction of the large air passages may be caused by tumours, or rarely by the inhalation of foreign bodies, and of the smaller air passages by inflammation. The process of collapse of lung tissue is fundamental to the development of many diseases of the lung.

The lung may be collapsed because it has never expanded, a condition called congenital pulmonary atelactasis.

SYMPTOMS: cough, shortness of breath and blueness, and pain in the chest.

TREATMENT: the treatment of acquired collapse of the lung is the treatment of its cause. Inflammations caused by micro-organisms will be treated by antibiotic drugs; tumours may in some cases be removed, and inhaled foreign matter, sticky sputum or blood clots can be removed through a bronchoscope.

• *Cancer of the lung.* This is one of the most important and common forms of cancer. It is a disease of men in their fifties and sixties. The incidence of the disease appears to be rising; it has been shown that cancer of the lung is more likely to develop in people who smoke cigarettes, and in people who live in towns. For every non-smoker who dies of cancer of the lung, five moderate smokers and fifteen heavy smokers die. A man who has smoked twenty cigarettes a day for twenty years is said to be forty times more likely to develop a cancer of the lung than a non-smoker.

SYMPTOMS: often the tumour is only discovered on routine X-ray of the chest, but in many cases the patient complains of a cough, a little pain in the chest, and a feeling of ill-health. He may cough up blood, and develop a low-grade fever. He becomes easily tired and loses weight. In some cases the symptoms of secondary malignant deposits bring the patient to the doctor; not infrequently the secondary tumour is in the brain, so that chest X-rays are carried out on all suspected cases of brain tumour. Other common sites for secondaries are in the bones.

TREATMENT: if possible, surgical removal. Unfortunately, the nature of the disease is to keep silent until it is too late.

Lupus: *Lupus vulgaris.* A tuberculous infection of the skin.
SYMPTOMS: a small nodule, the lupoma, develops in the skin.

It is only slightly raised from the surface and is described as looking like apple jelly; it is often found on the face, but it can occur on the rest of the body. It is commonest in young people, and more frequent in females than males. As the condition heals scarring may follow and lead to disfiguration of the face.

TREATMENT: isoniazid, para-aminosalicylic acid and streptomycin. When it is certain that the disease has been cured and is no longer active, plastic surgery may be able to reduce any deformity of the face. .

Lupus erythematosus. This is a disease which has general and cutaneous manifestations. It occurs most commonly in middle-aged women, and superficially looks like acne rosacea.

CUTANEOUS SYMPTOMS: red scaly patches of smooth skin develop on the exposed parts, often after exposure to a strong sun; the most commonly affected parts are the bridge of the nose, the cheeks, and the ears and backs of the hands. The reddened skin patches may run into each other, and the centres may heal up and scar while the edges of the lesions extend. The condition is chronic and disfiguring.

TREATMENT: treatment is not yet satisfactory. Anti-malarial drugs can be used, as can triamcinolone which is injected locally. Surface applications of betamethasone valerate (Betnovate) or fluocinolone acetonide (Synalar) may help. The skin must be kept shaded from strong sunlight and from the wind.

Systemic lupus erythematosus. This may or may not be associated with the cutaneous form of the disease. It is found in women more commonly than men between the ages of 30 and 50, and is more frequent in the U.S.A. than it is in Great Britain.

CAUSE: the patient's reaction of immunity is abnormal, and she forms antibodies which react with her own cell nuclei. Haemolytic anaemia, damage to the kidneys, the lungs, the heart and its valves, the spleen and the lymph glands are found; the disease processes are spread throughout the body.

SYMPTOMS: the symptoms are diffuse and vague; any organ of the body may be affected, and the disease can be present in the generalized form without there being any skin abnormalities to suggest the correct diagnosis.

TREATMENT: anti-malarial drugs, corticosteroids, and immuno-suppressant drugs are used in the treatment of the disease. The condition is very serious, and treatment may be difficult and the results disappointing.

Luxation: dislocation.

Lycanthropy: a condition in which a man changes into a wolf, the werewolf of legend. It is, of course, a delusion, but at one time in Central Europe it was widely believed to be possible.

Lye: a mixture of sodium hydroxide with sodium carbonate, once but no longer used freely in the household. It is extremely corrosive if drunk by mistake.

Lymph: the fluid found in the lymph vessels; it is clear, slightly yellow, contains lymph cells and, if it derives from the intestine, particles of fat. The name is also applied to any fluid which looks like lymph; the material from cowpox vesicles used to vaccinate against smallpox is called lymph, and so is the clear exudate from damaged tissues.

Lymphadenitis: inflammation of the lymph glands.

Lymphadenoma: another name for Hodgkin's disease (q.v.).

Lymphangitis: inflammation of the lymph vessels. It can sometimes be seen as thin red lines extending up the arm from infected wounds or other sources of inflammation on the fingers and hand.

Lymphatic Leukaemia: *see* Leukaemia.

Lymph Glands: *see* Glands.

Lymphocyte: *see* Leucocyte.

Lymphogranuloma: lymphogranuloma is another name for Hodgkin's disease. Lymphogranuloma venereum is a venereal disease caused by an organism resembling a virus, the main symptom of which is enlargement of the lymph glands in the groin.

Lymphosarcoma: a cancerous condition of the lymphatic elements in the body. It is not common, but occurs mainly in middle-aged men.

SYMPTOMS: painless swelling of the lymph glands, often in the neck. Enlarged groups of glands may press on neighbouring structures, for example in the chest, and so produce symptoms. There is anaemia with accompanying shortness of breath and fatigue, and there may be enlargement of the spleen and liver.

TREATMENT: this is by radiotherapy and cytotoxic drugs.

Lysol: a soapy solution of cresol once almost as popular in suicide attempts as it was as a general household disinfectant. It is now used far less in the home, and attempts at suicide with lysol have decreased. It is a very unpleasant poison, for it is caustic and burns wherever it touches.

TREATMENT: for lysol poisoning give egg white followed by large amounts of salt and water as an emetic, and then milk and olive oil. Wash out the stomach as soon as possible.

Lysozyme: an antibacterial enzyme found in tears and saliva.

M

McBurney's Point: named after a nineteenth-century New York surgeon, it is the point at which maximum tenderness is felt in the abdomen in cases of appendicitis. It lies on a line drawn from the umbilicus to the right anterior superior iliac spine – the bony point felt at the outer end of the fold in the groin – one-third of the way between the iliac spine and the umbilicus. It is quite possible to have appendicitis without having a great deal of tenderness at McBurney's point, but it is not common.

Maceration: the softening of a solid by fluid. In medicine, the softening and damaging of tissues by water as in a corpse some hours drowned.

Macula: a stain or spot, used in anatomy to mean a localized area distinguishable from its surroundings.

Macule: a macule is a flat discolored area of skin, as distinct from a papule, which is a raised spot. Rashes are often maculo-papular – they have raised areas of discoloration surrounded by flat areas.

Madura Foot: a tropical disease in which the foot swells and its tissues and bones become riddled with sinuses caused by a fungus; the disease is most commonly found in India.

Magnesium: used in medicine in the form of its salts; magnesium carbonate, hydroxide and trisilicate are used as antacid compounds in cases of peptic ulceration and gastritis.
'Milk of magnesia' has a slight aperient action; it is a suspension of about 8% magnesium hydroxide. Other laxative preparations are magnesium hydroxide and liquid paraffin emulsion, and magnesium sulphate – Epsom salts. A very small quantity of magnesium is essential in the diet, but it is present in many kinds of food. Magnesium deficiency may occur in chronic diarrhoea, and it leads to depression and fatigue.

Mal, Grand and Petit: *see* Epilepsy.

Malaise: a general feeling of being ill. It often goes before an acute fever.

Malaria: an infection with the parasite of malaria, the plasmodium. Four species of the genus infect man, and they are all carried by mosquitoes of the genus Anopheles. They flourish in tropical and subtropical countries.

The life-cycle of the malarial parasite. The mosquito bites a man and introduces into his blood sporozoites, small fusiform cells with one nucleus. They have to find the liver within one hour or they die; but if they do find their way to the liver they can there grow and reproduce. After a week, the parasites leave the liver as merozoites, which pass into the blood and invade the red blood corpuscles, where they start cycles of growth and reproduction. When the merozoite enters the red blood corpuscle, it takes the form of a ring and within a few hours fills the cell completely. Fission of the parasite takes place, and each one gives origin to 16 daughter cells. While the merozoite is growing it is called a trophozoite, and when fission starts it is called a schizont. The 16 new merozoites are liberated into the blood out of the red cells in which they developed, and the asexual reproduction cycle starts again as they penetrate new red blood corpuscles. The attacks of periodic fever characteristic of malaria coincide with the liberation of the daughter merozoites into the blood-stream. While the asexual merozoites start their reproductive cycle in the blood cells, sexual forms of the parasite called microgametocytes (males) and macrogametocytes (females) begin to appear in the blood. These can only survive and reproduce in a mosquito, and if one comes along and bites the infected man they pass into the stomach of the mosquito where macrogametocytes and microgametocytes join to produce a zygote, which pushes its way out of the stomach. On the outside of the stomach there is formed an oocyst within which many sporozoites develop. When fully grown the sporozoites travel through the mosquito into its salivary glands whence they hope to pass into another man when the mosquito bites him.

SYMPTOMS: there are four sorts of malaria, caused by the four species of plasmodium: Plasmodium falciparum, P.

vivax, P. malariae and P. ovale. All forms cause headache and shivering, sweating and pains in the limbs.

P. falciparum. Merozoites are liberated into the bloodstream 6 days after the sporozoites have entered the liver. All the parasites leave the liver at this time. The fever produced by the liberation of merozoites from red blood cells is not regular in falciparum malaria because the maturation of the parasites is not well synchronized. Falciparum malaria is called malignant malaria because clumps of P. falciparum may block capillaries in the vital organs – brain and spinal nervous system, lungs and suprarenals – at any time during the course of the disease, which may therefore prove quickly fatal.

P. vivax and P. ovale. Merozoites reach the blood 8 days after infection, and then are liberated from the red cells every 48 hours. The plasmodia do not all leave the liver, and cycles of asexual reproduction continue to take place there outside the red blood corpuscles. The fever is called tertian.

P. malariae. The merozoites reach the bloodstream some time after 8 days, and then the cycle takes 72 hours. Parasites remain in the liver and reproduce there as well as in the blood corpuscles. The fever is called quartan.

TREATMENT: *quinine*, which has been known as a specific drug for malaria since the seventeenth century, acts against the parasites while they are inside red blood cells, but it is not often used now because it affects the ears and may cause blackwater fever (q.v.). In acute emergency it can be given intravenously, especially in children.

Chloroquine, Amodiaquine (Nivaquine, Camoquine). Both these drugs are extremely effective. Chloroquine can be given intravenously, except in children. Some strains of P. falciparum are resistant. Dosage for non-immune adults is 6 tablets of 150 mg chloroquine on the first day followed by 2 tablets a day for 2 days. For partially immune adults, those who have spent their lives in malarious districts, 4 tablets are taken as a single dose. Amodiaquine is given as tablets of 200 mg, 3 the first day, then 2 a day for 2 days; or one dose of 3 tablets.

SUPPRESSION OF MALARIA: proguanil (Paludrine) and pyrimethamine (Daraprim) are compounds which destroy parasites while they are reproducing asexually in the red blood cells. In the case of malignant malaria they act upon the parasites before they reach the red blood cells. They also interfere with the reproduction of the parasite in the mosquito, so that if the mosquito bites a man who is taking the drugs and sucks his blood its infectivity is abolished. The prophylactic dose of proguanil is one or two tablets of 100 mg a day, and that of pyrimethamine, one 25 mg tablet a week. On the whole many people find it easier to remember to take a tablet a day than a tablet a week. The drugs should continue to be taken for a clear month after leaving a malarial country to be sure of avoiding an attack of malignant malaria.

Primaquine. This drug may have to be used to cure relapsing P. vivax and P. malariae infections caused by parasites surviving in the liver which escape the action of proguanil and pyrimethamine. The dose is 2 tablets of 15 mg a day for 2 weeks. The drug is to be taken under medical supervision because it may cause destruction of red blood cells. Relapses of benign tertian and quartan malaria may occur many months, even years, after the first infection.

PREVENTION OF MALARIA: because the disease is carried by the anopheles mosquito, all breeding-places for the mosquito have to be eradicated, which means draining all swamps and marshes and treating standing water. Houses must be kept free of mosquitoes, and such mosquitoes as there are must be killed. There are some places in the world where the task is nearly impossible, as in the delta of the river Niger, but there are many places where the efforts of the World Health Organization to stamp out malaria are proving successful.

Malathion: an insecticide, one of the organophosphorus compounds. It inhibits cholinesterase enzymes and so causes stimulation of the parasympathetic system. Symptoms of poisoning are headache, giddiness, nausea, disturbance of vision, muscular weakness and a slow pulse. The antidote is atropine sulphate given by intramuscular injection.

Male Fern: *see* Fern Root.

Malignant: of a tumour means cancerous, but it is also used of particularly severe forms of fever, for example malignant malaria, malignant smallpox.

491

Malingering: this is the feigning of illness of which there are many different degrees, ranging from pretence to a non-existent disease purely for reasons of financial gain as is common in the East on the part of beggars, and may occasionally be found in the civil courts of the West, to the kind of malingering which is virtually a sign of mental disorder, where patients will go from one hospital to another seeking operations for pretended illnesses the symptoms of which have been carefully studied beforehand. In between are those who malinger in order to obtain not money, but love and attention; this type of malingering may be entirely conscious or quite unconscious. Hysteria in one sense is a form of unconscious malingering.

Malleolus: the bony projections on each side of the ankle, formed by the lower end of the tibia on the inside and the fibula on the outside.

Mallet Finger: if the extensor tendon which normally straightens the tip of the finger is torn away from the base of the bone at the last finger-joint, the tip is left permanently half-flexed and is called mallet finger. It is treated by early plastering in an extended position, by fixation in the best position for the patient, or by open operation and repair of the tendon. Some people are not worried by the small disability and prefer to carry on without treatment.

Malleus: a small bone in the middle ear. *See* Ear.

Malnutrition: a term properly applied to diseases due to insufficient intake of particular substances essential for health, for example vitamins, proteins. It indicates deficiency in the quality of the diet rather than the quantity, but is often used to mean any deficiency in the diet of whatever kind.

Malta Fever: (Brucellosis). An infection with Brucella melitensis, a micro-organism that causes a fever in goats and is passed on to man in the goat's milk. Sheep may also become infected from the goats. *See* Undulant Fever.

Mamma: the breast; hence mammals, creatures that suckle their young.

Mandelic Acid: a drug used in the treatment of infection of the urinary tract.

Mandible: the lower jaw-bone.

Mandl's Paint: named after a nineteenth-century Hungarian physician who practised in France, an iodine solution for application to the throat.

Mandragora: Mandragora officinalis, the oriental mandrake, has properties which are like belladonna. It was therefore once used as a soporific:

> *Not poppy, nor mandragora,*
> *Nor all the drowsy syrups of the world,*
> *Shall ever medicine thee to that sweet sleep*
> *Which thou ow'dst yesterday.*

> OTHELLO, III, iii, 331.

Mandrake: not to be confused with mandragora, the mandrake was a forked root with magical properties. It shrieked when pulled out of the ground in such a way as to send men mad, so that it had to be rooted up by dogs. It was thought to be an aphrodisiac and a promoter of fertility in women; Donne the poet apparently believed that it could also be used in the contrary sense: 'His apples kindle, his leaves, force of conception kill.' ('The Progress of the Soul'). *See also* Genesis 30: 14–18.

Manganese: an element essential for life; no cases, however, are known of manganese deficiency in man, for only minute traces are necessary in the diet. It is used in medicine in the form of potassium permanganate as an antiseptic; if manganese fumes or dust are breathed in to excess, patients develop a condition very like Parkinson's disease.

M.A.O.: (Monoamine oxidase). An enzyme that acts upon amines and adrenaline to oxidize them; it is found largely in the kidneys, liver, intestines and brain, although it is present all over the body. Certain drugs used to treat depression – they include phenelzine (Nardil), nialamide (Niamid), isocarboxazid (Marplan), tranylcypromine (Parnate), and pargyline (Eutonyl) – stop the action of monoamine oxidase. They are called the monoamine oxidase inhibitors, and can be, in certain circumstances, dangerous and even fatal. Patients taking M.A.O. inhibitors must not take any drugs that imitate the action of adrenaline such as amphetamine or phenylephrine, a drug found in many proprietary cold cures; they must not take various articles of food, among which are cheese, yeast, beer, wine, broad beans and high-protein foods or concentrates; and they must be very careful in taking any other drugs, particularly morphine and pethidine (demerol).

Marasmus: progressive wasting, particularly in young children.

Marihuana: *see* Cannabis Indica.

Marrow: the marrow of the bones is red or yellow; red marrow is found in the skull, ribs, pelvis, breastbone, the bodies of the vertebrae and the ends of the long bones, and is actively engaged in making the cells of the blood. Yellow marrow is full of fat cells. It is in early life red, but by the end of the period of growth some of the bone marrow becomes inactive and yellow. In times of crisis it is still capable of making blood cells, in which case it turns red again.

Masochism: a sexual perversion in which satisfaction is gained from being cruelly treated. It takes its name from the nineteenth-century Austrian novelist, Sacher-Masoch.

Massage: is a manipulative treatment applied to the soft tissues in certain diseases mainly of the rheumatic type when the normal movements of the body which stimulate metabolism and the flow of lymph are difficult or impossible. The masseur or masseuse aids passive movements of the muscles, limbs and joints, and by such movements as stroking, pinching, pressing and kneading stimulates the tissues. Such movements are undoubtedly useful when limbs are paralysed or immobilized by fractures, having the effect of exercises; they are refreshing and have a considerable psychological effect, but, although they often hasten cure, they are not themselves a cure. The various movements are described as *effleurage* or stroking towards the heart, *stroking*, which is the same movement away from the heart, *pétrissage* or kneading, *frictions* or circular movements, and *tapotement* or percussion which is beating or whacking the tissue with the edge of the hand. The efficacy of a treatment is often to be measured by the vagueness or otherwise of the conditions it is supposed to benefit, and one which is concerned with 'rheumatism', 'nervous affections' (meaning neuroses), 'insomnia', etc., is likely to produce a good deal of its results psychologically rather than physically. There is a certain amount of hocus-pocus about massage, although nobody can doubt its value in the instances mentioned. Certified masseurs have to undergo a period of training.

Mast Cells: cells found in connective tissue. The name comes from the German *masten*, to feed, because they were once thought to feed on other cells. It is now thought that the granules which can be seen in mast cells are not the remains of other cells, but granules of carbohydrate which they themselves have manufactured. They also make histamine (q.v.) and a substance which prevents the clotting of the blood, heparin.

Mastectomy: removal of the breast. Simple mastectomy means the removal of the breast alone, but radical mastectomy, an operation carried out for cancer, means the removal of the breast together with the muscles upon which it lies and the lymph glands of the armpit. The purpose of such an extensive operation is to prevent if possible the spread of the disease, for the lymphatic vessels from the breast drain into the glands of the armpit and into the muscles of the chest wall. They also drain into glands lying inside the ribs – the internal mammary glands, which are also sometimes removed in the radical operation. The scope of any surgical operation is decided by the surgeon in the light of the special circumstances of each case, so that it is not possible to say that a radical operation should always be done in cases of malignancy; some cases do better with a simple removal of the breast combined with radiotherapy.

Mastic: a resin which comes from the tree Pistacia lentis. It is used as a skin dressing, and is also used in microscopy.

Mastitis (Acute): inflammation of the breast. It may

progress to form an abscess, and it is most commonly found in the period just after the birth of a baby in association with cracked or depressed nipples.

Treatment is by antibiotics, usually tetracycline; the breast is emptied manually, breast feeding is stopped and lactation arrested by administration of stilboestrol. The breast of a newborn baby may become inflamed, possibly because of hormones absorbed from the mother, but in most cases no treatment is needed and the condition clears up by itself. Somewhat similar cases occur in adolescent children which clear up spontaneously in a few weeks. Chronic inflammation is sometimes found after an acute infection has failed to heal completely, and rarely it turns out to be tubercular. For Chronic Mastitis *see* Breast Diseases.

Mastoiditis: infection of the mastoid cells of the temporal bone behind the ear. It usually follows middle ear infection, and has become increasingly rare since antibiotics came into use. At one time it was not uncommon, and was treated by immediate surgery to drain the mastoid cells; the operation was unpleasant and resulted in scarring behind the ear. Such operations today are rare, and are only carried out as a last resort in cases that do not respond to antibiotics. The necessarily crude technique that once was used to prevent meningitis and brain abscess by removing large amounts of bone so that pus would drain freely has given way to surgery carried out at leisure under the operating microscope.

Masturbation: self-stimulation of the sexual organs is almost universal and is in fact a normal stage in sexual development. It is found in nearly all boys and most girls (although the sexual impulse in women tends to be less conscious than in men until awakened). Masturbation produces no harmful effects physically and the only harm that can follow mentally is when a feeling of guilt is attached to the act. It is abnormal (*a*) if carried out to excess, when it indicates severe anxiety rather than excessive sexuality, and (*b*) if carried out in preference to normal sexual relations, when it indicates something seriously amiss with the individual's personal relationships. *See* Sex.

Maxilla: the cheek-bone, which also forms the upper jaw.

It takes part in the formation of the orbit or eye-socket, the nose and the hard palate. It contains the maxillary antrum, which drains into the nose and becomes inflamed in sinusitis. It is sometimes broken and depressed by direct violence, and has to be replaced in its normal position by an operation.

Measles: an infectious disease which appears in epidemics, often in the winter time.

CAUSE: infection with the measles virus, which is so infectious that in towns most children have the diease before they are five. A mother usually passes her antibodies to her child, passively immunizing it, but this protection does not last beyond the sixth month. The incubation period of the disease is 2 weeks.

SYMPTOMS: the virus produces a state which at first looks very like the common cold. The eyes are red, there is a cough, the nose runs, the patient sneezes, and exposure to strong light is uncomfortable. There is a headache and the temperature rises. Koplik's spots then develop inside the mouth – small, white, ulcerating papules surrounded by reddening of the mucous membrane. They appear three or four days before the red skin rash, which starts as macules behind the ears, on the neck, and on the forehead. It spreads quickly over the face, the limbs and trunk, and as it spreads it becomes maculo-papular; the red colour grows deeper. The formerly separate macules coalesce, and when the rash is at its height, about two days after it has started, the discoloured patches of skin are quite large. The rash then starts to fade, but may leave a brownish stain lasting for about a week. The lymph glands are generally enlarged. The danger of measles arises from the complications; because the mucous membranes of the upper respiratory passages are affected, the child is likely to develop secondary bacterial infection which leads to bronchitis and even broncho-pneumonia. The middle ear may become infected with bacteria, the appendix may become acutely inflamed, and the cornea of the eye may ulcerate. Encephalitis is a serious complication which occurs in a number of cases.

TREATMENT: the viral stage of the illness has no specific treatment, but the child feels ill and clearly must be put to bed. Infection is most likely to spread during the first two days of the disease – that is, while the condition still looks like

497

a severe cold – so that isolation once the rash has made the diagnosis clear is not much use. Antibiotics are used freely to combat bacterial infection and the resulting complications. Active immunization against measles is now possible, and it is given to children in their second year. They may develop a high temperature between five and ten days after the injection, and some have a minor rash. Passive immunization is conferred by doses of gamma globulin. One attack of measles confers immunity for life.

Meatus: any opening to a bodily passage, for example external auditory meatus, which leads to the ear.

Meckel's Diverticulum: a hollow blind appendage occasionally found growing from the small intestine about 50 cm from the ileo-caecal junction. It varies in size, the average length being about 5 cm. It is the remains of a structure in the embryo called the vitello-intestinal duct which joined the intestine to the umbilicus, and it may still be joined to the umbilicus by a fibrous cord, or very rarely may open at the umbilicus. It sometimes becomes inflamed and mimics the symptoms of appendicitis (the diverticulum is found at operation), and sometimes the intestine becomes twisted round the cord joining it to the umbilicus so that the gut is obstructed.

Meconium: the dark green semi-fluid material consisting of bile and debris discharged from the infant's bowels at birth or immediately afterwards.

Median Nerve: the median nerve is one of the nerves of the arm. It comes from the brachial plexus of nerves in the root of the neck, runs down the upper arm, in front of the elbow, down the forearm and ends in the palm of the hand. It has no branches in the upper arm, but in the forearm it supplies most of the muscles which flex the fingers and wrist, and in the hand the skin over the front of the thumb, index, obscene and half the ring finger, the palm, and the backs of the tips of the thumb and the first four fingers.

Mediastinum: the space in the chest between the two lungs. It contains the heart and great vessels, the oesophagus, the lower end of the trachea or windpipe, the thoracic duct, various nerves, the thymus gland and lymph glands.

Medinal: barbitone sodium tablets – not now often prescribed.

Mediterranean Fever: *see* Malta Fever, Undulant Fever.

Medulla: the inner part of a structure or organ. Also used to mean the marrow of a bone, the spinal cord, and that part of the brain which is continuous with the spinal cord – the medulla oblongata.

Megacolon: *see* Hirschsprung's Disease.

Megalomania: delusions of grandeur.

Megrim: another term for headache, migraine.

Meibomian Cyst: a cyst or swelling on the inside of the eyelid caused by blockage of the duct from one of the Meibomian glands which normally open at the edge of the eyelid. Treated by a simple incision made under local anaesthetic. Named after Meibom, a German anatomist, 1638–1700.

Meiosis: a type of cell division in which each daughter cell ends up with half the number of chromosomes in the original cell. This type of division occurs in the formation of the sex cells, so that while the cells of the human body each have 46 chromosomes, spermatozoa and ova have 23. If this were not so, the new individual formed by the fusion of spermatozoon and ovum would have double the number of normal chromosomes. *See* Mitosis.

Melaena: black motions caused by blood in the intestines or stomach, iron taken as medicine, bismuth, or some red wines.

Melancholia: *see* Mental Illness.

Melanin: the dark pigment of the skin, the choroid layer of the eye, and the hair. It is found in various tumours which are then referred to as melanotic; they are often malignant.

Melanuria: dark-coloured urine, or urine which turns dark if left standing, found in cases of jaundice, certain melanotic tumours, bleeding into the urinary tract, and the rather rare conditions of alcaptonuria and porphyria. *See* Porphyria.

Memory: defects of memory commonly result from (1) faulty perception during preoccupation with other matters – found often in neurosis; (2) structural damage to the brain as in senility, cerebral arteriosclerosis or poisoning from bacterial or other toxins, for example syphilis, carbon monoxide, alcohol (*see* Korsakow's Psychosis); (3) hysteria. There is nothing wrong with the memory of a neurotic person, but he possesses to an abnormal degree the common ability to forget what it does not suit him to remember, and of becoming panic-stricken at his 'poor memory' when his obsession with himself has prevented him from making proper contact with his environment; his retention of power of recall in the latter case is not at fault – his ability to take in impressions is. The vast majority of cases of 'poor memory' in younger people are of this type, which has nothing to do with memory and is in fact lack of attention. The type of memory defect common in organic conditions is described under Korsakow's Psychosis and ordinarily consists of clear recollection of the distant past combined with very poor memory for recent events.

So-called loss of memory is a form of hysterical dissociation, unconsciously produced, which nevertheless enables the individual to forget what he basically chooses to forget, for example when we read of the famous case of dual personality of the Reverend Ansell Bourne quoted by William James – how a respectable clergyman disappeared from a town in Rhode Island, only to turn up two months later as the owner of a small sweet shop in Pennsylvania with the name of A. J. Brown who 'came to' in a state of terror asking who and where he was – we do not for an instant doubt that the reverend gentleman was genuine in his lapse, but we do wonder what Mrs Bourne was like and whether the financial affairs of his church were quite in order. Patchy defects of memory may result from disease and occur after electroconvulsant treatment (q.v.) in a few cases; it is usually transient. Brain cells once destroyed cannot be replaced, but some kinds of organic memory defect are benefited or prevented from getting worse by the use of concentrated Vitamin B₁. *See* Retrograde Amnesia.

Menarche: the first appearance of the menstrual periods.

Mendelism: *see* Heredity.

Menière's Syndrome: an affliction of the balancing organ of the ear which causes giddiness.

CAUSE: the endolymphatic system of the inner ear is distended. It is not the result of other ear disease, nor of injury, unlike positional vertigo which makes the patient giddy when his head is in one particular position and follows head injuries and disease of the middle ear.

SYMPTOMS: the patient suffers from attacks of giddiness which are not associated with movement of the head. The disease may affect both ears, and the patient may in time go deaf and hear noises in his ears (tinnitus). Giddiness may become severe and make the patient vomit and collapse, but the natural course of the disease is that the attacks of giddiness become less as the deafness becomes worse; in the end the deaf patient suffers from no further attacks.

TREATMENT: various drugs have been recommended; prochlorperazine (Stemetil or Compazine) is one of the most useful. If the disease is very bad, it may be necessary to ask for a surgeon's opinion, for there are operations which can be performed on the labyrinth of the inner ear to relieve the symptoms although the hearing may suffer. Some surgeons recommend section of the sympathetic nervous system in the neck.

Meninges: the membranes surrounding the brain and the spinal cord. The outer membrane, the dura mater, is a firm fibrous sheet stuck to the inner periosteal membrane of the skull which splits to enclose various large blood spaces into which flow the cerebral veins. These blood spaces are called the intracranial venous sinuses, and they cannot either collapse or dilate. The dura also forms three large folds which project into the intracranial cavity: they are called the falx cerebri, the tentorium cerebelli and the falx cerebelli. The falx cerebri separates the two cerebral hemispheres, and the tentorium is a shelf which separates the inside of the skull into two compartments – the upper or supratentorial space containing the cerebral hemispheres, and the lower or infratentorial space containing the brain stem and cerebellum. The two spaces are connected by the tentorial notch which is occupied by the mid-brain. The falx cerebelli is a small fold beneath the tentorium. The biggest venous sinuses, the transverse, run in the edge of the tentorium where it is attached to the skull, and the other large sinus, the superior sagittal sinus, runs in the attached edge of the falx cerebri. The whole arrangement of the dural folds looks very much like the folds inside a walnut shell. Arteries, notably the middle meningeal, run in the substance of the dura. The membrane is not attached to the vertebrae as firmly as it is to the skull, and movements of the vertebral column can take place independently of the dura covering the spinal cord.

The arachnoid mater lies beneath the dura, and is separated from it by a space containing in health only a little tissue fluid. Beneath the arachnoid lies the pia mater, a soft membrane intimately adherent to the surface of the brain. Between the arachnoid and the pia run many fibres – from which the arachnoid is named, for the fibres look like a spider's web – and between the two membranes is a space occupied by the cerebro-spinal fluid and the arteries and veins running to the brain. Arachnoid granulations or valves extend into the venous sinuses through which the cerebro-spinal fluid is returned to the venous bloodstream. *See* Extradural and Subarachnoid Hemorrhage, Subdural Hematoma.

Meningioma: a fibrous tumour arising from the meninges; it is not malignant unless it is left to penetrate the skull, when the portion that breaks through may give rise to secondary tumours, but when it arises about the base of the brain it may be very difficult and dangerous to remove. It grows in relation to the venous sinuses of the skull, and produces symptoms according to its position both by direct pressure on the brain and by competing with the brain for the limited room inside the skull and thus producing the symptoms of increased intracranial pressure such as severe headache, deterioration of vision, and in extreme cases vomiting and disturbance of consciousness. The treatment is surgical removal, and the operation for the removal of a meningioma on the upper surface of the brain is one of the most satisfactory in neurosurgery.

Meningitis: inflammation of the meninges. It is possible for the dura mater to become inflamed as a result of injury to the skull or disease of the middle ear, but the term meningitis usually refers to leptomeningitis, inflammation of the soft membranes of the brain – the pia and arachnoid.

CAUSE: infection with micro-organisms. The commonest infection is meningococcal, which produces cerebro-spinal or spotted fever, but infection can also take place with streptococci, staphylococci, pneumococci and Haemophilus influenzae (acute suppurative meningitis). The organisms infect the subarachnoid space and usually spread from the base of the brain up over the surface and down the spinal cord. Infection appears to reach the inside of the skull from the throat and nose via the bloodstream.

SYMPTOMS: 1. *Meningococcal meningitis.* Most people who become infected with the meningococcus confine it to their throat, but if they are subject to damp and cold and over-crowding the organism is liable to pass into the bloodstream. The incubation period is short, being between one and five days, and the onset sudden. There is a high fever, and young children may go into convulsions, while adults may become delirious. There may be a skin rash. The patient starts to vomit, complains of severe headaches which make him cry out with pain, avoids the light and often insists on lying on his side, turned away from the light with his legs and spine extended. The neck cannot be flexed, and attempts to draw the chin down on the chest may make the spine extend even more. If the thigh is drawn up against the abdominal wall, and then an attempt made to straighten the leg, it will produce great pain (Kernig's sign), and the flexion of the thigh upon the abdominal wall will itself produce spontaneous flexion on the other side (Brudzinski's sign). If the patient goes into a coma the outlook is bad. Restlessness may be very obvious, but in some cases is due to retention of urine, and if this is relieved the patient will become quieter. The diagnosis is made certain by a lumbar puncture and examination of the cerebro-spinal fluid.

2. *Acute suppurative meningitis.* The symptoms of infection are

very much the same as those described above, and the diagnosis of the type of meningitis present usually rests upon finding the responsible organism in the cerebro-spinal fluid. TREATMENT: once the responsible organism has been identified, it can be tested for sensitivity to antibiotics and sulphonamides, but in all cases speed in treatment is vital and a valuable routine is to inject penicillin into the cerebrospinal fluid if the fluid withdrawn at lumbar puncture is turbid, to give intramuscular injections of penicillin, and to give a sulphonamide (sulphadimidine) by mouth. When the results come back from the laboratory the appropriate special drugs are given, for example ampicillin or chloramphenicol for H. influenzae infections, cephaloridine for pneumococcal meningitis. Response to energetic therapy is quick, and in a matter of days the patient should be on the way to recovery. It cannot be too strongly emphasized that the key to successful recovery is speed, and that it is delay in treatment that makes complications likely. If you think it is remotely possible that your child might have meningitis, lose no time in calling the doctor. *See also* Tuberculosis.

Meniscus: a semicircular or crescentic cartilage in a joint, used especially of the semilunar cartilages of the knee. Removal of such a cartilage is called meniscectomy.

Menopause: many women are troubled at the prospect of the change of life or menopause which may begin at any time from the late thirties to the late forties or early fifties, although it ordinarily occurs about the age of forty-five. At this time the menstrual periods cease, sometimes abruptly, but more frequently gradually with increasing intervals between. There is no necessary reason why any symptoms should arise, but women often resign themselves to a longer or shorter period of 'hot flushes', excessive bleeding, depression and general ill health, and there is no doubt that the expectation of these symptoms sometimes plays a part in bringing them on. It is advisable that a doctor should be seen if such symptoms appear, for they are usually capable of being treated, and if anything more serious is present this is the best time to deal with it. In particular bleeding after the periods have ceased should be reported immediately at whatever age it may happen. Most menopausal symptoms respond satisfactorily to sex hormones, although sometimes sedatives or tranquillizers may be necessary. It is worth while pointing out that although the period of fertility may have come to an end, sexual activity and desire are unaffected or may even be increased; the woman who has passed the menopause does not cease to be a woman even if she is no longer capable of being a mother. Normally the post-menopausal age should be one of comparative peace of mind in which depression is not natural, so its appearance to any disturbing degree should be mentioned to the doctor. Putting up with such symptoms is not being stoical, but simply giving in to foolish and unnecessary suffering and if other worries be present, however absurd, the woman will be wise if she unburdens herself of them to her medical adviser. The folklore of the change is extensive and for the most part so ill advised that exploding old wives' tales is both helpful and therapeutic to those burdened by them.

Menorrhagia: excessive blood loss at the monthly period. It may rarely be due to general conditions such as high blood pressure, but is more commonly due to local disorders, for example fibroids. It may be severe enough to cause anaemia; treatment depends on diagnosis.

Menstruation: this is a normal function of the female in man and the higher apes, and it consists of the monthly loss of blood through the vagina when pregnancy has not taken place. The lining of the womb (endometrium) is a soft velvety covering in which the fertilized ovum embeds itself, and this is grown monthly in the expectation of pregnancy only to be discharged with a varying amount of blood if pregnancy does not occur. The cycle is divided into four: the stage of quiescence, the constructive stage, the destructive stage, and the stage of repair. During the constructive stage the endometrium becomes greatly thickened, partly by increase in the number of cells, partly by engorgement of the glands and blood vessels. This is followed by a destructive stage during which the endometrium breaks down, blood leaks into the cavity of the womb, and soon the discharge of endometrial tissue and blood appears outside as the period. As soon as the menstrual flow has ceased, the repair of the endometrium begins; the remains of the blood are absorbed and the broken-down tissues replaced. Of the usual 28 days of the cycle about 5 are taken up by premenstrual congestion, 4 by the menstrual flow, 7 by the period of repair and 12 are spent in a state of quiescence, the whole being controlled by the hormones of the ovary and the pituitary gland at the base of the brain. During the first part of the cycle the ripening ovarian follicle containing the ovum secretes the hormone oestrogen; after ovulation the corpus luteum forms and both oestrogen and progesterone are secreted. When secretion of these hormones stops, as it does if pregnancy has not occurred, the endometrium breaks down. Ovulation occurs at some time about the mid-period, usually in a 28-day cycle on the fourteenth day before the beginning of the next period. Since fertilization can occur while the ovum is passing down the Fallopian tubes, there are about three days in a month during the mid-period when pregnancy can take place; it is unlikely (but not impossible) for it to occur in the week before, the week after, or during the period. It is important that girls should be given full information about the menstrual periods before they start, and that no feelings of disgust or guilt should be associated with them, for there is no doubt that a major cause of dysmenorrhoea (painful periods) is the individual's attitude towards this perfectly normal function.

A great deal of nonsense has come to be associated with the menstrual flow, originating in its apparently mysterious nature and the supposed connection (which is wholly imaginary) with the phases of the moon. Superstition and religion have combined to suggest that women are 'unclean' at this time, and among primitive (and not so primitive) people it is believed that contact with a menstruating woman is fraught with dire results or even that the woman herself is in some mysterious condition, so that she ought not to wash her hair or have it waved during her periods. This, of course, is absurd.

The periods should occasion as little upset as possible and no change of any kind in the daily routine. A mentally normal girl looks forward to the time when her periods will begin as the age when she is sexually mature; to ill-informed women it remains 'the curse'. Menstruation is very much under glandular control from the pituitary and this, in turn, is under the control of the hypothalamus in the base of the brain; since the hypothalamus is also concerned with the emotions it happens that emotions have a potent influence upon the periods. The association between painful menstruation and one's feelings about the function has already been mentioned, and it is possible for the periods to be stopped by fear or hope. Common causes of amenorrhoea (stopping of the periods) are the fear of being pregnant in those who have been in a position to become so, or in childless women, the hope that pregnancy has occurred. In pseudo-pregnancy the woman may show all the symptoms of pregnancy and have a distended abdomen or even go through a stage of imitated labour from purely psychological causes. As is well known, amenorrhoea is normally present before puberty, during pregnancy and lactation, and after the menopause (contrary to general belief, pregnancy can occur while the periods are absent, for example just before puberty, during lactation, and just after the menopause). Other causes of amenorrhoea are anaemia, debilitating diseases, change of environment and prolonged nervous strain.

One of the fallacies held about periods is that when they occur something 'bad' is being expelled from the body and that consequently when they do not occur the 'bad' is being retained. This is untrue, because the absence of periods nearly always implies that the material usually excreted has not been formed. The only circumstance when menstrual blood is actually retained is the form of primary amenorrhoea due to the blocking of the opening of the vagina by an imperforate hymen, i.e. the membrane that usually partially obstructs the opening and is (wrongly) regarded as an infallible sign of virginity.

Premenstrual tension is common and many women feel uncomfortable just before the period with pain, irritability and a feeling of fullness. It can be dealt with either by hormones or by diuretics, for example hydrochlorothiazide, since water retention seems to play a major part in premenstrual tension. Tranquillizers and Vitamin A have also been used. Ordinary dysmenorrhoea resulting in painful periods is usually due to psychological reasons, for example feelings of resentment or anxiety about the menstrual function inculcated by a stupid mother. It usually goes after the birth of the first child.

Mental Defect: the term means lack of intellectual development and is not to be regarded as a synonym for mental illness in general. Those whose intellectual development has been inadequate from the start are said to be suffering from amentia, whereas dementia results when a formerly normally equipped individual loses his intellect as the result of a disease process. There are certain well-defined types of mental deficiency, but others come into no special category other than the legal ones of idiocy, imbecility, and feeble-mindedness or moral deficiency which apply to all categories. Classification in the United States avoids the use of terms which might be regarded as stigmatizing. The idiot group corresponds to the severely retarded; the imbecile, moderately retarded; and the feeble-minded or moron, mildly retarded.

Although primary amentia is present from birth, it would be wrong to think that all such cases are inherited and we now know that many result from damage done within the womb as when the mother develops German measles during her pregnancy. Others appear to be due to glandular defects in the mother or child, metabolic defects, disease of the child, birth injury and other causes. Thus the belief that mental defect was caused by the child being dropped on the head in early life, although largely a fable, carried a grain of truth in its implication that inheritance was not necessarily at fault. By and large it is true to say that the grosser forms of idiocy and imbecility may occur in any family no matter how intelligent the parents may be. Minor degrees of backwardness become apparent only in delay in reaching the ordinary landmarks of growth, for example sitting up at 6 months or standing at 1 year, but the grosser forms are fairly obvious from the earliest months. There is general apathy to the surroundings combined with restlessness and repeated purposeless movements; inability to learn bowel and bladder control, dribbling and constant protrusion of the tongue. The inability to utter sensible syllables at the end of the first year while making strange noises is suggestive of idiocy, but may result from deafness and mutism. Fits are often associated with mental deficiency, being a sign of damage to, or malformation of, the brain.

The legal categories of mental deficiency are:

1. An idiot is one who is 'unable to avoid common dangers'

and is quite unable to exist unprotected.

2. An imbecile is one who is unable to manage himself or his affairs.

3. A feeble-minded person is one who in protected circumstances is able to provide for himself; he is, however, unable to compete with the normal person in most types of work and in life.

4. A moral imbecile is not a medical category at all but refers to those people who, in spite of training, require to be controlled for the protection of others, i.e. they are anti-social psychopaths who (let us admit) have become like this often because of faulty training.

See Mongolism, Goitre, Microcephaly, Hydrocephalus.

Mental Illness: mental illnesses are not illnesses in the usually accepted sense of the word, being forms of social maladaptation predisposed to in a greater or lesser degree by heredity and influenced by such factors as upbringing and physical disease. Insanity is largely a legal concept, not a medical one. Thus, if a man believes himself to have been harmed from a distance by one who intends his death and has pointed a bone at him he is quite normal in Australia among the aborigines and quite abnormal in England – but even in England one might take a different view of the case if one knew that he was a member of a strange community to whom this belief was natural. Insanity is also a social and cultural concept. Thus, in World War 2, a simple country boy from South Africa who while sitting in the desert had heard God call him by his Christian name of 'Willy' was regarded by the priests attached to a hospital as insane, whereas one of the doctors, an agnostic, found the boy wholly normal.

Nevertheless, there is always something that is inconsistent about psychotic or insane beliefs.

The most usual classification of mental disorders is as follows:

1. *Organic psychoses* caused by bacterial toxins in the acute fevers (delirium); infections of the brain (as in general paralysis due to syphilis); poisons such as alcohol, carbon monoxide, lead, etc.; disease of the arteries of the brain as in atherosclerosis; and the changes of senility or premature senility. Typical symptoms are disorientation for time, place

and person, loss of memory for recent events, hallucinations and delusions, and poor control over the emotions (*see* Korsakow's Psychosis).

2. *Functional psychoses* or insanity in which no organic disease has been found. (*a*) Manic-depressive psychosis in which there are moods of elation or depression. (*b*) Involutional depression or depression occurring at the change of life. (*c*) Schizophrenia, characterized by many varied symptoms, but usually by delusions, foolish behaviour and general deterioration, sometimes leading to dementia. Hallucinations are usually of hearing rather than of sight, as is common with the organic psychoses. Paraphrenia and paranoia (persecution mania) are forms of schizophrenia coming on later in life, so that there is less deterioration and the delusions are more integrated and less irrational than in the type with an early onset which used to be called dementia praecox.

3. *Psychopathic personality* is an ill-assorted group of which it would not be unfair to say that it includes all the people one happens to dislike, for example the abnormally aggressive, the sexually perverse, the inadequate, the brilliant, the drug-addict. There is no such disease as psychopathic personality: these are basically people who, although not psychotic, hurt society more than they hurt themselves.

4. *Neuroses* are divided into three groups: (*a*) anxiety neurosis in which anxiety and its physical accompaniments are the main symptom; (*b*) hysteria which mimics physical disease; (*c*) obsessional neurosis in which obsessions are the main feature, i.e. the compulsion to do or say or think certain things.

A major difference between the neurotic sufferer from 'nerves' and the insane patient is that the neurotic is very aware of his abnormality while the other is not; neurotic people go to doctors, psychotic people do not, or go for the wrong reason as did one patient who kept coming to his doctor for treatment for stomach trouble brought on, as he believed, by poisoned milk from a hostile dairy company. The neurotic patient has insight, the psychotic has none.

TREATMENT: the treatment of psychoses and neuroses has been revolutionized in recent years both by the discovery of new drugs and physical methods of therapy and by the greater understanding of mental illness which followed the work of Freud and others; but the most important change in the field of mental illness has been in the attitude of the psychiatrist and the staffs of the mental hospitals, who, in the last thirty years, have ceased to regard their work as largely one of diagnosis followed by the custodial function of a jailer, and have adopted an active and optimistic role in treatment. *See* also Psychoanalysis.

Menthol: an alcohol obtained from peppermint oil or prepared synthetically. It is mildly antiseptic, and has a slight local anaesthetic effect. It is used in medicine in inhalations and in various lotions and ointments which have a cooling effect on the skin; it is also used in cigarettes for its pronounced flavour.

Mephenesin: a substance which relaxes muscles by its central action on the spinal cord and has a sedative effect. It has been used in the treatment of spastic conditions and in states where muscular tension is secondary to tension with an emotional basis.

Meprobamate: (Equanil, Miltown, etc.). A 'tranquillizer' developed from the mephenesin group of substances. It is used to control mild anxiety states, and is prescribed in great quantities. It may produce a skin rash, clumsiness and sleepiness, but the greatest danger is the development of drug dependence.

Mercaptopurine: a drug used in the treatment of acute leukaemia in children, and to some extent in transplant surgery to reduce tissue reaction to the transplant.

Mercurochrome: Dibromohydroxymercuripropylsuccinylurea disodium salt, an antibacterial agent.

Mercury: this is not now often used in medicine, although at one time it was a major standby for physicians, particularly in the treatment of syphilis. In the form of calomel it was used as an aperient.

Mercury Poisoning: metallic mercury is not poisonous because it is not absorbed, but its soluble salts can be very dangerous. Poisoning may be acute or chronic.

Acute.

SYMPTOMS: severe burning pain of the mouth and gullet, vomiting, diarrhoea, abdominal pain, collapse.

TREATMENT: raw eggs beaten up in milk should be given at once, with the object of precipitating the mercury salts so that they are no longer soluble and cannot be absorbed. The stomach should be washed out as soon as possible. Dimercaprol is given over the next few days, and the patient is watched carefully for kidney failure which is treated as soon as any signs of it develop.

Chronic. Occurs in industry among people handling inorganic and organic mercurial compounds.

SYMPTOMS: 1. Inorganic compounds of mercury. The patient loses weight, his breath becomes foul because he develops inflammation of the gums, he is weak and shows a muscular tremor, and he may have the signs and symptoms of kidney damage. He may salivate excessively.

2. Organic compounds. The central nervous system is most affected; the patient's vision is disturbed, while he becomes clumsy and unsteady on his feet. His speech may be slurred.

TREATMENT: the patient must be removed from contact with mercury, given a good diet with plenty of fluids, and careful attention must be paid to the general state of his health. Dental treatment is carried out as necessary, and belladonna mixtures will dry up the excessive secretion of saliva. The condition may persist for a long time. In the case of poisoning with organic mercury compounds, the condition may prove to be irreversible. Dimercaprol, sodium calciumedetate and penicillamine have all been used to promote the excretion of mercury in cases of chronic poisoning. *See* Pink Disease.

Merozoite: *see* Malaria.

Mersalyl: a drug containing mercury used as a diuretic. It is given by intramuscular injection, and is effective and largely harmless; but it is being superseded by diuretics that can be taken by mouth. *See* Diuretics.

Mesantoin: (Mephenytoin). *See* Phenytoin Sodium.

Mescaline: a drug present in the cactus Lophophora

williamsii (Anhalonium lewenii). It is a 'psychotomimetic' drug and induces various symptoms of madness in those who take it. It changes the processes of perception so that the drugged man suffers from hallucinations, illusions, changes of time sense, and feelings of unspecified anxiety and perhaps persecution, according to his character. The Mexican drugs peyotl and mescal were used in religious ceremonies in which, it is said, communal hallucinations occurred, and mescaline has been used (like lysergic acid diethylamide) by various people in many countries to try to enlarge the bounds of experience – at least, that is what one understands they wish to do. Whether the induction of illusions and hallucinations in fact does this is open to argument. *See* L.S.D.

Mesencephalon: the mid-brain.

Mesentery: the double layer of peritoneum which supports the intestines by its attachment to the back of the abdominal wall.

Mesmerism: *see* Hypnosis. (Named after Anton Mesmer, 1733–1815, who practised hypnotism and invented the concept of animal magnetism.)

Mesoderm: the middle of the three primary germinal layers of cells in the embryo, from which are derived the bones, muscles, blood, kidney and gonads. *See* Ectoderm, Endoderm.

Mesomorph: the type of body in which there is a preponderance of the tissues derived from mesoderm, i.e. muscle and bone. *See* Ectomorph, Endomorph.

Metabolism: the total sum of all the processes by which the substance of the body is produced and maintained, and by which energy is supplied to the body to enable it to live and move and work. The 'basal metabolic rate' is a measure of the rapidity of the metabolic processes when the body is at rest, and it is estimated by measuring the exchange of oxygen and carbon dioxide during breathing under certain fixed conditions.

Metacarpals: the bones of the hand which at one end make the wrist joint with the small bones of the wrist, and at the other make the knuckle joints with the first bones of the fingers, the proximal phalanges.

Metastasis: a cancerous or malignant growth spreads both by direct extension and by the separation of small clumps of cells which make their way through the lymphatics and the blood vessels to other parts of the body, where they start to form secondary tumours. The process is called metastasis, and the tumours are called secondaries or metastatic growths.

Metatarsal Bones: the bones of the foot which run between the small bones of the ankle and the first bones of the toes.

Metatarsalgia: pain in the region of the metatarsal bones, usually caused by flat-foot (q.v.).

Meteorism: gas in the intestines, present in amounts sufficient to cause swelling.

Methadol: (Methyl alcohol). A poisonous alcohol which is drunk in methylated spirits by some, who run the risk of persistent vomiting, delirium and blindness. Methylated spirits are mostly ethyl alcohol, so that the fatal dose of methyl alcohol is not often reached (about 200 ml). Poisoning with methyl alcohol or with methylated spirits is treated by stomach washout, and general supportive measures. No treatment is known for the blindness.

Methadone: (Physeptone or Dolophine). A painkilling drug which, like morphine, may be classified as a drug of addiction. It has a very marked effect on the coughing centre and is used in small amounts to treat painful, dry coughing. It is used to treat drug addicts in the U.S.A.

Methedrine: (Methylamphetamine). Like other derivatives of amphetamine, this substance has fallen into disuse and disrepute because it has been misused by drug-takers in whom it can produce dependence.

Methicillin: a penicillin which is not very active against ordinarily penicillin-sensitive bacteria, but which has a high resistance to penicillinase and is therefore active against strains of staphyloccoci which resist other penicillins. It must be given by injection and quite large doses are needed. *See* Penicillinase.

Methylene Blue: a blue dye used in microscopy which is also used in cases of poisoning with cyanides or aniline compounds, being given intravenously for its effect in reducing methaemoglobin. Methaemoglobin is a useless compound into which a number of drugs and poisons convert haemoglobin so that the carriage of oxygen in the blood becomes inadequate.

Methylpentynol: (Oblivon). A drug with a short action which can be used for the rapid relief of fear and apprehension – it is, for example, useful to people who dread going to the dentist. It is only valuable in treating insomnia when the primary difficulty is getting to sleep, for the action is not prolonged enough to keep the patient asleep all night.

Methyl Testosterone: *see* Testosterone.

Methysergide: a substance derived from ergot which is used for the relief of migraine. It may produce nausea and vomiting, swelling of the ankles, or a curious reaction that resembles inflammation in the retroperitoneal tissues at the back of the abdominal cavity.

Metritis: inflammation of the womb.

Metropathia Haemorrhagica: a condition in which there is thickening of the lining of the uterus and irregular bleeding.
CAUSE: there is continued unopposed action of oestrogens, for the ovary (q.v.) apparently does not shed ova; no formation of corpora lutea takes place, and no progesterone is secreted. Presumably the condition is due to defective function of the pituitary gland, but the precise mechanism is not understood. In some cases there appears to be an

emotional underlay, and in some cases there is associated pelvic infection.

SYMPTOMS: a period of 6 to 8 weeks amenorrhoea is followed by irregular bleeding, which may be heavy, or cyclical bleeding.

TREATMENT: the diagnosis is made by examination of material obtained from the lining of the uterus by curettage, and the treatment is the administration of progestogens. In exceptional cases, particularly if the patient is over 40, removal of the uterus may be considered.

Metrorrhagia: irregular bleeding between the periods.

Meulengracht's Diet: a diet for the treatment of gastric ulcer.

Microbe: micro-organism, especially one capable of causing disease.

Microbiology: the study of micro-organisms; often used as a synonym for bacteriology.

Microcephaly: (pinhead). A congenital condition in which the head is abnormally small. There may be mental deficiency and convulsions.

Micturition: term for the act of passing urine.

Middle Ear Disease: *see* Ear, Mastoiditis.

Migraine: a particular sort of headache that is preceded by an aura (q.v.) and attacks in paroxysms.

CAUSE: migraine may, like epilepsy, be idiopathic, i.e. occurring for no known cause, or symptomatic – that is, secondary to another disease, such as an intracranial aneurysm, high blood pressure or atherosclerosis. Idiopathic migraine is often hereditary, and it is thought that the underlying change in an attack is spasm in a cerebral artery followed by dilation of blood vessels and intracranial oedema. Some think that attacks are manifestations of the allergic reaction.

SYMPTOMS: the premonitory aura is usually visual, consisting of flashing lights in the centre of the field of vision or in one-half of the visual field. Rarely there are odd sensations felt in the face or the hand, disturbances of speech or transitory weakness or paralysis. The aura lasts for about half an hour, although it may be shorter, and is succeeded by the headache, which may be accompanied by nausea and vomiting, is severe, and may last up to 6 hours. It is often felt only on one side of the head.

TREATMENT: because migraine is an affliction of intelligent and creative people, and is often associated with a degree of neurosis, particularly in women, treatment is not easy, nor is it possible to recommend one universal method of treatment. Each case has to be treated on its own merits. In general patients are better if they try to avoid excessive anxiety or tiredness, and in some cases they will find for themselves that they are better if they avoid certain articles of diet. The regular use of phenobarbitone or a mild 'tranquillizer' sometimes cuts down the number of attacks, and aspirin may be sufficient to cut the headache short. If, however, the attacks respond to nothing else, the drug ergotamine taken by mouth or in an inhaler is often specific. Because of the dangers of ergotism it has to be taken with caution. Migraine, which usually comes on about the time of puberty, is not dangerous to life or to the intelligence, and it normally disappears at the age of 50 or so.

Miliary: like a millet seed – used of small lesions, for example miliary tuberculosis.

Millions Fish: Lebistes reticulatus, cultivated in some parts of the world to live in areas of standing water and eat mosquito larvae, so helping in the control of malaria.

Miltown: a proprietary name for meprobamate.

Miosis: contraction of the pupil of the eye.

Miotic: a substance that causes the pupil of the eye to contract.

Miscarriage: the term used for expulsion of the foetus before the child is capable of life (i.e. before the 28th week);

later expulsion is described as premature labour. About one in five pregnancies end in miscarriage and 37% of child-bearing women miscarry before 30 years of age, most commonly before the end of the fourth month.

The symptoms of miscarriage are unmistakable and the appearance of vaginal bleeding with periodic pains in the lower abdomen in a woman known to be pregnant should receive immediate attention from the doctor; prior to his arrival all she can do is rest in order to discourage further bleeding.

TREATMENT: the treatment of a threatened miscarriage is a matter for the doctor, who may use hormones and sedatives. In incomplete but inevitable abortion the remains of the pregnancy will have to be removed by a minor operation. Habitual abortion requires prolonged treatment, but the outlook is quite good. The great dangers of a miscarriage, whether accidental or deliberately induced, are haemorrhage and sepsis; these are very considerable risks and no unprofessional interference with pregnancy is ever justifiable. *See* Abortion.

Mite: a minute member of the order Acarina. It is possible for men to become infested with them, for they normally live in sugar, flour and other materials which are handled in quantities. Examples of such infestation are miller's itch and grocer's itch. The Demodex folliculorum is known as the face mite or the hair mite from its living quarters, but the mite that makes its presence most felt is the Sarcoptes scabiei, that burrows into the skin and causes scabies (q.v.). The family Ixodidae, although members of the Acarina order, are not properly referred to as mites, but rather as ticks.

Mithridatism: King Mithridates tried to acquire an immunity to poisons by eating minute amounts of them and increasing the dose slowly. The process has been named after him.

Mitosis: the process by which a cell divides in such a way as to produce two daughter cells each with the same number of chromosomes as the original cell. *See* Meiosis.

Mitral Stenosis: *see* Heart.

Mixture: a combination of different drugs usually put up in water. The modern tendency in prescribing is to use one specific drug in the form of a tablet or capsule, but there are many conditions, particularly those in which a precise diagnosis proves elusive, in which variously coloured mixtures are curative. Mixtures are also very useful in stomach troubles and intestinal upsets, and when treating children who do not like tablets; moreover the dose is easily varied.

M'Naughton Rules: In 1843 a man named M'Naughton was acquitted on a charge of murdering the private secretary of Sir Robert Peel on the grounds of insanity. The reasons for acquittal have since then been used in the defence of many cases of murder on the grounds of insanity, and may be quoted thus: 'To establish a defence on the grounds of insanity it must be clearly proved that at the time of committing the act the party accused was labouring under such a defect of reason from disease of the mind as not to know the nature and quality of the act he was doing, or, if he did know it, that he did not know he was doing what was wrong.'

Mole: a pigmented spot on the skin, usually raised above the surrounding level, and sometimes hairy. Moles should not be interfered with except by a surgeon, and if they appear to change or to be irritated by the clothes a doctor's opinion should be sought. It is of especial importance to ask for the doctor's advice if the mole starts to bleed. The technical name for a mole is benign melanoma; melanomata may also be malignant.

Molluscum Contagiosum: a skin condition usually seen in children.
CAUSE: a virus infection, often caught in the swimming-baths.
SYMPTOMS: small, round, nodular tumours develop to about the size of a split pea. They have a little dent on top, and contain a creamy soft material. They are painless and harmless, but may be ugly.
TREATMENT: they can be scraped off painlessly with a sharp

519

curette, removed by squeezing out the contents and cauterizing, or abolished by the application of 12% salicylic acid in collodion or on adhesive tape.

Molluscum Fibrosum: (Von Recklinghausen's disease). Tumours may form in the skin in this disease (otherwise called neurofibromatosis) which may enlarge to 3 or 4 in (75 or 100 mm) across. Fibrous tissue tumours may also grow on the nerves, and brown pigmented areas appear on the skin. There is no specific treatment for the disease, which is familial and appears as a Mendelian dominant, but tumours which are causing trouble can be removed surgically. Tumours of the meninges of the brain are sometimes associated with von Recklinghausen's disease, and the fibrous tumours on nerves may occur within the skull and give rise to symptoms.

Mongolism: a congenital defect associated with mental deficiency.
CAUSE: children with this condition tend to be the offspring of older mothers. It is found that the cells show 47 chromosomes instead of the normal 46. Mongolism may be familial.
SYMPTOMS: the face is said to look 'mongoloid' – it shows slanting eyes, a protruding tongue and retroussé nose; the head looks round (brachycephalic). The child seems to be weak. There is in about one-third of the cases an abnormality of the heart, which may produce symptoms, and the brain in mongolism is small, the mentality being retarded.

Monitor: it is possible to pick up various physiological measurements from patients, such as the pulse rate or the electrocardiogram, and show them as a continual display on an instrument at a distance. The process is called monitoring and the instrument, usually a cathode ray tube, a monitor. The theory is that a nurse can sit in a central office and observe her patients continuously without having to go and carry out separate intermittent observations. Other theoretical applications include the suggestion that an anaesthetist could sit in a central office, perhaps looking down through the windows at the operating theatres, and watch the progress of more than one unconscious patient, relaying instructions as necessary to the staff in the theatre or even controlling the supply of anaesthetic gases and agents from a central panel. The techniques are roughly those used to watch the physiological activities of astronauts, although signals from space must be transmitted by radio, whereas in the case of hospital monitoring the signals can be sent by wire.

Monoamine Oxidase Inhibitors: *see* M.A.O.

Monocyte: the largest of the white cells circulating in the blood, and the least common. Its nucleus is single, irregular and pale; it is formed by cells called monoblasts in the blood-forming tissues. Monocytes are able to pass through the walls of capillaries to scavenge in the connective tissues of the body and they pick up fragments of old cells, waste substances and microscopic foreign bodies. *See* Leukocytes, Reticulo-endothelial System.

Mononuclear: a cell having one nucleus; a monocyte.

Mononucleosis: infectious mononucleosis is also called glandular fever (q.v.).

Morbidity: the condition of being sick; the sickness rate.

Moron: a feeble-minded individual, with a mental age of between 8 and 12 years at maturity. In the United States this degree of deficiency is termed mildly retarded.

Morphine: *see* Opium.

Mosquito: an insect of the order Diptera, the family Culicidae; the medically important tribes are anopheline and culicine. About 250 separate species of culicine mosquitoes are known, and most of them are capable of carrying the organisms of malaria, although only about twelve are normally implicated in the spread of the disease. Anopheline mosquitoes can also carry filariasis (Wuchereria bancrofti and Brugia malayi) as can some culicine mosquitoes; but the most deadly disease carried by the culicine insects, notably Aedes aegypti and Culex pipiens, is yellow fever.

They also carry dengue fever and types of encephalitis caused by arbo-viruses.

Motion Sickness: nausea and vomiting caused by the effect of angular and linear acceleration and deceleration on the inner ear, these being caused by the motion of the ship, aircraft, or car in which the victim is travelling. Hyoscine is the traditional drug used to prevent seasickness, but the newer antihistamines have the same action. Some recommend the combination of hyoscine (0.3 mg hyoscine hydrobromide by mouth) before the voyage or flight with an antihistamine, for example promethazine theoclate (Avomine) in doses of 25 mg repeated every 6 hours. It is difficult to know what avoiding action to recommend to those prone to seasickness, except to say that a heavy meal is dangerous, and to remind them that it is said that the best position in which to sail is lying down amidships.

Motor System: that part of the nervous system which is concerned with movement, as opposed to the sensory system, which is concerned with sensation.

Mould: an appearance caused by the growth of various fungi, of which the common ones are Aspergillus, Rhizopus, Penicillium and Mucor. They are filamentous, and the filaments weave together to make the visible part of the fungus. Some of these organisms are very useful, and antibiotic drugs are derived from them; some are a nuisance, for they grow where they are not wanted; and some can produce disease in man by setting up reactions in the lungs when they are breathed in. *See* Farmer's Lung, Bagassosis.

Moulding: a term used in obstetrics to describe the adaptation of the shape of the baby's head to the confines of the birth canal.

Mouth: common diseases affecting the mouth are described under their own headings. *See* Gumboil, Lips, Teeth, Tongue, Thrush, etc.

Moxibustion: the burning of a little bundle of inflammable material on the skin to provide counter-irritation.

M.P.D.: the maximum permissible dose of ionizing radiation – the greatest amount that will not lead to permanent damage or the subsequent development of disease.

Mucomembranous Colitis: a type of colitis largely brought on by the excessive use of purgatives in neurotic people. It is now much less common than it was at the turn of the century.

Mucous Membrane: membranes which secrete mucous form the internal lining of the body surface and are composed of various sorts of epithelial cells according to the different functions they have to carry out. *See* Epithelium.

Multipara: a woman who has borne more than one child.

Multiple Sclerosis: (Disseminated Sclerosis). A disease of the nervous system in which patches of sclerosis (hardening) appear in the spinal cord and the brain.
CAUSE: unknown. The disease affects people between the ages of 20 and 40, but can start before 20 or after 40; it is virtually never found for the first time in those over 50 or before adolescence. It is a disease of temperate climates.
SYMPTOMS: the areas of hardening are named plaques, and they interrupt the fibres of the spinal cord and brain. The onset of the disease can easily be mistaken for other conditions, among them hysteria, for the patient commonly complains of tingling in a limb or of clumsiness which seems to recover. One of the characteristics of the disease, however, is its dissemination or scattering both in space and time, so that in the early and middle stages of the condition there are relapses and exacerbations lasting for a while, followed by remissions in which the symptoms may clear up to a great extent. The general course of the disease is to worsen over a period, perhaps of years, although it is not possible to say how long the development of the last, chronic, stage will take. The symptoms vary a great deal according to the site of the plaques, but almost all cases show blurring of vision, clumsiness of movement, double vision, tingling and patches of numbness in the limbs or over the body. In the early stages of the disease these symptoms may seem to recover completely, but in the end less and less relief is afforded by

remissions and the symptoms become permanent. The patient cannot walk properly, being stiff and unsteady, control of the bladder and bowels is uncertain and the arms are clumsy and shake when they are used. Very often the brain is affected so that the patient is much more cheerful than one would expect, but this is not the rule.

TREATMENT: no treatment is known which will cure the disease, but this is not to say that nothing can be done. The patient can be helped a great deal both by the medical attendants and by the family, for the worst thing that can happen is for invalidism to sap the will-power. Patients should continue to do what they can as long as it is humanly possible for them to carry on, and they must be given every possible encouragement to keep going. In the later stages of the disease regular physiotherapy is extremely valuable.

Mumps: (Epidemic parotitis). A virus infection of the salivary glands, gonads and occasionally other parts of the body.

CAUSE: (incubation period two to three weeks). The infecting organism is a paramyxovirus. Spread is by direct infection.

SYMPTOMS: the parotid gland, in front of and below the ear, is most commonly affected. In children, among whom the disease is common and sometimes epidemic, swelling is usually the first sign, but adults sometimes run a temperature and feel ill a couple of days before the glands enlarge. The swelling is often at first uncomfortable or painful. If the disease occurs after puberty, the testicles may be affected; although the ovary may be infected, it is far commoner to find the gonads swollen in the male. If the disease spreads to the testicles the swelling and pain are very considerable; there is a high fever, and the patient may become depressed and even a little confused. Mumps can also lead to meningitis and encephalitis with delirium, severe headache and other signs of irritation of the meninges, or it may spread to the pancreas when the symptoms include pain in the abdomen and loss of appetite. The patient may vomit.

TREATMENT: little is needed in the way of treatment in the ordinary uncomplicated case of mumps; no attempt should be made to prevent children, particularly boys, catching the disease if they are under the age of 12, for while it is of little consequence in the child, mumps is a fairly serious condition in the adult. There is no need to confine children to bed, but adults should remember that inactivity will reduce the risk of the infection spreading to the gonads. If inflammation of the testicle develops corticosteroids are used, the testicles are slung in cotton wool between the thighs and analgesic drugs are given. The patient who is depressed needs to be told that in two-thirds of cases no permanent damage is done, and that even if one testicle does become atrophic it is very rare for both to become sterile. Moreover, sterility following mumps does not mean that sexual power is lost. A mumps vaccine is available (*see* Immunization).

Murmur: the noise heard through a stethoscope placed over the heart when disease of the valves is present; the noise is thought to be due to the passage of blood over roughened areas or through narrow orifices. Murmurs are of varying significance; much more important are the other signs of heart disease such as breathlessness and reduced tolerance to exercise.

Muscle: there are three types of muscle in the human body differing both in structure and function. These are: striate or striped, which is the type found in the ordinary voluntary muscles of the body (i.e. the ones over which we have voluntary control); the smooth or involuntary muscle of the intestines, bladder and the lining of the larger blood vessels over which we have no control; and the muscle of the heart, or cardiac muscle, which is in a category of its own.

Striped muscle is seen under the microscope to be composed of a large number of fibres held together by loose connective tissue, which also surrounds the whole muscle; the fibres are built up from even more minute fibrils embedded in a semifluid substance and surrounded by a delicate sheath. The fibrils are seen to be marked with alternate bands of dark and light (hence the name striped muscle). Each end of a muscle is attached to a bone, and contraction draws the two ends together, thus producing either flexion (bending) or extension (straightening) of a limb. The process which causes a muscle to contract is very complex and involves several biochemical reactions. It must be sufficient here to say that a muscle to which oxygen is not supplied in sufficient quantities becomes the seat of painful spasm or cramp. When a muscle is at rest it remains slightly contracted and, since all contractions give off heat, the maintenance of posture and tone in muscle plays a large part in maintaining the body heat as well as enabling movements to take place more rapidly than would otherwise be the case. Plain or unstriped muscle is found in the alimentary canal, the respiratory and urinary tracts, the pupil of the eye and the skin, where it causes the involuntary phenomenon of 'gooseflesh'. Cardiac or heart muscle is partly striped, but differs from voluntary muscle in not being under voluntary control and in being in constant regular action.

Muscles with and without stripes receive their nervous supply from a different source; the voluntary muscles are supplied by the motor and sensory nerves and the involuntary ones by the autonomic nervous system (*see* Nervous System). Pressure and stretching give rise to a feeling of pain if carried to excess, but cutting produces no effect on muscle, and it is therefore possible to operate without anaesthetic on the internal organs if the skin of the abdominal wall is anaesthetized. The attachment of a muscle to a less movable bone is known as its origin, its attachment to the more movable one is its insertion. Thus the deltoid muscle of the top of the shoulder arises from the collar-bone and shoulder blade and is inserted into the humerus.

Muscle Relaxants: a number of drugs when injected into the bloodstream act upon the junction between the muscle fibres and the nerves in such a way as to prevent the muscles contracting, and others act upon the central nervous system to produce the same effect. These drugs are spoken of as muscle relaxants, and they include the South American arrow poison curare. Muscle relaxants are used by anaesthetists to produce sufficient relaxation to enable the surgeon to expose deep structures without giving an increased concentration of anaesthetic agent, which might be dangerous to the patient although convenient for the surgeon. Those with a short action are used when a tube is being passed into the trachea or windpipe in order to prevent muscular spasm, and those with a longer action are used in the treatment of tetanus. While the muscles are paralysed the anaesthetist has to assist the patient to breathe, for the action of the relaxants includes the muscles of respiration.

Mustard: made from the seeds of Brassica nigra and B. alba, which contain volatile oils. From them mustard obtains its characteristic taste and stimulating properties, which are still used to provide counter-irritation to the skin as well as the tongue.

Mustard Gas: sulphur mustard was used as an agent of chemical warfare in World War 1, but it was found 20 years later that its nitrogen derivatives could be used in the treatment of cancer, for their action upon cells is similar to the action of ionizing radiations, attacking the chromosomes and stopping growth. They are among the group of cytotoxic drugs now used in combination with radiotherapy and surgery to treat various malignant diseases.

Mutation: chromosomes, which are responsible for the passing on of inherited characteristics, are made of the substance D.N.A. An alteration of the D.N.A. at a particular place in the chromosome (the gene) will result in a change of inherited characteristics so that the character of the offspring is different from that of its parents. The offspring that shows such a change is called a mutation, and the process of change is also called mutation. Mutations can be natural, or can be brought about by such external agents as radiation or the administration of nitrogen mustards; most are not an advantage to the offspring, and some indeed are lethal, but a very few strengthen the offspring in some way and so become established in time by the process of natural selection.

Myalgia: muscular pain.

Myasthenia Gravis: a rare condition in which the muscles become fatigued abnormally quickly. It is found most often in young adults.
CAUSE: at present not fully understood. There is a defect of function at the junction between the nerve and muscle fibres caused by a lack of acetylcholine, the substance necessary for transmission of nerve impulses. This is thought

to be due in some way to disorder of the thymus gland in the upper part of the chest, possibly through an immune reaction.

SYMPTOMS: the disease begins by producing weakness of the muscles supplied by the cranial nerves, so that the upper eyelid droops, there is double vision, and difficulty in speech, swallowing and breathing. Later any muscle may become involved.

TREATMENT: edrophonium chloride is injected intravenously to make the diagnosis, for it has a dramatic action on the disease. It is not, however, used in treatment because the action only lasts a short time. Longer-acting drugs are neostigmine and pyridostigmine, which are taken in doses varying according to the patient's condition. The thymus gland is removed surgically in many cases, of which about one-third may be expected to show a marked improvement; but the operation is not usually carried out in patients over 50.

Mycobacteria: thin, slightly curved, rod-shaped micro-organisms, two kinds of which cause tuberculosis and leprosy.

Mycotic Disease: disease caused by vegetable micro-organisms, for example ringworm, actinomycosis and Madura foot.

Mydriatics: drugs such as belladonna which cause dilatation of the pupil of the eye.

Myelin: the substance forming the sheath round certain nerve fibres.

Myelitis: inflammation of the spinal cord, or inflammation of the bone marrow.

Myelocele: the spinal cord may protrude or herniate through a congenital defect in the bones of the spinal column called a spina bifida to form a swelling known as a myelocele. The condition may be associated with hydrocephalus.

Myelocyte: a cell of the red bone marrow which gives rise to the granular white cells of the blood.

Myelogram: an X-ray of the spinal cord made by injecting a radio-opaque oil (Myodil) into the subarachnoid space (normally filled by fluid) by lumbar puncture. The radio-opaque material is heavier than the cerebro-spinal fluid, and can be run up and down the spinal column by altering the position of the patient. X-ray plates are exposed to show the cord at various levels, and if there is a block to the passage of the Myodil or an enlargement of the spinal cord it will be seen.

Myeloid Leukaemia: *see* Leukaemia.

Myeloma: a tumour of the bone marrow. Multiple myeloma is a disease in which many myelomata form and destroy bone tissue, commonly in the ribs, the skull, the vertebrae and the pelvis – the bones which contain active blood-forming marrow. In this disease the urine shows the Bence-Jones protein, which when the urine is heated precipitates at 50–60 °C., dissolves as the urine comes to the boil, and precipitates again on cooling. The treatment for a solitary myeloma is radiotherapy, and for multiple myeloma radiotherapy and cytotoxic drugs. Multiple myelomatosis is a malignant disease.

Myiasis: the condition of being infested with maggots. The ox suffers from warble-fly, and the horse from bot-fly, but man is only infested by accident; there is no maggot which cannot breed without man. The commonest conditions for producing maggot infestation are found in the tropics, although in any climate open wounds and discharges may attract flies to lay their eggs. (The infestation of wounds with maggots is not as bad as it might appear, for they scavenge freely and a maggoty wound is a clean wound. Nevertheless it takes a brave surgeon to suggest such treatment and a brave patient to submit to it.)

In Africa the tumbu- or mango-fly lays its eggs on the ground and they are sometimes picked up by human beings, into whose skin the larvae burrow to produce painful swellings, and in tropical America the 'human' warble-fly attaches its eggs to mosquitoes who pass them on to man. The bot-fly and the cattle warble occasionally lay their eggs on man, and the larvae creep into the skin.

Myocarditis: inflammation of the heart muscle.
CAUSE: usually rheumatic fever; it may be secondary to acute virus infections, among them smallpox, influenza and glandular fever, or acute bacterial infections such as diphtheria, typhoid and scarlet fever.
SYMPTOMS: the pulse may be irregular, there may be a fainting fit, the patient may feel pain in the chest or angina, and he may become unduly fatigued or even breathless.
TREATMENT: strict rest and the treatment of the causative condition. *See* Rheumatic Fever, Rheumatism.

Myoclonus: involuntary contractions of a group of muscles, one muscle or a portion of a muscle. The contractions may be associated with various diseases. Clonus is a condition of alternate contraction and relaxation of a muscle or a group of muscles in which the tone is raised. A condition in which there is spontaneous clonic movement of the muscles of the face, often at first round the eye but in time spreading to involve one side of the face, is not uncommon among the middle-aged and the elderly.

Myodil: *see* Myelogram.

Myoma: a tumour, nearly always benign, which consists of muscle fibres. Myomata are common in the uterus, where they contain fibrous as well as muscular tissue and are known as fibromyomata or fibroids.

Myopathy: disease of muscle not due to a defect in the nervous system. The myopathies are rare, and are described as progressive muscular dystrophy, for the muscle fibres are gradually replaced by fat and fibrous tissue. The disease falls into three groups according to the clinical picture. In pseudo-hypertrophic muscular dystrophy the muscles of the legs appear to be large, but are weak; the child, almost always a boy, fails to walk or ceases to be able to walk. The muscular weakness spreads and the muscles waste; the child may eventually succumb to intercurrent infection, particularly of the respiratory system. In facio-scapulo-humeral dystrophy the wasting and weakness is confined to the face and the shoulder muscles, and in limb girdle muscular dystrophy the pelvis and shoulders but not the face are affected. These two latter diseases are found in both sexes, and remissions occur. Progressive muscular dystrophy has no known specific treatment; orthopaedic appliances may help the legs. The condition is hereditary.

Myopia: short sight. *See* Eye, Spectacles.

Myositis: inflammation of the muscles. Myositis ossificans is a condition in which ossification (bone formation) occurs in muscles and interferes with their power of contraction. The condition is in many cases thought to be due to repeated small injuries, and it may follow a fracture where there has been extravasation of blood into the tissues. True infective inflammation of the muscles is rare, but includes gas gangrene, tuberculosis and myositis purulenta tropica in which there is fever, pain and abscess formation in the muscles.

Myotonia Congenita: a rare disease in which the patient's muscles do not relax after they have contracted, so that he cannot easily let go after shaking hands and may burn himself because he cannot let go of hot objects. The difficulty wears off on exercise, and the disease is otherwise harmless.

Myringotomy: incision into the eardrum, commonly made for the relief of pus in the middle ear before the advent of antibiotics made such cases rare.

Myxoedema: the condition that results from lack of the thyroid hormone. *See* Goitre, Thyroid Gland.

Myxoma: tumour of mucous tissue.

Myxovirus: viruses characterized by their affinity for mucus. The three groups of myxoviruses that afflict humans produce influenza; the viruses that produce mumps, measles and respiratory disease in infants are larger than the myxovirus and are called paramyxoviruses.

N

Naevus: *see* Nevus.

Nails: common diseases affecting the nails are:
1. *Purulent infection.* It is common to find collections of pus forming in relation to the nail folds and under the nails as the result of bacterial infection of minor cuts and abrasions. The infection may be acute or chronic, and it is called a paronychia. In acute infection the nail fold is red and tense, and there is considerable pain; the condition is treated by antibiotics and if necessary the pus is let out by the removal of part of the nail. Chronic infection is common among people whose hands are continually damp, and it may be associated with fungus infections. Treatment is not easy, and impossible unless the hands are kept dry and clean.
2. *Injury.* Injuries may result in the formation of a collection of blood under the nail, which may be very painful until it is evacuated and may lead to the loss of the nail, which, however, soon grows again. If the nail bed from which the nail grows is crushed or otherwise damaged, the new nail may be deformed. (The nail grows out from under the nail fold, and the nail bed visible outside the fold takes no part in its formation.)
3. *Ingrowing toe nail.* The nails of the toes – mostly the great toe is affected – sometimes grow forwards into the nail bed at one or both corners because the shoes fit badly or the nail has been cut too short. The growth of the nail into the flesh is painful and may give rise to infection. Treatment is to trim the nail away from the nail fold and to make sure as it grows out that it does not grow into the flesh again. The nail should be cut straight across when it eventually grows free of the fold, and the shoes must be changed if they fit badly. If the nail bed and folds are badly infected it may be necessary to remove the nail.
4. *Ringworm.* This fungus infection affects the toe nails and sometimes the finger nails. It discolours, thickens and deforms them, spreading into the nail from its free edge. Treatment is by the antibiotic griseofulvin, which has to be

taken for several months until the infected nail has been renewed.

The nails have much to tell about a person's health; in heart or lung disease they may be slightly blue rather than pink, and the finger tips may be 'clubbed'; in anaemia they are spoon-shaped, and a serious illness leaves a groove across the nail (the date can be calculated because it takes about six months for the nail to grow from the nail bed to the tip of the finger). Bitten nails in the adult are a strong indication of neurosis.

Nalorphine: (Lorfan). A specific antidote for morphine poisoning, to be used with caution in cases where it is suspected that the patient is an addict, for he may become uncontrollable. Nalorphine is itself an analgesic if it is given without any other drug being present, and can produce mild respiratory depression, yet it counteracts the respiratory depression produced by morphine and reverses its analgesic effect. Nalorphine should not be used in barbiturate poisoning.

Napkin Rash: dermatitis of the area covered by the napkin is due to irritation by the urine, which is found to be ammoniacal, having been chemically broken down by a micro-organism occurring in the faeces. The reddened skin should be covered by zinc compound paste, and the napkins sterilized by boiling and the use of a very mild antiseptic.

Narcissism: love of self, usually regarded as a normal stage of development which becomes abnormal if it is carried to excess in later life.

Narcoanalysis: the technique of using a narcotic drug to aid in psychoanalysis.

Narcolepsy: in this condition the patient has from time to time an irresistible desire to fall asleep. In children it may follow encephalitis, but it may develop in adults spontaneously with no known cause. It is one of the few conditions in which amphetamine may prove useful.

Narcotics: a term applied in the legal sense to certain drugs which produce stupor or unconsciousness.

Nasopharynx: the part of the pharynx above the level of the soft palate: that part of the back of the throat which lies behind the nose.

National Health Service: inaugurated in July 1948 under the National Health Service Act of 1946 in England and Wales, and under separate acts in Scotland and Northern Ireland. The service is open to everyone in the Kingdom regardless of insurance qualifications and the Act was intended 'to promote the establishment ... of a comprehensive health service designed to secure improvement in the mental and physical health of the people' by the prevention, treatment, and diagnosis of illness. It provides hospital and general practitioner services, dental, pharmaceutical, ophthalmic and local health authority services.

Naturopathy or Nature Cure: there are people who believe that 'natural' cures are possible by such methods as eating 'natural' foods, which may simply mean a largely vegetarian diet or in the case of extreme purists food which is not only vegetarian but 'compost-grown', i.e. on which modern artificial fertilizers, insecticides, or methods of cultivation have not been used. There are also people known as herbalists who believe that 'natural' medicines made from herbs are better, healthier or safer than those used by orthodox medicine. Although it is beyond doubt that many people suffering from a surfeit of high living and low thinking are likely to be benefited by a Spartan diet from time to time, that any sort of diet in itself – except in such diseases as diabetes and other conditions where the diet necessary needs to be scientifically worked out by a skilled dietician – is likely to cure a disease, is improbable in the extreme. It is true that some of the food we eat has been spoilt or even made dangerous by modern methods of farming, such as the use of poisonous fertilizers and insecticides or the giving of sex hormones to animals to fatten them up for killing. This, of course, is a matter which requires stricter legal control. But that naturopathy accomplishes anything worthwhile is incredible and its beliefs often verge on the ridiculous.

In the first place, we must ask ourselves what is meant by 'natural' food or methods? The Eskimos 'naturally' live on blubber for the reason that there is very little else to eat, and hunting tribes in many cases exist almost wholly on lean meat – the only thing we can say with certainty is that no primitive tribe has ever been exclusively vegetarian. Indeed, man's teeth show that they were designed for a mixed diet, so it is vegetarianism which is unnatural. Then there is the argument that civilization is unnatural and that we should turn to a life which is closer to nature; but, if this is so, why is it that it is precisely those who live closest to nature whose lives are 'nasty, brutish, and short'? Nobody nowadays believes in the noble savage, but what we do know is that among primitive peoples the average expectation of life is something like 30 years while in our 'unnatural' civilization it has advanced to more than 70 years. We have seen within seven years the death-rate in Ceylon halved by modern medicine plus D.D.T., which together have practically wiped out malaria. How does a herbalist or naturopath cure malaria or syphilis, how does he deal with yaws and leprosy? Even G. B. Shaw as an enthusiastic vegetarian only lived to the great age he did with the aid of injections of liver extract for his pernicious anaemia. Finally there is the odd argument that herbs are not only more natural than, say, penicillin used in the treatment of syphilis, but that they are safer, that even when they do not cure they at least do no harm. This is plain nonsense, because everybody with a smattering of knowledge about drugs knows that the most deadly poisons in existence are the vegetable ones – strychnine, prussic acid, and the alkaloids in general. In so far as naturopathy or the art of the herbalist claims to be a complete system of medicine in opposition to orthodox medicine – doubtless only the extremists would claim this – to that degree the public is being deceived.

Nausea: the unpleasant sensation that precedes vomiting; 'feeling sick'.

Navel: umbilicus, the scar in the centre of the abdominal wall where the umbilical cord joined the body to the placenta in the womb.

535

Near Sight: *see* Spectacles.

Nebulizer: an apparatus for administering a drug in the form of a spray or cloud.

Necator: a genus of nematode parasites; hookworms, Necator americanus being the New World hookworm. *See* Hookworm, Worms.

Neck: the part of the body joining the upper part of the chest to the base of the skull. Its main contents are the throat, the thyroid gland, the tubes for air and food (i.e. the windpipe or trachea and the gullet or oesophagus), the great blood vessels going to and from the head and brain, the muscles and the seven cervical vertebrae. The cervical nerves which leave the spinal cord in this area supply the muscles and skin of the neck and arms. The pharynx, the cavity of the throat, lies in front of the spinal column from the base of the skull to the sixth cervical vertebra, at which point the oesophagus continues it below. The larynx opens out in front at the level of the fourth to sixth cervical vertebrae, and the thyroid cartilage can be felt just beneath the skin. The larynx is continued below by the trachea, which is crossed by the narrow part or isthmus of the thyroid gland, the lobes of the gland being easily felt on either side. The main muscle in front is the sterno-mastoid, passing from the mastoid process behind the ear to the top of the sternum or breastbone and the inner end of the clavicle or collar-bone. This covers the sheath containing the carotid artery, the internal jugular vein, and the vagus nerve (q.v.) and also a chain of lymph glands. More superficially lie the external jugular vein passing from the angle of the jaw almost straight downwards, and the smaller anterior jugular vein which passes down near the mid-line on either side. All these structures occupy only the front one-third of the neck: the two-thirds remaining behind them is made up of the cervical part of the spinal column and the large mass of muscles that move it and move and support the head.

Necropsy: an autopsy or post-mortem examination.

Necrosis: the death of a small part of the tissues, for example in gangrene.

Needling: the old operation for cataract whereby the lens was torn by a needle in order to let the opaque material escape and be absorbed with the fluid of the anterior chamber of the eye.

Negativism: in psychiatry, the refusal of a patient to attend to the examiner, or a tendency for him to do the opposite of what he is asked or what his normal feelings would indicate.

Neisseria: a genus of micro-organisms named after Albert Neisser, a German physician (1855–1916). Neisseria include in particular the organisms of gonorrhoea and meningitis.

Nematode: a roundworm or threadworm. *See* Worms.

Neoarsphenamine: (Neosalvarsan). An arsenical compound which was used before the discovery of antibiotics in the treatment of syphilis. It is more soluble and less toxic than Ehrlich's original Salvarsan.

Neomycin: this antibiotic is derived from bacteria of the streptomyces group. It is mainly active against Gram-negative organisms, but is very toxic and cannot be given by injection. It is not absorbed from the intestines, and can therefore be used in bowel infections such as bacillary dysentery. It is also used on the skin in powders, ointments and creams, and neomycin drops are used to deal with ear and eye infections.

Neonatal: applied to matters arising in the first four weeks after birth.

Neoplasm: a tumour or new growth, malignant or simple.

Nephrectomy: the operation for removal of a kidney.

Nephritis: strictly, nephritis means inflammation of the

537

kidney, but the diseases to which the word is applied are not primarily caused by inflammation.

A synonym for nephritis is Bright's disease, for Bright (1789–1858) described examples of many different diseases which can be included under the term.

A convenient classification which will be used here divides the medical diseases of the kidney into acute nephritis, chronic nephritis, and the nephrotic syndrome.

Acute nephritis.

1. Acute glomerulonephritis.

CAUSE: this disease follows infections with haemolytic streptococci, which used to give rise to scarlet fever but now that antibiotics are so promptly used are nearly always confined to causing a sore throat. A week or two after the patient has recovered from his sore throat he develops acute nephritis because of the collection within the glomeruli of the kidney of combinations of antigen and antibody.

SYMPTOMS: blood in the urine, swelling of the face and legs, pain in the small of the back, headache, and a rise of blood pressure. As the disease progresses the patient may become a little breathless, may develop a cough and in some cases suffer from nausea and even vomiting. The output of urine is diminished.

TREATMENT: the patient is put to bed and given a salt-free diet; fluids are restricted, and the intake of protein cut down. After a week to ten days the patient passes normal quantities of urine again and begins to feel better. He should be kept in bed for another two or three weeks in mild cases and for longer if the symptoms have been severe.

2. Recurrent haematuria. Men and boys sometimes pass blood in the urine after excessive exercise or during the course of an infection of the nose or throat, and the urine may be found to contain protein. The condition may recur; it may be of little significance but may go on to chronic nephritis.

3. Anaphylactoid purpura. In this condition, which follows a sore throat or other infection by haemolytic streptococci in children, a rash comes out on the skin and the joints swell up, particularly those of the leg. There may also be pain in the abdomen and vomiting, and the passage of blood in the urine. The condition usually clears up but may exceptionally progress to chronic nephritis.

538

4. Radiation nephritis. In this condition the damage to the kidneys is caused not by the deposition of an antibody-antigen complex nor by hyper-sensitivity as is believed to be the case in anaphylactoid purpura, but by the action of X-rays. It is now uncommon, but at first occurred because it was not recognized. The nephritis develops about six months after the radiation injury – the period may be as long as a year – and the symptoms are similar to those of acute nephritis, although some cases may progress to a state of chronic nephritis without passing through an acute phase.

5. Polyarteritis nodosa (q.v.) may damage the kidney.

Chronic nephritis. This is the state into which patients pass who do not make a complete recovery from acute nephritis. SYMPTOMS: many patients have no symptoms, and the condition is only discovered because there is protein in the urine. Others, however, go on to some degree of renal failure and develop a high blood pressure which in time produces its own symptoms (*see* Hypertension). Failure of the kidney is accompanied by deficient excretion of waste products containing nitrogen, so that the level of urea in the blood rises, and there is also a loss of salt in the urine, which becomes very dilute because the kidney cannot concentrate it. Because the volume of urine is increased the patient has to pass water more frequently than usual. Some patients become anaemic.

TREATMENT: patients who have no symptoms need no treatment, and can lead a perfectly normal life. If the kidney starts to fail, retention of nitrogenous waste matter is treated by attention to the diet, and the loss of salt and water made good by giving enough to balance the loss. A rise of blood pressure is treated by giving the appropriate drugs. Selected cases may benefit from dialysis of the blood on an artificial kidney machine, and in some cases transplantation of a kidney may be considered, but it is clear that for the foreseeable future such treatment can only be offered to carefully chosen cases.

The nephrotic syndrome. Many diseases of the kidney result in a condition in which there is such a great loss of albumin in the urine that the level of protein in the blood falls and there is oedema – wet swelling of the tissues. The condition that accompanies the passage of large quantities of albumin

539

in the urine is called the nephrotic syndrome. The diseases which lead to it include: acute nephritis, other types of glomerulonephritis, diabetes, lupus erythematosus, and poisoning with drugs, particularly those containing mercury. Some patients develop the nephrotic syndrome without the kidney showing obvious anatomical abnormality, and these patients include most of the cases that occur in childhood. SYMPTOMS: the syndrome is most common in children aged between 2 and 4, and occurs more often in boys. There is swelling of the face and legs, which obscures the wasting of muscles that also takes place, and the urine is found to be full of protein. Intercurrent infections are common and may be dangerous. The condition may persist for a long time, perhaps years, before it passes into the stage of chronic nephritis. In children the condition may clear up spontaneously, but in some cases it recurs.

TREATMENT: if an underlying condition can be treated this is the first line of defence; in particular noxious drugs can be stopped. The oedematous swelling is treated by the use of diuretics such as frusemide (Lasix) and ethacrynic acid (Edecrin), which are given with covering doses of potassium salts, and the adoption of a sodium salt-free diet. The diet should also be high in protein, but the protein may have to be made up with substances such as sodium-free milk powders because a normal high-protein diet includes too much sodium. In cases where little or no disease is obvious in the kidney (a fact which may be discovered by biopsy of the kidney) corticosteroids are beneficial, but in other cases they may produce no change. If patients develop a high blood pressure it should be treated with the appropriate drugs, but kidney failure may complicate the condition.

Nephrolithiasis: stones in the kidney.

Nephropexy: an operation carried out to fix the position of the kidney in cases where undue mobility is thought to produce pain or discomfort. Symptoms are, however, only very rarely due to a 'floating kidney' and the results of such an operation are liable to be disappointing.

Nephrosis: *see* Nephritis; the nephrotic syndrome is what is meant by the term nephrosis.

Nephrostomy: the operation of making an artificial opening into the pelvis of the kidney in order to drain it.

Nephrotomy: the operation of cutting into the kidney to remove stones or for any other reason.

'Nerves': a popular term for neurosis (q.v.), which has nothing to do with the nerves.

Nervous Diseases: diseases affecting the structure and therefore the function of the nervous system. The word is often used in a confusing sense as a euphemism for mental diseases which may not have very much to do with the nervous system. A physician who specializes in nervous diseases in the proper sense of the term is a neurologist, and one who specializes in the study of mental afflictions is a psychiatrist; one who studies the normal operation of the mind, especially by a study of the behaviour, is a psychologist. The diseases of the nervous system are discussed under their several headings, and for psychiatric conditions *see* Mental Illness, Neurosis, etc.

Nervous System: divided into the central nervous system, which includes the brain and the spinal cord, the peripheral nervous system, and the autonomic nervous system which comprises the sympathetic and parasympathetic systems.
Central nervous system: The brain, which is contained in the skull, is divided into cerebrum, cerebellum and brain stem. Together with the spinal cord it is made up of neurones – nerve cells having very long processes by which they interconnect – and the cells of the neuroglia, the supporting tissue. The central nervous system weighs 1.5 kg. The structure is of the utmost complexity, and no attempt will be made here to describe it in any detail; it is a matter for specialists. Roughly speaking the brain is the seat of consciousness and the originator of the nervous impulses upon which the life of the body depends. If the brain is destroyed the man cannot survive, a self-evident fact which has become very important since artificial hearts, lungs and kidneys came into common use and techniques of transplanting organs emerged from the laboratories into operating

theatres (*see* Death). The nature of consciousness and the
philosophical basis of behaviour are so little understood that
it is better to confine any discussion of the central nervous
system to observed facts, and to keep them simple.

ANATOMY: the brain has an outer cortex or rind which is
grey; it covers a mass of white matter, which forms the bulk
of the brain, and has buried deep in it the basal ganglia and
the thalamus, large areas of grey matter which are cell
relay stations and have many intricate connections with
each other and the cortex. The bulk of the brain is formed
by the cerebral hemispheres; below them emerges the brain
stem, and to the rear of the brain stem is the cerebellum.
The brain stem is continuous with the spinal cord. Very
roughly, the cortex of the cerebral hemispheres, which is
convoluted like a walnut so that its surface area is greater
than is apparent, contains the cell bodies, while the white
matter is made up of connecting fibres and supporting
tissue. Inside the brain are cavities called ventricles, which
are normally full of cerebrospinal fluid, formed inside them
by masses of small blood vessels (the choroid plexuses).
There are two lateral ventricles, one inside each cerebral
hemisphere, and between and below them is the third
ventricle, which connects above with the two lateral
ventricles and below through a passage called the aqueduct
with another mid-line ventricle, the fourth. From the fourth
ventricle the cerebro-spinal fluid is discharged into the
subarachnoid space to flow up over the surface of the brain
and down over the spinal cord. The brain is covered by three
membranes, the dura, arachnoid and pia, and it derives its
blood supply from the carotid and vertebral arteries which
join together to make up a remarkable arterial ring at the
base of the brain called the circle of Willis, through which
the major cerebral arteries communicate with each other.
The veins of the brain drain into large venous spaces in the
dura mater called venous sinuses, which conduct the blood
out of the skull into the internal jugular veins of the neck.
From the brain stem emerge the 12 cranial nerves, and from
the spinal cord in the vertebral column originate 31 pairs of
mixed nerves which run to all parts of the body.

FUNCTION: sense organs in the skin, muscles and joints, and
the internal organs, as well as the organs of sight, hearing
and smell, set up impulses when they are stimulated which

are carried by sensory nerves to the brain through the spinal column or the cranial nerves. Some of the impulses are recognized in consciousness through mechanisms which are only partially understood, and some without rising to the conscious level set in progress reflex responses. (Reflex pathways, connections between the sensory and motor nerves, occur in the spinal cord as well as higher in the brain.) The result is that stimuli acting upon the sensory system result consciously or unconsciously in observable action. Impulses travel back along the motor nerves to set in motion muscles (or to stop the motion of muscles). In a primitive organism the process is fairly obvious – poke it and it moves – but the complexity of man will sustain as many theories as there are brains to form them. Nevertheless, it is useful to regard the brain as functioning on more than one level – the lower, the old brain, regulating the mechanical and vegetative functions of the body, and the higher, the new brain, being the seat of the intellect. The cerebral hemispheres may be thought of as being essential to the functioning of the intellect, and the middle and the base of the brain as being essential for the processes of life. The cerebral hemispheres spend a good deal of their time in keeping the 'old brain' in check.

Autonomic nervous system. A system of nerves that carries impulses to and from the internal organs, blood vessels and glands of the body. It has two components, separated according to their anatomy and function, called the sympathetic and parasympathetic systems. The parasympathetic nerves emerge from the head and tail ends of the nervous system – through the cranial nerves and the sacral nerves – and find their way all over the body, while the sympathetic nerves emerge from the spinal cord between the first thoracic and upper lumbar segments. The sympathetic fibres form a chain of ganglia, or relay stations, beside the spinal column on both sides of the body, from which connections pass to the sweat glands of the skin, erector muscles of the hairs, the heart, lungs, intestines and other internal organs and the blood vessels. Both systems are regulated by the brain but the manner of their central connection is far from clear. The function of the sympathetic system is to prepare the body for action – to stiffen the sinews and summon up the blood. The function of the parasympathetic system is the opposite.. It has been said that it corresponds to the state of an old man after dinner – sleepy, slow and snoring.

No satisfactory model of the brain exists; although its activity is accompanied by changes of electrical potential this does not mean it works by electricity, and the analogies of telephone exchange and computer leave many of its functions unexplained. In general, attempts to explain the action of the central nervous system on physiological grounds end up by postulating a 'biological computer', and those founded on psychology seem to imply that there is a 'little man inside'. *See* Spinal Cord.

Nettle-rash: *see* Urticaria.

Neuralgia: a term implying pain along the course of a nerve. Usually nothing abnormal can be seen, but sometimes there is evidence of mild inflammation in a nerve or ganglion, and sometimes there has been a preceding attack of herpes zoster. The term is not precise except when it is applied to trigeminal neuralgia, a disease which has a well-defined course. The cause of this condition is not understood, but it occurs in age and is not seen before the fifties.

SYMPTOMS OF TRIGEMINAL NEURALGIA: attacks of severe paroxysmal pain start on one side of the face in one of the divisions or branches of the trigeminal nerve, the sensory nerve of the face. The first division of the nerve supplies the eye, the forehead and the front of the head; the second division supplies the cheek and the upper jaw, and the third supplies the lower part of the face and the lower jaw. The pain comes in spasms that last less than a minute, and during the spasm the victim screws his face up, often cries out and tries to shield the affected part with his hand although in most cases he cannot bear to touch it. The pain is set off by various stimuli; a draught of cold air, blowing the nose, eating, washing the face – the disease may sometimes be recognized because the affected side of the face is discoloured and unshaven. The pain spreads as the disease progresses from one division of the trigeminal nerve into the next. At first the pains come at infrequent intervals, and there may be remissions of the disease lasting months, but the progress of the condition is steady and the attacks start to strike at decreasing intervals. The agonized contortions of the face during a paroxysm of pain have given the disease its alternative name, tic douloureux.

TREATMENT: phenytoin sodium (Epanutin) or carbamazepine (Tegretol) may be tried with success, although a sharp look-out must be kept for signs of adverse reactions in old people to carbamazepine, for they may take the drug in doses greater than advised and develop nausea, vomiting and skin rashes. If drug therapy becomes ineffective, the root of the nerve can be divided surgically inside the skull – an operation which most patients stand well – or alcohol can be injected into it. This last procedure is often very useful, but it is not as reliable as the operation.

Neurasthenia: an old-fashioned term which can be very useful in filling up medical certificates when the doctor wishes to avoid mentioning the fact that a patient is neurotic, a word which has social implications.

Neurectomy: the operation of removing part of a nerve.

Neurilemma: the thin covering which surrounds nerve fibres.

Neuritis: inflammation of a nerve. The condition referred to sometimes as neuritis, but more often as polyneuritis or, preferably, polyneuropathy – for strictly speaking the condition is not an inflammation – is a change in the state of the nerves resulting in weakness, loss of the reflexes, and changes of sensation.

CAUSE: it has many causes, which include diphtheria and diabetes mellitus, poisoning with insecticides, mercury, lead, arsenic, alcohol, and isoniazid (the drug used to treat tuberculosis), and vitamin deficiency – in particular deficiency of the Vitamin B complex. Cancer of the lung also produces polyneuropathy.

SYMPTOMS: numbness and tingling in the hands, legs and feet, with cramp in the calf, followed by weakness, clumsiness especially in walking, and wasting of the muscles of the legs and the hands. In diphtheria patients develop double vision before they find the arms and legs abnormal, and they may have difficulty in swallowing.

TREATMENT: this is the treatment of the primary condition and the provision of a good diet rich in vitamins, especially of the B complex. It is very important that the affected muscles should not be allowed to stretch and that the joints should be kept moving, if necessary being moved passively, to prevent them becoming stiff.

Neurofibroma: a tumour formed from the connective tissue surrounding the nerve fibres.

Neuroglia: the supporting and connective tissue of the central nervous system.

Neurology: the specialty which deals with the nervous system in disease and in health. It does not deal with mental diseases that have no known anatomical or physiological basis.

Neuroma: tumour of a nerve. There is some difference of opinion about the precise origin of the cells that form the tumours found along the course of nerves and nerve roots, and so although tumours grow from the connective tissue supporting the nerve fibres, and not from the nerve fibres themselves, they are known by a variety of names – neuroma, neurinoma, neurofibroma, neurilemmoma, Schwannoma. Some neuromata are single, but in some cases they are found all over the body in association with patches of brown pigmentation. This condition is called von Recklinghausen's disease. The tumours are usually innocuous, but when they grow on the auditory nerve in the skull they not only make the patient deaf but may by pressure on the brain stem produce grave illness and incapacity.

Neurone: the nerve cell, with its processes long and short. Sometimes the term is used to mean the long process of a nerve cell which forms a nerve fibre.

Neurosis: mental diseases are either (*a*) physical diseases with 'mental' symptoms, or (*b*) forms of social maladjustment especially in the sphere of interpersonal relations which, of course, may produce real or apparent physical symptoms. The neuroses are in group (*b*). Group (*a*) requires medical treatment, and group (*b*) a prolonged process of adjustment and analysis which can in some cases be avoided by the use of drugs which suppress the symptoms, although this is unlikely to lead to permanent results.

The neuroses are the result of social maladjustment learned in the individual's early life with heredity as a factor; but although neuroses often run in families they are usually handed on by unconscious training rather than heredity; for example it is hardly surprising that obsessional neurosis runs in families as no habit is more readily acquired than the obsessional one. Some of the factors thought to cause neurosis may be briefly summarized as follows:

1. In Freudian theory (*see* Psychoanalysis) the main cause is the difficulty in controlling primitive impulses by the more socialized ones, for example neurosis manifesting itself as fear of the intentions of men who might be found hiding under the bed is a clear indication of an unsatisfactorily repressed wish on the part of an elderly spinster.

2. In the theory of Alfred Adler (as also in that of Freud) an important part is played by the individual's desire for significance or power and the fear of being shown up. A neurotic in this view is a person who, worried by his feelings of inferiority, tries to cover them up or use them as an 'illness' to get out of difficult situations.

3. In more recent schools of thought the neurotic's failures in personal relationships have been emphasized; neurosis is simply the expression of a wrong attitude to such relationships. The neuroses are divided into the following rough categories: *Anxiety states* in which symptoms are anxiety, which takes the form of generalized apprehension without apparent cause; the appearance of the physical concomitants of fear, for example palpitation, nameless dread, attacks of breathlessness and sweating; the thought of going mad; tremor of the hands and body; the appearance of phobias which are irrational fears (claustrophobia in enclosed spaces, agoraphobia in open ones, fear of animals, heights, crossing the road, etc.). In *conversion hysteria* the main symptom is an apparently physical one without physical basis (for example paralysis, blindness, deafness, inability to write, etc.). This is now rather rare, and furnishes an example of the unconscious duplicity of neurosis, since these naïve physical manifestations have disappeared with increasing popular

knowledge of medicine and the realization that paralyses and the rest are not popular when no physical disease is there to account for them. *Obsessional states* manifest themselves as the compulsion to carry out or think certain (usually absurd) actions or thoughts, for example touching the lamp-posts one passes, counting numbers which are invested with a magical significance. In all these there exists the idea 'if I do this then . . .' or 'if I don't do this then . . .' and some event is supposed to follow for better or worse. To these may be added the *personality disorders* in which relationships with others are disrupted to an extent which causes inconvenience to the individual or his associates (for example the sort of woman who always 'by fate' marries the wrong man), and the *psychosomatic diseases* where tension, perhaps at a much deeper level, leads finally to a serious and sometimes fatal physical disease (for example duodenal ulcer).

TREATMENT: the treatment of the neuroses or psychoneuroses is, by choice, psychotherapy, which gives the patient a chance to look himself in the face and understand his problems with a view to dealing with them. He must also understand his problems in relation to those of others; for we are all neurotic in varying degrees and it is simply a medical convenience to describe as neurotic someone who is a trouble to himself or others. Many gross neurotics are overlooked because their failing is in a direction approved of in general by society; thus it is neurotic and a nuisance for a housewife to keep on cleaning unnecessarily or for a man to think of nothing but money and his work, but although these types need a psychiatrist's help as much as anyone else who is neurotic, they are often commended for their behaviour. There is no such thing as a nerve tonic, nor does the neurotic need rest or a holiday, unless it is of such nature as to take him away from the task he is busy evading through his illness, when he will naturally recover almost instantaneously until the day he has to return. Sedatives and the tranquillizing drugs have some effect upon symptoms but do not alter the fundamental state.

Neutropenia: a fall in the number of neutrophilic white cells circulating in the blood to an abnormally low level. *See* Leucocyte.

Nevus: term applied to a birthmark consisting of blood vessels or pigmented cells. The blood vessel naevus is called a haemangioma, and the pigmented naevus a melanoma or mole. A common form of naevus is the 'port-wine' stain, which persists throughout life, but may be treated by plastic surgery. *See* Birthmark.

Nicotinamide: the amide of nicotinic acid.

Nicotine: an alkaloid with pharmacological actions on the conduction processes of nerve impulses.

Nicotinic Acid: part of the Vitamin B complex; it is essential to life and health, for a deficiency in the diet leads to pellagra. This disease is characterized by dermatitis, diarrhoea and dementia, and is associated with the cultivation and exclusive use of maize, which is a poor source of nicotinic acid. The vitamin is present in wheat, but is removed during the processes of making fine flour, just as it is removed from rice during the process of polishing. This is well understood, and nicotinamide is added to finely ground flour. A diet of polished rice does not produce severe cases of pellagra, for rice contains the amino acid tryptophan from which the body can make nicotinic acid.

Niehan's Cell Therapy: Dr Niehan's particular form of treatment is based on the belief that if any organ of the body is not functioning properly it can be revitalized by the injection of fresh cells taken from the corresponding organ of a young or preferably unborn animal. The new healthy foetal cells, it is claimed, inevitably find their way to the affected part of the body. There is said to exist a natural affinity between the embryonic heart cells, for example, of a chicken, mouse or man, In practice, the organs are collected at the local slaughter-house where a pregnant animal is killed, and the required parts extracted from the foetus. They are then rushed as quickly as possible to the patient, passed through a sieve to reduce them to a 'cellular state' and, suspended in a normal salt solution, injected into him.

In spite of the many famous people who are said to have benefited from this method, it is rejected by most orthodox medical bodies; most medical men believe that the whole rationale is highly dubious, and that sometimes the treatment may be dangerous.

Night Blindness: caused by lack of Vitamin A in the diet, which shows itself as an inability to see in dim light although the vision in bright light is normal. The visual purple of the retina is built up from the vitamin. *See* Rhodopsin.

Nightmares: unpleasant dreams which, if they are very frequent or severe, may be an indication that the victim should consult his physician, who may send him to the psychiatrist.

Night Sweats: characteristic of tuberculosis, and found in various low fevers.

Nikethamide: (Coramine). A substance used to stimulate the respiratory centre. It is usually given by injection; an overdose may set up convulsions. It has no action on the heart, but in grave emergency an intravenous injection of 2 ml may be used to sober up a fit patient who is dead drunk.

Nipples: *see* Breast.

Nit: a louse egg. *See* Louse, Parasites.

Nitrites: nitrites and organic nitrates have an important action in dilating the blood vessels. The most commonly used compounds are amyl nitrite, a liquid supplied in a capsule which the patient breaks to inhale the drug for a very quick effect; glyceryl trinitrate, which is put up in tablets to be sucked; and sorbide nitrate, which is weaker but has a longer effect. The drugs are used in treating coronary thrombosis and angina pectoris.

Nitrofurantoin: (Furadantin). A drug used in the treatment of infections of the urinary tract. It is active against the Gram-negative organisms, but not uncommonly produces the side effects of nausea and vomiting.

Nitrogen: an almost inert gas, not able to support life (although its compounds make life possible), which makes up about four-fifths of the air we breathe. It is soluble in the blood, and when it has been dissolved under increased pressure during diving, injudicious speed in rising to the surface may decrease the pressure too quickly so that the gas forms bubbles in the blood and causes various severe symptoms. Sudden decompression in high-flying aircraft can have the same effect. *See* Caisson Disease.

Nitroglycerin: Glyceryl trinitrate. *See* Nitrites.

Nitrous Oxide Gas: the first general anaesthetic. It is more of an analgesic than an anaesthetic, a property which makes it very useful when used for short operations like opening an abscess or extracting a tooth, for the patient does not have to be made deeply unconscious. It is difficult to produce general anaesthesia with nitrous oxide gas and air without depriving the patient of oxygen, so that if the gas is used for any length of time it must be given with oxygen. It is often used in combination with volatile anaesthetic drugs and oxygen, the proportions being chosen to give the effect needed. *See* Anaesthetics.

Nocturnal Enuresis: *see* Enuresis.

Non-union: a very serious state in a fractured bone, caused by infection, too much traction, interference with the blood supply, poor immobilization, or disease of the bone. Treatment is difficult and long.

Non-viable: not capable of independent life; used of the foetus under 28 weeks.

Noradrenaline: (Norepinephrine). The substance believed to be responsible for the transmission of impulses in the sympathetic nervous system. *See* Nervous System.

Normoblast: the immature red blood cell, which still has a nucleus. As it matures and enters the circulation the nucleus disappears in normal circumstances, but in conditions in which new red cells are being formed at a great rate normoblasts are seen on examination of the blood.

Nose, Diseases of: tonsils and adenoids, sinusitis, and

epistaxis or nose bleeding are dealt with separately, and here it is only necessary to mention polypi, foreign bodies in the nose, and loss of the sense of smell (anosmia). *Polypi* are soft jelly-like masses usually found in the area of the middle turbinate bone. They are shiny and grey and arise from an overgrowth of the mucous membrane due to chronic inflammation. The main symptom is an awareness that the nose is always blocked, but the condition can only be diagnosed for certain after an examination by the doctor, who will recommend a simple operation for removal. *Foreign bodies* are often found in the noses of children and sometimes adults. They should be removed by the doctor if blowing the nose will not dislodge them; poking in the nose should be strongly discouraged. *Anosmia* or loss of the sense of smell is always present in any condition which causes blockage of the nose; it is also present in some cases of fracture of the skull affecting the olfactory nerves, and in other conditions including intracerebral tumours and the common cold.

Nosology: the scientific classification of diseases.

Notifiable Diseases: those diseases which by law must be notified to the Local Authorities or the Board of Health.

No-touch Technique: a technique used in the operating theatre particularly by orthopaedic and neurological surgeons, but applicable to any sort of surgery. It is designed to cut down the risk of passing infection from the surgeon and his staff to the operation site, for in these branches of surgery infection of the operation wound and underlying structures is a disaster. In essentials, neither the surgeon nor anybody else touches the 'business' end of the instruments that are to be used, the ligatures and needles, the swabs, or the tissues upon which the operation is being carried out. The technique is quite easy with practice, and is well worth using, for it is known that however careful the surgeon is in preparing his hands he cannot sterilize them, and surgical gloves often develop small punctures during an operation.

Novarsenobenzol: Neosalvarsan or neoarsphenamine (q.v.).

Novobiocin: an antibiotic introduced in 1955. It can be taken by mouth and is active against staphylococci, preventing their multiplication but not killing the organisms, which easily develop an immunity to it. Its use is further limited by the side effects it may produce, which include urticaria and diarrhoea, and it is only prescribed when specially indicated by sensitivity tests.

Nuclein: a substance formed from the breakdown of nucleoprotein. It has been used in medicine to try to stimulate the formation of white cells in agranulocytosis, a dangerous condition in which they are absent or very scarce in the blood.

Nucleus: the body inside a cell which contains within a membrane the sex chromatin, the nucleoplasm and the nucleolus. This last is a concentration of R.N.A. (ribonucleic acid, q.v.); the bulk of the nucleus is taken up by D.N.A., which controls the formation of R.N.A. It is only when the cell is ready to divide that chromosomes become visible inside the nucleus (*see* Cell). Another meaning of nucleus is a collection of nerve cells with a special function in the central nervous system. In chemistry nucleus means the central basic framework of the molecule of a class of compounds.

Nucleus Pulposus: the soft centre of the intervertebral disc, formed by white and yellow connective tissue fibres and surrounded by the annulus fibrosus. *See* Slipped Disc.

Nullipara: a woman who has not borne children.

Numbness: may result from damage or disease of the nervous system or of the blood vessels.

Nursing: as we know it today the profession of nursing dates from Florence Nightingale and the Crimean War, although in quite early times there were hospitals for the sick poor in Egypt, India, Greece and Rome. The nursing system as an organized state of affairs and a branch of medical treatment originated with the deacons and deaconesses of the early Christian Church, and from the fourth century onwards hospitals were managed by the clergy, and male and female nurses were recruited from monastic orders; in England the oldest surviving institutions are St Thomas's and St Bartholomew's hospitals. It was not until the Reformation that nursing came to be separated in some measure from religion, but properly trained nurses, as contrasted with those who simply learned their work by experience in the wards, are a creation of the mid-nineteenth century. The system developed in Germany under Pastor Fliedner, whose institute at Kaiserswerth was founded in 1836 and was the training-school of Florence Nightingale. Two years later an institute was founded in Philadelphia, and in another two Elizabeth Fry had founded one in London, the nurses of which were trained at Guy's and St Thomas's hospitals. The appalling conditions of the Crimean War to which Florence Nightingale brought a band of trained nurses led to new reforms in nursing and played a large part in raising the profession in the public esteem.

Nursing is usually thought of as a feminine profession, but the number of male nurses has greatly increased in recent years.

Nuts: a valuable substitute for meat in a vegetarian diet, for they contain not less than 50% of vegetable fats and oils.

Nux Vomica: obtained from the dried seed of Strychnos nux-vomica, a West Indian tree. It contains strychnine and is used in small doses as a tonic, for it stimulates the appetite.

Nyctalopia: night-blindness.

Nystagmus: a condition in which the eyeballs show an involuntary rapid movement from side to side, or less commonly up and down, or a rotary motion which is a combination of the two.

Nystatin: named after the New York State Department of Health, nystatin is a drug obtained from the fungus Streptomyces noursei, active against fungus infections. It is most effective when it can be applied directly to the infected area; it is not absorbed from the intestines. It is particularly useful in treating infections caused by Candida albicans (q.v.).

O

Oath: for Oath of Hippocrates, *see under* Hippocrates.

Obesity: in the strict sense there is only one cause of being overweight: eating too much (or eating too much of the wrong kind of food) so that the intake of calories is greater than the output. This is not invalidated by the fact that glandular factors may play a part or that there are some people who can eat as much as they like without becoming overweight since their basal metabolic rate increases to deal with the excess; for the overweight person's diet is unsuitable for him or her in the circumstances. It is now recognized that a major factor in the production of obesity is a psychological one, and that some individuals can be addicted to food (and especially to sweet and starchy foods) as others are addicted to drink. In practice dieting means taking a low-calorie diet high in protein and low in fat and carbohydrate. Such a diet would be somewhat as follows: coffee or tea with milk but no sugar at breakfast, accompanied by crispbread or starch-reduced rolls and a small amount of butter but no jam or marmalade and no brown or white bread or toast. At lunch, grilled lean steak, grilled fish, or an egg dish and salad followed by jellies or fruit or crispbread and cheese – but no potatoes, peas or beans (with the exception of French beans). The evening meal may consist of grilled or steamed fish, clear soup, cheese and fruit, but there must be no fried food or sweets at any time. The basic principles of this diet are obvious: lean meat, non-fatty fish, eggs, fruit, crispbread or starch-reduced rolls but no fried foods, fat meat or fish, bread, potatoes, sweets or cakes. Small amounts of butter and quite a lot of milk are permissible.

This is a conventional diet, but of recent years a new theory has sprung up which takes the view that fat people are those who have some innate difficulty in dealing with carbohydrates and that a diet which cuts out carbohydrates almost entirely and allows as much fats and protein as desired – in fact the more fat the better – is indicated. It is pointed out that people such as the Eskimos who live on a fat-high diet do not become overweight whereas those whose diet has a high carbohydrate content very well may unless their basal metabolic rate is capable of increasing to deal with it. A specimen diet of this type (which has proved very successful in suitable cases) is as follows: a large breakfast of bacon, eggs, kidneys, etc. fried in plenty of fat, or kippers, ham, or Continental sausage, starch-reduced rolls and butter, but no jam or marmalade. Midday meal of steak with fat or any other fat meat, omelette or Continental sausage, salad but no potatoes, tomatoes as desired, French beans or other green vegetables, high-fat cheese (cream, Camembert, Wensleydale, etc.), apple or orange. Main evening meal as for breakfast and lunch combined. Cheese, tomato, water, are unrestricted and dry alcoholic drinks may be taken, for example dry sherry, dry white wine, gin and bitters, but no beer, rum or sweet wines or liqueurs. The great benefit of this diet is that it works, that it can be carried on without discomfort even after the weight has been reduced, and that it is safe – although it is not for people who are suffering from chronic illness or whose digestion is poor. According to this view the total intake of calories is less relevant than the form in which they are taken and the conventional slimming diet is only a form of slow starvation. To be avoided are bread and root vegetables, potatoes, anything from the baker's or confectioner's, soups other than clear soups, beer and sweet drinks. Leading authorities on nutrition do not deny that this diet works but hold that it is, in fact, merely a low-calorie diet since those who eat much fat (*a*) do not eat a great deal of it and (*b*) do not desire carbohydrates.

Obsession: *see* Neurosis.

Obstetrics: that branch of medicine concerned with midwifery.

Obstruction: a blockage of the intestines.
CAUSE: it may come about as the result of a tumour, inflammatory processes, by the twisting of the gut upon itself (volvulus) or round adhesions, or because the gut is caught in a hernial sac.

SYMPTOMS: acute obstruction shows itself by colicky pain in the abdomen, vomiting, constipation, distension of the abdomen and collapse.

TREATMENT: the patient's condition is improved as much as possible by gastric suction and intravenous fluids, for the incessant vomiting results in loss of salts as well as water, and then the abdomen is opened and whatever operation proves necessary is carried out. In cases of acute obstruction the hernial orifices in the groin and the upper part of the thigh must always be inspected carefully, for if an obstructed hernia is present there is also strangulation (obstruction to the blood supply of the gut), and unless operation is speedy gangrene may develop. In chronic obstruction there is a place for conservative treatment. The patient is observed carefully while the gastric suction and intravenous fluids continue, and the effect of an enema may be tried. If flatus or faeces are passed, then it may be thought that the obstruction is incomplete; but operation must only be withheld while the patient is making obvious progress. Operations for the relief of obstruction include short-circuits, colostomies, and the removal of part of the intestines, but it is rare to be able to perform a definitive operation in cases where there is a tumour. Usually the obstruction is first relieved, and the tumour removed at a later time when the patient's general condition is satisfactory.

Occiput: the back of the head.

Occupational Diseases: few trades or even professions are free from the risk of specific diseases, although until recently the main concern of the practitioner of industrial medicine has been with the manual worker. It was with the manual worker in mind that Paracelsus in 1567 published his monograph on *Miners' Sickness and Other Miners' Diseases*; possibly the first specialist in industrial medicine was the Italian Bernardino Ramazzini (1633–1714), who wrote the textbook *Diseases of Tradesmen*. But today, two hundred years after the beginning of the Industrial Revolution, the scope of the specialist is much wider, for he can argue that the director's duodenal ulcer or coronary thrombosis is as much an occupational disease as caisson sickness. Of course, one may play safe with the observation that many people

557

may get a duodenal ulcer who have never worked at all, whereas caisson disease can only be contracted in a diving bell, but the modern industrial medical officer rarely takes this attitude; for the fact is that a better understanding of 'tradesmen's diseases' has played a large part in wiping them out.

Some of the more obvious conditions may be mentioned here, taking the apparently safest professions first – and what could be safer and healthier than working on the land? The agricultural worker may develop epithelioma or cancer of the skin from exposure to sun and weather, actinomycosis (a serious fungus infection) from working with grain, anthrax from working with horses or hides, tuberculosis from cattle, spirochaetal jaundice from working in muddy ditches, and an endless number of aches and pains from physical stress. Pet-shop dealers may develop ornithosis, telegraphists cramps, workers with cosmetics dermatitis, housewives housemaid's knee, clergymen and politicians laryngitis, doctors angina pectoris from prolonged mental stress (although the misguided will say that a diet rich in cholesterol is the main cause). The more specifically industrial diseases include the following: caisson disease in divers, cataract in glassblowers, and spirochaetal jaundice in miners and sewer workers (who may also be affected with hookworm or ankylostomiasis). Poisons employed in various trades which may harm workers include arsenic, antimony, mercury, lead, nickel, and such non-metallic substances as phosphorus, carbon disulphide, carbon tetrachloride (in cleaners and dyers), the coal-tar products and various insecticides and pesticides. Other very important occupational diseases are silicosis, asbestosis, byssinosis, dermatitis, chrome ulceration, cancer induced by irritant chemicals and the consequences of overexposure to radioactive substances in medical work and atomic research stations.

Most large concerns now have their own medical and welfare workers, whose work extends from the prevention of physical hazards to the worker or hazards to the consumer (for example in food factories) to the application of industrial psychology in respect of particular tasks in a given environment and morale in general. The factory medical officer is not exploiting his full potential if he restricts his work solely to the physical hazards facing workers, for at the best he can be a liaison point between workers and management acting on his knowledge that nothing which harms the worker physically or psychologically can be good for either the firm or its customers in the long run.

Occupational Therapy: occupational therapy originated in mental hospitals as a means of taking the patient's mind off his own problems and rehabilitating him into society, but today it takes all forms from the aspect of designing work to exercise specific groups of muscles to the encouragement of free expression painting in psychiatric cases which may give insights into the patient's problems. Much is being learned not only about specific skills but also about the emotional and social aspects of employment from hobbies to hard work.

Oculentum: an ointment for the eye.

Oedema: *see* Edema.

Oedipus Complex: Oedipus, a famous king in Greek mythology, was brought up by a foster parent. Later in life he killed his real father and married his mother. On finding out what he had done, he blinded himself. The Oedipus complex is the sexual desire of a son for his mother.

Oesophagus: *see* Esophagus.

Oestradiol: *see* Estradiol.

Oestrogen: *see* Estrogen.

Oidium Albicans: an older name for Candida albicans, the organism that causes thrush.

Ointment: a preparation for external application, semi-solid and usually medicated.

Olecranon: the tip of the elbow.

Olfactory Nerve: the nerve which conveys the sensation of smell from the nose to the brain. It is the first cranial nerve,

559

and it runs from the interior of the nose through the cribriform plate, a part of the ethmoid bone perforated by many small holes, to relay in the olfactory bulbs which pass back into the brain. It may be damaged in head injuries involving a fracture of the ethmoid bone, or by pressure from tumours of the brain or the meninges. The sense of smell is then lost.

Oliguria: the passage of small amounts of urine.

Omentum: the apron of peritoneum containing fat which hangs down in front of the intestines.

Omphalos: the umbilicus.

Onchocerca: a filarial worm that infests the skin and subcutaneous tissues and may cause blindness (African river blindness). It is found in Africa and Central America, and the vector is Simulium, the blackfly or buffalo gnat. *See* Filariasis, Worms.

Oncology: the term for the study of tumours.

Onychogryphosis: gross thickening, overgrowth and deformity of a toe nail due to chronic inflammation or to injury of the nail bed. The treatment is removal; if the deformity recurs, the nail bed must be cut away.

Onychomycosis: ringworm of the nails.

Oophorectomy: the removal of an ovary.

Oophoritis: inflammation of the ovary. It may be due to salpingitis, other infections in the pelvis such as appendicitis, or mumps. There is discomfort and pain, the ovary may become sterile, and excessive menstruation occurs. The treatment for this condition is rest and antibiotics; in severe cases an operation may have to be carried out.

Operable: term applied by the surgeon to cases in which an operation is technically possible and has a good chance of curing the condition.

Ophthalmia: inflammation of the eye or the conjunctiva; the term is usually only applied to severe infections, for example ophthalmia neonatorum, which is gonorrhoeal conjunctivitis of the newborn.

Opthalmic: to do with the eye.

Ophthalmoplegia: paralysis affecting one or both eyes. It is *external* when the muscles moving the eye from outside the eyeball are affected, *internal* when there is interference with the movements of the pupil or lens.

Ophthalmoscope: an instrument for looking at the back of the interior of the eyeball. It has a system of lenses through which the examiner looks along the path of a beam of light projected from the instrument. Ophthalmoscopy – the act of examining the back of the eye – can also be carried out if the examiner wears a head-mirror with a small hole in the centre, through which he looks. A lamp is placed to one side of the patient's head, and the examiner adjusts the mirror so that the reflected light enters the pupil of the eye. He holds a lens between his eye and the patient's. The doctor often puts eyedrops into the eye to be examined to dilate the pupil and make the examination more effective, and these may take a little time to wear off.

Opisthotonus: the position assumed in certain forms of seizure where the tensed body curves backwards with the spine and hips fully extended. It is characteristic of tetanus and strychnine poisoning, and is the position which is taken up if all the muscles of the body contract, for the extensor muscles are more powerful than the flexors except in the arms, which are flexed at the elbow. In extreme cases the patient rests on the back of his head and his heels.

Opium: the effects of opium are largely due to its content of morphine, so the two drugs will be dealt with together. Opium is the dried juice of the unripe seed capsule of the poppy Papaver somniferum. It contains about 10% of morphine as well as codeine, thebaine, papaverine and narcotine. Papaverine has no analgesic activity, but is a powerful relaxant of smooth muscle, and narcotine is used

561

in cough medicines. The actions of morphine are: it calms those suffering from pain and diminishes the pain felt; it brings sleep; it relieves anxiety; it depresses the respiratory centre; it depresses the cough centre; it may produce nausea and vomiting; and it quickly produces physical as well as mental dependence. It also produces constipation, spasm of the small air passages in the lungs, and retention of urine. The pupil of the eye is contracted by the drug, and an overdose depresses the breathing so far that the patient may die. The antidote is nalorphine. Morphine is used in medical practice for a variety of reasons, but always with caution because of the possibility of drug dependence. Opium is one of the most valuable drugs we have and one of the oldest; in the last century laudanum was as commonly used as aspirin is today, and many men have used opium freely and been none the worse for it. Unfortunately this is not always true, and we may deny the truth of De Quincey's words, 'Thou hast the keys of Paradise, oh just, subtle and mighty opium!'

Opsonization: antibodies alter the state of antigens so that they are more easily engulfed by the large white cells of the blood and tissue spaces. This process is called opsonization.

Optic Nerve: the second cranial nerve through which sensory impulses travel from the retina of the eye to the brain. It is sometimes the seat of optic atrophy, caused by injury, tumours, drugs, among which are quinine and tobacco, disseminated or multiple sclerosis, and tertiary syphilis. It is affected by increased pressure inside the skull which makes it swollen (the head of the nerve can be seen by ophthalmoscopy as it emerges into the eye), a state called papilloedema. Its function is sometimes partially affected by tumours pressing upon it in its course, and in such cases a careful consideration of the pattern of vision loss may make it possible for the neurologist to locate the tumour accurately.

Oral Contraceptive: *see* Contraception.

Orbit: the bony socket in the skull that contains the eye.

Orchidectomy: removal of the testicle.

Orchidopexy: an operation by which the undescended testicle is fastened in the scrotum, usually carried out when the boy is about 5.

Orchitis: inflammation of the testicle.

Organic Disease: essentially this means structural or chemical disease of the body which can be demonstrated by clinical examination, special investigations such as microscopy, or chemical examination of the blood. It is contrasted with functional disease, in which only the functions of the body are disordered and there is no demonstrable structural or chemical abnormality. 'Functional' was once regarded as synonymous with 'neurotic', but modern opinion holds that functional disease may readily pass into organic disease, as in the psychosomatic conditions.

Organic Substances: roughly speaking, substances which are derived from living matter, or related to compounds found in living matter.

Organo-phosphorus Compounds: these compounds are used as insecticides, and some are in fact so dangerous that they are used as war gases, for they block the action of the enzyme acetylcholinesterase which is essential for the proper functioning of the nervous system. The symptoms of poisoning by the compounds are: weakness, sweating, a slow pulse, excessive secretion of saliva, and spasm of the small air passages of the lungs which may cause wheezing. These symptoms are followed by twitching of the muscles, constriction of the pupils, which may interfere with vision, convulsions and cessation of breathing. Treatment of poisoning: atropine is given by injection, preferably intravenous, in doses of 2 mg every 20 minutes until the pupils dilate, and Pralidoxime is given slowly into the veins, the dose being about 2 g. Recovery is usually complete, but some of the organo-phosphorus compounds, such as tri-orthocresol phosphatex, used as an anti-corrosion agent, can produce lasting damage in the nervous system.

Orgasm: the climax of sexual pleasure accompanied in men by the emission of semen and in women by reaching a height of excitement with contractions of the vagina followed in both cases by a sudden decline in tension. In men failure to reach orgasm or reaching orgasm too soon (premature emission) is a sign of partial impotence which will probably disappear in time as the couple become adjusted to each other, although the condition may need to be referred for advice. On the whole, few men fail to reach orgasm on some occasion or another. In the case of women the situation is rather different and in Britain and America few women reach orgasm every time and some – perhaps as many as 60–70% – never do so at all. The main reason for mentioning this is that whereas in Victorian days and even earlier women were thought to be licentious if they showed any sign of sexual pleasure, in our own day the attitude has been entirely reversed and, as every doctor knows, many women worry themselves sick because they either obtain little pleasure or do not achieve orgasm. Complete frigidity needs expert advice, but the failure to reach orgasm while still obtaining some pleasure is perfectly compatible with a happy married relationship. It is society which makes many women feel 'bad' in these circumstances by causing them to feel that there is something shameful about not being completely sexually satisfied. Society is wrong, and it is time we grew out of the silly idea derived from the early sex reformers (many of whom, like Havelock Ellis and Marie Stopes, themselves had serious marital difficulties) that sexual technique is everything in a happy marriage. Many couples who have orgasms every time end up by divorcing each other, while the majority who do not achieve in most cases perfectly satisfying relationships. Sex and affection can never be entirely separated from each other in marriage, but affection and mutual understanding are far more important than sex. *See* Sex and Sexual Problems.

Oriental Plague: *see* Plague.

Oriental Sore: *see* Kala-azar.

Ornithosis: a disease which, like psittacosis, is carried by birds and can infect man.

CAUSE: micro-organisms called Bedsoniae, which are larger than viruses but smaller than bacteria. (Bedsoniae also cause trachoma and lymphogranuloma venereum.) In ornithosis the organisms are carried by pigeons, sea-birds and domestic poultry; psittacosis is spread by parrots and budgerigars, although the regulations affecting their importation have almost stamped the disease out in the United Kingdom.

SYMPTOMS: incubation period ten days. The patient begins to feel generally ill, and has a headache and loss of appetite. There is a moderate fever, and a cough may develop, for the lungs often become inflamed.

TREATMENT: the Bedsoniae are, unlike viruses, sensitive to tetracycline and other antibiotics.

Orthodontics: that part of dentistry which is concerned with treating irregularity and inaccurate opposition of the upper and lower teeth.

Orthopaedics: that branch of surgery concerned with the treatment of diseases, injuries and deformities of the bones, joints and muscles.

Orthopnoea: term applied to the state of a patient who is unable to breathe unless he is sitting up. It is a symptom of severe left heart failure (*see* Heart).

Orthoptics: a method of exercising the eyes in cases where there is a squint, in order to align their axes.

Ossicles: small bones; usually applied to the small bones of the middle ear.

Ossification: the process whereby bones are formed. It takes place by the action of cells called osteoblasts, which are closely related to the cells which form fibrous connective tissue and cartilage. Bone which has been laid down by the osteoblasts is shaped by the action of osteoclasts, cells which can absorb bony tissue, and included in the bony tissue as it is formed are cells called osteocytes, which are responsible for the nutrition of the bone. *See* Bone.

Osteitis: inflammation of bone.

Osteo-arthritis: *see* Rheumatism.

Osteoarthropathy: any disease affecting the bones and joints.

Osteochondritis: (1) An inflammation of the bone and cartilage. (2) A change in the centres of growth in the bones of children often referred to as osteochondrosis. This condition leads to necrosis or degeneration in the affected bone which may produce grave deformity unless it is recognised and treated. The condition affects various bones, and according to its site is known by various different names: in the tuberosity of the tibia it is called Osgood-Schlatter's disease, in the head of the femur or thigh-bone Legg-Calvé-Perthes' disease, in the semilunar bone of the wrist Kienböck's disease, and so on. The most important sites are in the head of the femur, where lameness and later arthritis of the hip may ensue, and the vertebrae, where it may produce hunchback or other deformity. (3) Osteochondritis dissicans is a condition in which loose bodies are found in the knee joint, the ankle, elbow and shoulder. It is thought to be due to injury, which makes a small piece of bone underlying the cartilaginous joint surface break away. The condition is found in young people.

Osteochondrosis: *see* under Osteochondritis.

Osteoclast: 1. A cell which is able to absorb bony tissue, and which plays a large part in the shaping of bone according to the lines of stress. Osteoclasts are active after fractures in reshaping the bony tissues roughly laid down by the osteoblasts. *See* Bone.
2. A surgical instrument for fracturing bones.

Osteoclastoma: a tumour of bone which behaves midway between a malignant and a benign tumour. It tends to invade tissues round about it, but rarely forms metastatic deposits in other parts of the body. The treatment is removal of the tumour with the surrounding tissue.

Osteogenesis Imperfecta: also known as Fragilitas ossium, a condition in which the bones are abnormally brittle, the sclera of the eyes blue rather than white, and the ears deaf. The cause is unknown, but the disease may be inherited; in some cases the child dies in the womb.

Osteology: the study of bones.

Osteoma: a benign or simple tumour of bone, which grows on the skull or on the long bones. It is as hard as ivory, and need only be removed if it is ugly or blocking an air sinus or the orifice of the ear, for it does not become malignant.

Osteomalacia: a condition in which the bones are soft.
CAUSE: lack of calcium in the diet or lack of Vitamin D; osteomalacia is virtually adult rickets. It is found principally in the East, in women who are affected during pregnancy.
SYMPTOMS: the bones become grossly deformed, and in particular the pelvis becomes triangular because of pressure exerted by the spine and the two thigh-bones: the deformity may progress to such a degree that childbirth through the natural passages is impossible.
TREATMENT: the correction of the diet. In certain cases the condition follows disease of the kidneys or disease of the parathyroid glands causing loss of calcium: if these conditions are present treatment may not be straightforwardly dietetic.

Osteomyelitis: inflammation of the bone marrow.
CAUSE: the infection may be carried from a distant focus of infection in the bloodstream to the bone, or it may follow an injury in which the bone has been exposed – an open fracture or wound, or an open operation. Poor health and poor nutrition predispose to the disease, which is therefore commoner in the less well-endowed parts of the world and among the poorer people, especially the children. The micro-organism responsible is usually the Staphylococcus aureus.
SYMPTOMS: the disease may be acute or chronic.
1. *Acute.* The affected limb becomes painful, and the area of

567

inflammation is extremely tender. There is fever, and the patient feels generally ill. As the disease progresses a swelling develops over the infected bone, and the skin becomes red.
2. *Chronic.* This type of inflammation is more likely to follow wounds and open fractures than blood-borne infection. There is pain, and much discharge of pus. The course of the disease is irregular, with exacerbations of inflammation and then apparent recovery.

TREATMENT: 1. Antibiotics are given as soon as the condition is diagnosed; if pus has formed the area must be opened up surgically, and if necessary holes drilled into the bone through which the pus can escape. The development of acute osteomyelitis in an open fracture or an operation site is a very dangerous complication. Before antibiotics it often ended in amputation – there are to this day middle-aged men who lack a limb because in World War 2 there were theatres of action in which it was considered better to amputate for an open fracture than to wait until infection cost a life.

2. Chronic osteomyelitis is usually associated with the presence of dead bony tissue or foreign bodies, which may be bullets or shell fragments or plates and screws put in by the orthopaedic surgeon. Dead bony tissue is called a sequestrum, and it must be removed by operation, as must all foreign bodies. The cavity in which the dead tissue is found is curetted and allowed to heal from the bottom, the limb is put in plaster, and antibiotics are given according to the sensitivity of the organisms present.

Osteopathy: 'A complete science of healing based on the normalizing of the body and its functions on the assumption that a structural derangement of skeletal parts known as the "osteopathic lesion" is the significant factor in all disease.' Osteopathy has no connection whatever with manipulative surgery, although its procedures involve manipulation, and its theory that defect in structure is at the root of all pathological conditions is not accepted by orthodox medicine, which does not believe that diseases are caused to any significant degree by obstruction of arteries or nerves by the pressure of maladjusted bones in the vertebrae of the spinal column. The system originated with the American physician Andrew Taylor Still in 1874, and numerous colleges teaching osteopathy exist in America. In London the British School of Osteopathy is at 16 Buckingham Gate, S.W.1. From the orthodox point of view the main fallacy of osteopathy is that of any similar branch of 'fringe medicine', namely the assumption that diseases have any one basic cause or can be cured by a single basic method. But nobody doubts that most practitioners are sincere and capable men who may in many cases have a better knowledge of bones and joints than most orthodox practitioners. *See* Fringe Medicine.

Osteophyte: an excrescence growing from a bone.

Osteoporosis: increased porousness of bones, often found in old age. It causes the bones to fracture more easily than they should, and when present in the spine may lead to collapse of the vertebral bodies and consequent deformity and loss of height. It may be accompanied by severe pain, and is sometimes a consequence of steroid therapy. Anabolic steroids – which are quite different from corticosteroids, being fundamentally derived from the male sex hormone – may control the pain and improve the patient's condition.

Osteosarcoma: one of the most commonly occurring bone tumours. It is malignant.
SYMPTOMS: it often affects young people and children, and develops in one of the long bones of the limbs, producing a tender swelling which has on occasion been mistaken for osteomyelitis. It may make its presence known by producing a pathological fracture of the bone.
TREATMENT: the limb is first treated by intensive radiotherapy, and if in about three months' time there is no indication that secondary growths have developed, particularly in the lungs, amputation may be considered.

Osteotomy: the operation of cutting a bone. It is sometimes performed to try to straighten the spine especially in cases of ankylosing spondylitis, to improve the position of badly set fractures, or to make a false joint especially at the hip. In cases where the hip joint has become useless or very painful the femur may be divided at the top of the shaft, which is displaced towards the mid-line to engage with the lower lip of the acetabulum.

Otitis: inflammation of the ear. Otitis externa involves the external opening and the passage to the eardrum, otitis media involves the middle ear, and otitis interna is inflammation of the inner ear.

Otolaryngology: the study of the structure, function and disease of the ear and the throat.

Otology: the study of the ear considered as a single specialty.

Otorhinolaryngology: the same as otolaryngology with the nose added.

Otorrhoea: discharge from the ear; a running ear, usually caused by chronic middle ear infection.

Otosclerosis: the formation of spongy bone in the labyrinth of the inner ear, which results in the footplate of the stapes becoming fixed in the oval window (*see* Ear) and consequent deafness, which may in some cases be helped a great deal by operation.

Ouabain: a substance obtained from the bark of Acokanthera ouabaio or schimperi and used as an arrow poison in East Africa. It is chemically the same as Strophanthin (which comes from a different source), and it has a similar action to digoxin, but very much shorter; it is sometimes used for its rapid action in acute heart failure. *See* Digitalis.

Ovaries: these are the female sex-glands.
Anatomy. The ovaries are shaped like almonds, about 4 cm long by 2 cm by 1 cm. In women who have not had children they lie applied to the wall of the pelvis in front of the division of the iliac arteries, attached to the broad ligament, the fold of peritoneum which covers the uterus and the two uterine tubes which run from the upper corners of the uterus to a position near the ovaries. In women who have had children the position of the ovaries varies, but the openings of the tubes are always nearby. The ovaries have a cortex and medulla, and the cortex, which forms the bulk of the organ, contains the germ cells. The blood supply is from the ovarian arteries, which branch directly from the abdominal aorta and run down into the pelvis. The right ovarian vein drains into the inferior vena cava and the left

runs into the left renal vein. The lymphatic vessels from the ovary drain into the lymph glands lying at each side of the abdominal aorta.

Function. The ovaries show a cycle of activity centred round the development and fate of the germ cells that persists throughout the child-bearing time of life. A single follicle containing an ovum comes to full development each month by an obscure mechanism, and breaks so that the ovum is discharged from the surface of the ovary to find its way into the uterine tube and so into the uterus. The follicle from which the ovum was discharged now forms the corpus luteum, the yellow body, which secretes steroid hormones for about ten days; then, if the ovum in the uterus is not fertilized, it ceases to produce any hormone and degenerates into a scar called the corpus albicans. The production of an ovum is regarded as the middle point of the ovarian cycle; the first day is taken to be the day of onset of monthly bleeding from the uterus, the first day of menstruation. The developing ovarian follicle secretes the hormones known as oestrogens, under the influence of which the lining of the uterus is replaced by regeneration of the endometrial cells. On the fourteenth day after menstruation began the ovum is released from the ovary, and the hormones of the corpus luteum, the progestogens, are added to the oestrogens. Under the influence of the corpus luteum the lining tissue of the uterus, the endometrium, changes again and develops a deep spongy layer and a superficial compact layer ready for the implantation of a fertilized ovum. If fertilization does not occur, the corpus luteum degenerates and there is a quick fall in the amount of oestrogen and progestogen circulating in the blood. The endometrium breaks down and menstruation begins. The whole cycle usually takes 28 days. In addition to the hormones described, the ovaries secrete small amounts of the male hormone testosterone.

The ovarian cycle is influenced by the hypothalamus at the base of the brain acting through the pituitary body, which secretes F.S.H., the follicle stimulating hormone, and L.H., the luteinizing hormone. It is thought that a feedback mechanism is involved, so that when the blood level of oestrogens goes up the hypothalamus stimulates the pituitary body to secrete L.H., while progestogens stop the production of L.H.; F.S.H. is secreted when the levels of oestrogen and progestogen fall at the onset of menstruation. One ovary is enough to maintain full function.

DISEASES OF THE OVARY: 1. *Inflammation* (see Oophoritis).

2. *Endometriosis.* A condition in which there are abnormal deposits of tissue identical with that normally lining the uterus. Such deposits are commonly found on the ovaries, but may also occur in the tissues dividing the vagina and rectum, at the umbilicus, in the scars of operations on the lower abdomen, on the intestinal contents of the pelvis or on the bladder.

CAUSE: thought to be migration of tissue through the uterine tubes on to the ovaries, whence the tissue may spread to other pelvic structures.

SYMPTOMS: the disease is not usually found in patients under the age of thirty. There may be pain, particularly at the time of the periods. If the ovary is badly affected the patient may be sterile because of scarring and adhesions, and for the same reasons obstruction of the intestines may occur. There may be excessive blood loss at the periods.

TREATMENT: treatment is by operation. In younger women the surgeon tries to preserve as much functioning tissue as possible, but when the patient is older and does not wish to have any more children all the organs affected that can safely be taken away are removed – ovaries, uterine tubes and uterus. The condition is not malignant, nor does it become malignant. Hormone treatment is of limited value.

3. *Cysts.* Cysts of the ovary are common. They may be found to be benign or malignant; the majority are benign. They may attain an enormous size, and usually occur between the 30th and 60th years.

SYMPTOMS: they may grow quietly, and only be noticed because of the abdominal distension, and because they take up so much room in the pelvis that there may be frequency of passing water or obstruction to venous drainage which causes swelling of the legs. Sometimes they become twisted on their pedicle, or stalk, and then there can be considerable pain and vomiting so that the condition is mistaken for appendicitis. The diagnosis soon becomes clear at operation. Intermittent twisting may occur, producing obscure symptoms. Bleeding may take place into a cyst, or it may burst; both conditions may be painful and give rise to fever and abdominal tenderness.

TREATMENT: surgical removal.

4. *Malignant tumours*. These are far less common in the ovary than simple tumours, but rapid growth with pain and irregular bleeding coming on after the periods have stopped suggests the diagnosis. The treatment if possible is by operation, which may be combined with cytotoxic drugs. If there is any doubt about the nature of a tumour of the ovary the surgeon prefers to remove the whole organ; and if the patient is over 45 any sign of abnormality in the other ovary is taken as an indication that it is advisable to remove both, as there is a considerable risk of bilateral disease.

Ovulation: the shedding of an ovum, or egg, from the ovary (q.v.).

Ovum: Latin for egg. *See* Ovary.

Oxalic Acid: an irritant poison. The symptoms of poisoning with oxalic acid or oxalates are: burning pain in the mouth and throat, vomiting, convulsions, the passage of blood in the urine, or the suppression of urine. Treatment is the administration of magnesium sulphate, calcium lactate or calcium gluconate intravenously. At least five litres of fluid are to be taken a day unless there is suppression or diminution of the passage of urine.

Oxalates are sometimes found in the urine after a meal of strawberries or rhubarb, and some people normally pass oxalates in the urine. Oxalates are very commonly found in kidney stones.

Ox-gall: used to stimulate the flow of bile when this is considered necessary.

Oxidase: oxidases are enzymes of various sorts which have to do with the oxidation of a number of biochemical substances.

Oxophenarsine: an organic compound containing arsenic which was at one time used in the treatment of syphilis, and is still used if for any reason the patient cannot tolerate penicillin.

Oxycephaly: a condition in which the head is more pointed

573

than normal; also named steeple head, the condition may have to be relieved by surgical decompression. Patients with this deformity are not necessarily feeble-minded.

Oxygen: a colourless, odourless gas which forms one-fifth of the air we breathe and is essential for life. Atomic number 8; it exists in three isotopes with atomic weights 16, 17 and 18. Oxygen is given for medical purposes to those suffering from diseases of the lung, circulation and blood, either through a mask or by means of an oxygen tent.

Oxymel: a home-made medicine compounded of vinegar and honey used for coughs, colds and sore throats; at one time recommended as a cure-all without any justification, it is harmless.

Oxytetracycline: *see* Tetracyclines.

Oxytocin: the anterior lobe of the pituitary body secretes under the influence of the hypothalamus at the base of the brain a hormone called oxytocin which stimulates the pregnant uterus to contract. The hormone may be given by intravenous injection or as a tablet in cases where labour is slow, or in order to induce labour. It can also be used to hasten the third stage of labour, delivery of the placenta. Other drugs with the same action are called oxytocic agents.

Oxyuriasis: infestation with threadworms (pin-worms). *See* Worms.

Ozaena: chronic disease of the nose in which there is atrophy of the lining with the formation of foul-smelling discharge and crusts.

Ozone: a gas which is chemically O_3 in contrast to oxygen's O_2. It has a typical salty odour but is poisonous in large amounts and, although its existence has been publicized in travel pamphlets as appearing in the air of mountain and seaside resorts, it is doubtful whether any large amount is really present or whether any benefit would arise if it were. Ozone is a powerful deodorant and germicide in suitable amounts and is probably found in the highest concentrations in the dynamo rooms of power-stations.

P

Pacemaker: in complete heart-block the impulses which should travel to the ventricles from the atria of the heart, where they are set up in the sinuatrial bundle of conducting fibres by the atrio-ventricular node (*see* Heart), are blocked by disease so that the atria and the ventricles beat independently. The ventricle takes up a slow rate of beating between 30 and 50 a minute, and heart failure may supervene. Moreover, the patient may become subject to attacks of fainting called Stokes-Adams attacks because the supply of blood to the brain is inadequate. To remedy this state of affairs an artificial pacemaker is used which delivers electrical impulses to the muscle of the ventricle. Usually an electrode is introduced into the heart through a vein, often the external jugular, and it conducts impulses at about 70–80 a minute set up by a small apparatus and battery which is inserted into the armpit. Modern developments are to power the apparatus by an atomic battery, and to arrange a feedback mechanism so that impulses are only fed into the heart when they are needed.

Pachymeningitis: inflammation of the dura mater of the brain. *See* Meningitis.

Pacinian Corpuscle: a very small structure, about 4 mm long, found just below the skin and in other parts of the body, which in section is rather like an oval onion. It is attached to a sensory nerve fibre and it is sensitive to pressure.

Paediatrics: *See* Pediatrics.

Paget's Disease of Bone: (Osteitis deformans). A disease of bones in advancing age.
SYMPTOMS: the bones become thickened and soft, so that the thigh-bones bend outwards and the shins forward. The collar-bones are prominent and enlarged, and the skull itself becomes obviously bigger. The patient may complain that he can no longer wear his hat. He may also become deaf

575

from bony changes affecting the ear, and the bones may be painful. They may be more prone than normal to fractures, and occasionally malignant tumours develop in them.

TREATMENT: no effective treatment is known, but pain is relieved by suitable drugs.

Pain: the precise nature of pain is not understood. It is easy to say that it is an unpleasant sensation which arises when the body is damaged, but this is not always true; it is a matter of common observation that those who are injured in war or in an accident may feel little pain for a considerable time although their injuries might be expected to be very painful, and that sensitivity to pain depends a great deal upon the state of mind. In general it appears that the sensation of pain is not originated by particular nerve-endings or sensory organs, unlike touch, temperature and stretching; and that it arises as the result of some analysis made in the central nervous system of many incoming sensory impulses. Experimental work on pain is unsatisfactory for a number of reasons which stem from the fact that an animal with a nervous system has to be used as the experimental subject, and that the experiment cannot be carried out when the subject is anaesthetized for anaesthesia abolishes pain.

Anatomy of pain. It is known that the sensory nerves responsible for producing sensations of pain travel in the peripheral sensory nerves to the spinal cord; injection of local anaesthetic abolishes pain in the area supplied by the anaesthetized nerve. The impulses then travel in the spinothalamic tracts – bundles of fibres that run up in the antero-lateral part of the spinal cord to end in the thalamus – on the other side of the cord to the point of entry, so that impulses set up in the right side of the body travel in the left side of the spinal cord, and vice versa. The neurosurgeon can cut the spinothalamic tracts and so relieve pain in various parts of the body, for the sensory nerve fibres run in a particular order. The operation is called cordotomy and is carried out for intractable pain, particularly in cases of malignant disease. The spinothalamic tracts also carry the impulses that underly the sensation of temperature. When in the basal area of the cerebral hemispheres the tracts reach the thalamus, it is not possible to be precise about the onward path of pain impulses. Sensations of various sorts are localized in the thalamus, and although the neurosurgeon can with stereotaxic apparatus stimulate different points in the thalamus and produce sensations seeming to come from the body, attempts to relieve sensations of pain by destroying discrete areas of the thalamus have been disappointing. Nor is it possible to modify the sensation of pain for more than a few days by operations on the cortex of the brain.

Localization. In general the localization of pain on the outside of the body presents no problem; the pain is acute and referred to the site of the injury or disease, which is clearly visible. In pain coming from the inside of the body this may not be the case; not only may it be impossible to see or detect the lesion, but the pain may be referred to a different part of the body. Pain arising in the diaphragm, for example, may be referred to the neck; pain from the heart may go to the tip of the shoulder.

Character of the pain. The character varies according to the place of origin. Pain caused by damage to the skin is sharp, and makes the subject move away from the source of the injury; there is nothing like a pin for making someone move quickly. Pain coming from structures deep under the skin is different; moreover, although any stimulus that damages the skin is felt, only certain stimuli give rise to pain from deep structures – stimuli that in general may be expected to be signs that all is not well with function. Intestine can be cut without pain, although it cannot be stretched without very unpleasant sensations; and the worst pain from the hollow tubes of the body is caused by spasm of the muscle of their walls (colic) which may be expected to arise from obstruction or irritation. The character of pain sometimes gives a clue to the best first-aid treatment; the pain arising from a broken bone, for example, makes the injured man keep still and above all keep the injured bone still. Similarly the pain coming from the inflamed peritoneum in peritonitis serves to keep the patient immobile.

Treatment. The treatment of pain is the treatment of the underlying condition and it is worth remembering that it is not very sensible to treat any sort of pain until a diagnosis has been made. It has been said that most of us suffer at least one severe twinge of pain a day for which no reason can be found, although a consideration of the sales of aspirin and similar popular 'pain-killers' prompts the conclusion that most people are in pain all the time. The action of drugs on pain is fortunately in most cases satisfactory, although in severe chronic cases they lose their effect and doses may have to be increased. If pain becomes intractable the operation of cordotomy outlined above may be advisable, but most doctors prefer to avoid it because it has certain sequels which may be unpleasant for the patient.

Painter's Colic: colic arising from lead poisoning.

Palaeopathology: the study of disease processes shown in prehistoric remains.

Palate: the roof of the mouth, which is also the floor of the cavity of the nose lying above. It consists of the hard palate in front made of bone and covered by the mucous membrane of the mouth below and that of the nose on the upper side, and the soft palate behind – which is composed of muscle similarly covered. When food or air passes through the mouth the soft palate rises to shut off the nose. For Hare Lip *see* Cleft Palate.

Palpation: the method of examining the surface of the body, and such of the deeper structures as can be felt, by touching gently with the hands.

Palpebrae: the eyelids.

Palpitations: a state in which the heart beats forcibly or irregularly so that the individual becomes aware of its action. This is nearly always a condition which has very little to do with the heart itself and it is extremely doubtful whether tobacco, alcohol, coffee, tea or even 'excesses' have anything to do with it as was formerly thought. Although palpitations do occur among other symptoms in serious heart disease, the vast majority of cases are due to anxiety and have no direct connection with heart disease whatever. The treatment is that of anxiety; reassurance after a careful examination of the heart (usually more for the patient's than the doctor's benefit), and tranquillizers or sedatives as necessary.

Palsy: this is an archaic word for paralysis.

Paludrine: (proguanil). A drug taken to suppress malaria (q.v.).

Panacea: a fabled remedy to cure all diseases.

Pancreas: a large mixed gland lying on the back wall of the upper abdominal cavity; the main secretion is passed through the pancreatic duct into the intestine, while the endocrine secretion (insulin) passes directly into the bloodstream.

Anatomy. The gland is about 15 cm long; it has a large head, and a long body and tail. The head fits into the curve of the duodenum, and is on the right; the body passes to the left across the aorta, the left suprarenal gland and the left kidney, renal artery and vein. The tail continues up towards the spleen. The pancreas takes its blood supply from the splenic, hepatic and superior mesenteric arteries, with each of which it comes into close relationship. It contains a duct which runs the length of the body, collects the secretions of the various lobules of the gland, and opens into the duodenum at the same place as the bile duct, with which it is joined just before both ducts come to a common orifice on the duodenal papilla about 10 cm from the pyloric end of the stomach. There is sometimes an accessory duct which drains the head of the gland.

Functions. 1. The exocrine part of the gland. This part of the gland consists of many lobules which contain a number of passages coming to blind ends called acini, lined with secreting cells. Through the passages and into the small ducts which join the main pancreatic duct drain the secretions of the acini, called the pancreatic juice. The juice is alkaline, and contains the forerunners of the enzymes trypsin and chymotripsin, which are activated by the intestinal juice, the enzymes amylase and lipase, and the chlorides and bicarbonates of sodium, calcium and potassium. These substances play a large part in the digestion of food in the duodenum and small intestine.

2. Endocrine secretion. *See* Insulin.

Pancreatitis: inflammation of the pancreas.
CAUSE: commonly associated with disease of the biliary system, pancreatitis is most often due to infection travelling up the pancreatic duct from its common opening into the

duodenum with the bile duct. Occasionally a gallstone blocks the duodenal papilla (*see* above) and bile enters the pancreatic duct as a reflux.

SYMPTOMS: 1. *Acute haemorrhagic pancreatitis*. Trypsinogen, forerunner of the enzyme trypsin, is thought to be activated by the entry of bile into the pancreatic duct. The enzyme digests the pancreas and its vessels, so that the patient collapses with acute upper abdominal pain, vomiting and failure of the circulation. The condition may be severe enough to render the patient unconscious.

2. *Subacute pancreatitis*. Like acute pancreatitis, but with a far less catastrophic onset. There is fever, pain and tenderness in the upper abdomen. The condition may resolve of itself, only to recur.

3. *Chronic pancreatitis*. Pain is felt in the upper abdomen and often in the back, and there may be jaundice. Sometimes there is diarrhoea, with rather bulky, foul-smelling motions; the disease may be associated with an excessive intake of alcohol.

TREATMENT: in the case of acute and subacute pancreatitis, operation is avoided if possible, but sometimes a laparotomy has to be carried out because the diagnosis is obscure and the patient is extremely ill. Fluids are given intravenously, gastric suction is set up, and antibiotics are used to combat peritonitis. In chronic pancreatitis the situation is different, and the abdomen must be opened in order to rule out the possibility of a cancerous growth of the pancreas. If there are gallstones or gall-bladder disease in association with pancreatitis, operative treatment may be found necessary to correct the condition of the biliary tract.

4. The pancreas may be affected in mumps.

Pandemic: an epidemic affecting a large area, for example a continent.

Panhysterectomy: complete removal of the womb and its appendages.

Panophthalmitis: inflammation of all the structures of the eyeball.

Papilla: a small elevation shaped like a nipple.

Papilloedema: swelling and congestion of the head of the optic nerve as it enters the back of the eye, due to increased pressure inside the skull.

Papilloma: a tumour growing on a free surface of epithelium (q.v.). It may be found on the skin, in the bladder or in the colon, in which places there are commonly multiple growths, upon the penis under the foreskin (infective warts), in the pelvis of the kidney and in the rectum. A papilloma may undergo malignant change to become a papillary adenocarcinoma. Treatment is according to site; a simple papilloma on the skin is of little consequence, whereas papillomata in the bladder may bleed and have to be treated by fulguration (q.v.); those in the large intestine are best treated by removal.

Papule: a small, solid, discrete elevation of the skin.

Para-aminosalicylic Acid: (P.A.S.). A synthetic drug, used in the treatment of tuberculosis. It is given by mouth; it may have the disagreeable side effects of nausea and vomiting, with perhaps some diarrhoea, but the usefulness of the drug makes it worth while to persevere. If, however, sensitivity reactions appear – a skin rash, with fever and, sometimes, enlargement of the lymph glands – the drug must be stopped. *See* Streptomycin, Isoniazid.

Paracentesis: the puncture with a hollow needle of any body cavity in order to withdraw abnormal fluid either for the relief of symptoms or for pathological examination.

Paracetamol: an aminophenol derivative used as an analgesic drug. It is very like aspirin in its action, but does not irritate the lining of the stomach to such an extent. At the last count it had 15 proprietary names differing according to which drug company moulded the substance into a tablet. *See* Drugs, The Commercial Aspect.

Paracusis: any alteration in the sense of hearing.

Paraesthesia: *see* Paresthesia.

Paraffin: (Petrolatum). A mixture of hydrocarbons obtained from petroleum, used in medicine when solid as a base for ointments and when liquid as a laxative. Chronic irritation from paraffin can produce a granulomatous tumour called a paraffinoma: it occurs sometimes in the lungs.

Paraganglioma: a rare tumour made up of cells normally found in the medulla of the adrenal gland occurring in different parts of the body. The cells secrete norepinephrine, and can cause paroxysmal attacks of high blood pressure.

Paragonimus: the lung fluke, common in the East; it needs two intermediate hosts, the first being a snail and the second a crab. If the infected crab is eaten raw, the paragonimus escapes into the man's small intestine, makes its way through the wall of the gut, and journeys up through the abdominal cavity to penetrate the diaphragm and creep into the lungs. *See* Fluke, Worms.

Paraldehyde: a colourless liquid of ethereal odour and burning and nauseous taste used as a safe and powerful hypnotic. It leaves a strong smell on the breath, and because of this and its unpleasant taste it is used far more in institutions than in home or hospital practice.

Paralysis: loss of muscular power and the capacity to move, due to disturbance of the muscles or nerves.

Paralytic Ileus: a condition of the small intestines in which there is paralysis of the muscle of the gut due to inflammation, injury or bleeding into the abdominal cavity. There is distension of the abdomen, but the condition is not painful of itself. It is treated by rest; nothing is given by mouth; the stomach is aspirated and fluids are given intravenously.

Paramnesia: distortion or falsification of memory or recognition.

Paranoia: this term describes a mild form of schizophrenia that is more of a character disorder than a mental disease. The patient's personality does not change, but he has delusions of persecution and may falsify memory and maintain that situations and words have a meaning far from their true significance. The condition is not uncommon, and does not stop the subject from carrying on a profession or doing a job, although it can be trying for his colleagues.

Paraphimosis: if the foreskin is tight, and it is drawn back beyond the corona of the penis, it may happen that the end of the penis becomes engorged and swollen so that the foreskin can no longer be replaced. As the swelling increases so the constriction at the site of the drawn-back foreskin becomes worse, and a vicious circle is set up. The only treatment is replacement of the foreskin by steady pressure; if this is not possible it may have to be divided under general anesthetic. Circumcision is usually carried out later when the swelling has gone down.

Paraphrenia: some patients, although they suffer from the paranoid type of schizophrenia with delusions and hallucinations, still retain their original personality. The condition is found among older people, and is called paraphrenia; it is midway between paranoid schizophrenia and paranoia. *See* Mental Illness.

Paraplegia: paralysis of both sides of the body, usually both legs from the waist down. It may be high enough in cases of lesions of the cervical part of the spinal cord to affect the arms as well as the legs in which case the condition is known as quadriplegia. Hemiplegia is paralysis that affects one side of the body only, and results from injury or disease in the brain; paraplegia is usually the result of disorder of the spinal cord.

Paraquat: a weedkiller. It is only dangerous if it is continually inhaled in full concentrations, when it may cause nose bleeding and congestion of the lungs.

Parasites: man may form the living quarters for a number of other organisms which feed upon him and are therefore parasites. These organisms include viruses, bacteria, protozoa – one-celled organisms – and fungi, which are said to infect man, and worms and insects which are said to infest him. It is only the worms and insects that are usually referred to as parasites, the best-known insects being lice, fleas and bed-bugs, and the best-known worms threadworm, round-worm and tapeworm. All these organisms are discussed under their own headings.

Parasympathetic Nervous System: *see* Nervous System.

Parathion: an organic phosphorus insecticide. *See* Organo-phosphorus Compounds.

Parathormone: the hormone secreted by the parathyroid glands.

Parathyroid Glands: there are four parathyroid glands. They are found in relation to the thyroid gland in the neck, two on each side of the trachea or windpipe on the back surface of the thyroid gland, one at the level of its mid-point and one at its lower margin. They are small – about 5 by 4 mm – and yellow, and their function is to regulate the use of calcium in the body. When the parathyroid glands are re-moved, as has happened in the past accidentally in the course of surgical removal of the thyroid gland, the patient finds that his forearm muscles go into spasm, that his arms, feet and face tingle and are numb, and that he has pain in the abdomen because of muscular cramps and difficulty in breathing because of spasm of the vocal cords. The condition is called tetany, and is cured by the administration of calcium. If the condition is allowed to continue it may lead to convulsions and even to paralysis of the muscles used in breathing. Overfunction of the parathyroid glands leads to disturbance of calcium metabolism, which is shown by lack of calcium in the bones and possibly formation of stones in the kidney. It is commonly caused by tumours of the parathyroid glands. Treatment is surgical removal of the tumour.

Paratyphoid Fever: *see* Typhoid Fever.

Paregoric: camphorated tincture of opium. Used in cough mixtures, and to treat diarrhoea.

Parenchyma: the functional tissue in an organ or gland, as distinct from the framework (stroma).

Parenteral: a method of administering drugs other than by the mouth and the intestines, for example by injection.

Paresis: weakness, as opposed to paralysis which means total loss of function.

Paresthesia: an abnormal sensation, for example burning in the absence of heat, or formication – the feeling that ants are crawling over the skin.

Parietal: concerned with the walls of a cavity – the parietal bones form the walls of the skull, the parietal pleura is the membrane that lies against the chest wall.

Parkinson's Disease: (Paralysis agitans). A disease of the nervous system in which the patient's muscles become stiff, and he has a continual tremor or shake.

CAUSE: unknown. Some cases follow severe attacks of encephalitis, but in most the disease begins to show itself in later middle age, and is thought to be a consequence of 'degeneration', particularly in the basal ganglia. It is a disease of the extra-pyramidal system (q.v.).

SYMPTOMS: the patient shows a combination of tremor of the limbs and muscular stiffness; the description originally given by Dr James Parkinson of Shoreditch in 1817 runs: 'involuntary tremulous motion, with lessened muscular power, in parts not in action and even when supported; with a propensity to bend the trunk forwards, and to pass from a walking to a running pace, the senses and intellect being uninjured.' The face has little expression, and the voice becomes weak. In the last stages of the disease the patient is not able to move, and presents a distressing spectacle, for his mind may be uninjured while he cannot speak or write (one of the characteristic signs of the disease is that the writing becomes progressively smaller and more tremulous).

TREATMENT: there is no single effective treatment for Parkinson's disease. A number of drugs exist which will to a certain extent reduce tremor and rigidity, such as atropine, benzhexol (Artane), orphenadrine (Disipal), and others;

and this disease is one of the few conditions in which the amphetamines are without doubt justifiably used to combat depression and muscular fatigue, for in advanced cases the possibility of drug dependence ought not to weigh against the possible benefit that the drugs can bring. L-dopa is a new drug given to treat Parkinsonism, and it seems promising, but it cannot be used in all cases, for in some it produces nausea and in others various bizarre involuntary movements and disturbances of mental equilibrium which limit the dosage. In carefully chosen cases operation by sterotaxic surgical techniques on the thalamus at the base of the brain produces dramatic results, but not all cases can be improved by operation.

Paronychia: infection occurring in the folds of tissue beside the nail. *See* Nail.

Parotid Gland: the largest of the salivary glands. It is situated just in front of the ear and behind the angle of the lower jaw, and has a duct which enters the mouth opposite the second last tooth of the upper jaw. The gland may be enlarged by mumps, when it forms the characteristic swelling, by other inflammation or because the duct is blocked, usually by a stone.

Paroxysmal Tachycardia: any part of the heart muscle is capable of setting up rhythmic impulses which may be conducted through neighbouring tissue to make the heart give an extra beat. Sometimes this irritability of the heart muscle causes the heart rate to double, a condition called paroxysmal tachycardia because it appears in attacks which start and finish of themselves. It is not associated with any disease of the heart in most cases, although it must be carefully distinguished from cases of tachycardia, or abnormally rapid pulse rate, due to disease. There is in some cases a family history; no treatment is generally necessary, and the only significance of the condition is that it may make the patient slightly breathless and uncomfortable in the chest and neck. It is very rarely found in infants but when it is, it must be treated promptly.

P.A.S.: *see* Para-aminosalicyclic acid.

Pasteurization: a process named after Louis Pasteur (1822–95), the Frenchman who founded the science of bacteriology and upon whose work an enormous amount of medical theory and practice is based. Pasteurization involves heating milk to a temperature short of boiling, for example 60 °C. for a fixed period, often 30 minutes, in order to destroy the organisms of disease and delay the development of other bacteria, thus prolonging the keeping time of the milk and rendering it harmless.

Patella: the knee cap.

Patent Ductus Arteriosus: a congenital condition of the heart in which the communication between the pulmonary artery and the aorta which bypasses the lungs in the foetus persists after birth. Normally it closes at birth when the baby begins to breathe. The treatment is surgical; the open duct is tied off.

Pathogenic: capable of producing disease.

Pathognomonic: characteristic of a particular disease.

Pathology: the study of the changes brought about in the body by disease.

Pectoral: relating to the chest.

Pediatrics: that branch of medicine dealing with the diseases of children.

Pediculosis: infestation with lice.

Pellagra: a deficiency disease.
CAUSE: it was shown by Dr Goldberger, working in the southern part of the United States between 1913 and 1928, that pellagra was due to a dietary deficiency of a substance that was soluble in water and unchanged by heat. Goldberger died before the substance was identified as nicotinic acid in 1937. Pellagra is found in places where the main diet is maize, which is not only deficient in nicotinic acid but contains no tryptophan, an amino acid from which the body can

587

produce nicotinic acid. Pellagra is now found only in patients with digestive conditions that prevent them absorbing nicotinic acid, and in those whose diet is abnormally poor – for example, alcoholics.

SYMPTOMS: the three Ds – diarrhoea, dementia and dermatitis.

TREATMENT: nicotinic acid or nicotinamide.

Pelotherapy: the medical use of mud.

Pelvimetry: measurement of the pelvis, particularly of its outlet, made by the obstetrician in order to estimate the likelihood of a normal birth in cases where there may be disproportion between the head of the baby and the bony part of the birth canal.

Pelvis: the pelvis is a bone shaped like a basin connecting the legs with the spine and consisting of the haunch-bones on either side and the sacrum and coccyx behind. The haunches are made up of three bones, separate in the child, but fused together in the adult: the ilium, the crest of which can be felt when one puts one's hands on one's hips, the ischium with a rounded tuberosity upon which one sits, and the pubis in front. The lower opening of the pelvis is closed in life by the two levator ani muscles and the sacro-iliac ligaments, leaving gaps only for the urinary and genital passages and the rectum. Within the pelvis are the urinary bladder and rectum in both sexes, the seminal vesicles and prostate gland surrounding the bladder's neck in the male, and the womb, ovaries and their appendages in the female, together with varying lengths of small intestine.

Pemphigus: pemphigus neonatorum is a condition in which the skin of newborn, or recently born, babies develops large infected blebs. The cause is lack of cleanliness in handling the babies; the infection is spread by the attendants. The treatment is antibiotics and strict asepsis.

Pemphigus vulgaris is a much rarer disease occurring in middle age. It starts with blisters on the skin or on the mucous membranes, and slowly progresses.

CAUSE: a defect in the skin itself allows spaces to form in its substance.

SYMPTOMS: the appearance of blisters on the skin or the mucous membranes, often of the mouth, leaving ulcerated areas which do not heal up when they burst. Secondary infection complicates the disease, which is slowly progressive and very serious.

TREATMENT: corticosteroids and antibiotics.

Penicillin: the original antibiotic discovered in London in 1929 by Sir Alexander Fleming in the mould Penicillium notatum (first described by a Scandinavian in 1911 without its healing properties being known). Florey and Chain of Oxford, who shared a Nobel Prize with Fleming in 1945, showed how penicillin could be produced in bulk, a discovery without which it might have been useless. Penicillin (apart from allergic reactions) is practically non-toxic to human beings, but capable of killing a large number of disease-producing organisms. It is now supplied in many different forms.

Penicillinase: an enzyme produced by some micro-organisms which renders penicillin inactive; the ability to make the enzyme is handed down from generation to generation of bacteria so that in time penicillin-sensitive organisms in a community are eliminated, leaving a growing number of penicillin-resistant strains. This is particularly likely to happen in hospitals, which have become notorious for harbouring antibiotic-resistant bacteria.

Penis: the male sex organ through which semen and urine are discharged by way of the urethra. The shaft of the penis contains spongy tissue which fills with blood when the owner is sexually excited; the ensuing erection makes sexual intercourse possible.

Pentothal: proprietary name for thiopental or thiopentone, a substance of the barbiturate group used as an intravenous anaesthetic because of its short action.

Pepsin: an enzyme in the gastric juice which breaks down protein.

Peptic Ulcer: *see* Stomach Diseases.

Peptones: substances derived from the digestion of protein by acids or enzymes. They are soluble in water and are not precipitated by heat.

Percussion: the procedure of 'thumping' the chest or other parts with the fingers which is carried out by doctors in order to find out what is going on beneath. The principle behind percussion is simple, being a matter of resonance; thus if a cigar-box filled with sand is percussed a dull, flat note will be given out, but if the box is empty the note will be hollow and resonant. Similarly the lung filled with exudate in pneumonia will give a dull note and the normal lung a resonant note. What is distinguished is the difference between hollow and solid or semi-solid organs, whether they are normally so or by disease have become so.

Perforation: term commonly applied to the development of a hole in one of the hollow structures in the abdomen, usually the stomach or intestine. Perforations may be produced by disease, as in the case of a gastric or duodenal ulcer, or by wounds which penetrate the abdominal wall. The patient suffering from a perforation becomes progressively more ill and shocked as peritonitis spreads; the treatment is by gastric suction, intravenous fluids, and, as soon as feasible, by operation.

Periarteritis Nodosa: *see* Polyarteritis Nodosa.

Pericarditis: inflammation of the pericardium.
CAUSE: there are many causes, which include rheumatic heart disease, tuberculosis, bacterial infection, virus infection, infarction of the heart muscle, wounds, including operation wounds, and cancerous deposits.
SYMPTOMS: often the patient feels pain, which may spread to the back, the shoulders or the abdomen. It is made worse by movement and by deep breathing. Fluid may develop within the two layers of the pericardium, in which case the action of the heart may be impeded, so that the patient becomes breathless and begins to cough. After a long period of chronic inflammation, the pericardium may become scarred and constricted, and this so interferes with the heart's action that the liver becomes enlarged, fluid collects in the abdo-

men, and eventually there is generalized oedema and breathlessness.

TREATMENT: this is directed towards the underlying condition, but when fluid has collected it must be drawn off by puncturing the chest wall with a needle. Constrictive pericarditis is relieved by open operation.

Pericardium: the membranous sac which contains the heart. It has two layers, between which is a capillary space containing a film of fluid which provides lubrication to assist in the free movement of the heart in relation to neighbouring structures. The outermost part of the pericardium is fibrous.

Perichondrium: the fibrous membrane which covers cartilage.

Pericranium: the membrane covering the outer surface of the skull.

Perilymph: fluid found in the inner ear. It separates the membrane of the labyrinth from the bone, and is separate from the endolymph fluid inside the membranous labyrinth.

Perimetry: the measurement of the outer limits of the fields of vision of each eye.

Perinephric: surrounding the kidney. Applied to the perinephric fat, and also to pus round the kidney, which forms a perinephric abscess.

Perineum: the fork; the region between the pubic bone in front and the coccyx behind.

Periodic Syndrome: *see* Cyclical Vomiting.

Periods: *see* Menstruation.

Periosteum: the membrane which surrounds the bones.

Periostitis: inflammation of the periosteum. It is caused by injury, when the membrane is stripped off the bone by the extravasation of blood, by bacterial infection spreading from the underlying bone or the overlying tissues, by syphilis and by tuberculosis.

Peripheral: a term applied to structures in the outer part or towards the edge of the body or an organ of the body, for example the peripheral nervous system, as opposed to the central nervous system.

Peristalsis: the process by which food is moved along the intestines. The muscle of the walls of the gut contracts and relaxes in slow waves which pass along the length of the stomach and the intestine, the contractions being set up by the nervous plexus present in their walls. Peristalsis occurs in response to distension of the gut or stimulation of the nervous plexus. *See* Paralytic Ileus.

Peritoneum: the membrane which covers the inner walls of the abdominal cavity and the organs contained in it. The membrane covering the walls of the abdomen is called the parietal layer, and that covering the internal organs the visceral layer. Between the layers is a thin film of fluid which acts as a lubricant and allows the organs to move about in relation to each other and the abdominal walls. The peritoneum forms various folds by which organs are suspended, and one large fold in front called the omentum, an apron full of fat hanging down from the stomach. To the back of this is applied the transverse colon. The small intestine is attached to the back wall of the abdomen by a fold of peritoneum called the mesentery, in which run the blood vessels and lymphatics of the intestine, but the kidneys, ureters, and bladder all lie outside the peritoneum, with only part of their surfaces covered by the membrane. The peritoneal sac is closed in the male, but in the female the two uterine tubes form passages through which the cavity communicates with the exterior of the body. The peritoneum is well able to deal with bacterial infection, and usually localizes infections and collections of pus by forming adhesions; the omentum in particular adheres to the site of any inflammation. The peritoneum has been called 'the surgeon's friend', and the omentum 'the abdominal policeman'.

Peritonitis: inflammation of the peritoneum.

CAUSE: perforation of an internal organ, the spread of bacterial infection, or interference with the blood supply of an internal organ. Peritonitis may be acute or chronic.

SYMPTOMS: 1. *Acute.* Severe pain, spreading all over the abdomen. The patient lies still, is pale, has a quick thready pulse, bad breath, dry mouth and clammy skin. He is often apprehensive. The breathing is shallow, and constipation is absolute. There are no bowel sounds because the gut in peritonitis becomes paralysed. The muscles of the abdominal wall are rigid.

2. *Chronic.* In children the cause is often tuberculosis; the patients lose weight, develop a protruding belly, may have colic, and may suffer from intestinal upsets. In adults the peritoneum may become chronically inflamed because of the presence of cancerous deposits which sometimes provoke an outpouring of fluid sufficient to distend the abdomen.

TREATMENT: depends upon the cause. In general, the stomach is aspirated in acute cases and an intravenous infusion set up. Antibiotics are given. Pain should not be relieved until a diagnosis has been made, but in most cases this will resolve itself into a decision whether to operate or to wait. Once this has been decided morphia may be given to quieten both the pain and the patient's characteristic apprehension. The treatment of tuberculous peritonitis is the treatment of tuberculosis, but collections of fluid (ascites) caused by malignant deposits can only be removed by aspiration as necessary, for no effective and lasting treatment is possible in the majority of cases.

Peritonsillar Abscess: (Quinsy). An abscess behind the tonsils.

CAUSE: usually acute tonsillitis; the abscess itself tends to form behind the upper part of the tonsil.

SYMPTOMS: the tonsillitis causes a sore throat and fever, perhaps with painful swellings in the neck. As the quinsy develops there is increasing difficulty in swallowing, acute pain, a rise of temperature and considerable swelling of the structures at the back of the throat so that the patient may be in fear of choking.

TREATMENT: the abscess may burst of itself, or may have to be opened by a slight operation which can be carried out under local anaesthetic. Antibiotics are given according to the sensitivity of the infecting organism.

Quinsies may recur, and if they do consideration must be given to the advisability of removing the tonsils after the infection has settled down.

Pernicious Anaemia: (Addison's anaemia). A type of anaemia in which there is an abnormality in the formation of the red blood cells.

CAUSE: deficiency of Vitamin B_{12}. Basically the stomach becomes atrophied, and ceases to secrete either hydrochloric acid or a substance essential for the absorption of Vitamin B_{12} from the intestines called the intrinsic factor. In a very few cases, mostly among vegetarians, there is a deficiency of Vitamin B_{12} in the diet, and in cases where a large part of the stomach has had to be removed there will be too little intrinsic factor. It is possible that underlying the atrophy of the stomach is an antibody-antigen reaction. Without a supply of the vitamin the maturation of red blood cells in the bone marrow cannot occur properly, and the circulating blood shows reduced numbers of red cells, most of them abnormal although they usually have the full complement of haemoglobin. A very similar state of affairs follows deficiency of folic acid (q.v.) in the diet.

SYMPTOMS: slowly developing breathlessness and fatigue, angina and palpitations. The appetite is lost, and the patient depressed. The skin takes on a peculiar lemon colour and the tongue becomes red and sore. Because Vitamin B_{12} is essential for the preservation of the substance myelin, which forms the sheath of nerve fibres, signs and symptoms of trouble in the nervous system may develop, and the patient has tingling and pins and needles in the feet and hands, clumsiness and weakness, and loss of position sense, touch and pain. The knee jerks disappear, the Babinski reflex becomes extensor, and eventually mental changes may supervene. The nervous manifestations of deficiency of Vitamin B_{12} are called subacute combined degeneration of the cord. The firm diagnosis of pernicious anaemia is made upon examination of the blood under the microscope.

TREATMENT: Vitamin B_{12} by intramuscular injection. The injections must be given regularly once a month for life.

Pernio: chilblain.

Peroneal: the name given to the nerves, muscles and blood vessels of the outer side of the leg. The outer bone of the leg is called the fibula, which in Latin is a pin; perone is the corresponding Greek word.

Peroxide of Hydrogen: or H_2O_2, is a colourless and odourless liquid, the antiseptic properties of which are due to its ability to give up oxygen and turn into water in the process. It is therefore very safe, and the strength of a solution is measured in terms of the amount of oxygen it is capable of releasing; for example the usual 10-volume strength is capable of releasing 10 times its bulk of oxygen. Hydrogen peroxide is most commonly used in cleaning wounds (but not as a dressing), in extracting wax from the ears – when it should be washed out by water subsequently as impurities in the solution may cause irritation – as a mouth-wash, and as a bleach for the hair. A solution in warm water is very useful for removing dressings that have stuck, without disturbing the wound.

Perspiration: sweat is a watery fluid secreted by tiny sweat glands scattered all over the surface of the body. Over half a litre of water is lost unnoticed every day by evaporation from the skin, a loss called insensible perspiration, but when the external or internal temperature rises sweat can be seen forming on the surface of the skin, whence it evaporates and in so doing cools the surface of the body. This mechanism is one of the most important that man uses to keep his temperature constant, and in a dry atmosphere the skin temperature can by this means be kept down to 35°C. while the body temperature is 37°C. The sweat glands are controlled by fibres of the sympathetic nervous system which work by the release of acetylcholine at the nerve-endings; the central control of sweating is in the hypothalamus at the base of the brain. The sweat itself is water with 0.5% solids. It contains sodium chloride, so that when sweating is profuse it is sensible to take salt tablets with water during the day. Sweat may be coloured blue by taking indigo by mouth.

There is a tendency on the part of manufacturers of soap and other toilet products to proclaim that sweat and the secretion of the apocrine glands – large glands very like sweat glands which secrete a thicker material in the armpits, the external passage of the ear and the perineum – are offensive, and should be prevented or washed away at once, and it is even suggested that unless we take chlorophyll by mouth we shall stink. In fact there are rare conditions in which the odour of the body may be disagreeable, and there is no doubt that people are the better for washing regularly, but it is well to remember that the smell of sweat and the apocrine secretions have a greater sexual significance than the perfumes of the advertiser.

Perthes' Disease: a disease of the hip-joint in which there is flattening or fragmentation of the head of the femur. *See* Osteochondritis.

Pertussis: term meaning whooping cough (q.v.).

Pes Cavus, Pes Planus: pes cavus is a foot with an exaggerated arch in the longitudinal axis, often associated with claw toes. It is usually congenital, but may be associated with disease of the nervous system, for example poliomyelitis. Surgical treatment may be required in very severe cases of pes cavus, but a great many patients have only one real difficulty – finding shoes to fit them; if this can be done, there are no further symptoms. Pes planus: *see* Flat-foot.

Pessary. 1. Instruments in various forms, commonly a ring, designed to support a displaced womb from inside the vagina. 2. A medicated substance made up usually with a glycerine base and shaped like a bullet to be inserted into the vagina, where it releases the drug with which it has been impregnated.

Pestis: plague (q.v.).

Petechiae: small spots in the skin due to tiny haemorrhages which form a red or brown rash, turning blue and yellow later. The causes range from acute infections to fragility of the capillaries.

Pethidine: (Demerol). A powerful, synthetic analgesic

which can be taken by mouth, and has a fairly short action – three or four hours – producing less depression of the respiratory centre than morphine. Unfortunately patients often develop a tolerance to the drug, so that doses have to be increased, and it is undoubtedly a drug of addiction. It is used as a short-acting pain-killer and a premedication for general anaesthesia.

Petit Mal: *see* Epilepsy.

Peyotl: a drug produced from the Mexican cactus Anhalonium lewenii. *See* Mescaline.

Phaeochromocytoma: *see* Pheochromocytoma.

Phage: bacteriophages, or phages, are viruses which attack bacteria. Although they have not proved useful in therapeutics they are of great assistance to the bacteriologist in identifying and typing micro-organisms.

Phagocyte: any cell which eats other cells or micro-organisms. Phagocytes may be fixed or free; the cells of the blood which are phagocytic are the monocytes and the polymorphonuclear cells. *See* Leucocytes, Reticulo-endothelial System.

Phalanx: the phalanges are the small straight bones of the fingers and toes.

Phalloidin: the toxin of the fungus Amanita phalloides which produces rapid and complete necrosis of the liver when eaten in mistake for an edible mushroom. *See* Poisonous Plants.

Phantom Limb: after a limb has been amputated, the patient often has the sensation that it is still there. Usually the phantom disappears in the course of time, but in rare cases it becomes painful and presents a difficult problem. There is, however, a natural tendency for the pain to go.

Pharmacology: the study of the nature and action of drugs. Although these matters have been of considerable interest to physicians and others since ancient times, modern pharmacology has little in common with the remedies of our forefathers:

> *Anything green that grew out of the mould*
> *Was an excellent herb of our fathers of old*
> (Kipling: *Our Fathers of Old*)

Medicines of the past have included excrement, vegetables both fresh and dried, all manner of dead creatures and other curious substances. There are only three major drugs which have been known for centuries: opium, digitalis and quinine. Alcohol may be considered to be a fourth. A hundred years ago modern pharmacology began to emerge from the mass of untidy and often useless formulae that had accumulated over the centuries, and as the chemical industry grew so did the drug firms. By the turn of the century an ever-increasing stream of drugs began to pour from the laboratories which has never stopped – and does not look like stopping. Pharmacology is now big business, and this besides bringing up a number of ethical difficulties means that every drug has as many names as there are drug firms making it, as well as a chemical name and an 'approved' official name; the doctor has to keep his wits about him in threading the maze of advertisements and advertising promotions in order to find sensible remedies for his patients.

Pharmacopoeia: the official list of drugs. The *United States Pharmacopeia* is published by the United States Pharmacopeial Convention, Inc., and is legally recognized; in Great Britain there is a Pharmacopoeia Commission, the *British Pharmacopoeia* and the *Pharmaceutical Codex* are recognized, and there is a *British National Formulary*.

Pharmacy: the technique or art of preparing medicines or the place where they are prepared or sold.

Pharynx: in front, the pharynx is continuous with the nasal cavity and the mouth. Above, the pharynx reaches to the base of the skull behind the nose, and it is continuous with the larynx and the oesophagus or gullet below. The Eustachian tubes from the middle ear open into it on each side in its upper part, and the adenoids, masses of lymphoid tissue, grow from its back wall. It has three constrictor muscles which run round it; when food is swallowed the soft palate cuts the nasal cavity off, the larynx is shut and guarded by the epiglottis, and the constrictor muscles direct the food into the oesophagus. Pharyngitis is inflammation of the pharynx, a common accompaniment of upper respiratory infections.

Phenacetin: a mild analgesic drug similar to paracetamol, but having a slightly slower action and more severe side effects, which include damage to the kidneys and reduction in the oxygen-carrying capacity of the blood; it causes haemoglobin to form compounds (methaemoglobin and sulphaemoglobin) which are stable and cannot take up oxygen from the lungs. Paracetamol is to be preferred.

Phenazone: (Antipyrine). A substance derived from coal tar which is used as an analgesic and antipyretic. It is dangerous, and has no advantage over aspirin or paracetamol.

Phenergan: (Promethazine hydrochloride). An anti-histamine drug which has a slightly longer action than some others, so that an adequate level can be kept up in the blood on two instead of three doses a day. It is used in hay fever, serum sickness, urticaria and angio-neurotic oedema; it makes the patient feel sleepy, and can be dangerous to those who have to manage machinery. It is not advisable to drive if this drug is being taken; moreover, the sleepiness is made worse by alcohol.

Phenindione: (Dindevan, Davilone). A drug which interferes with the clotting of the blood. It can be taken by mouth and is used in conditions such as venous thrombosis, coronary thrombosis, strokes and sometimes in angina pectoris. There are side effects which include skin rashes, diarrhoea, and damage to the liver and kidneys, so that the use of phenindione has decreased.

Phenobarbitone: an old-established barbiturate used in the treatment of epilepsy and as a sedative. *See* Barbiturates.

Phenol: (Carbolic acid). An extremely poisonous crystalline derivative of coal tar; when water is added it becomes a powerful disinfectant and antiseptic. It was the substance used by Lord Lister in his original antiseptic technique, but it is now used less in medicine than in the manufacture of plastics.

Phenolphthalein: a laxative substance which acts six hours after it has been taken. It can cause skin reactions, and turn urine pink.

Phenylbutazone: (Butazolidine). An analgesic and anti-pyretic drug which is particularly useful in cases of inflammation of the joints, for example acute gout and acute arthritis. Unfortunately it may have undesirable side effects which include the aggravation of peptic ulcers, and the production of disorders of the blood, skin rashes and diarrhoea, although irritation of the stomach is to a certain extent avoided by the use of tablets coated with aluminium hydroxide. Phenylbutazone is an excellent drug when used with care, but it must not be used freely as an aspirin substitute.

Phenylketonuria: a disease frequently associated with mental retardation, characterized by impaired metabolism of the amino acid phenylalanine. The enzyme which acts upon this amino acid is absent from the body, causing phenylalanine to accumulate in unusually high amounts. The affected person tends to be fair, with blond hair and blue eyes, because conversion of phenylalanine to pigment is less than normal. There appears to be an increasing deterioration in intellect and many victims develop seizures. The disease is inherited on a recessive basis, indicating that both parents carry the trait and have one chance in four of having an affected child from each pregnancy.

TREATMENT: is to reduce the dietary intake of phenylalanine, especially during infancy and early childhood. Research studies suggest that keeping the phenylalanine levels low will halt the decline of mental ability. The disease can be detected by urine and blood tests after the third day of life, and such testing is mandatory by law in some states of the U.S.A.

Phenytoin Sodium: (Epanutin or Mesantoin). An anticonvulsant drug used in cases of epilepsy, in which it is useful because it makes the patient less sleepy than phenobarbitone. In many cases phenobarbitone and phenytoin are used in combination, the proportion of each drug being adjusted to suit the particular case. Phenytoin is effective in some cases of trigeminal neuralgia. It has one common side effect, thickening and swelling of the gums.

Pheochromocytoma: a rare tumour of the medulla of the adrenal gland, associated with paroxysmal attacks of high blood pressure, headaches and palpitations. *See* Paraganglioma.

Phimosis: Tightness of the foreskin, which prevents it being drawn over the end of the penis. This is not uncommon in little boys, but it must be remembered that the foreskin may not be entirely free from the underlying glans penis until the child is three or four, and that this is quite normal. Phimosis is often thought to be an indication for circumcision, but without infection it rarely is. Nevertheless, cancer of the penis is not found in men who have been circumcised, and it is thought that the occurrence of cancer of the neck of the womb is less in their wives. If in doubt it is better to have boys circumcised.

Phlebitis: inflammation of a vein, usually applied to the condition of superficial venous thrombosis, clotting of the veins near the surface. It is commonest in varicose veins in the leg, where it may follow injury or infection. It is also a method of curing varicose veins, for phlebitis or clotting is followed by scarring of the vein which eventually becomes a fibrous cord; an aseptic phlebitis can be induced by injecting the varicosities with an irritant solution. *See* Varicose Veins. TREATMENT: elastic support and if necessary aspirin or phenylbutazone, which must be used with care. There is no need for the patient to cut down normal activity.

Phlebolith: a stone in a vein. Concretions are not very uncommon, especially in the pelvic veins, where on an X-ray plate they may look to the unwary like stones in the ureter.

Phlebotomus: the sandfly. It carries the organisms of

leishmaniasis, the trypanosomes Leishmania donovani and L. tropica, which are injected into people the sandfly bites and from whom it sucks blood. It also carries the arbovirus of sandfly fever. The fly breeds in cracks and crevices, in old houses and rubble, but spraying with D.D.T. is effective.

Phlebotomy: the incision of a vein in blood-letting.

Phlyctenula: a tiny blister or ulcer on the conjunctiva or the cornea.

Phobia: the word is applied to any abnormal fear, and often a compound word is made with phobia as the suffix to the name of the thing feared, for example, agoraphobia, fear of being in the open, or claustrophobia, fear of being shut up.

Phonocardiogram: a record of the vibrations produced by the heart sounds and by cardiac murmurs. The record may be taken through a pick-up on the chest wall or by a very small instrument on the end of a catheter passed into the chambers of the heart through the great veins.

Phosgene: (Carbonyl chloride). An irritating and lethal war gas.

Phosphorus: phosphorus was at one time the cause of the condition known as 'phossy jaw', when poisoning in chemical or match works led to necrosis of the lower jaw. This is almost unknown today, but illness and death still occasionally occur from swallowing rat poison where the typical symptoms are those of ingesting an irritant substance followed by grave liver damage. Phosphoric acid is a constituent of many tonics where it has no effect whatever; the idea that it had, as in the case of the glycerophosphates, arose from the observation that nervous tissue contains phosphorus. Neurosis was thought to be due to exhaustion of nerve tissues, and it was therefore thought that neurotics needed phosphorus. The argument hardly needs refuting. Phosphates constantly appear in the urine, as phosphorus is one of the commoner elements in the body and in food; they have no particular significance, but the cloudy appearance caused by them when the urine becomes alkaline often causes much needless anxiety to unqualified urine-examiners.

Photophobia: fear of the light. It is a symptom of some eye diseases and of meningitis, i.e. infection and irritation of the membranes surrounding the brain.

Phrenic Nerve: the nerve which supplies the muscle of the diaphragm. Because the diaphragm develops from the tissues of the neck, and during the course of development passes down to lie between the chest and the abdomen, the phrenic nerve takes its origin from the plexus of nerves in the neck called the cervical plexus. Surgeons used to cut the nerve to paralyse the diaphragm in cases of tuberculosis, so that the movement of the lung was diminished, but now indications for operating on the nerve are rare, except in some cases of intractable hiccough.

Phrenology: the pseudo-science founded about 1800 by Gall and Spurzheim and based on the notion that the 'bumps' on the skull could be read to give an analysis of the individual's character, for example his 'amative' or 'possessive' propensities. This is based on two fallacies (1) that such faculties are located in the brain, and (2) that the shape of the brain influences the shape of the skull (unfortunately the reverse is more often true). Today belief in phrenology is limited to the uneducated, but it had a considerable influence in its time and aided the development of the study of personality by more scientific means.

Phthirus Pubis: the crab louse.

Phthisis: wasting. Because it so often used to accompany pulmonary tuberculosis, the word phthisis was frequently used by the profession as a synonym for the disease.

Physeptone: trade name for methadone (q.v.).

Physiology: the science which deals with the normal workings of the human body or those of animals and plants, when it is preceded by the appropriate adjective.

Physiotherapy: therapy by means of physical processes, usually active and passive bodily movements, although a well-equipped physiotherapy department has a variety of apparatus. Physiotherapy is of great importance particularly in surgery, where good results in terms of function are often dependent on good physiotherapy.

Physostigmine: a substance derived from the Calabar bean of West Africa, where it was once used as a poison. Physostigmine is otherwise called eserine and is described under that heading.

Pia Mater: the innermost of the three membranes that cover the brain. It dips down between the convolutions of the cortex, and forms a sheath round the blood vessels of the brain as they enter its substance. *See* Meninges.

Pica: a perversion of appetite supposed to be typical of neurotic children or pregnant women; unusual substances such as coal are eaten. Dirt eating is common in mentally defective children but in others, and in pregnant women, it is most likely to be due to the desire to attract attention. There are places in the United States where white clay (or kaolin) and laundry starch are eaten in large amounts as a peculiar dietary habit. Ordinarily no treatment is needed.

Picric Acid: an explosive which was once used in solution in order to produce a protective coat over a burn or other injury by its capacity to coagulate proteins. It is now out of fashion.

Piles: (Haemorrhoids). Varicose veins of the anus and rectum. External piles are those which are outside the anus, and covered by skin; internal piles arise at the junction of the rectum and the anal canal, so that they are covered with mucous membrane.

CAUSE: overweight, chronic constipation and straining at stool, the use of powerful laxatives, pregnancy, tumours of the rectum and adjacent structures, and very rarely disease of the liver resulting in high pressure in the portal vein, so that in places where the intestinal or portal system of veins joins the systemic or general venous system there is liable to be a 'blow-out'. There is probably a hereditary factor involved in the development of piles.

SYMPTOMS: 1. *Internal piles.* Haemorrhoids are classified according to the extent to which they intrude upon the patient's comfort and consciousness – first-degree piles are those which never appear at the anus, but may bleed from time to time; second-degree piles protrude beyond the anus but return by themselves; third-degree piles having protruded do not return spontaneously but have to be replaced inside the anus. All of them are liable to complications, usually thrombosis (clotting) which is at the time painful but may in the case of first- and second-degree piles be curative. Third-degree piles are particularly liable to infection and strangulation. In all cases there is liable to be bleeding from time to time, usually on passing motions, itching round the anus, discharge and, when the piles thrombose, strangulate or become infected, pain.

2. *External piles* are not noticed unless they thrombose; they then become very painful.

TREATMENT: the commonest trouble is itching round the anus. There are a number of ointments on sale to relieve itching; but by far the best remedy is to keep the anus and skin round it clean by washing with water after every motion, or more often if much discharge is present and the skin becomes sodden. The bowel habits should be regulated and the motions kept soft. When bleeding is the trouble first- and second-degree piles may be injected with an irritating solution to make them thrombose and shrivel up, an operation which is a little uncomfortable but not painful. If third-degree piles give trouble they are best removed by operation; if they prolapse and then become strangulated and infected the patient must be put to bed, and the piles replaced with the help of cold compresses. The condition may be very painful. After the inflammation has subsided the piles are removed. If external piles become painful, it usually means that they have thrombosed. Although with patience they will scar up and so be cured, the pain sometimes makes it advisable to incise them and turn the clot out.

Pilocarpine: an alkaloid derived from the leaves of the plant Pilocarpus microphyllus or jaborandi. Its action mimics stimulation of the parasympathetic nervous system; it constricts the pupil of the eye and improves drainage in glaucoma. It is sometimes used in hair tonics, for which purpose it is entirely useless.

Pilonidal Sinus: a small abnormal opening in the skin in the mid-line about 3 cm behind the anus, which contains dead hairs. It is often infected and becomes painful and swollen. Never seen in children, its development is in some way dependent on the growth of body hair, but the precise way in which it forms is obscure. It may be like the sinuses which form on the hands of barbers because hairs are driven into the skin; it may be congenital; but whatever the cause, the treatment is surgical removal.

Pineal Body: a small structure in the brain, formed by a projection of the back wall of the third ventricle (*see* Nervous System). It was thought by Descartes to be the seat of the soul; recent experimental work in rats indicates that it secretes a hormone called melatonin which has a profound influence upon the sexual cycle and its development. Children who develop a pinealoma (a rare tumour of the gland) are retarded sexually, while damage to the gland may provoke precocious puberty.

Pinguecula: a yellow patch of fat which forms in the eyes of elderly people in the conjunctiva on the nasal side of the cornea. It is harmless.

Pink Disease: (Erythroedema). A disease of young children of between six months and three years in which a mild feverish illness led in about five weeks to redness and swelling of the hands and feet. Redness also occurred on the nose, ears and cheeks, and the child was extremely miserable with sweating, itching, loss of appetite, and photophobia (distaste for light). The cause was related to the use of mercury in teething powders, and when this was stopped the disease disappeared.

Pinkeye: a type of conjunctivitis which is epidemic and contagious.

Pinta: a disease caused by spirochaetes which is very like syphilis; it has three stages, and the organism, Treponema carateum, is identical with the organism of syphilis, T. pallidum. In pinta, the skin becomes discoloured in red, white or blue spots; it is spread by direct contact, but is not necessarily venereal. The disease is found in the Caribbean and tropical America.

Piperazine: the salts of piperazine are active in infestations with threadworms and roundworms. They paralyse the parasites, which are passed in the motions.

Pituitary Gland: (Hypophysis). A small gland about the size of a pea at the base of the brain, just above the back of the nose; it got its name from the Latin word for mucus, 'pituita', for it was once thought that the gland secreted mucus from the brain into the nose. It in fact elaborates several hormones and influences many distant parts of the body, and its importance is reflected in the anatomical arrangement whereby it has its own well-protected bony cavity, the pituitary fossa or sella turcica, named for its resemblance to a Turkish saddle. The gland is divided into four different parts, and is connected to the hypothalamus at the base of the brain by a stalk. The four parts of the pituitary gland are: the pars anterior, pars intermedia, pars posterior and pars tuberalis. Their functions are: (1) the adenohypophysis, which consists of pars anterior, intermedia and tuberalis, secretes growth hormone (G.H.), thyroid-stimulating hormone (T.S.H.), adrenocorticotrophic hormone (A.C.T.H.), luteinizing hormone (L.H.), follicle-stimulating hormone (F.S.H.), and prolactin. (2) The posterior part, otherwise called the neurohypophysis, secretes the antidiuretic hormone (A.D.H.), which is also called vasopressin, and oxytocin.

Growth hormone. This hormone is necessary for the normal growth of the body, although the tissues can grow without it at a diminished rate. The hormone conserves the body's stores of protein by mobilizing fat to be used as fuel and decreasing the breakdown of amino acids. Over-production of growth hormone associated with acidophil tumours of the pituitary gland produces gigantism or acromegaly (q.v.) and under-secretion produces the pituitary dwarf.

607

Thyroid-stimulating hormone. This is responsible for the normal functioning of the thyroid gland. The level of T.S.H. in the blood is raised in cretinism (caused by underaction of the thyroid) and diminished in thyrotoxicosis (over-secretion of thyroid hormone).

Adrenocorticotrophic hormone. This hormone maintains normal activity in the adrenal cortex, and stimulates the secretion of corticosterone and cortisol. In Addison's disease (q.v.) the level of A.C.T.H. in the blood is raised.

Luteinizing hormone and follicle-stimulating hormone. Both these hormones are concerned in regulating the secretions of the sex glands, and are named for their effect on the ovaries. L.H. also stimulates the interstitial cells of the testis so that its alternative name is interstitial cell stimulating hormone (I.C.S.H.), and F.S.H. controls spermatogenesis.

Prolactin. This hormone regulates the development of the breast and the secretion of milk after pregnancy.

The secretion of these hormones is under the control of the hypophysis, the part of the brain just above the pituitary gland; although the anterior part of the pituitary, the adeno-hypophysis, is not directly connected with the hypothalamus like the posterior part, various 'releasing factors' are carried in blood vessels that run between the hypothalamus and the adenohypophysis. The known releasing factors are: growth hormone releasing factor, corticotropin R.F., thyrotrophic hormone R.F., luteinizing hormone R.F., and follicle stimulating hormone R.F. There is in this way direct control of the functions of the body's ductless glands by the central nervous system.

Antidiuretic hormone. This hormone, secreted by the posterior part of the pituitary gland, is also called vasopressin. It raises the blood pressure by a direct action upon the smooth muscle of the walls of the arteries, but only in doses much greater than could occur in nature. Its action on the kidney is more important than its experimental action on blood vessels, for it regulates the amount of water that is lost in the urine. The secretion of A.D.H. is depressed by alcohol, which therefore produces in drinkers a large amount of dilute urine, and increased by nicotine, which may lead to the production of a concentrated urine and water retention in very enthusiastic smokers. (Water retention is commonly held to be depressing.) The destruction of the posterior pituitary leads to the development of diabetes insipidus, a condition in which a great deal of urine is passed so dilute that it looks like water.

Oxytocin. This hormone makes the muscle of the uterus contract. It has an important part to play in labour but the mechanism by which labour is controlled is not clear.

The posterior part of the pituitary gland, the neurohypophysis, is connected directly to the hypothalamus by the pituitary stalk, and the secretion of A.D.H. and oxytocin can be influenced by the central nervous system through the nerve fibres that run in the stalk.

Pityriasis: 1. *Pityriasis alba* is a dry dermatitis found in the young and caused by exposure to the wind and sun, or sometimes by soap. It is of little consequence.
2. *Pityriasis rosea* is a skin affliction of adults which produces quite large brownish-red patches of dry scaling skin. It may irritate, and the best symptomatic treatment is calamine lotion. It is self-limiting and there is no specific treatment.
3. *Pityriasis capitis* is a name for dandruff.

Placebo: a drug given not for its real pharmacological effect, but, as the name indicates, to please the patient. It is therefore usually inert. Two points must be made about the doctor's occasional use of placebos which, no doubt, many laymen regard as a deceitful practice. The first is that, as medicine now is, many patients come to the doctor in a frame of mind which positively demands 'a bottle' (in fact, in some parts 'a bottle' is still the only real medicine and the patient may feel that pills or tablets are fobbing him off the genuine article). This is wrong; the doctor's proper function may very well be to give advice rather than a prescription, but it can well be imagined in what frame of mind most people would leave the doctor's surgery if they were simply given advice. People hate advice, which is, by implication, a criticism of the way they have been leading their life; they prefer to feel that the doctor is like a watch-repairer to whom they take the offending part and demand that it be fixed as if it had nothing at all to do with their real self. Since the doctor cannot re-educate everyone, he must in some cases comply with his patient's often unspoken wishes so long as these do not go too much against the grain. Secondly, placebos are really little doses and symbols of faith. It does in fact have a remarkable effect on a man when he knows that regularly, three times a day, in water, after meals, he must take a particular dose, and even the most intelligent among us is the better for this symbol of the persisting influence of the doctor in our home. Many tests have shown what extraordinary effects can be produced by an inert pill plus belief and, indeed, the effect may be so potent as to nullify trials of a new drug.

Placenta: the placenta is the organ through which the developing foetus in the womb is nourished by its mother. It is a fleshy disc about 3 cm thick and about 20 cm across; when fully developed it weighs about 500 g. The umbilical cord runs from it to the foetus, and is about 50 cm long. The blood from the foetus runs in the umbilical cord to spread out in the foetal side of the placenta; it is always separated from the mother's blood on the maternal side of the placenta by the placental membrane. The placenta is part of the foetus, and before birth it has to act as its lungs, intestines and kidneys, transferring waste matter into the mother's circulation and taking in food and oxygen. Some foetal cells do pass the placental membrane into the mother's blood, and they may be important if the mother is Rhesus negative and the foetus Rhesus positive, for they can then sensitize the mother against her child and produce the condition of icterus gravis neonatorum (q.v.). The placenta is known to produce hormones (steroids and gonadotropins), but little is known of its detailed physiology because the placenta is a difficult organ to investigate; it lasts only for the length of a pregnancy, and then quickly degenerates and is detached and expelled from the womb in the third stage of labour.

Various abnormalities are liable to affect the placenta; it may separate before its time, or fail to separate when it should. It may cover the outlet of the uterus (placenta praevia) or be split into two lobes. Some disease organisms can pass through the placental membrane to affect the foetus, the best known being syphilis and rubella, or German measles, and some drugs can reach the foetal circulation.

Plague: CAUSE: infection with the micro-organism Pasteurella pestis, which is endemic in South America, India, China and some parts of Africa, and the United States west of the Mississippi River. The organism normally affects rats and other rodents, but when they die and the rat flea, which harbours P. pestis, cannot find another rat, it may find a man to live on. This starts an epidemic, for plague is then passed from man to man both by fleas and bedbugs. In countries which are liable to the disease dead rats in the streets herald an outbreak.

SYMPTOMS: the three main types of plague are:

1. *Bubonic*. Named because buboes, or swellings in the groin, are the distinguishing characteristic. In this very fatal form of the disease a spreading rash appears on the skin after painful enlargement of the lymph glands of the groins, armpits and neck.

2. *Pneumonic*. This is the name given to the disease when the organism enters the lungs and multiplies there, producing broncho-pneumonia. The sputum becomes blood-stained, being full of organisms and highly infective. Infection is spread by coughing and sneezing.

3. *Septicaemic*. In this type of case the infection spreads so rapidly in the blood that there is no time for swollen lymph glands to develop.

TREATMENT: plague was endemic in Europe from the fourteenth to the end of the seventeenth centuries; the dreadful Black Death was the most deadly of all diseases, and no treatment was known. There are still outbreaks of plague on a smaller scale, and still reservoirs of infection among rats; but cleaner habits make the spread of plague less likely, and sulphonamides and streptomycin have been used successfully in treatment. It can never be wiped out until all the infected rats have been killed, but precautions can be taken nowadays to contain it and limit its spread.

Plaque: a plate, flat area or patch. It is the name given to a patch of disease process in multiple or disseminated sclerosis.

Plasma: in medicine, the fluid part of the blood in which the blood cells are suspended (the fluid left after blood has clotted is called serum). Plasma can be dried, and made up again with water to be used as an intravenous infusion when whole blood is not available, but in the past dried plasma has been responsible for the spread of hepatitis and it is less used than it might be; modern methods of preparation are making dried plasma a safer substance.

Plasmodium: the organism of malaria (q.v.).

Plaster of Paris: desiccated calcium sulphate dihydrate which, if mixed as a powder with water, sets hard and can be used for making casts for fractured bones and for immobilizing various parts of the body.

Plastic Surgery: the reconstruction and repair of damaged or deformed tissues. Deformities may be congenital or acquired, for example cleft palates, birthmarks, and the scars of burns, extensive surgical removal of growths, or accidents involving the face and neck. Plastic surgery has in some places acquired a slightly dubious reputation because undue emphasis has been placed on 'cosmetic' surgery.

Platelets: small, round, colourless bodies in the blood, having no nucleus. They are smaller than the red blood cells, and are concerned with the formation of clots. There are about 300,000 per cubic millimetre and they are produced in the bone marrow from cells called megakaryocytes; they last about ten days. When a blood vessel is damaged platelets stick to the damaged part of the vessel wall and, if it is a small vessel, plug the defect. They then liberate fibrinogen and a phospholipid concerned with the train of reactions necessary for the formation of a blood clot. *See* Thrombocytopenic Purpura.

Plating: (1) a technique used by orthopaedic surgeons in treating an unstable fracture by fastening a plate of metal to the bone to hold the broken ends in place; (2) the technique of inoculating a plate of nutrient medium with bacteria.

Platysma: a thin sheet of muscle lying just under the skin running from the lower jaw to the upper part of the chest. It is thought to correspond to the 'panniculus carnosus', a muscle which is found in animals just under the skin.

Pleura: the membranes that cover the lungs. The outer (parietal) membrane is applied to the inner wall of the thorax, and the inner (visceral) membrane covers the substance of the lungs. Between the two membranes is a capillary space filled with fluid, which enables the lungs to move freely in the chest. The parietal membrane is reflected from the chest wall to cover the upper surface of the diaphragm, and in the midline it covers the mediastinum, the partition which separates the two sides of the chest and contains the heart, great vessels and other structures which run through the thorax.

Pleurisy: inflammation of the pleura.

CAUSE: infection spreading from the lung, for example in tuberculosis, pneumonia or abscess of the lung; or irritation without infection in cases of cancer of the lung or injury to the lung or the chest wall.

SYMPTOMS: in 'dry' pleurisy, breathing produces a sharp pain in the chest which may spread to the neck or the tip of the shoulder. The patient takes small breaths and tries not to move the wall of his chest more than he must. There is a fever, due to the underlying cause, and a painful cough. One type of dry pleurisy which is not associated with a cough or with inflammation of the lung is called Bornholm disease (q.v.); in this condition there is pain in the diaphragm and the intercostal muscles as well as the pleura, but it is not serious and passes within a few days.

In 'wet' pleurisy, otherwise pleurisy with effusion, which may follow dry pleurisy, there is little pain because the inflamed pleural membranes are separated by an effusion of fluid, which may be sterile or infected. When the fluid is infected and becomes purulent the effusion may be localized as an empyaema by the formation of fibrous tissue. Although there may be little or no pain in 'wet' pleurisy, the patient feels ill, runs a fever, and may, when there is much fluid in the pleural cavity, become breathless. Large sterile effusions of fluid are associated particularly with cancer of the lung.

TREATMENT: consists of the treatment of the underlying condition in cases of tuberculosis, pneumonia, lung abscess, cancer, etc. In Bornholm disease no treatment is necessary. Large collections of fluid can be aspirated by puncture of the chest wall under local anaesthetic, but a well-localized and encapsulated empyaema may require the removal of a section of the overlying ribs before it drains properly.

Pleurodynia: pain on taking a deep breath felt in the muscles between the ribs (the intercostal muscles) and thought to be a manifestation of rheumatism. Pleurodynia is sometimes used as another name for Bornholm disease or devil's grip (q.v.).

Plexus: a network of structures, the term usually being applied to a network of nerves, veins or lymphatic vessels.

Plumbism: lead poisoning.

Pneumoconiosis: an occupational disease of the lungs, found in miners and others who work with dusty substances.
CAUSE: inhalation of certain sorts of dust over a number of years leads to fibrosis of the lungs, increased susceptibility to infection, and consequent tuberculosis, chronic bronchitis, emphysema and even cancer. The dust that causes most trouble comes from coal, and is a mixture of coal, silica and silicates; pneumoconiosis is also caused by silica alone, asbestos, talc, kaolin, mica, beryllium, cadmium, iron, cotton (byssinosis), and other fibrous substances.
SYMPTOMS: cough, shortness of breath, loss of appetite, loss of weight, and the symptoms of tuberculosis, chronic bronchitis and emphysema as they develop. Those who are exposed to asbestos dust are particularly liable to develop cancer of the lung.
TREATMENT: removal from exposure to dust. Pneumoconiosis is well recognized as an industrial disease liable to affect people who work with rock containing silica, or with sand, as in sand-blasting, grinding or the manufacture of abrasives, or with the other substances mentioned above. Many regulations are in force which are designed to cut down the risk of the disease and compensate those who develop it, but no effective treatment is known. Patients must be followed up and periodic X-ray examinations of the chest carried out because of the risk of subsequent respiratory disease, which is treated as it arises. *See* also Occupational Diseases.

Pneumonectomy: removal of a lung.

Pneumonia: inflammation of the lungs. There are basically two types, lobar pneumonia and broncho-pneumonia, but they run into each other and are treated in the same way.

CAUSE: infection with bacteria, viruses and similar organisms, or with funguses, and irritation by worms, inhaled matter, irritant dust or noxious gases.

1. *Bacterial pneumonia.* Micro-organisms found in the sputum of infected cases are the Pneumococcus, Streptococcus pneumoniae, Staphylococcus pyogenes, Klebsiella pneumoniae, and Mycobacterium tuberculosis. Haemophilus influenzae is also found, and rarely Pasteurella pestis (plague) and Bacillus anthracis (*see* Anthrax).

SYMPTOMS: the patient suddenly feels ill, runs a temperature, shivers, and may have a dry cough. The most striking thing about early pneumonia is that the symptoms do not point to the lungs; the patient is more likely to have a headache than a pain in the chest, and he often complains of feeling terribly ill, but has no idea what is wrong. Over a few hours, however, the cough becomes worse, and pleurisy may develop with its characteristic pain on breathing to make the diagnosis clear. Before antibiotics the disease was full of drama, with a week's fever and delirium preceding the 'crisis', in which the patient would suddenly sweat, the fever would fall, and a peaceful sleep and recovery follow.

TREATMENT: as soon as the diagnosis is made, the patient is put to bed, and given penicillin by injection, or ampicillin or tetracycline by mouth. It may be necessary to give oxygen, and sometimes patients, especially the elderly, become restless; nursing may not be easy. Bacterial pneumonia is still a severe and in some cases dangerous disease, but the majority of patients respond quickly to treatment. The diet should be light, with plenty of fluids.

2. *Virus pneumonia.* There are a number of viruses that may infect the air passages and the lungs; they include measles, influenza, smallpox, adenoviruses, and the Bedsoniae of ornithosis and psittacosis which are perhaps not strictly speaking viruses but may be included with them. Another organism like a virus is the Eaton agent, Mycoplasma pneumoniae, one of a group of micro-organisms called P.P.L.O. (pleuro-pneumonia-like organisms). Pleuropneumonia is a well-known disease of cattle; Mycoplasma pneumoniae causes in man the patchy pneumonia often called atypical pneumonia.

SYMPTOMS: the symptoms of atypical pneumonia are very much like those of bacterial pneumonia, but are less dramatic; the fever is less, and the patient though feeling ill is not overwhelmed; the disease lasts for three weeks or more. Virus infection of the lungs by the smallpox virus occurs during the course of a generalized infection, and not by itself, and the same is true of the measles virus. The influenza virus can produce a fatal infection of the lungs, but this is uncommon; the pneumonia that sometimes follows influenza is usually the result of secondary bacterial invasion.

TREATMENT: the antibiotic used in cases of atypical pneumonia and ornithosis is tetracycline.

3. *Fungus infections* of the lungs include blastomycosis, aspergillosis, infection with Candida albicans, the organism of thrush, actinomycosis, histoplasmosis and torulosis.

4. *Worms and parasites*. The lungs may be affected by the lung fluke, Paragonimus westermani, by schistosomiasis, by the organism of malignant malaria, Plasmodium falciparum, and by amoebae in amoebic dysentery. The treatment is the treatment of the general disease.

5. *Inhaled matter*. Pneumonia arising from this cause is called aspiration pneumonia, and it is found in patients who cannot clear their air passages of mucus or other substances by coughing. Mucous secretions in chronic bronchitis may be sucked farther down into the lungs in old people, to turn bronchitis into broncho-pneumonia, and others who cannot clear the air passages by coughing include those under general anaesthesia and the half-drowned.

6. *Irritant dust* may provoke bronchitis and broncho-pneumonia. *See* Pneumoconiosis.

Pneumoperitoneum: air in the peritoneal cavity. It may be induced for diagnostic purposes, and was once used in cases of tuberculosis to raise the diaphragm and so rest the base of the diseased lung. It may be caused by injury or rupture of an internal organ.

Pneumothorax: air in the pleural space of the thorax. It was formerly induced in tuberculosis to rest the lung and prevent the spread of infection, but now the commonest causes of pneumothorax are injury to the chest wall or spontaneous rupture of an enlarged air sac in young men or asthmatic subjects. One form of pneumothorax is insidiously dangerous – the tension pneumothorax, caused by injury to a lung, often by the fractured end of a rib; as air is drawn into the lungs by the expansion of the chest, it is also drawn through the injured lung into the pleural space. The expiratory movement of the chest wall may then put up the pressure in the pleural space and close the opening in the lung, so that a non-return valve is in effect pumping air into the space between the chest wall and the lung. Pressure builds up, the lung collapses, and the structures in the chest are displaced. They include the heart and great vessels in the mediastinum, and unless a needle is put through the chest wall and the pressure let down the patient may die. A valvular injury of the chest wall may have the same effect.

Podagra: gout in the great toe.

Podophyllin: if the root of the plant Podophyllum peltatum is dried and powdered the resin can be used to shrivel up certain papillomas and warts growing on the skin.

Poison Ivy Rash: (Rhus dermatitis). The inflammatory condition of the skin which occurs when a sensitive person has contact with the North American plants poison ivy (Rhus toxicodendron) or poison oak (Rhus diversiloba). A few hours to several days after exposure, the skin develops a burning, itching rash characterized by redness, blistering, and swelling. This rash may spread from the initial point of contact so that extensive areas become inflamed. Some people are so sensitive that they develop the dermatitis from mere closeness to the plant, or from handling a pet or object which has touched it. Others appear relatively unaffected by poison ivy, but this degree of immunity may change during a lifetime.

TREATMENT: the primary treatment is aimed at relief of the itching, for more harm is done by scratching than by the actual rash. Corticosteroids, especially if used at the onset, are effective in making the sufferer more comfortable and in shortening the course of the rash. The drug may be used directly on the skin, as an ointment or cream, or may be taken by mouth or injection. Hot compresses of liquor

617

aluminium acetate (Burrow's solution), 4 tablespoons of the concentrated solution to 1 quart of hot water, are helpful in relieving the itch, pain, and swelling of the acute phase. Various cooling lotions, such as calamine lotion, may be applied in the less severely affected areas. Antihistamines may be beneficial through their sedative action.

Immunization with an extract of poison ivy and oak has been attempted; prevention by this means has not been particularly successful.

Similar allergic skin reactions may occur in sensitive persons from contact with the poison sumac, primrose and dogwood plants of North America.

Poisonous Plants: *Mushrooms.* The genus Amanita is very poisonous, and some members of it can be mistaken for edible mushrooms. Amanita phalloides, the death cap, not only looks like an edible mushroom, but also has an attractive taste. In general, it is true to say that all mushrooms with white gills are to be avoided.

SYMPTOMS: the symptoms of poisoning by the death cap are severe abdominal pain coming on from 6 to 36 hours after the fungus has been eaten, diarrhoea and vomiting, and jaundice. Death follows from failure of the liver. The symptoms of poisoning by Amanita muscaria and pantherina develop much more quickly, and diarrhoea and vomiting accompanied by acute pain in the abdomen are present only an hour or two after eating the fungus. The victim begins to sweat, and may be delirious and hallucinated.

TREATMENT: if there is any doubt at all about the toxicity of a fungus that has been eaten the doctor must be called at once, for the success of treatment for poisoning by the death cap depends on quick and thorough action which includes removal of the stomach contents by washing out, the administration of corticosteroids and the use of transfusions.

Deadly Nightshade: (Atropa belladonna). The berries of this plant are sometimes eaten by children in mistake for blackberries, and the result is belladonna poisoning. The child becomes flushed and hot, the pupils of the eyes dilate so that he cannot see properly, and he is confused and excited. Other wild plants that can cause similar poisoning are Datura stramonium (thornapple or Jimson weed), Solanum nigrum (black nightshade) and Solanum dulcamara (woody nightshade or true bittersweet), whose seeds or berries may be mistakenly eaten.

TREATMENT: the stomach is washed out and an injection given of neostigmine 1.0 mg.

There are many other plants whose seeds, leaves and roots may poison the individual who eats them. Children of an enquiring nature are likely to chew on plants and may accidentally find a harmful species. The adult searching for 'nature' medicines may concoct a poisonous extract if his knowledge of botany is inadequate. Some such plants are: yew (Taxus baccata), whose leaves and seeds produce abdominal pain, diarrhoea and vomiting; water hemlock, the root of which causes convulsions and muscle paralysis; laburnum, whose seeds cause vomiting, confusion, clumsiness and drowsiness; meadow saffron (Colchicum autumnale), whose leaves and seeds may be included in salads and cause gastrointestinal upset; monk's hood root (wolf bane) and larkspur, whose leaves and roots contain a poison which paralyses the heart; and mountain laurel, whose shoots and leaves may cause convulsions and paralysis. Treatment of such poisoning should be promptly undertaken by a physician.

Poisons: the most important thing to do in a case of poisoning is to send for the doctor and keep anything that may give him a clue to the poison – this includes vomit. It is best to forget any thought of an 'antidote', for very few exist, and it is far more important to support the patient's general condition by keeping him warm and if he is unconscious keeping his air passages clear. He should be turned on to his side with his face turned towards the ground; in certain cases of barbiturate poisoning artificial respiration may be necessary.

If there is likely to be much time before the doctor comes or the patient can be got to hospital it may be possible to make the patient vomit by tickling the back of his throat with a finger; this should not be done in the case of poisoning by corrosive substances, when milk or water should be given in large quantities. If you are in difficulty in the United States, specific advice may be obtained from Poison Centers, located in emergency rooms of hospitals, and in the United Kingdom, dial 999 for emergency medical services.

There is no satisfactory definition of poison, but it is usually taken to mean a substance which in relatively small amounts is dangerous to life or at any rate injures health, its effect being produced chemically and through absorption into the bloodstream (ground glass, for example, which produces any result it might have by physical means, is not a poison). There is hardly any substance which could not, in sufficient amounts, produce poisonous effects, and it is well known that in allergy (q.v.) comparatively innocuous foods may prove deadly to those who are sensitized to them. Two of the many possible classifications of poisons are: (1) according to source we may describe them as animal, vegetable or mineral, and further according to chemical type as organic, inorganic, acid, alkaline; (2) according to effect they may be classified as narcotic, corrosive, convulsant and irritant.

Narcotics cause giddiness, headache, drowsiness, and weakness of the muscles by acting directly upon the brain and spinal cord, often after initial excitement. Examples: opium and its derivatives, hyoscine, chloral and chloroform, the barbiturates, etc.

Corrosives include strong acids and alkalies such as carbolic acid, lysol and corrosive sublimate; they stain and blister the mouth and the area surrounding it, damage the gullet and the stomach lining, and affect swallowing and breathing. There is vomiting, diarrhoea, intense colic, and subsequently perforation or gangrene of the intestinal tract.

Irritants are many and include oxalic acid, arsenic preparations, copper sulphate, phosphorus, zinc and lead salts, croton oil, cantharides, etc. There is indigestion when these substances are given in continued small doses, wasting, and many of the appearances of a chronic infection of the intestines (hence their appeal to the poisoner who does not realize how easily most of them can be traced after or before death).

Convulsant poisons like strychnine produce fits; the symptoms of strychnine poisoning are very similar to those of tetanus. Death is due to suffocation or exhaustion, but consciousness is ordinarily unaffected.

Food poisoning is usually caused by infection of the individual with germs which continue to multiply in his body causing gastro-enteritis (inflammation of the stomach and intestines), but the rare condition of botulism and the common one of staphylococcal food poisoning are caused by the toxins of a specific germ which has multiplied in food.

Poliomyelitis: A paralysing disease of the nervous system.
CAUSE: virus infection of the anterior horn cells of the spinal
cord and the nuclei of the motor cranial nerves. The infection is spread by droplets from the nose and mouth, by
contamination of water and food with sewage or human
ordure, and by spread of infected matter by flies.

SYMPTOMS: in the mildest form of attack the patient develops
a sore throat, a slight fever, tiredness and a headache. In
more severe attacks there is pain and stiffness in the neck,
and in the full-blown disease on the fourth or fifth day
paralysis develops and proceeds to its full extent in about
thirty-six hours. These times may vary, but the paralysis
usually affects the limbs and the muscles become painful
and tender, beginning to waste about three weeks after the
onset of paralysis. If the muscles of respiration are affected
breathing may be embarrassed, and in severe cases where
the cranial nerves are affected as well as the spinal cord – the
bulbar form of the disease – swallowing, speaking and coughing may be difficult.

TREATMENT: all patients who are suspected of having the
disease must rest, for it is clear that paralysis is more likely to
occur in muscles which are active. If paralysis develops pain
is treated by aspirin and similar drugs, and the muscles are
not allowed to stretch. If necessary artificial aids to breathing
are used. After about three weeks, when the tenderness has
gone, the muscles are gradually moved and physiotherapy
becomes more active. It is not for a long time possible to tell
which muscles are going to recover and to what extent, but if
they begin to contract within the first month it is almost
certain that they will recover. If they do not, it does not
mean that they will be useless; six months or more must pass
before a final judgment can be made. A very few cases are
left with difficulty in breathing, and fewer still have to
depend on artificial aids to respiration for the rest of their
lives. Death in poliomyelitis comes about because of aspiration pneumonia or circulatory collapse. Most patients recover, but have scars in the shape of wasted muscles, which
are often subject to cramp in the night.

PREVENTION OF THE DISEASE: vaccines have cut the incidence
of poliomyelitis to a fraction of what it was in Great Britain

and North America. Epidemics do not now occur, although sporadic cases are seen particularly in late summer and autumn; but the disease still afflicts tropical countries where flies are a pest. Oral vaccines are commonly used, the first dose being given before the sixth month, a second dose after 2 months and a third after a further 6 months. Subsequent doses are given at 5 and 15 years. The oral vaccine (Sabin type) contains living virus; dead virus vaccine (Salk type) can be given by injection. Patients with poliomyelitis must be isolated, and contacts observed and kept away from children for 3 weeks; if an epidemic should break out, measures of general hygiene must be enforced, flies killed as far as possible, and communal bathing forbidden.

Polyarteritis Nodosa: a disease of connective tissue in which the walls of the arteries undergo a process that results in clotting of the blood and blockage of the arteries with, in some cases, bleeding through diseased parts of the artery into the surrounding tissues. The cause is not known; because any part of the arterial tree can be affected, the disease may give rise to damage in any of the organs. Most commonly affected are the kidneys, in which case a high blood pressure and uraemia develop; the heart is often affected, with the development of coronary thrombosis and perhaps heart failure; the lungs, liver, intestines, muscles, joints, the eye and the nervous system may all be affected, and the skin may be diseased. Treatment is by steroids, which may prolong the patient's life considerably if started early.

Polycystic Kidneys: a condition in which cysts form in the kidneys, which grow to a considerable size. It is thought that the cyst formation is congenital, and there is some evidence that the condition runs in families. The disease often does not show itself until adult life, and then it may be found that the liver, spleen and pancreas are also affected. The condition may give rise to pain, and may interfere with the proper function of normal kidney tissue so that kidney failure follows. It cannot be set right.

Polycythaemia: increase in the number of circulating red blood cells. This may follow conditions in which the circulation is impaired, such as congenital heart disease, or in which the oxygen exchange in the lungs is inefficient – for example emphysema or chronic bronchitis. It may also be found without any obvious cause, in which case it is called polycythaemia rubra vera, or primary polycythaemia. This disease is not common; it is a condition of middle age. The blood becomes thick and viscous because of the abnormal number of cells, and the patient is liable to thrombosis and blockage of the blood vessels. The face has a high colour, and the veins are distended.

Treatment of primary polycythaemia includes blood-letting and the use of radioactive phosphorus, which is taken up by the bone marrow and depresses the formation of red cells.

Polymastia: the condition in the human female of having more than two breasts.

Polymorph: *see* Leucocytes.

Polymyxin: an antibiotic obtained from the soil bacterium Bacillus polymyxa which, unlike most antibiotics, is active against the Pseudomonas genus of bacteria, an organism which may be very difficult to eradicate from infected wounds or the urinary tract.

Polyneuritis: peripheral neuritis. *See* Neuritis.

Polypus: a growth originating from mucous membrane. Usually applied to the greyish overgrowths from the mucous membrane of the nose and the accessory nasal sinuses which may follow chronic infection. Polyps may occur in the bladder or the bowel, in the uterus and in other places where there is mucous membrane. If they are troublesome – usually they show themselves by bleeding – they are removed.

Polyuria: the passage of a great deal of urine.

Pons: that part of the brain which lies in front of the cerebellum and below the cerebrum. Below, it is continuous with the medulla, above, the cerebral peduncles emerge from it and run into the cerebrum, and behind it forms the front wall of the fourth ventricle.

Population: the population of the world is increasing to an unprecedented degree, and the rate of increase becomes greater with every year that passes. This has a number of significant consequences: (1) the great benefits made possible by science of better health, better nutrition and higher standard of living are being nullified as quickly as they are being developed; (2) population pressure is not only a serious problem in itself but a major cause of war (the basic cause of the Sino-Japanese War was the desperate attempt of the grossly overcrowded islands of Japan to find an outlet for their excess population); (3) in the words of Julian Huxley, '. . . beyond his material requirements, man needs space and beauty, recreation and enjoyment. Excessive population can erode all these things. The rapid population increase has already created cities so big that they are beginning to defeat their own ends, and even in the less densely inhabited regions of the world open spaces are shrinking and the despoiling of nature is going on at an appalling rate. Wildlife is being exterminated; forests are being cut down, mountains gashed by hydroelectric projects, wildernesses plastered with mine shafts and tourist camps, fields and meadows stripped away for roads and airports.'

A century and a half ago, the Reverend Thomas Malthus pointed out that population always increased more rapidly than the available food supply, and that consequently there was likely to be widespread misery and starvation in some parts of the world for any foreseeable time to come. Expressed more scientifically, population increase is based on a geometrical or compound-interest progression, whereas food production only increases by arithmetical progression. During the late nineteenth century and the early twentieth, this was shown to be only partially true; for at that time food production increased by more than arithmetical progression. But we now realize that there is an inevitable limit to this rate of increase, and that Malthus was basically right. The growth of the population of this planet has accelerated from a very slow beginning until it has now become explosive, each phase of increase following some major invention or discovery. Before hunting gave way to an agricultural way of life, about 6000 B.C., the number of people in the world was about 22 million, and each new technological revolution –

the building of the first cities, the harnessing of wind and water to do the work of man, the Industrial Revolution, and in our own time the revolution in medical techniques – has led to a fresh burst. In Shakespeare's day the world population was 500 million, but by the middle of the nineteenth century it had become 1,000 million and in the early 1920s 2,000 million. That is to say, it doubled itself twice over between 1650 and 1920, but the first doubling took two centuries, the second less than one. In primitive civilizations the average expectation of life is something like 30 years, and as late as 1880 the average expectation of life in civilized Massachusetts was only 40 years; today all technically advanced societies have life expectancies of about 70 years. In the brief period since World War 2 the introduction of modern medicine and hygiene to Ceylon has halved the death-rate, largely by virtually wiping out malaria with drugs and D.D.T.; but the birth-rate remains the same and, at the present pace, the population will more than double every 25 years. The same is true of such countries as India, Malaya and Thailand together with many others where death-rates have been reduced by a third.

It is in the poorest and most backward countries that people have the largest families: European couples average two or three children, but most Asiatic countries average about six and some as many as eight. The basic reason for this decrease in the technically advanced countries is industrialization and the spread of knowledge. Agricultural societies tend to have more children, partly out of ignorance, but also because children are an economic asset as they help their parents on the land from a very early age; but in an industrial society children are unable to work until they are 15 and often older, and because they are an economic liability, families become smaller. We cannot hope that industrialization will have any significant effect in the world as a whole in the near future, and at the present rate of population increase in countries such as Ceylon the inevitable result, without interference, will be a 64-fold increase in less than two centuries.

The main cause of the present predicament is death control without birth control, and whether we like it or not the introduction of a birth control plan is the only possible solution. This solution is opposed, of course, by the Roman

Catholic Church, and, oddly enough, by many Communists, but few experts believe that there is any other way out.

Porencephaly: a condition associated with mental deficiency in which there are cysts in the substance of the brain arising from developmental errors or damage at birth.

Porphyria: a defect of metabolism in which porphyrins, the substances with which iron and the protein globin unite to form haemoglobin, are excreted in the urine; the defect is inherited.

CAUSE: unknown. There are two main types, congenital and acute intermittent.

SYMPTOMS: 1. *Congenital.* Usually seen in boys; the child's skin is sensitive to light, becoming blistered and infected if exposed to the sun, the teeth may be coloured red, and from time to time the urine becomes pink or purple.

2. *Acute intermittent.* Usually seen in adult women, the symptoms are brought on after the patient has taken barbiturates or sulphonamides. She develops curious symptoms that are often mistaken for hysteria; pain of various sorts in the abdomen, peripheral neuritis with changes in sensation, and confusion. The pain in the abdomen may be so severe that the condition is mistaken for a surgical emergency, and the abdomen opened. This unfortunate accident can only be prevented if the urine is carefully examined; it may not be red, and may only darken if left in the light.

TREATMENT: no specific treatment is known. Obviously, if a child's skin is sensitive to light it must be kept as far as possible in the shade and the skin must be covered, and it is important that known adult cases should not be given sulphonamides or barbiturates. If the condition is known to occur in one member of a family, the other members should be examined to make sure that they, too, are not suffering from porphyria. In addition to sulphonamides and barbiturates, patients must avoid alcohol and contraceptive pills. In an acute attack corticosteroids may help.

Portal Vein: the vein which carries the blood that drains from the intestines to the liver.

Porto-caval Shunt: an operation carried out in cases where

626

because of liver disease the flow of blood in the portal vein is obstructed and pressure in the portal system rises, so that varicosities, which may bleed, develop where the portal system forms anastomoses with the systemic veins – at the lower end of the oesophagus, or in the rectum, or in some cases at the umbilicus. To effect a bypass of the liver the portal vein is joined to the inferior vena cava.

Port-wine Stain: a birthmark whose name is descriptive, the port-wine stain persists throughout life, but may be treated by the plastic surgeon.

Positive Pressure Ventilator: an apparatus which inflates and oxygenates the lungs of a paralysed or anaesthetized patient. If it is to be used for any length of time, as in the case of a severe head injury, the machine is connected through a tracheostomy or artificial opening in the windpipe.

Post-mature: overdeveloped; used of an infant born after its time.

Post-partum: after childbirth.

Post-traumatic: following injury.

Postural Drainage: used in conditions where there is a collection of mucus or sputum in the main air-passages in the lungs, postural drainage means putting the patient into such a position that the main bronchi drain by gravity. The patient usually has to hang head-downwards over the side of the bed, or may be tipped by raising the foot of the bed. Postural drainage is helped by breathing exercises, and is used as a first-line treatment in cases of bronchiectasis (q.v.).

Potassium: deficiency of potassium causes thirst, giddiness and confusion; it has a weakening effect on the heart and other muscles. It follows the loss of salts suffered in vomiting and diarrhoea, and may also follow enthusiastic use of diuretics.

Pott's Disease: curvature of the spine due to tuberculous disease, which collapses the vertebrae. Tuberculosis of bone is mainly acquired from infected milk, but has become progressively less common as milk supplies have become cleaner and tuberculosis in cattle has decreased. Infected milk can be sterilized by pasteurization (q.v.) in places where milk is still suspect, and tuberculosis of the spine can now be treated by drugs and surgical techniques which minimize the deformity.

Pott's Fracture: a fracture or fracture-dislocation of the ankle. Named after Percival Pott, 1713–88, who sustained such a fracture while walking across London Bridge and wrote a full description of it.

Poultice: a soft, moist preparation which retains heat and is applied to a part of the body in order to warm it and keep it from drying up. The most satisfactory poultice is one of kaolin, which can be made up with various antiseptics or irritant substances, is not messy, and can be heated under the grill; it is used on boils and carbuncles and to furnish counter-irritation in various painful conditions.

Pralidoxime: this substance reactivates acetylcholinesterase after it has been attacked by the organophosphorus compounds (q.v.). It is therefore used in cases of poisoning with these chemicals, and is given intravenously or by intramuscular injection in doses of 1–2 g.

Precordium: the region in front of the heart, i.e. slightly to the left side of the chest.

Prednisolone: a synthetic corticosteroid. It has five times the anti-inflammatory activity of natural steroids but the same power of retaining salt, and it is therefore used for anti-inflammatory purposes in preference to hydrocortisone. *See* Corticosteroids.

Pre-eclampsia: eclampsia is a state of convulsions and coma, associated with high blood pressure and protein in the urine, found in pregnancy and childbirth. Pre-eclampsia is the state which unless controlled may lead to eclampsia. It usually comes on after the 28th week of pregnancy; the patient's blood pressure starts to rise, her weight increases more than it should, there may be puffiness of the hands or face, and protein is found in the urine. If the condition progresses, the patient is put to bed, preferably in hospital, and if necessary labour is induced. The foetus is nearly always viable unless the condition has developed unusually early in pregnancy, and in severe cases stands a much better chance of survival if the pregnancy is not allowed to continue to full term.

Pre-frontal Leucotomy: *see* Leucotomy.

Pregnancy: the average duration of pregnancy in the human being is from 274 to 280 days, the commonest early signs of its existence being amenorrhoea or cessation of the periods, enlargement of the breasts, and occasionally nausea in the mornings or evenings and frequency in passing urine. The nipples and the surrounding areola begin to get darker about the third month, and 'quickening' or movements of the foetus may be felt from about the 18th week. From the third month onwards the pregnant womb begins to rise out of the pelvis and can be felt through the abdominal wall. None of these signs is absolutely diagnostic of pregnancy, however, and it is even possible for a woman to have them together with progressive enlargement of the abdomen without being pregnant at all. Positive signs are the hearing of the heartbeat at about the sixth month, agreement on the part of experienced doctors from vaginal examination that a pregnancy has occurred, and positive results from one or other of the biological tests.

Although pregnancy is a normal state of affairs, it is important that regular antenatal examinations should be carried out so that if any abnormalities are present they can be corrected in time. Data collected during the first examination will include the patient's family, personal, and obstetric history; her general medical condition; measurements of the pelvis and blood pressure; urine tests and blood tests for kidney disease and the presence of Rh-antibodies (*see* Blood Groups); and in addition, tests for syphilis will be carried out and the blood group determined. The mother is advised about health and diet, and may be put in touch with an antenatal clinic or a hospital where arrangements for her confinement can be made. Subsequent regular examinations enable the doctor to make sure that the pregnancy is progressing normally or to deal with difficulties as they arise.

Premature Birth: a baby that weighs less than $5\frac{1}{2}$ lb, or 2,500 g, at birth is regarded as premature, however many days the pregnancy is thought to have lasted. If a baby weighs less than $2\frac{1}{2}$ lb, or 1,100 g, (the expected weight at 28 weeks) at birth, it very rarely survives. Of babies that weigh over $4\frac{1}{2}$ lb, or 2,000 g, 96% are expected to survive with proper care. The causes of premature birth are in many cases not understood, but in about two-thirds of the 7% of births that are premature the onset of labour is hastened by conditions such as multiple pregnancy, bleeding and pre-eclampsia. Prematurity is associated with poverty. Premature babies must be guarded against infection by being nursed in special units where they can be isolated; they must be kept warm, if necessary in incubators, and they must not be fed until it is obvious that they are able to suck and swallow, for otherwise there is a grave risk of them developing lung infections from milk that has 'gone down the wrong way'. *See* Respiratory Distress Syndrome.

Premedication: various drugs may be used to prepare a patient for general anaesthesia; they usually include atropine, or a similar substance to dry up the secretion of the lungs and lessen the risk of aspiration pneumonia, and an opium derivative or similar drug to allay anxiety and induce somnolence.

Prepatellar Bursitis: housemaid's knee.

Presbyopia: the changes which occur in eyesight after the age of 40. They are largely caused by decreasing elasticity of the lens, and necessitate the use of glasses for reading and close vision.

Prescription: the directions written by a doctor to the pharmacist about the preparation and the administration of a drug or medicine. A prescription is required by law for many substances, particularly poisons and drugs of addiction, and before a doctor can legally write a prescription he must satisfy the authorities in the country in which he proposes to practise about his competence. The prescription is written in a particular form; it bears the patient's name and address, the date, and the doctor's name and address. The directions about the supply and dosage of the medicine are preceded by the symbol ℞, an abbreviation of the Latin word *recipe*, or 'take'; the name of the drug or the formula for the medicine follows; the amount of each dose is specified, and when it is to be taken; and the total amount of drug or medicine to be supplied is clearly stated.

Presentation: the 'presentation' describes that part of the foetus which will pass first into the birth canal. It changes during pregnancy; normally the head is the presenting part, and the foetus has its neck bent so that the back of the head, the occiput, is first seen as the baby is born. The face normally points backwards, but in a number of cases it is applied to the mother's pubic bone and delivery may be difficult. If the face is the presenting part delivery progresses reasonably well if the chin is to the front, but may be complicated if it is to the rear. In about 3% of cases the baby does not stand on his head, but rather sits down to be born, so that his rear is the presenting part – a state of affairs known as breech presentation. Sometimes the obstetrician is able to turn the baby before birth, for a breech birth is a little more dangerous to the child than the normal head-first position, sometimes he prefers to deliver the mother by Caesarean section, particularly if she is no longer young or has a deformity of the pelvis, but in most cases a breech delivery is successfully accomplished.

Priapism: a condition in which there is a persistent erection of the male organ without any sexual desire; it is caused by thrombosis of the veins of the penis or by various blood diseases, one of which is leukaemia.

Prickly Heat: when there is unaccustomed profuse sweating and the surface of the skin becomes and remains damp, as may happen when people go to hot climates and wear inappropriate clothes, the sweat glands become blocked and little blisters form in the skin. The duct from the sweat gland ruptures, and as a result the skin begins to go red and starts to itch.

TREATMENT: because the sweat glands are put out of action the patient is affected more than usual by heat, and until he

can sweat normally again he must not expose himself to the
hot humid conditions that brought on the attack of prickly
heat. He is transferred to an air-conditioned room, and loose
clothes are worn. Washing should be carried out if possible
without using soap, unless it is of the first quality, but a light
dusting powder may be used on the skin, which must under
no circumstances be scratched; if necessary a sedative drug
should be taken. Baths of tepid water containing a little
hexachlorophane are helpful, and the condition should
recover in about three weeks. The same care would apply to
infants, who seem more susceptible to heat rash than adults.
Care should be taken to keep all skin folds dry, such as in the
neck, armpits, groin, and back of the knees, because moisture
quickly causes the infant's skin to break down.

Primidone: (Mysoline). An alternative to phenobarbitone
in the control of epilepsy.

Primipara: a woman who has given birth, or is in the process of giving birth, to her first child.

Probenecid: (Benemid). A drug originally synthesized for
its effect in diminishing the excretion of penicillin through
the tubules of the kidney, probenicid is used both to lengthen
the action of penicillin where necessary (for example in
subacute bacterial endocarditis) and to increase the excretion of uric acid in cases of gout. For this latter purpose it
should only be given in the absence of an acute attack; it
may bring one on, which has to be treated with other drugs,
but in the end the use of probenecid or a similar drug will
cut down the number of attacks or even stop the gout entirely.

Procaine: a fairly weak local anaesthetic, used less now
than it used to be, for it has been supplanted by more potent
preparations. A complex of penicillin G and procaine is
called procaine penicillin; the active drug is slowly released
from the compound, so that one injection will keep a satisfactory level of penicillin in the blood for 24 hours instead of
the 3 hours of the simple penicillin G.

Procidentia: term meaning complete prolapse of the womb.

Proctalgia: pain in the rectum. No cause is known for the

632

spasmodic attacks of severe pain (they may last for 10 minutes) which are called proctalgia fugax.

Proctitis: inflammation of the rectum or anus. It may occur in a variety of conditions which include haemorrhoids, dysentery, ulcerative colitis, bilharzia and venereal disease.

Proctoscope: an instrument for inspecting the interior of the anal canal and the lower part of the rectum.

Prodromal: a symptom or sign that precedes the full development of a disease.

Progeria: premature old age.

Progesterone: a naturally occurring hormone secreted by the ovary (q.v.).

Prognosis: a forecast of the probable course of an illness.

Progressive Muscular Atrophy: a disease of the motor neurones.
CAUSE: unknown; it occurs more commonly in men than women, and is a disease of late middle age.
SYMPTOMS: clumsiness and weakness of the hands, followed by wasting of the muscles of the hand so extensive as to produce a 'claw hand'. The muscles of the arms and shoulders become weak and wasted, and occasionally the legs follow suit.
TREATMENT: no effective treatment has yet been found.

Proguanil: (Paludrine). An anti-malarial drug that stops the development of Plasmodium falciparum in the stage before it enters the red blood cells, and the development of the other malaria parasites after they have entered the red cells. It is widely used as a prophylactic drug, being taken in a daily dose of 100–200 mg beginning the day of entering a malarious area and continuing for a month after leaving it. *See* Malaria.

Prolactin: a hormone secreted by the anterior part of the pituitary gland (q.v.). It stimulates the flow of milk in nursing mothers.

Prolapse: the falling down or forwards of a part, usually used of the womb, which may fall in later life as a result of injuries suffered in childbirth, or of an intervertebral disc, as when the discs in the lower lumber region protrude and press on the emerging nerves.

Promazine: (Sparine). A centrally acting sedative, which is useful in the treatment of morphine addiction and alcoholism. It is used particularly in the sedation of the elderly.

Pronation: the movement of turning the hand palm down. The opposite movement is called supination.

Prophylaxis: treatment undertaken to prevent disease; the prevention of disease.

Proptosis: a protrusion, usually used to mean prominence of one or both eyeballs.

Prostaglandins: substances which are found in seminal fluid and to a lesser extent in the kidneys, lungs, brain and other tissues. They have a stimulating action on smooth muscle, and make the uterus contract. They are currently under active investigation because they are thought to be concerned with the regulation of the action of other hormones, and because it is possible that they might provide the long-looked-for method of procuring an early abortion by taking a pill.

Prostate Gland: the gland that surrounds the neck of the bladder and the beginning of the urethra in men. It is about $3 \times 2.5 \times 4$ cm, and has three lobes – two lateral and one middle. The most common malady affecting it is benign enlargement; other diseases include cancer, inflammation, tuberculosis and stones.

Benign enlargement. CAUSE: unknown.

SYMPTOMS: difficulty in starting to pass water, poor stream, dribbling and frequency, and predisposition to infection of the urine. Eventually the urethra may be entirely blocked, so that no urine will pass.

TREATMENT: removal of the enlarged gland either by an open operation through the lower abdominal wall or by a closed operation carried out through an operating cystoscope, in which part of the enlarged gland is cut away by diathermy. The open operation is preferable, but is not always possible. After removal of the prostate men are usually sterile, but not impotent. In cases of acute retention of urine the bladder is if possible emptied by means of a catheter, but if this cannot be done the bladder is drained through the abdominal wall under local anaesthetic.

Cancer of the prostate. The symptoms are the same as those of benign enlargement, with the addition that metastatic spread of the cancer may produce symptoms elsewhere – very often in the bones, so that an abnormal fracture or one that will not heal properly may be the first indication of the disease.

TREATMENT: if possible – if the disease has not spread too far, and the patient is fit enough – the prostate is removed. If not, then the condition is treated by doses of the hormone stilboestrol which makes the cancer in the gland diminish and the secondary deposits shrink and become painless. The effect is unfortunately not permanent, but it may last a long time.

Prostatitis: acute. The gland may become infected in the course of an inflammation of the urethra – for example in gonorrhoea – or after the passage of an instrument into the bladder. It may also become infected for no obvious reason. The commonest micro-organisms that infect the prostate are Neisseria gonorrhoeae, Escherichia coli and Staphylococcus aureus.

SYMPTOMS: pain in the perineum and on passing motions, with frequency of passing urine and sometimes obstruction.

TREATMENT: antibiotics and surgical drainage of any abscess that might form.

Chronic. Follows urethritis, gives rise to pain and frequency of passing urine and is treated by antibiotics and prostatic massage.

Tuberculosis. Nearly always found with other foci of disease in the genito-urinary system, and treated by drugs rather than by surgery.

Stones. These form as a result of chronic inflammation, and may not be harmful. If it appears that they are causing trouble the whole or part of the prostate may be removed either by open operation or through the operating cystoscope.

Prosthesis: any artificial part used to replace one that has been removed, for example false eye, leg or teeth.

Prostigmine: (Neostigmine). An anti-cholinesterase drug which is used in the diagnosis and treatment of myasthenia gravis. It is also used in the treatment of megacolon (q.v.).

Protamines: basic, simple proteins, used in combination with insulin and zinc to prolong the action of insulin, and also used as protamine sulphate to stop the action of the anti-coagulant heparin. The protamines are obtained from the sperm of fish.

Proteins: complicated nitrogenous compounds made up of about twenty amino acids which are the main constituents of the substance which forms an animal or plant cell.

Proteolysis: the breakdown of proteins into simpler compounds by the biological action of enzymes (q.v.).

Prothrombin: a substance in blood plasma that is converted into thrombin when blood clots. *See* Blood Clotting.

Protoplasm: the material of living tissues.

Protozoa: micro-organisms with one cell which form the lowest division of the animal kingdom. They differ from bacteria, for the characteristics of the protozoan cell resemble closely the characteristics of the cells from which the multi-cellular mammals are made. About thirty types of protozoon are known to exist as parasites on man, but about half of these are harmless. The others are responsible for such diseases as malaria, amoebic dysentery, sleeping sickness and kala-azar. Of the pathogenic protozoa some are passed from man to man by insects, some by contamination of food and water, some in other ways. They can provoke the formation of antibodies, but vaccination is not yet possible nor is the production of passive immunity. Protozoa are found as parasites throughout the animal and plant kingdoms and in any place where there is moisture – the sea, fresh water and the soil.

Proximal: the word is used to describe anything which is nearer to a given point of reference; things farther away are called distal. The knee, for example, is spoken of as proximal to the foot and the foot is distal to the knee, for in anatomy the centre point of the body is taken as the reference point.

Prurigo: an itching condition characterized by papules deep in the skin.

Pruritus: itching; a sensation which makes the subject want to scratch himself, found in a number of conditions ranging from insect bites to old age. In general the treatment depends upon the underlying condition, but in simple cases calamine lotion, if necessary fortified by 1% phenol, is effective; in more severe cases corticosteroids applied in an ointment are often very useful, and in intractable cases it may be justifiable to give corticosteroids by mouth. Sedatives are often used, and antihistamines are given by mouth for their tranquillizing effects – they should not be used on the skin for they sensitize the patient, and are disappointing as a local application.

Pseudocyesis: false pregnancy, a curious condition in which the signs of pregnancy are present but the womb is empty.

Pseudomonas: Pseudomonas pyocyanea is a Gram-negative bacillus which infects wounds, burns and the urinary system. It is resistant to most antibiotics and common disinfectants and is therefore found flourishing in hospitals, as well as in the intestines and on the skin of healthy people. Once an infection has become established it is remarkably difficult to abolish.

Psittacosis: *see* Ornithosis.

Psoas: the fillet, a muscle which runs from the lumbar vertebrae to the upper part of the thigh-bone.

Psoriasis: a very common skin disease, in which red scaly spots and patches appear on the elbows and knees and other parts of the body, usually symmetrically on the two sides. The cause is unknown, but the disease tends to run in families and is first seen in adolescents or even earlier, although it may come on in middle or old age. It does not itch very much, but is disfiguring; it has spontaneous remissions but appears again after intervals of greater or lesser duration. Treatment

637

is by external applications of tar and salicyclic acid ointment or dithranol, zinc and salicylic acid paste. The patient must be careful not to overtreat his skin, and not to be unduly depressed if progress is slow. The disease is not dangerous.

Psychedelic: from the Greek word *psyche*, the soul, and *delos* – obvious, clear; applied to the process of making the soul manifest by taking certain drugs which confuse the perception and thereby, it is thought, release the soul from the imprisonment of reality. Others would say that the drugs produce hallucinations and delusions.

Psychiatry: that branch of medicine which deals with mental illness.

Psychoanalysis: refers (*a*) to the theories of Sigmund Freud and (*b*) to the method of treatment based thereon. Freud showed that mental illness (and normal behaviour, too) can be explained in terms of a conflict between primitive emotions in the unconscious mind and the more civilized and learned tendencies in the conscious mind. The personality is divided into the 'id', which is the unconscious, containing primitive and repressed impulses, the conscious 'ego', and the half-conscious, half-unconscious 'superego' which may roughly be equated with the conscience. Thus all behaviour is the result of a three-cornered struggle between the ego (representing reality), the super-ego (representing the social impulses) and the id (representing the primitive desires). Initially the child is entirely primitive, but his growing up is a process of slowly putting away childish ways and learning to repress unsuitable behaviour or sublimate it into something more useful; if this process fails, neurosis may develop in later life and the individual's relationships with others suffer. The first persons to whom the child has to relate himself are, of course, the parents, and psychoanalysis attaches great importance to this as the prototype of all later relationships, for example a child who hates his father may grow up with an unreasoning hatred of all authority, or a child who is unloved will be unable to form any genuine love relationships later. The main instincts are the sexual and aggressive ones from which all the others arise, the word sexual being used in the widest possible sense to include, for

638

instance, the infant's pleasure in sucking or in its bowel movements. Psychoanalysis is a form of psychotherapy (q.v.) which is suitable in certain selected cases only, i.e. in those whose personality is on the whole good, who are young and of high intelligence, and who are capable of affording the time and money for treatment which takes about an hour on five days a week, during which the patient's problems are analysed by the method of free association. The patient lies on a couch and says whatever comes into his head, and this enables the analyst to unravel the sources of his troubles. Although free treatment can be obtained at the various institutes throughout the great cities of the world, it is ordinarily necessary to obtain private therapy, which can be quite costly. Psychoanalysts must be trained in an institute.

Psychology: that branch of science as opposed to medicine which deals with the workings of the normal mind and is concerned with the study of normal behaviour.

Psychoneurosis: synonymous with neurosis (q.v.).

Psychopathic: an adjective applied to any form of abnormal behaviour; a psychopath is one who is in some respects at odds with society – his disturbance takes the form of antisocial actions. In this way he is a trouble to others rather than to himself.

Psychopharmacology: the branch of pharmacology that concerns itself with the study of the actions of drugs on the psychological functions.

Psychosis: insanity as ordinarily understood.

Psychosomatic Diseases: these are physical diseases in which a major factor in causation is clearly mental. The mind acts through the autonomic nervous system (*see* Nervous System) by means of its sympathetic and parasympathetic divisions and by hormones to produce effects which may ultimately influence the structure of the body and lead to such troubles as peptic ulcer, essential hypertension and many skin diseases. One major rediscovery of twentieth-century medicine has been that all diseases are in some degree psychosomatic, i.e. they happen to persons, not to inanimate objects; what the person thinks and feels will have an immense influence upon his health. It is incorrect, except in a very loose sense, to speak of this as the influence of mind over matter because the individual is a unified being, even if the medicine and science of the nineteenth century thought of him as a ghost in a machine.

Psycho-surgery: surgery performed on the brain in order to modify psychiatric disease. *See* Leucotomy.

Psychotherapy: a general term used for any kind of mental healing. It may take many forms, which can be described briefly under the headings of autosuggestion, heterosuggestion and analysis. *Autosuggestion* was much popularized in the early years of this century by Emil Coué whose 'every day and in every way I am getting better and better' became famous. It is, in fact, true that some results can be obtained by this sort of self-hypnosis, but they are unlikely to be lasting and only comparatively trivial conditions can be so treated. *Heterosuggestion*, either in the form of persuasion, telling with authority or by hypnosis, is a good deal more potent, but has disadvantages which stem from the fact that every symptom has a cause; the symptom can only be removed permanently by the removal of that cause. If someone has a fear of closed spaces there must be a reason why this is so which will not be removed by telling him even under the deepest hypnosis that he has no such fear; the symptom may go, but another will take its place. Most schools of *analytical psychotherapy* today are under the influence of Freud (*see* Psychoanalysis) and depend upon a rational examination of the causes of the trouble, but it is impossible to assess the parts played by faith and the therapist's personality.

Pterygium: a fold of membrane that is the shape of a wing on the conjunctiva, extending from the cornea across the sclera or white of the eye.

Ptomaine: a substance otherwise called a putrefactive alkaloid formed by the action of bacteria on animal matter, once held to be responsible for food poisoning.

Ptosis: the falling of an organ or part as in visceroptosis;

applied particularly to drooping of the upper eyelid as the result of paralysis of the third cranial nerve.

Ptyalin: an enzyme contained in saliva which breaks starch down into dextrose and maltose.

Puberty: the period between the appearance of the secondary sexual characteristics and the attainment of full growth. The onset of puberty usually occurs at the age of 12 years in girls and 14 years in boys, with a 3-year range on either side being normal. There are what may be termed early developers and late developers, either difference in onset of maturation often becoming a source of alarm to the oversensitive person in this age group. Appearance of secondary sex characteristics earlier or later than the average age range, as above, should be appraised by a physician.

Pubis: the os pubis, the pubic bone, is the bone felt at the bottom of the abdomen; it is the bone through which the hipbone or os coxae joins its fellow on the other side. The midline joint between the two pubic bones is called the pubic symphysis.

Puerperal Fever: childbirth fever, a septicaemia which was, up to the middle of the last century, a widespread killer. Oliver Wendell Holmes of Boston observed and described the fact that the disease was contagious, and Semmelweiss of Vienna showed that it could be caused by attendants at a lying-in coming to the case without washing their hands, in some instances having been engaged in dissections and similar septic activities. Washing the hands and the use of antiseptics have greatly reduced the incidence of the disease, which is in fact caused by bacterial infection of the raw area where the placenta was attached to the uterus or of lacerations in the birth canal. Although infection following childbirth is by no means unknown, puerperal septicaemia is now rare; it is most often seen after a long neglected labour or after criminal abortion. It is treated with antibiotics.

Puerperium: the lying-in period after childbirth, usually regarded as lasting a month.

Pulmonary: to do with the lungs.

Pulmonectomy: the surgical removal of a lung.

Pulp Infection: the pulp meant in this term is the pulp of the finger-tip; infection is common here and can have serious consequences if it is not dealt with quickly and adequately. The fact that treatment is not entirely straightforward is shown by the existence of more than one school of thought – one holds that early incision is necessary, another that the knife must wait until pus has clearly formed and is pointing. One opinion favours poulticing, the other simple immobilization of the finger and hand. There is no doubt that antibiotics should be used, nor is there any doubt that neglect will lead to infection of the bone of the tip of the finger and serious trouble. All septic fingers require a doctor's attention.

Pulse: the expansion and contraction of an artery in response to fluctuations of blood pressure between high systolic and low diastolic levels as the heart beats. It can be felt at the wrist where the radial artery lies over the bone just below the base of the thumb, and can also easily be felt at the temple. The pulse should be regular, and in health the resting rate in men is about seventy-two, in women about eighty. A great number of variations are described, many dating from the years before electrocardiography and other more refined methods of examining and analysing the heart's action were possible; the type of pulse, for example, that is found in disease of the aortic valve, where the blood can run back into the heart after each beat, is called 'water-hammer pulse', 'Corrigan's pulse', 'cannon ball pulse', 'locomotive pulse', 'trip-hammer pulse' and 'collapsing pulse'.

Pupil: the opening in the centre of the iris (q.v.).

Purgatives: *see* Constipation.

Purpura: a condition in which purple spots appear under the skin due to the escape of blood from small blood vessels. It is caused by a number of diseases, among which are anaphylactoid purpura, a disease of children which follows severe infection with haemolytic streptococci or is sometimes associated with allergic reactions; scurvy, caused by lack of vitamin C; various blood diseases and fevers such as measles and smallpox, in which severe forms are purpuric; and drug sensitivity. Purpura may also be caused by a lack of platelets in the blood in the condition called idiopathic thrombocytopenia, which is thought to be an auto-immune disease; antibodies are produced by the individual against his own platelets.

Pus: tissue fluid containing the products of inflammation – white cells, bacteria and broken-down tissue.

Pyaemia: a state in which the blood contains pus or pieces of septic clot. Multiple abscesses form in various parts of the body.

Pyelitis: inflammation of the pelvis of the kidney. It is rarely found on its own, but is usually associated with inflammation of the substance of the kidney. *See* Pyelonephritis.

Pyelography: X-ray examination of the pelvis of the kidney after it has been outlined by a radio-opaque substance. A compound containing iodine, for example Urografin, is injected into a vein after plain X-ray photographs have been taken of the abdomen, and further pictures are taken after 5, 10, 15 and 30 minutes. The kidney concentrates the compound and secretes it into the renal pelvis, and as it runs into the bladder through the ureters these structures are outlined. Some idea of the function of the kidney can be obtained from the time taken to concentrate the iodine and the degree of concentration achieved. If the kidneys are not seen clearly another way of filling the bladder, ureters and renal pelves is to pass a cystoscope into the bladder and introduce fine catheters up the ureters through which the contrast medium can be injected. The method whereby contrast medium is injected into a vein is called intravenous pyelography, or I.V.P., and the second method by direct injection into the ureters is called retrograde pyelography.

Pyelonephritis: inflammation of the kidney and the renal pelvis.
CAUSE: the commonest infecting micro-organism is Escherichia coli, which normally lives harmlessly in the gut. Other organisms may be implicated, among which are streptococci,

staphylococci and Bacillus proteus. Infection may reach the kidneys through the bloodstream or by spreading up the ureters from the bladder and urethra, and is commonly associated with pregnancy in women and enlargement of the prostate gland in men, for in both conditions there is obstruction to the passage of urine and consequent stagnation. Other causes are congenital abnormality and stones.

SYMPTOMS: fever and shivering, pain in the small of the back and sometimes in the abdomen, scalding on passing water and frequency of urination. The disease may be recurrent, especially in women, and chronic disease may produce a high blood pressure.

TREATMENT: sulphonamides or antibiotics, according to the sensitivity of the infecting organism. If an enlarged prostate or other abnormality is found it must be set right or the infection will become chronic.

Pyknolepsy: petit mal. *See* Epilepsy.

Pyloric Stenosis: narrowing of the outlet from the stomach.
CAUSE: *Congenital.* The direct cause is unknown, but the condition is found usually in baby boys between the second and the sixth weeks and is inherited. The muscle surrounding the pylorus is overdeveloped.

Acquired. Narrowing in adults usually results from the scarring that follows a duodenal ulcer near the pylorus, or is caused by a carcinoma of the lower end of the stomach.

Acute duodenal ulcers may cause apparent narrowing by setting up a spasm of the pyloric muscle and by provoking oedematous swelling of the mucous membranes and underlying structures.

SYMPTOMS: *Congenital.* The baby starts to bring its food back, at first gently but soon by violent vomiting which is sometimes described as projectile vomiting, loses weight, becomes dry and is unmistakably ill. There is no diarrhoea with the vomiting.

Acquired. The patient has a history of indigestion leading to attacks of vomiting. The vomiting is characteristic; large amounts of undigested food are brought up at a time, and the remains of meals taken some little time ago may be identified. The patient loses weight, vomits about once a day, and becomes dry.

TREATMENT: in both types of pyloric stenosis the first step is to restore water and salt balance in the patient by giving intravenous fluids. The stomach is aspirated through a tube and washed out with normal saline, and when the patient's condition is as good as it can be the abdomen is opened. In babies, the muscle of the pylorus is cut through until the mucous membrane lining the stomach and duodenum can be seen; it is allowed to swell up into the incision through the muscle, which is left open, the abdomen is closed and the child takes food again in a matter of hours. In adults the operation of choice is partial removal of the stomach, but this is not always possible, and the surgeon may have to restrict his operation to a short-circuiting gastro-enterostomy.

Pylorospasm: spasm of the muscle at the pylorus usually caused by a duodenal ulcer. Treatment is medical.

Pylorus: the opening at the end of the stomach through which food passes into the duodenum.

Pyogenic: anything which produces pus, usually applied to micro-organisms.

Pyorrhea: the discharge of pus; pyorrhoea alveolaris is a disease of the gums and teeth in which pus is continually discharged; eventually the teeth become loose in the jaw.

Pyrethrum: a powder lethal to insects, obtained from the plants Chrysanthemum cinerariaefolium or Chrysanthemum occineum.

Pyrexia: fever.

Pyridoxine: Vitamin B_6. A deficiency of this vitamin may cause convulsions in infants.

Pyrogen: any substance which provokes a fever.

Pyuria: the passage of pus in the urine.

Q

Q Fever: an acute illness with fever and pneumonia.
CAUSE: infection with a micro-organism called Coxiella burnetii, which normally is found infecting sheep, cattle and goats, and is passed on by ticks and lice from animal to animal. The infection may be passed to man through contaminated milk. It may also be passed on by the contamination of food with infected dust, or the dust may be inhaled.
SYMPTOMS: very like influenza, but the disease may be prolonged by the ability of the organism to infect the valves of the heart.
TREATMENT: tetracycline.

Quadriceps: the large muscle at the front of the thigh which is really a combination of four muscles called the vastus medialis, vastus intermedius, vastus lateralis and rectus femoris. The quadriceps is inserted into the top of the tibia through the patellar tendon, in which lies the knee-cap, and its main action is to extend the leg at the knee.

Quadriplegia: paralysis of all four limbs.

Quarantine: the isolation of people who are suspected of having a communicable disease, or who have been in contact with one. Ships may be held in quarantine if they arrive from ports where a severe infection is rampant, or if they have cases of infectious disease aboard. *See* Incubation Period.

Quartan: one type of malaria is called quartan because the paroxysms of fever recur every third day. The organism is Plasmodium malariae, which completes its cycle in 72 hours. *See* Malaria.

Quassia: a bitter-tasting wood from which an infusion can be made which was once used as a remedy for fevers; it can also be incorporated in an enema for the treatment of threadworms. *See* Worms.

Quickening: the first movements of the foetus, felt by the mother at about the 20th week.

Quinidine: a drug like quinine obtained from the cinchona; it is in chemical terms the dextrorotatory isomer of quinine. It is used to diminish the excitability of heart muscle.

Quinine: an alkaloid obtained from the bark of the cinchona tree of South America which was for many years used as a remedy for malaria. It is still used in certain cases of malignant malaria, for it can be given by injection to small children, and it is given to adults when Plasmodium falciparum proves resistant to other drugs. It is poisonous if taken in an overdose, producing ringing in the ears, headache, vomiting, blurring of vision or even blindness, and damage to the heart which may end in circulatory collapse. *See* Cinchona.

Quinsy: *see* Peritonsillar Abscess.

Quotidian: used of a form of malaria where the paroxysms recur every day. This can occur when the infection is mixed.

R

Rabies: a disease occurring in certain animals, notably the dog and the wolf, which can be passed on to man. Rabies is endemic in skunks, racoons, foxes and bats in America. In parts of South America rabies exerts tremendous economic toll as a result of vampire bat transmission to cattle.

CAUSE: infection of the central nervous system by a rhabdovirus. The disease is transmitted to man by a bite from an infected animal; the incubation period is anything from a week to six months, being shortest when the bite is on the face and longest when it is on the foot, for the virus travels up the nerves to the brain.

SYMPTOMS: in the dog, irritability and excitement; the dog runs about snapping, and barks on a characteristic high note. It becomes paralysed and dies within ten days. As the animal sickens, it becomes limp, it cannot swallow and chokes on saliva. The owner may attempt to aid the animal by searching for the cause of choking, putting his hand into the mouth and thus inoculating his own skin with the saliva. In man, the first signs are depression and restlessness; the name hydrophobia arises from the spasms of the pharynx that occur when the patient tries to drink. The painful muscle spasms spread, and the patient suffers general convulsions and becomes mad. Within a few days he is paralysed and he dies in a coma.

TREATMENT: once the disease has appeared it is certain to be fatal; treatment must be preventive. In Great Britain rabies is now a disease of the past, because all susceptible animals are kept in quarantine on arrival in the country for a period of time long enough for the disease to appear if the animal is in the incubation period. In other parts of the world which are not surrounded by sea it is not possible to control rabies in the same way. It is said still to cause 20,000 deaths a year in India. Domestic dogs can be inoculated, and where they flourish wild dogs and jackals must be kept away from pets and if necessary shot. If a man thinks he has been bitten by a rabid animal he must at once start treatment, and the animal must if possible be caught for examination. The bite is surgically cleaned, and hyperimmune rabies serum injected. Active immunization is started with injections of killed rabies virus. Methods of immunization vary slightly, but all are founded on the principle that the patient must acquire active immunity before the incubation period of the disease has finished.

Rachitic: rickety. *See* Rickets.

Radiculitis: inflammation of a root; applied to inflammation of the root of a spinal nerve.

Radioactivity: *see* Ionizing Radiation.

Radiography: the production of X-ray pictures. The radiographer is responsible for taking and developing the films; the radiologist is medically qualified and examines and reports on the appearances of the films.

Radiology: the branch of medicine concerned with the use of radiation in the treatment and diagnosis of disease.

Radiotherapy: the use of radiation in the treatment of disease.

Radium: a metal which is a source of spontaneous radiation. It was discovered in 1898 by Mme Curie, who isolated it from pitchblende; it emits alpha, beta, and gamma rays, which are similar to X-rays, and it is warm, always being at a temperature from 2 °C. to 5 °C. above the surrounding atmosphere. It has for a long time been used in medicine for its gamma radiation, for it can be implanted into diseased tissues in the form of needles or seeds. *See* Ionizing Radiations.

Radius: the bone of the forearm which lies on the outer side when the arm is by the side and the palm turned to face forwards. It is able to rotate round the ulna, the other forearm bone, so that the movements of pronation and supination are possible. It plays a small part in the formation of the elbow joint, but a larger part in the wrist joint, where it is the bigger bone, for the ulna tapers somewhat from its size at the elbow.

It is often fractured at the wrist by falls on the outstretched hand (Colles' fracture). *See* Ulna.

Râle: a sound heard through the stethoscope in diseases of the lung and air passages. *Râles* are said to be moist or dry, and are produced by the passage of air over or through dried-up or wet secretions or into air-sacs the walls of which stick together. *Rhonchi* are very coarse snoring or wheezing noises caused by partial obstruction to the air passages.

Ranula: a cyst which develops underneath the tongue on one side or the other, thought to be the result of a blocked duct and consequent enlargement of a small salivary gland. It is not dangerous, and the treatment is surgical.

Rash: a temporary eruption or discoloration of the skin, usually associated with an infectious fever. Salient characteristics of various rashes are as follows:

Measles. Before the rash appears on the skin, small white spots develop inside the mouth (Koplik's spots). The skin rash starts as small red spots behind the ears and on the forehead which spread on to the face and so down on to the trunk and over the whole body. The rash is fully developed in about two days. As it develops it darkens, and the spots become raised, running together to form large blotches. It lasts about a week.

Chickenpox. The rash starts on the trunk and is most marked on those parts of the body which are normally covered. It begins as small flat spots, which quickly become pimples and then small blisters which turn purulent, burst and form scabs. The rash itches a great deal, and lasts about a week. The pocks form in crops and take a day to turn from small flat spots into pustules.

Smallpox. In this disease the rash may be preceded by small haemorrhages into the skin (petechiae) or generalized reddening roughly over the area covered by a pair of trunks. The main rash, which starts about the third day of the disease, appears in the opposite way to the rash of chickenpox; first it develops on the forehead and the face, then on the hands and the wrists, and then on the feet and the legs. It is more marked on those parts of the body which are least covered, and is sparse on the trunk. The rash is at first pink, and composed of small flat spots. These harden into pimples within a day and the pimples turn into blisters over the next two days. The blisters become purulent and after about a week break down and form scabs, which may persist for a further few weeks. All the elements of the rash change at the same time, and may run into each other; but the appearance and character of the rash may be changed by partial immunity following previous vaccination, so that the rash seems to appear in crops like the rash of chickenpox and is less severe.

Scarlet fever. Red, flat, irregular spots or blotches appear on the second day of the illness, and last for about a week before they disappear. The rash avoids the area round the mouth and is attracted to the folds of the skin at the elbows, groins and arm-pits. The tongue goes through a series of characteristic changes; at first it is covered with a white deposit, then this starts to go and the papillae of the tongue become enlarged and stick up through the white fur so that the tongue is said to look like an unripe strawberry, then the white deposit goes leaving the red tongue looking like a ripe strawberry. These changes take about four days. If the rash has been severe, a day or two after the tongue has become red the skin starts to scale.

Rubella. The rash in this disease, also known as German measles, is formed of tiny red spots, starting on the face and spreading to the trunk, but only lasting about two days. The spots do not run together, nor are there any white spots inside the mouth.

Rat Bite Fever: rats may by biting infect man with Streptobacillus moniliformis, in which case the patient after about five days develops a severe fever with a skin rash and pain and enlargement of the joints, or with the Spirillum minus, which produces local enlargement of lymph glands with an intermittent fever and a red skin rash about a month after the bite. Both micro-organisms are sensitive to penicillin, but in the case of infection with Spirillum minus the disease may become chronic, recurring for many months.

Rauwolfia: a substance obtained from the root of the plant Rauwolfia serpentina, which is widely found in South-East Asia. Its use to quieten excited patients, known for hundreds of years in India, spread to Europe by the eighteenth century. In the years following World War 2, reserpine, one of the rauwolfia alkaloids, was used not only in psychiatry but also in general medicine to lower high blood pressure; it was in its time a revolutionary drug, but has been superseded by a number of new compounds.

Raynaud's Disease: a disease in which the fingers and toes become pale and dead, especially in cold weather.
CAUSE: unknown. Similar conditions are found running in families, or may be produced by compression of the subclavian artery between the collar-bone, the first rib and the anterior scalene muscle – the costoclavicular syndrome – and by certain occupations, such as handling pneumatic drills. Conditions which resemble Raynaud's disease are described as showing Raynaud's phenomenon.
SYMPTOMS: the disease is most commonly found in women of early middle age. If the hands are exposed to cold the fingers go blue and then dead and white, and in time little ulcers may form at the finger tips, for the arteries may be in spasm for as much as half an hour at a time, and thrombosis may develop.
TREATMENT: the hands must be protected from cold. Various drugs are made and advertised as improving the circulation in the hands and feet; one of the best is alcohol. In very severe cases surgical removal of the sympathetic nervous ganglia which supply nerve fibres to the blood vessels of the arm or foot may be considered.

R.B.C.: abbreviation for red blood cell.

Rectum: the last part of the intestinal canal before the anal canal. It begins at the third part of the sacrum, being continuous with the pelvic colon. It is most of the time empty, for the passage of faeces into the rectum sets up the desire to defaecate. The rectum is about 12 cm long.
Diseases which affect the rectum and anal canal include piles or haemorrhoids, proctitis, prolapse, pilonidal sinus, pruritus ani, fissure, and fistula, which are dealt with under their own headings. Tumours include polypi and papillomas, which are removed by surgery, and cancer of the rectum. This shows itself usually in middle age by bleeding,

constipation alternating with diarrhoea, and discomfort. It is treated by removal of the rectum, often with restoration of the continuity of the bowel. If this is not possible the patient is left with a colostomy (q.v.), but this is infinitely preferable to the terminal stages of cancer of the rectum.

Reflex Arc: *see* Nervous System.

Refraction: in medicine, the determination of refractive errors in the eye, and their correction by spectacles.

Regional Ileitis: *see* Ileitis.

Rehabilitation: the restoration of a patient after injury or illness to a state in which he or she can be self-sufficient even if the occupation has to be changed. It includes re-training for employment as well as physiotherapy, and is begun as soon as possible.

Reiter's Disease: non-specific urethritis. A condition in which there is discomfort on passing water, some discharge, arthritis, and inflammation of the eye (irido-cyclitis). The treatment is not easy, but antibiotics and cortisone may be used.

Relapsing Fever: (Famine fever). A fever with characteristic periods of high temperature alternating with remissions.
CAUSE: the spirochaetes Borrelia recurrentis or Borr. duttonii. Borr. recurrentis is spread by lice, and is found in India, North America, China and Eastern Europe, while Borr. duttonii is spread by the soft tick Ornithodorus and is found in West Africa and other tropical and subtropical places.
SYMPTOMS: the fever rises to about 39 °C. or 40 °C. or even higher for a day or two, then falls for a few days only to rise again. The periods between the bouts of fever are variable. There is headache, sometimes diarrhoea, a skin rash or mild jaundice, and the disease can be fatal.
TREATMENT: tetracycline is now used.

Relaxant: a drug that reduces tension; a muscle relaxant is a drug used by anaesthetists to supplement the action of

653

general anaesthetics and produce relaxation of the muscles without the need for excessive doses of anaesthetic drugs.

Remission: an abatement of symptoms during the course of a disease.

Renal Calculus: stone in the kidney.
SYMPTOMS: pain and the passage of blood in the urine. The stone that stays in the pelvis of the kidney may be painless, even when it is very big; but a small stone that passes into the ureter produces severe colic which is quite unmistakable. Large stones may produce pain in the loin because they lead to chronic infection of the kidney, but they may remain undetected until an X-ray is taken.
TREATMENT: renal colic is relieved by injections of atropine and morphine, and if the patient passes the stone out of the ureter into the bladder and so to the exterior the colic will not recur unless there are still stones left, or the condition which gave rise to the stones gives rise to more. It is therefore important that all cases of renal colic should be carefully investigated to identify the underlying cause and detect remaining stones.
Sometimes stones enter the ureter but will not pass into the bladder; they tend to stick where the ureter passes through the bladder wall, and they must be dislodged by manipulations carried out through the operating cystoscope or by open operation. When large stones are discovered in the pelvis of the kidney they can in some cases be removed by the surgeon without removal of the whole kidney, and if there is any appreciable amount of functioning kidney tissue still undamaged efforts are always made to preserve it. Very large stones are sometimes left, particularly when they are present on both sides, because efforts to remove them might destroy the little kidney tissue left.

Repellants: usually applied to substances used to drive off insects, such as dimethylphthallate (D.M.P.) and diethyltoluamide (D.E.T.).

Reserpine: *see* Rauwolfia.

Resolution: in medicine, the process of healing, for

example: 'The pneumonia resolved quickly, and the patient is now well.'

Respiration: the process of breathing. It includes the muscular movements of the chest wall and diaphragm whereby the lungs are filled with air, and the exchange of gases in the lungs between the air and the blood. In health the normal resting respiratory rate is 18 to 20 breaths a minute.

Respirators: machines which help paralysed patients to breathe. They can be divided into two groups, those which pump air or oxygen into the lungs – the positive pressure respirators – and those which produce a diminution of atmospheric pressure outside the chest wall and so draw air into the lungs through the normal air passages, the mouth and nose being outside the box in which the partial vacuum is induced. This type of respirator is the 'iron lung', and is used for cases of chronic paralysis; the positive pressure machines, which deliver their air through a tube passed through the mouth and larynx, or through a tube passed into the trachea through a tracheostomy, are in general used for acute cases. The word is also applied to a gas mask.

Respiratory Distress Syndrome: this is the name given to a lung condition of uncertain cause, occurring in infants who are born under abnormal circumstances – prematurely, by Caesarean section, or from a diabetic mother.
CAUSE: the air-sacs of the lung are coated with fluid which blocks the exchange of gases between air and blood. Although extensive study has been made, there has been no satisfactory explanation of how this occurs or why it is found only in this group of infants.
SYMPTOMS: the illness develops shortly after birth, and is characterized by rapid, laboured breathing, blueness of the skin, and exhaustion of the baby. If the infant survives the first few days of life, gradual recovery occurs within the week, leaving no permanent changes in the lung.
TREATMENT: these babies require highly specialized and constant care in hospital nurseries. They need moist oxygen, incubator environment, and regulation of body chemistry and nutrition through intravenous feedings. Antibiotics may

655

be used if lung infection is feared. This condition has been called pulmonary hyaline membrane disease because of the appearance of the coating material when seen through a microscope.

Resuscitation: the process of reviving a patient. Properly applied to bringing an apparent corpse back to life, the term is extended to cover the treatment of surgical shock.

Retention: the process of keeping back or holding in position; usually applied to the involuntary retention of urine because of an obstruction to urination. In dentistry it is applied to the keeping of a prosthesis in position within the mouth.

Reticulocytes: newly formed red blood cells, so called because they show on staining a network which is thought to be the remains of the nuclear apparatus; a mature red blood cell has no nucleus. Increased numbers of reticulocytes are seen in the blood in cases where red blood cells have been lost in large numbers or where they are being destroyed, for example in lead poisoning.

Reticulo-endothelial System: a name given to cells scattered throughout the body which have the special function of phagocytosis, that is, the eating up of other cells, bacteria and fragments of foreign material. The cells which carry out this function are the endothelial cells lining the blood vessels, the connective tissue cells, the cells found in the blood spaces of the spleen, the liver, the bone marrow and the adrenal bodies, and the wandering cells of the blood and tissue spaces called monocytes and macrophages. The cells of the reticulo-endothelial system are concerned also with the formation of antibodies and the immune reaction, with the formation of lymphocytes or 'small round cells', and with the formation of the cells of the blood.

Retina: *see* Eye.

Retinitis: inflammation of the retina, with consequent impairment of vision. It is caused by many diseases, including kidney disease, diabetes, eclampsia, leukaemia and syphilis. Retinopathy is a name that is used for any disease of the retina which is not inflammatory.

Retrobulbar Neuritis: inflammation of the optic nerve behind the eyeball.

Retroflexion: the backward bending of an organ or structure, especially that of the bending backward of the body of the uterus upon the cervix.

Retrograde Amnesia: loss of memory for a period of time extending back from a particular incident. It is usually applied to the type of memory loss that follows a severe blow on the head resulting in unconsciousness. The patient cannot remember events leading up to the accident; he may remember, for example, leaving home in the morning, but not getting into his car to drive to work nor any details of the drive that led up to the accident. The period of time covered by retrograde amnesia varies very roughly according to the severity of the concussion, and tends to shrink as the patient recovers. The old idea that another blow on the head would bring back a lost memory is false; another blow on the head only brings back the headache.

Retropharyngeal Abscess: an abscess behind the back wall of the pharynx, rarely seen, which is the result of tuberculosis of the vertebrae of the neck.

Retroversion: a turning backwards; usually applied to the uterus which when retroverted lies with the fundus directed backwards. This may happen as the uterus develops at puberty, and about one in five healthy women have their uterus retroverted for this reason. The condition is normal and gives rise to no trouble except rarely at the beginning of pregnancy, when the uterus may fail to rise out of the pelvis easily and have to be assisted to do so by manipulation. Retroversion may follow pregnancy, but in this case, unless the uterus was retroverted before, it may give rise to discomfort; the uterus is better replaced and supported by a pessary while it settles in its normal position. Operations are sometimes carried out in chronic cases to replace the uterus in the forward position.

Rheumatism: a term loosely applied to inflammation of the joints and connective tissue which causes pain and stiffness on movement. It is best considered under the headings of the separate diseases which commonly affect the joints and connective tissue, which are rheumatic fever, rheumatoid arthritis, osteoarthritis, gout, and arthritis occurring in the course of other illnesses.

Rheumatic fever. A disease of children and adolescents, which affects the joints, heart, and nervous system.

CAUSE: an abnormal response to infection of the throat by Streptococcus pyogenes. The organism provokes the formation of antibodies which react not only with the streptococci but with normal constituents of human heart muscle and joint membranes.

SYMPTOMS: about two weeks after the development of a sore throat, the patient begins to have pain in the joints, sometimes a rash, feels generally ill and runs a temperature. The joints involved are usually the ankles, knees, and wrists, and over the elbows and wrists nodules can be felt under the skin. The pulse becomes rapid, heart murmurs are heard and the electrical activity of the heart recorded by the electro-cardiograph changes. If the disease affects the nervous system the patient becomes irritable and excitable, and his movements are clumsy. Spontaneous movements develop, mostly in the face and arms (chorea, St Vitus' dance).

TREATMENT: the patient is put to bed until the fever settles and the pulse rate is down to normal. He is nursed carefully and not allowed to exert himself; the streptococcal infection is treated with penicillin. Rheumatic fever is a disease of overcrowding and poverty, and the diet may need attention. Aspirin is given for the joint pain, and corticosteroids may be used if the heart is badly affected. It is often recommended that penicillin should be given continuously for 5 years after an attack, and it is sure that children who have suffered from rheumatic fever should be watched carefully; if they show any signs of heart disease they should not over-exert themselves, nor take up an occupation that demands severe physical exercise. The commonest heart condition to follow rheumatic fever is mitral stenosis, which may take some years to show itself.

Rheumatoid arthritis. This is a disease usually found in women between 18 and 40 years old.

CAUSE: not understood; but thought to be a disorder of the immune reaction. The disease is chronic but there are remissions.

SYMPTOMS: the small joints are affected in the hands and feet, and not uncommonly the joint between the lower jaw and the skull just in front of the ear and the sterno-clavicular joint between the collar-bone and the top of the breast-bone show signs of disease. The joints swell and are stiff and painful. Sometimes the large joints are involved, and then the muscles acting upon them quickly waste; the joints are particularly stiff after a period of rest, and the pain eases off as they are used. The joints are affected symmetrically, small nodules may appear under the skin, and the active phase of the disease is accompanied by a low-grade fever. In time the tissues round the joints become thickened, movement is increasingly difficult and deformity develops.

TREATMENT: rest is essential in the acute stage; cortisone at one time seemed to be very effective in combating the disease, but subsequent observations have not confirmed early impressions. Drugs now used include phenylbutazone, aspirin, and gold, which is given by injection. Indomethacin is also used, but like phenylbutazone it should not be taken by patients who have had trouble with peptic ulcers. If necessary hypnotic drugs are used to ensure sleep. It is important to prevent the onset of deformities, and to maintain as much movement as possible. Physiotherapy and the use of splints prevent the limbs becoming fixed in the flexed position which the patient always finds most comfortable. As the disease passes from the acute to the chronic state physiotherapy becomes even more important, for the patient must be helped to make the best use of what function remains; occupational therapy is invaluable in starting rehabilitation. The disease can be crippling, and a great deal of ingenuity on the part of the medical attendant and determination on the part of the patient may be needed.

Osteoarthritis. This condition affects men more commonly than women, and is seen above the age of 50. It is thought to be a degenerative condition, and is the commonest form of arthritis.

CAUSE: osteoarthritis accompanies increasing age, and the site is often determined by old joint injuries either suffered over a period of time in the course of the patient's normal occupation or the result of accident.

SYMPTOMS: the joints, especially the large weight-bearing joints, become increasingly painful and stiff. Exercise makes the pain worse, and rest relieves it. The joints at the end of the fingers are affected, and small bony knobs develop there which are called Heberden's nodes. The joints may swell, and may be felt to grate as they are moved.

TREATMENT: is directed towards the relief of pain. This will often involve rest, reduction of weight, change of occupation, and physiotherapy; in cases of any severity the advice of an orthopaedic surgeon will prove invaluable, for there are various surgical operations and appliances that can bring relief to patients who otherwise might become crippled. *See also* Gout.

Rh Factor: *see* Blood groups.

Rhinitis: inflammation of the mucous membrane lining the nose. In the acute form it is very common, occurring in the common cold; when it is chronic it may lead to the formation of polypi and may be associated with infection of the nasal sinuses.

Rhinophyma: a condition in which the nose becomes red and swollen. It is associated with acne rosacea (q.v.) and is disfiguring.

Rhinoscopy: inspection of the interior of the nose.

Rhodopsin: visual purple. It is derived directly from Vitamin A, and is present in the rods of the retina; in the dark it is purple, but is bleached by light. Deficiency of Vitamin A leads to night-blindness. *See* Adaptation.

Rhonchi: snoring noises produced in the air passages by partial blockage; they are easily heard through the stethoscope. *See* Râles.

Rhubarb: the root of Rheum officinale or palmatum was once popular as a purgative, especially for children.

Rib: the curved, long, thin bones, 12 on each side, that run from the thoracic vertebrae behind towards the breastbone in the middle line of the front of the body; they form the walls of the chest. Below each rib runs an intercostal nerve, an artery and a vein; the ribs are connected by the intercostal muscles, and the ends in front are made of cartilage. The ribs are fairly easily broken by direct violence, and the broken ends may in some cases be driven inwards to lacerate the lung, so that cases in which the chest wall is injured must be watched to make sure that any signs of bleeding into the chest or of escape of air from the lungs into the pleural cavity are recognized. *See* Pneumothorax.

TREATMENT: the treatment of broken ribs has changed, for it used to be thought they should be strapped up; it is now thought that this restricts breathing too much, and an injection of local anaesthetic into the intercostal nerves is used to diminish the pain without restricting breathing, which might lead to pneumonia especially in those inclined to bronchitis. Where a number of ribs are fractured, particularly if they are fractured in two places, rapid surgical treatment is needed, and the possibility of underlying injuries to the liver, spleen or intestines must not be forgotten.

Riboflavin: Vitamin B_2, or Vitamin G.

Rickets: formerly known as the English disease, probably because of the part that lack of sunlight plays in its production, rickets is caused by deficiency of Vitamin D. Sunlight prevents the disease by irradiating the skin, which contains a provitamin which is changed into Vitamin D by ultraviolet light.

CAUSE: lack of Vitamin D is often caused by poverty; the vitamin is found in dairy produce, eggs and fish liver oil. Smoke in the towns prevents the sunlight shining in the streets, but, curiously, in many tropical places where the sun shines regularly the custom is to cover infants from its rays and so to make them rickety.

SYMPTOMS: the child's abdomen protrudes, it is weak, suffers from diarrhoea, and may be anaemic. Its bones are soft, and the long bones bend; the limbs become deformed.

TREATMENT: administration of Vitamin D and exposure to sunlight. Rickets is sometimes due to deficiency of absorption from the intestines or to disease or abnormality of the kidney, and these cases require more extensive treatment.

Rickettsiae: micro-organisms which are somewhere between bacteria and viruses; they are like bacteria in many ways, but cannot survive outside living cells. They cause typhus, Rocky Mountain spotted fever, scrub typhus and Q fever, and are sensitive to tetracycline; they are spread by lice, fleas, mites and ticks.

Rigor: 1. An attack of shivering and sweating accompanied by a sensation of cold, suffered during spikes of fever. 2. Rigor mortis is the stiffening of the muscles after death. Very roughly, it starts in the face six hours after death, is complete in twelve hours, lasts for twelve hours and takes twelve hours to pass off.

Ringworm: fungus infection of the skin.
CAUSE: the fungi commonly infecting human skin come from three groups: Microsporon, Trichophyton and Epidermophyton. The class to which these genera belong is that of Fungi Imperfecti. The fungi are passed on by direct contact; ringworm is contagious, and is picked up in schools, swimming baths and so on.
SYMPTOMS: ringworm of the scalp is usually a disease of children, and it produces no disability although it is socially a nuisance. The patches of skin affected are round, red at the edges where the disease is advancing, and pale at the centre. The fungus grows into the hairs, which become dull and brittle, so that they break off and the child develops round patches of comparative baldness. Under ultraviolet light the infected hairs are fluorescent. There is one severe form of ringworm of the scalp – favus – which is found in adults as well as children. Fungus infection of the spaces between the toes is very common, and is popularly called athlete's foot; infection of the crutch area is found in adolescent boys; the toe and finger nails may be infected; the beard area sometimes develops a fungus infection, particularly in people who look after cattle; and ringworm may occur anywhere on the body, often being caught from domestic animals.
TREATMENT: undecylenic acid cream or powder is used locally on the skin, and the drug griseofulvin is given by mouth. Those who suffer from fungus infection between the

toes will find that it is almost impossible to get rid of the infection entirely, but frequent changes of socks, the use of dusting powder, and washing the feet twice a day in soap and water will keep the disease at bay. Shoes should be light and well ventilated.

Rinne's Test: a test made by alternately placing the foot of a tuning fork on the bone behind the ear and then holding it in the air half an inch away from the ear until it can no longer be heard in one of the two positions. If it is heard longer through the air, the test is said to be Rinne positive; when it is heard longer on the bone, the test is Rinne negative. The other ear is closed while the test is being carried out. Normally the sound is heard longer in the air than through the bone, but when there is some impediment to the conduction of sound in the outer or middle ear and the inner ear and auditory nerve are normal the reverse is true, and Rinne's test is negative. *See* Ear, Weber's Test.

R.N.A.: Ribonucleic acid, the substance by which information contained in the D.N.A. (deoxyribonucleic acid) handed down from cell to cell is used in the formation of protein. D.N.A. is found in the cell nucleus; R.N.A. transfers the information to the ribosomes outside the cell nucleus where amino acids are strung together to form proteins. It is through this mechanism that hereditary characteristics are handed down from generation to generation.

Rocky Mountain Spotted Fever: a fever caused by Rickettsiae which is carried by dogs and rodents and passed on to man by ticks. It was originally described in the Rocky Mountains, but has since been recognized in many other parts of North America. It is treated by tetracycline.

Rodent Ulcer: a malignant tumour of the skin arising from the basal cells (*see* Skin). It is usually found on the face, particularly in those who have been exposed to the sun, and it looks like a small raised ulcer. It is only locally malignant, and does not give rise to metastatic growths in other parts of the body, but it is capable of eating through skin and bone as it enlarges slowly over a period of years. It is treated by complete surgical removal or by radiotherapy.

Rombergism: Romberg's sign is said to be present when a patient cannot stand without swaying when his eyes are closed and his feet close together. It is classically found in tabes dorsalis (locomotor ataxia).

Röntgen: international unit of radiation, named after the German physicist Wilhelm Röntgen (1845–1923) who discovered X-rays in 1895.

Rorschach Test: the 'ink-blot' test devised for investigating intelligence and personality.

Rosacea: *see* Acne Rosacea.

Round Ligament: the round ligament of the uterus corresponds to the gubernaculum testis in the male. It runs from the ovary as the ovarian ligament to the uterus, and then continues as the round ligament to the deep inguinal ring. It runs through the inguinal canal and into the labium majus; rarely an indirect inguinal hernia follows its course.

Roundworm: *see* Worms.

Rubefacient: a substance that produces reddening of the skin by increasing the blood flow.

Rubella: German measles. An acute infective fever with a skin rash.

CAUSE: a virus infection. Incubation period about three weeks.

SYMPTOMS: headache, enlargement of the lymph glands behind the ear and down the side of the neck, sore throat and general malaise. The rash is pink, and consists of small raised spots which remain discrete and are most numerous on the face and trunk. They only last for two or three days. Adults may complain of pain in the joints lasting for two or three weeks.

TREATMENT: none is needed. It is best for girls to catch rubella while they are young, and so develop an immunity to it, for if it is acquired during early pregnancy – within the first three months – the virus passes across the placenta and damages the foetus so that the child may be born with cataract, deafness, heart defects and microcephaly. If a pregnant mother thinks she has come into contact with the disease she should at once go to the doctor. No attempt should be made to prevent young girls catching the disease, but rather they should be encouraged to do so. A vaccine is available to produce active immunization against the disease.

Rupture: hernia (q.v.).

Ryle's Tube: a thin tube that has a metal olive incorporated in the tip and is used for withdrawing fluid from the stomach. There are four holes 2 cm above the olive; the tube is swallowed by the patient, often being passed through the nose, and is marked with rings – one at 14 in, two at $20\frac{1}{2}$ in, three at 26 in and four $30\frac{1}{2}$ in from the tip.

S

Sabin-type Vaccine: a vaccine given orally and consisting of live but attenuated poliomyelitis viruses. *See* Salk-type Vaccine. *See also* Immunization.

Saccharomyces: the yeasts.

Sacro-iliac Pain: pain felt in the lower part of the back just to the right or left of the mid-line over the joint between the sacrum and the ilium. It is not uncommon, and is usually caused by osteoarthritis, rarely by other bone disease. It is often found to be part of a general osteoarthritis, and the treatment is that of osteoarthritis. Occasionally sacro-iliac disease gives rise to pain spreading down the leg.

Sacrum: a triangular bone formed by the fusion of the five sacral vertebrae. It is massive because it transfers the weight of the body from the spinal column to the pelvis; it forms the back wall of the bony pelvis, binding the two hip-bones together. Above, it joins the lumbar spine, articulating with the fifth lumbar vertebra, below it forms a joint with the coccyx, and on each side an articular surface takes part in the formation of the sacro-iliac joint. The fifth lumbar nerve emerges from the vertebral canal between the fifth lumbar vertebra and the sacrum, and the upper four sacral nerves emerges from the sacral foramina. The fifth sacral nerve emerges between the sacrum and the coccyx.

Sadism: a sexual perversion in which pleasure is attained by inflicting pain on others.

Safe Period: a method of contraception that is based on the assumption that a woman is only capable of becoming pregnant on certain days of the menstrual cycle. Ovulation (q.v.) normally takes place about fifteen days before the next period is due; if five days are allowed for errors each side of this date, the fertile period is likely to be from the 8th to the 18th days of the ordinary 28-day cycle. Any time outside this is said to be in the safe period, but because menstruation tends to be irregular and because emotional and other factors influence ovulation the idea of a safe period is a misconception.

St Vitus' Dance: chorea. *See* Rheumatism.

Salicylates: the bark of the willow Salix alba is an old remedy for fevers, and during the first half of the nineteenth century the active principle was found to be the substance salicin, from which salicylic acid was obtained. Salicylic acid can also be prepared synthetically from phenol, and by the last half of the nineteenth century sodium salicylate was widely used both to reduce fever and to relieve pain. The acetyl ester of salicylic acid is aspirin, which was first made in Germany at the turn of the century and has since become the standby of millions of people. Aspirin was called after the German name for salicylic acid, *Spirsäure*.

The actions of salicylates are: antipyretic – that is, they reduce a high temperature; analgesic – they dull mild pain; anti-inflammatory – they diminish the inflammatory reaction. They are used particularly in rheumatic fever, but must not be given to people who suffer from asthma or are prone to peptic ulceration. Those who are sensitive to salicylates, and a surprisingly large number of people are, develop skin reactions, spasm of the bronchioles, or angio-neurotic oedema; the symptoms of salicylate poisoning are nausea and vomiting, noises in the ears, headache, confusion and delirium, and if a large enough dose has been taken, sleepiness. The only people who are likely to be poisoned accidentally by aspirin are children.

Saliva: the secretion of the parotid, submandibular and sublingual glands, as well as many smaller glands in the mouth. Saliva contains ptyalin, which breaks down starch to sugar and water, and mucus, which lubricates the inside of the mouth and gullet and makes swallowing possible. It is secreted in response to the presence of food or in anticipation of it by a nervous reflex.

Salk-type Vaccine: a vaccine made from poliomyelitis virus which has been treated with formalin. It is given by injection. *See* Sabin-type Vaccine, Immunization.

SALMONELLA

Salmonella: *see* Food poisoning.

Salpingitis: inflammation of the Fallopian, or uterine, tubes.
CAUSE: infection following abortion or associated with some other pelvic inflammation such as acute appendicitis, gonorrhoea, or tuberculosis.
SYMPTOMS: in acute salpingitis, usually caused by gonococcus or streptococcus, there is severe pain in the lower part of the abdomen, usually on both sides, frequency of passing water perhaps with discomfort, a vaginal discharge and menorrhagia. In chronic disease the symptoms are similar but less severe.
TREATMENT: rest in bed, antibiotics, and, if the condition fails to improve, surgical operation. In chronic conditions operation may be advisable if there are recurrent attacks; in tuberculous salpingitis chemotherapy is the treatment of choice.

Salt: sodium chloride, a substance essential for life. When it is deficient the blood volume and blood pressure fall, there are muscular cramps, dizziness and fainting, and sometimes confusion. Normally there is a comfortable excess of salt in everyday food, but in a hot climate, especially after a good deal of sweating or a bout of diarrhoea, it is sensible to take salt tablets.

Salvarsan: (Arsphenamine). Ehrlich's original 'magic bullet', which he designed to destroy trypanosomes. It proved to be specific for the spirochaetes of syphilis in man, and the work paved the way for modern concepts of chemotherapy.

Sanatorium: a special open-air hospital for the treatment of tuberculosis.

Sandfly Fever: (Phlebotomus fever). A virus fever transmitted by the sandfly or Phlebotomus on the shores of the Mediterranean. There is intense headache, redness of the conjunctivae, and a fever of 39 °C.–40 °C. which lasts for three or four days. There is no specific treatment.

Saphenous Vein: the internal saphenous vein can be seen
668

running up the inside of the leg from the ankle to the groin, and the short saphenous vein from the outer side of the foot to the back of the knee. The veins, particularly the internal or great saphenous vein (which is the longest vein in the body), are the site of varicosities in about one in five people. *See* Varicose Veins.

Saprophyte: any micro-organism that lives upon decaying or dead animal matter.

Sarcoidosis: a chronic disease in which granulomata are formed in many parts of the body.
CAUSE: unknown. The formation of the granulomata may be an abnormal immunological response. In many cases the granuloma looks very much like a tuberculoma, the granulomatous lesion found in tuberculosis; in others it looks like a syphilitic lesion, or even like the lesions found in leprosy, but sarcoidosis is not identical with any of these diseases.
SYMPTOMS: the disease is usually chronic and occurs in women slightly more often than in men; the patients are usually between 25 and 30 years old. The symptoms depend on which organs and parts of the body are involved – perhaps the lungs, when the symptoms include coughing and shortness of breath, perhaps the eyes, when there is disturbance of the vision. If the skin is involved various papules and nodules form which may be associated with fever, pains in the joints, and enlargement of lymph glands.
TREATMENT: corticosteroids are used, but they may have to be continued for a very long time.

Sarcoma: a malignant tumour of connective tissue. It may be named after the tissue in which it originated, for example osteosarcoma (sarcoma of bone), or it may, if it does not resemble any normal tissue, be named for the type of cell it contains, for example round cell sarcoma. The tumour usually spreads by metastasis through the bloodstream, very often to the lungs; sometimes it metastasizes through the lymphatics, and in other cases it spreads a long way by direct invasion of neighbouring tissue. Malignant tumours of connective tissue are not very common, but when they do occur they are difficult to treat; surgery, radiotherapy and the use of cytotoxic drugs may all have to be tried.

Sarcoptes: Sarcoptes scabiei is the mite of the skin disease scabies. *See* below.

Scabies: a disease of the skin.

CAUSE: infestation with the mite Sarcoptes scabiei.

SYMPTOMS: the disease is popularly known as the itch, and it is extremely irritating. The mites are spread by direct contact – in some cases scabies is virtually a venereal disease – and they burrow into the skin, leaving a streak about half a centimetre long ending in a little blister, near which the mite can be seen as a tiny dot. The burrows are found on the sides of the fingers, on the wrists or on the penis, where the patient may mistake scabies for syphilis, and in the burrows the female Sarcoptes lays her eggs. The mites wander about on the skin when they are warm – they take about a week to hatch out and become mature – and they set up intense itching, particularly when the skin is hot, so that the patient tends to be covered with septic scratches on the wrists, elbows, waist, arm-pits, the genitalia and the backside, but not on the face or neck.

TREATMENT: emulsion of benzyl benzoate is painted on to the skin after the patient has had a warm bath, and is left there for a day, after which the treatment is repeated. People who come into intimate contact with the patient should also be treated.

Scaphoid: one of the eight small bones of the wrist. It articulates with the radius, and is the largest member of the nearer row of wrist bones. Its particular importance is that it is sometimes fractured by falls on the outstretched hand or severe blows on the palm. Fractures of the scaphoid bone are often very hard to see in an X-ray, and if the surgeon thinks there might be a fracture he will usually plaster the wrist and take another X-ray after a week or so, when the fracture line shows up because the bone round it becomes rarefied. The fracture takes anything up to three months to heal in most cases, but in a few it does not heal at all and the bone has to be grafted or removed.

Scapula: the shoulderblade.

Scarlet Fever: (Scarlatina). A sore throat with a specific skin rash.

CAUSE: infection of the tonsils by Streptococcus pyogenes, which in susceptible patients, usually children, produces a toxin which provokes a skin reaction.

SYMPTOMS: an acute sore throat, with exudate on the tonsils and swelling of the lymphatic glands of the neck, brings with it a fever, shivering, nausea and vomiting. The pulse rate is high. On the second day a rash develops, which consists of red spots all over the body except round the mouth, and the tongue is covered with white furring which in the course of three days disappears and leaves the red papillae on the glossy tongue surface looking like the outside of a strawberry. The skin spots begin to fade in a few days, and in a week or so the skin begins to scale. The patient in an uncomplicated case recovers in two or three weeks. The most important complications are nephritis (q.v.) and rheumatic fever.

TREATMENT: penicillin, continued for a week to ten days. The disease is not now as severe as once it was.

Schistosomiasis: *see* Bilharzia.

Schizomycetes: class name for one-celled organisms which multiply by cell division and are considered to be plants. The class includes micro-organisms pathogenic to man.

Schizont: a stage in the development of the malaria parasite. *See* Malaria.

Schizophrenia: *see* Mental Illness.

Sciatica: a pain running down the course of the sciatic nerve, which supplies sensation to the back of the thigh and outer side of the leg and foot. (The sciatic nerve is the largest nerve in the body, and as well as carrying sensory fibres it carries motor fibres to the hamstring muscles and to all the muscles of the leg and foot.) Pain felt in the distribution of the nerve may be provoked by a number of conditions, but the most common are osteoarthritis of the lower lumbar spine and lumbosacral region and prolapse of an intervertebral disc in the same part of the vertebral column. Other conditions causing sciatica are osteoarthritis of the sacro-iliac joint or of the hip joint, and there are a number of uncommon diseases such as tumour and tuberculosis of the spine which have to be taken into consideration. In some cases no underlying cause can be found. The treatment is that of the cause, but if this cannot be discovered symptoms are treated as they arise by various forms of physiotherapy and analgesic drugs.

Scintiscan: a diagram of the gamma radiation of an isotope concentrated in a tissue or organ such as the thyroid gland or the brain.

Sclera: the white fibrous outer coat of the eyeball, continuous behind with the sheath of the optic nerve and in front with the margin of the cornea. It forms the white of the eye.

Scleroderma: an uncommon disease in which the skin becomes thickened and hard, and there is associated change and malfunction of parts of the gullet and intestines which makes swallowing difficult and leads to discomfort and disturbance of the bowels.

Sclerosis: hardening of a tissue, used particularly of the nervous tissue in disseminated or multiple sclerosis, and of the walls of the arteries in atherosclerosis.

Scolex: the head and neck of a tapeworm; the part with which it attaches itself to the wall of the gut.

Scoliosis: a deformity of the spine due to curvature and rotation to one side.

CAUSE: paralysis of the muscles that normally support the spine consequent on such diseases as poliomyelitis; congenital abnormality or acquired disease of the vertebrae or ribs; and chronic conditions of one side of the chest. In some cases, perhaps the majority, no underlying abnormality can be found.

SYMPTOMS: in early life none, but the deformity predisposes to degenerative disease of the joints of the spine and of other weight-bearing joints because the lines of weight transfer are not normal, and the patient may in later life be crippled by osteoarthritis.

TREATMENT: physiotherapy, which includes exercises to improve posture and the strength of the muscles of the spine, and observation. Only in very severe cases is operative interference recommended, but the surgeon may recommend a brace.

Scopolamine: trade name for hyoscine, which is used as a premedication before general anaesthetics to reduce the secretions from the lungs, salivary glands and stomach. *See* Premedication.

Scorpion: the scorpion is a venomous nocturnal arachnid carrying a sting at the end of its tail. *See* Bites and Stings.

Scotoma: a patch of diminished vision inside the visual field, which may be seen as a shadow.

Scrofula: tuberculosis of lymph glands, especially in the neck, in which the disease slowly progresses to the formation of fistulous openings. *See* King's Evil.

Scruple: a unit of weight in the apothecaries' system, equal to 20 grains or 1.296 g.

Scurvy: a vitamin deficiency disease.
CAUSE: deficiency of Vitamin C.
SYMPTOMS: bleeding from the gums, into the skin, where large bruises may form, and into the vital organs. Bleeding beneath the membrane covering the bones may cause extreme tenderness of the limbs.
TREATMENT: Vitamin C is found in fresh fruit and vegetables but is largely destroyed in cooking especially if baking soda is used. The amount of the vitamin required is between 10 and 20 mg daily, much less than is contained in a normal diet; it can if necessary be taken as a tablet of ascorbic acid. At one time the disease was widespread among sailors who were kept at sea without fresh food for weeks at a time, and the Royal Navy used lime juice as a prophylactic – hence the name 'Limeys' for the British which dates from the eighteenth century.

Seasickness: a form of motion sickness (q.v.).

Sebaceous Cyst: sebaceous cysts are formed directly under the skin by enlargement of the sebaceous glands (*see* below). The cysts may form wherever there are sebaceous glands, which is everywhere on the body except the soles of the feet and the palms of the hands, but they are most common on the scalp, where they may be multiple. The treatment is surgical removal, usually carried out while the patient is under local anaesthetic.

Sebaceous Glands: glands set in the skin, usually in the angle between a hair follicle and its arrector pili muscle, which secrete a fatty substance called sebum to protect and lubricate the surface of the skin. The glands become more active at puberty, and their development is complete by the twenty-fifth year. Abnormalities affecting the sebaceous glands include the formation of sebaceous cysts (*see* above), and seborrhoea (*see* below), a condition in which there is an excessive secretion of sebum. A microscopic mite called Demodex lives in the ducts of the sebaceous glands and in the hair follicles, especially on the face, but it does no harm of any kind.

Seborrhoea: a condition in which there is excessive secretion of sebum from the sebaceous glands. It does not occur in children, for the secretion of sebum depends on the presence of sex hormones. In seborrhoea oleosa the skin and hair become greasy; in cystic seborrhoea plugs composed of sebum and keratin, the horny substance that is part of the skin, form in the hair follicles from which they can be squeezed; and a very common form of seborrhoeic disturbance is acne (q.v.). It was once thought that dandruff was a manifestation of seborrhoea, but it is now clear that the scales which form on the scalp are from the horny layer of the skin and are not dried sebum.

Seconal: trade name for quinalbarbitone, a barbiturate that is used as a sedative and hypnotic.

Secretion: the process by which a gland elaborates its specific hormone or other special substance; the word is also applied to the material secreted by the gland.

Sedative: a drug used to quieten a patient.

Sedimentation Rate: if a specimen of whole blood is prevented from coagulating by the addition of an anticoagulating agent – usually sodium citrate – and allowed to stand, the red cells will fall to the bottom of the container, leaving a clear column of plasma above them. The rate at which the cells fall is the sedimentation rate; it is increased in certain conditions, and whereas in health it is not more than 5 mm in men and 7 mm in children in one hour (tested by Westergren's method), it may rise to five or six times that figure in active infections, cancer, or pregnancy. The sedimentation rate is a rough indication of the blood levels of fibrinogen and globulins, and is a valuable way of following the progress of chronic infections such as tuberculosis as well as being an aid to diagnosis.

Sella Turcica: the pituitary fossa in the base of the skull; it is formed in the sphenoid bone, and is thought to look like a Turkish saddle. *See* Pituitary Gland.

Seminoma: this is a malignant tumour of the testicle.

Senna: the dried leaf of Cassia acutifolia, which is used as a purgative or cathartic. It is safe, and may be obtained in either standard granules or capsules.

Sensitivity: a state in which there is an abnormal reaction to stimulation; patients who react abnormally to drugs are said to be sensitive to them, for example if penicillin produces skin rashes the patient is said to be sensitive to penicillin. It is also used to indicate the reaction of a micro-organism to a drug which kills it or retards its growth, e.g. staphylococci are sensitive to penicillin.

Sepsis: (1) poisoning of a part or of the whole of the body by toxins formed in decaying matter. 'Septic' is commonly used in connection with infections resulting in the formation of pus, but to be correct it should only be applied to the products of putrefaction. (2) Sepsis violacea, the dungfly.

Septal Defect: a deficiency in a septum (q.v.); the term is often applied to congenital defects in the septum dividing the right from the left atrium of the heart or that dividing the right and left ventricles. A defect in the inter-atrial septum will result in blood passing from the left to the right side of the heart because of the pressure differential, so that the right ventricle becomes enlarged. Such a defect is often associated with other cardiac abnormalities, but when it is isolated there are few indications of trouble apart from the fact that the child does not grow properly. Abnormal sounds are heard on examination of the chest, but full investigations are needed to make firm diagnosis. The treatment is by open operation. Defects in the septum dividing the two ventricles are not uncommon; they too are often associated with other congenital heart abnormalities, although the defect may be found by itself and is then in some cases not dangerous. Most cases, however, should be submitted to operation, for there is every prospect that the surgeon will be able to make a satisfactory repair. *See* Heart.

Septicaemia: a condition in which toxins arising from decay are free in the blood, the term being commonly used of the toxins elaborated by bacteria. *See* Blood Poisoning.

Septum: a partition; for example, the nasal septum, which divides the two sides of the nasal cavity.

Sequestrum: the name given to a piece of necrotic bone which has become separated from the main bone and its blood supply and has died. Sequestra are formed in osteomyelitis, and must always be removed, for otherwise the condition will not heal and pus formation and discharge through sinuses in the skin will persist.

Serum: the clear fluid which separates when whole blood is allowed to clot and stand, as opposed to plasma, which is the fluid remaining when the cellular element has been removed from unclotted blood. Serum contains antibodies, and serology is the study of antibody-antigen reactions.

Serum Sickness: a reaction which may develop in patients who are given injections of horse serum, usually for the prophylaxis of gas gangrene or tetanus; antibodies against these diseases are prepared by active immunization of horses and used in the passive immunization of susceptible human beings. The reaction comes on from five to ten days after the injection, and there is fever, pain in the joints, and urticaria of the skin. The skin rash is very irritating but can often be relieved by adrenaline or similar drugs; sometimes prednisone must be used. Because of the occurrence of serum sickness in something like one case in twenty, and because of the risk of anaphylaxis (q.v.), the use of horse serum is if possible avoided. In the case of tetanus it is far better to produce active immunization in children by the routine use of tetanus toxoid.

Sex and Sexual Problems: it was for long the custom to think of sex as an impulse arising at puberty and dying out in women at the change of life and in men a little later. This totally false belief caused many to feel that any manifestations of sex before or after these ages must be abnormal, but it is now realized that the impulse is present in various forms from the earliest months until the end of life. Infants (quite apart from the Freudian theory that sucking and defaecation are both forms of sexuality in the widest sense) evince interest in their sexual organs, and their interest is carried on throughout childhood with the special characteristic that at this age the main interest is autoerotic, i.e. centred on the child's own body. Masturbation is a feature of this stage and an almost universal one which causes no physical or mental harm in spite of warnings dating from Victorian times. It is, however, necessary to note that masturbation carried to excess may well be a sign of something wrong, usually indicating extreme anxiety rather than overdeveloped sexuality. Just before puberty there is a brief homosexual stage which may or may not be marked by physical manifestations of interest in the same sex. Ordinarily this is the time when schoolgirls develop 'crushes' for older girls or schoolteachers, and schoolboys similarly have their heroes. There are few people who have not at one time or another manifested homosexual tendencies and there is nothing necessarily abnormal about this, since the natural development of sex is from the self through the similar to the quite different, i.e. the other sex.

Puberty is the stage when the interest becomes heterosexual (directed towards the other sex) and at the same time the body matures so that parenthood becomes possible, the menstrual periods beginning in girls and seminal emissions in boys. Such emissions are normal and it is wrong to believe – as indeed a little thought would make obvious – that emissions are weakening. Clearly they are no more so than sexual intercourse in adults. The periods need equally be no cause for distress in girls, and it is worth while noting that a great deal of dysmenorrhoea (pain with the periods) is related to faulty teaching which associates them with guilt or shame (*see* Menstruation). The proper way to educate children in sex matters is (*a*) to answer from the earliest days every question the child asks about sex and to answer truthfully; (*b*) to answer only what has been asked without elaborating or giving lectures; (*c*) to ensure that lectures are given at the proper time and place, i.e. in school as a part of biology lessons. Parents who fail to do this are living in a fool's paradise, since nearly all children learn the 'facts of life' in a garbled form from their comrades, and the choice is not between some information or none but between accurate and inaccurate information. Faulty upbringing has much to do with later difficulties in sexual relations during married life, which in nearly all cases are difficulties of personal relationships showing themselves in sexual guise. Thus although impotence in men is occasionally the result of a general disease such as advanced diabetes or Addison's disease, it is much more usually the expression of unconscious or conscious conflict such as fear of failure or lack of genuine interest in the partner. Frigidity in women ranges from total frigidity to the very common inability to reach orgasm which in our own civilization is perhaps more often the rule than the exception. Both these disabilities, if they trouble the individual, should be referred to a doctor who deals with such problems.

Sterility, the inability to have children, is often mistakenly thought to be the fault of the woman although a large number of cases concern the man; problems of sterility should be discussed with the doctor, who will probably arrange a consultation and treatment at a fertility clinic. Problems associated with the menopause are discussed under that heading. Sexual perversions are cases of failure to develop beyond a certain level of childish sexuality or the replacement of normal sexual feeling by tendencies which, although not necessarily abnormal in themselves, are abnormal when they become the whole aim of the act. Homosexuality, as mentioned above, is a normal stage of development through which everyone passes; it becomes abnormal when it is retained into adult life. The cause of homosexuality is psychological and may be related in the male to a dominating mother. Lesbianism, or homosexuality in the female, has various and complex origins, such as fear of assuming a mature woman's role, overdependence upon the mother or mother substitute, and undue apprehension concerning the sexual act itself, bred from misinformation. The outlook for treatment in a confirmed case is not good as few homosexuals have any desire to be 'cured'. Those wishing to be unburdened of a socially stigmatized sexual maladjustment, however, may find help in psychiatric treatment. Sadism and masochism, the obtaining of sexual pleasure from hurting and being hurt respectively are examples of a normal component of sex which has got out of hand and become the main aim, as is fetishism, which is sexual satisfaction associated with inanimate objects such as shoes, brassières, and hair. It is not abnormal to feel attraction to articles associated with the beloved, but it is quite abnormal to make them the sole object of sex. Such perversions require treatment, and the outlook is reasonably good in cases where there is a real desire to achieve normality. *See* Impotence, Orgasm.

Shaking Palsy: Parkinson's disease, or paralysis agitans.

Shell Shock: the name given to a war-neurosis in World War I under the false impression that it was caused by the physical effect of shell explosions rather than emotional stress.

Shigella: a genus of micro-organisms that cause dysentery (q.v.).

Shingles: *see* Herpes.

Shock: two kinds of shock are ordinarily described; surgical shock and 'nervous' shock. The latter means mental distress caused by some disagreeable event, and is quite different from surgical shock, with which we shall be concerned here. The characteristics of surgical shock are low blood pressure, a cold, sweaty, pallid skin, and prostration. Shock may follow a haemorrhage or an extensive injury involving the loss of fluid, as for example a burn, and in such cases it is due to loss of fluid from the circulation. Treatment consists of replacing the fluid by intravenous infusion and stopping the loss; it is usually possible to combine these activities, except in the case of massive arterial bleeding. The patient's state is made worse by pain, which can produce an over-all drop in blood pressure, and by cold; morphine is the best analgesic drug to use in these circumstances, and the patient should be kept warm – but not hot. Other conditions which produce a state of shock are coronary thrombosis, acute and powerful bacterial infections, and septicaemia. In anaphylactic shock hypersensitivity to the injection of a foreign protein produces a profound fall in blood pressure and the escape of fluid into the tissues, and the treatment is immediate injection of adrenaline and steroids. The first-aid treatment of surgical shock is to keep the patient lying down, with the legs higher than the head if he feels faint, keep him warm, and unless he has an abdominal injury encourage him to drink any fluid he fancies except alcohol.

Shunt: in medicine, the term is applied to operations which are designed to join blood vessels in order to divert the flow of blood, for example porto-caval shunt, in which blood is diverted from the portal venous system to the inferior vena cava in cases where the blood pressure in the portal system is high because of liver disease.

Sialitis: inflammation of a salivary gland.

Sialolithiasis: the formation of stones in the duct of a salivary gland. They cause the gland suddenly to swell up, but can often be persuaded to pass out of the duct if the patient perseveres in sucking acid-drops and lemons.

Sickle-cell Anaemia: an inherited blood disease.
CAUSE: the presence of an abnormal haemoglobin called haemoglobin S in the red blood cells, which when it is reduced (de-oxygenated) becomes a gel. Red blood cells containing reduced haemoglobin S become deformed; because under the microscope they look like crescents they are named sickle-cells. They are quickly destroyed in the bloodstream.
SYMPTOMS: the fully developed disease usually shows itself before a child is two years old. It produces symptoms of anaemia with recurrent pains in the abdomen and the bones

which may resemble an acute abdominal condition or osteo-myelitis. There may be defects of vision resulting from haemorrhages in the eye, and blood may be passed in the urine; the kidneys in this condition are often unable to con-centrate the urine properly. Ulcers are prone to develop in the legs. In many cases the disease is not fully developed, and patients are found whose red cells only show sickling from time to time – when flying in a poorly pressurized aircraft, for example, they may develop abdominal pain, or they may pass blood in the urine, which may not be properly con-centrated. Normally such patients, who are said to have a sickle-cell trait, keep in good health.

TREATMENT: no specific treatment is yet known, so that treat-ment must be symptomatic. There is often a deficiency of folic acid, which suggests daily doses of 5 mg, and because sickling is thought to occur most readily when the blood reaction tends towards the acid side, enough sodium bi-carbonate can be given by mouth to keep the reaction of the urine alkaline. Iron should if necessary be given to prevent the development of iron-deficiency anaemia. There is one benefit which the disease brings; those who show sickling of their red blood cells are resistant to infection with Plasmo-dium falciparum, the organism of malignant malaria, and as many people who have sickle-cell disease are West Africans the benefit is by no means purely theoretical.

Side Effect: an effect produced by a drug other than that for which it has been given; usually the side effect is not wanted, for it may be damaging to the patient.

Sigmoid: a structure shaped like an S, for example the sigmoid colon.

Sigmoidoscope: an instrument for inspecting the sigmoid colon. It is a hollow tube carrying a light at its far end and a lens through which the surgeon looks, and it is passed into the rectum through the anus and so up into the colon under direct vision. A pneumatic bulb is provided so that the gut can be gently distended with air to make the passage of the instrument possible. A long pair of forceps can be used to take a specimen for subsequent microscopy from any ab-normal structures that may be seen.

681

Silicosis: *see* Pneumoconiosis.

Silver: in general silver compounds are used externally in medicine in the form of silver nitrate (lunar caustic), which is used as a stick for cauterizing warts or in very weak solutions for treating conjunctivitis, or silver proteinate (argyrol, etc.) for infections of the eyes, throat and nose, or urethra.

Sinus: (*a*) the cavities or venous spaces within the skull, or air spaces in the skull bones (*see* below); (*b*) an abnormal opening through which pus is discharged.

Sinusitis: inflammation of the mucous membrane lining the sinuses, the air spaces in the bones of the skull which open into the nose.
CAUSE: sinusitis is usually secondary to an infection of the nose, although the maxillary sinus in the upper jaw can be infected by a carious tooth. Nasal deformities and polyps are contributing factors, and swimming and diving may drive infection from the nose into the sinuses.
SYMPTOMS: the symptoms vary with the sinus affected; in addition to the maxillary sinuses of the upper jaw, there are frontal sinuses above the eyebrows and ethmoidal sinuses on either side of the root of the nose. There is pain and swelling over the affected part, fever, a blocked nose with some discharge, and headache.
TREATMENT: most cases clear up with rest in bed, inhalations designed to shrink the swollen mucous membrane and let the pus escape from the sinuses through the canals which connect each with the inside of the nose, the use of nasal sprays or drops for the same purpose, and treatment with antibiotics. In only a few cases is operation necessary, its aim being to establish drainage from the affected sinus.

Skeleton: the bony framework which supports the soft parts of the body.

Skin: the skin covers the outer surface of the body, and is continuous with the mucous membranes which cover the interior surface of the body at the nose, mouth, urethral meatus, vagina and anus. It is tied loosely down to the underlying connective tissue except over the joints, where the attachment is firmer on the flexor side. The skin has two layers, a surface layer called the epidermis, and a deeper part called the dermis.

In the dermis, the deeper layer which supports the epidermis, there is a papillary layer, which looks like a great number of minute hills and valleys upon which the epidermis lies, and a reticular layer. The dermis contains fibrous tissue and fibroblasts which multiply rapidly after an injury and elastic fibres which give the skin its elasticity. The dermis also contains the nerves, blood vessels and lymphatic vessels of the skin. The epidermis has in its thickest parts – over the soles and palms – five layers, and in the other parts of the body four. The five layers are called the strata corneum, lucidum, granulosum, spinosum and basale. The stratum basale is attached to the dermis over the papillary processes and it contains pigment cells which are more numerous in people with dark skins. The next layer is the stratum spinosum, named from its appearance under the microscope, then the stratum granulosum over which in the soles and palms lies the stratum lucidum. The outer layer of the skin is called the stratum corneum, because it is horny; it consists of dead cells made of the substance keratin, a fibrous protein, which is impervious to most substances. Keratin also forms the nails and hair, and in animals forms the hooves, claws, horns and feathers. It is produced by the cells of the epidermis.

In the skin are sweat and apocrine glands (*see* Perspiration) and hair follicles, which are all appendages of the epidermal layer, as are the sebaceous glands (q.v.) and the nails. The sweat glands are part of the heat regulating system of the body, and are supplied by nerves from the sympathetic nervous system, while the apocrine glands secrete a thicker substance than sweat round the hairs. The hairs themselves grow out of follicles formed by ingrowths of the epidermal layer, and associated with them are the sebaceous glands which lubricate the skin and hairs. The hair, which is dead keratin, grows from a small 'hair bulb' at the bottom of the hair follicle. To the side of the hair follicle is attached a small strip of smooth muscle called the arrector pili. When these muscles contract the skin comes up in goose pimples. The skin has a rich blood supply, and the vessels loop up into the papillary processes of the dermis. The function of the blood vessels of the skin is less to nourish the skin than to act as a surface radiator or heat exchange system, and the arterioles have muscle in their walls so that they can be shut off when heat must be conserved. There are also a number of short-circuits between the arterioles and the venules in the face and ears, fingers and toes, and palms and soles. These are known as glomus bodies and have to do with temperature regulation. As well as protection and heat regulation another prime function of the skin is the provision of sensory information about the surroundings of the body, and it therefore has a rich nerve supply. Some of the nerves end in specialized sensory organs, others in beads in the dermis, and the network of fibres picks up sensations of touch, pressure, pain, temperature, and itching. It is not fully understood how the sensation of itching is produced, but it is thought to be caused by stimuli which are sufficient to damage the skin but not to produce pain.

Although the skin is impervious to most substances, those which are soluble in ether and water will pass through it to a certain extent; absorption through the skin is augmented by damage, by an increase in blood flow, or by a rise in surface temperature.

Skull Fractures: these injuries are not important in them-selves; they are only significant in terms of accompanying damage to the brain, its membranes and blood vessels, and the cranial nerves. *See* Concussion.

Sleep: for about 8 hours of the 24 we withdraw from the world of consciousness and movement into sleep, a state which is far from understood. It is not unconsciousness, for we can be woken up; the mind is not inactive, for we can selectively pick up signals that will wake us – a mother will in her sleep recognize the cry of her child, picking it out from any number of other noises. Lack of sleep is not fatal, but the longer one stays awake the more irritable and slow one is liable to become, and after about 48 hours one tends to have delusions of a minor sort. During sleep the electroencephalo-gram alters, showing large slow waves; after about an hour of uninterrupted sleep the waves are reduced in amplitude and the eyes begin to make rapid movements, and it is at this time that the sleeper dreams.

Dreams, as is well known, can be stimulated by many

factors, for example an uncomfortable or unfamiliar bed, a heavy or indigestible meal, a worrying day just past or a possibly worrying one to come, and the dreams which ensue are disguised forms of our own personal problems. In some cases they are an attempted solution to such problems, but for the individual the main issue is whether they are pleasant or unpleasant. Unpleasant dreams are what we describe as nightmares in which primitive impulses from the unconscious seem about to break into awareness, and if these are frequent, especially in children, it is best to see a psychiatrist or child psychologist. In children nightmares often take the form of night terrors, where the child wakes in a state of fear and may not be pacified or capable of recognizing his surroundings for some minutes after waking. Possibly due to a lag in the awakening of different parts of the brain is 'paralysed wakefulness', where the individual wakes up intellectually but finds himself unable to move for some minutes or seconds after attaining full consciousness. This, if unpleasant, is of no serious significance. *See* Insomnia.

Sleeping Sickness: (Trypanosomiasis). A tropical disease caused by a genus of protozoa called trypanosomes. It is spread by the tsetse fly and must not be confused with sleepy sickness, otherwise encephalitis lethargica (q.v.).
CAUSE: trypanosomiasis is found in West and East Africa, the Congo and Rhodesia, Trypanosoma gambiense being spread by the fly Glossina palpalis and Trypanosoma rhodesiense by Glossina morsitans.
SYMPTOMS: the most characteristic feature of the disease is its long-latent period, the early stage of periodic rises in temperature, swelling of the spleen and lymph glands, and oedema (swelling) of the legs lasting up to three years before the next stage of tremors, vacant expression and slow speech. Later, the patient becomes increasingly sluggish and weak and sleeps or dozes during the day; there is wasting, apathy and a subnormal temperature, and the victim becomes comatose and bedridden before death.
TREATMENT: treatment is with suramin (Bayer 205) and pentamidine in early cases where the trypanosome has been found in the blood; later melarsoprol (Mel B) gives good results.

Slimming: *see* Obesity.

Sling: the one important thing about a sling for the arm is that the hand should always be higher than the elbow.

Slipped Disc: popular term for prolapse of a lumbar invertebral disc.

CAUSE: the inside or nucleus of the intervertebral disc is made of spongy but firm elastic tissue which acts as a shock-absorber for the spinal column, being held in place by a strong ring of fibrous tissue (the annulus fibrosus). If this gives way for some reason, the nucleus of the disc is able to slip out at the back of the vertebral body and press upon one or other of the spinal nerve roots, causing very severe pain.

SYMPTOMS: slipped disc is one of the commonest causes of pain in the back and, usually occurring in the lumbar region, it involves the nerves going to the buttocks, thighs, calves and feet; it is a cause of 'sciatica' and of 'lumbago'.

TREATMENT: the usual treatment is rest in bed, but even with traction (stretching) and other measures full recovery may take six weeks to six months. In about 20% of cases recovery does not follow conservative treatment and it is necessary to carry out a laminectomy. In this operation a portion of the arch of the vertebra is removed and the protruding part of the nucleus of the disc is taken away. It is possible to get out of bed a few days after the operation and to go home in about two weeks.

Slough: dead tissue which separates from healthy tissue as the result of ulceration or inflammation. It is to soft tissue what a sequestrum (q.v.) is to bone.

Smallpox: (Variola). An acute infectious fever; it attacks people of all ages and is equally prevalent in males and females. There are two varieties, variola major and variola minor. They are very much the same, except that in variola major the death rate is about 15%, but in variola minor not more than 0.2%.

CAUSE: infection is spread by contact, by articles handled by the infected person, by third persons, and probably by flies and air, the virus being inhaled. The cause is a filterable virus found in the fluid of the pocks, and the incubation period is 10–14 days.

SYMPTOMS: the onset is usually sudden with headache, vomiting, backache, and a rigor as the temperature rises to 103 °F.; often there is a 'prodromal' reddish rash rather like scarlet fever before the true one makes its appearance on the third day. When the true rash appears the temperature falls to normal, and initially the rash takes the form of spots and papules which turn into blisters and then pustules. During the pustular stage the temperature begins to rise again and the pustules burst about the twelfth day, forming crusts on the sixteenth. When the crusts separate in 2–3 weeks depressed scars are left behind. The rash makes its first appearance on the peripheral parts of the body, slowly moving towards the trunk, i.e. it arises on the forehead and scalp, the legs and the wrists before spreading inwards. (This is the opposite of chickenpox where the rash begins on the trunk and moves outwards.) Three types of the disease are usually described: (a) discrete, the ordinary type where the pustules remain more or less separated from each other and the outlook is fairly good; (b) confluent, where there are many pustules which coalesce, sometimes forming superficial abscesses, and usually there is great prostration and delirium with a correspondingly grave prognosis; (c) haemorrhagic, where there is bleeding into the pustules and haemorrhages from the mucous membranes and into the conjunctivae. Haemorrhagic smallpox is the most fatal type.

TREATMENT: there is no specific treatment, but the patient must be put to bed, the hair is best cut short, and the skin should be bathed with 1% potassium permanganate solution; it is important to protect the eyes and face as much as possible, and the eyes should be bathed frequently. The patient must be isolated for 6 weeks or until all the scabs have separated. Prophylactic treatment is to vaccinate in infancy, thereafter at intervals and again if there is an epidemic. Contacts should be vaccinated and observed for 16 days. The drug Marboran (N-methylisatin B-thiosemicarbazone) has a prophylactic action on contacts, and is given in 2 doses of 3 g. Individuals who have been in contact with the disease can be treated prophylactically with hyperimmune vaccinia gamma globulin.

Smoking: the term generally refers to the smoking of tobacco and it is in this sense that it will be employed here, although many other substances can also be smoked, for example various herbs, opium, and stramonium, which some use in the form of cigarettes in the treatment of asthma. Tobacco has been used by the American Indians from remotest antiquity and was introduced into Europe by Francisco Hernandez de Toledo, a physician to Philip II of Spain, in 1559. It reached the French court in the following year through the medium of the ambassador Jean Nicot (who thus gave his name to the botanical term for the plant, Nicotiana, and to the alkaloid nicotine which is found in tobacco). Sailors returning from the Americas first introduced smoking to England about 1565 and Sir Walter Raleigh brought it to the notice of court circles. Tobacco, of course, was not only smoked but also chewed or taken in the form of snuff, and it was at one time administered by physicians as an enema, for initially tobacco was thought to be of great medicinal value – in fact, almost a cure-all. At a later date laws supported by heavy punishments and even the threat of excommunication by the Church were introduced to exterminate the practice of smoking; these had as little success as the propaganda of today.

Enough has been said about the dangers of lung cancer; it is probably true that most of the heavy smokers we have known did not develop cancer, but these were among the lucky seven out of eight and perhaps we did not meet the eighth, the man who died of it. What concerns us here are the other real or alleged consequences of smoking, and what can be done by those who wish to give up the habit. Perhaps it is best to begin with those conditions which are known for certain to be either caused or worsened by smoking, and here it is necessary to remember that the death-rate of middle-aged people who smoke more than twenty cigarettes a day is more than twice that of non-smokers, taking all diseases into account. Although rare now, tobacco used to be a common cause of cancer of the lips and tongue in people who smoked clay pipes, the edge of the stem causing a sore which became cancerous when the hot tobacco smoke incessantly came into contact with it. Thromboangitis obliterans, a disease in which the arteries of the leg become narrowed and thickened, is believed by some authorities to be a form of allergic response to tobacco and is always associated with heavy cigarette-smoking. The well-known 'smoker's cough' is usually of local origin, being a form of pharyngitis or laryngitis brought on by irritation, and bronchitis is certainly made worse by smoking. Patients with a peptic ulcer usually feel better if they stop smoking (at least on an empty stomach) and regain their appetite. Nicotine stimulates the heart to beat faster (although this effect is much less noticeable in those who smoke habitually) and by some is believed to be a cause of tachycardia and palpitations; the bowels are stimulated and the smoker often finds that his first pipe or cigarette of the day brings on the desire to defaecate. Whether coronary thrombosis is linked with smoking is still a matter for debate.

Smoking cures come under three, or perhaps four, general headings: (1) the use of mouth-washes containing, for example, a dilute solution of silver nitrate, which make smoking taste so unpleasant that it is supposed to turn the smoker against the habit; as with most aversion treatments, the 'cure' is more likely to be given up than the habit. (2) The use of a dummy cigarette which may contain something to give it a taste such as menthol; whether this helps or not one would not be prepared to say, but there is some evidence that menthol itself can occasionally produce unpleasant symptoms or illness. (3) The use of lobeline or one of its derivatives. Lobeline is an alkaloid which produces effects on the body when taken by mouth similar to those produced by nicotine, and the theory is that it can be used to tide the smoker over the initial stages of deprivation. (4) Simply stopping smoking abruptly, which is probably the only effective way. Smoking is undoubtedly a dangerous habit and the best solution is not to begin. If a man has already started then one can only say that he must decide, according to his own temperament, whether he wishes to take a calculated risk or not. If he wants to stop smoking he should stop now – suddenly.

Snakes: *see* Bites and Stings.

Soap: a compound made of an alkali and fatty acids. Providing the quality is good, no one soap has an advantage over any other; all soap is antiseptic, so that the addition of another antiseptic is of doubtful value, but it is true that some cakes of soap smell better than others.

Sodium: a soft white metal which is normally only found in combination with other elements. It is essential for life, and forms the chief cation in the fluids of the body outside the cells. It is usually taken in the form of sodium chloride (common salt) for it is not present in the diet in any great amount; it is normally retained by the body only in the quantities required, so that the intake of salt is balanced by the output, but there are abnormal conditions in which a fairly large intake of salt is necessary, such as incessant diarrhoea or vomiting and some kidney diseases. The symptoms of lack of salt are weakness and fainting, with some mental confusion; muscular cramps are liable to affect people who have lost a large amount of salt by excessive sweating.

Soft Sore: (Chancroid). An acute venereal infection.
CAUSE: Haemophilus ducreyi, a bacillus. Incubation period 5 days.
SYMPTOMS: a blister appears on the genitals which quickly becomes purulent and ulcerates. The ulcer is soft, as opposed to the chancre of syphilis which has a hard base, and there is a profuse foul discharge. The regional lymph glands in the groin are swollen and tender and may break down and discharge in a bad case.
TREATMENT: the condition is best treated in the first instance with sulphadiazine or streptomycin, for neither of these drugs affect the organisms of syphilis, and it is important to know whether the patient acquired syphilis at the same time that he became infected with Ducrey's bacillus. If the passage of time makes it clear that there is no syphilis, and the soft sore has not healed, tetracycline may be used.

Solar Plexus: the largest of the sympathetic nervous plexuses. It lies behind the stomach at the level of the first lumbar vertebra, and takes its name from its radiating branches which are thought to be like the rays of the sun. Its fibres unite the two large coeliac ganglia.

Somatotype: a particular type of body, the classification being made on certain physical appearances. *See* Ectomorph, Endomorph and Mesomorph.

Sonne Dysentery: dysentery caused by the micro-organism Shigella sonnei. *See* Dysentery (bacillary).

Sore Throat: *see* Throat.

Spanish Fly: *see* Cantharides, Aphrodisiac.

Spastic: term applied to that type of paralysis in which the muscles are stiff rather than limp, a condition caused by damage to the upper motor neurones of the brain either in the cortex or in the internal capsule, where the motor nerve fibres are gathered together as they pass downwards from the cortex towards the brain stem and spinal cord. Because many birth injuries result in spasticity, the word spastic is often used popularly to mean a child suffering from a spastic type of paralysis.

Spatula: a blunt flat tool used for mixing substances; often used to mean the flat piece of metal or wood a doctor uses to keep the tongue down when he is inspecting the back of a patient's throat.

Spectacles: there are four types of refractive errors which require the use of glasses: myopia (short-sightedness), hypermetropia (long-sightedness), astigmatism, and presbyopia. *Short-sightedness* is due to the refractive power of the eye being too strong so that the image is brought to a focus in front of the retina, producing blurred vision. This is often a problem in children who are unable to see objects at a distance such as the blackboard at school and it is important that suitable glasses should be supplied as early as possible. *Long-sight* is the reverse condition in which the refractive power of the eye is reduced and the image of near objects is brought to a focus behind the retina; whereas in myopia a concave lens is used for viewing distant objects, in hypermetropia convex lenses are used for near work and distant vision is not affected. In *astigmatism* (q.v.) the curvature of the cornea or lens is not symmetrical, so that rays of light in one place cannot be focused at the same time as those in the plane at right angles to it. There is distortion of both near and distant vision; a circle is seen as an ellipse and is blurred at two points opposite each other. The lens for this type of defect must be cylindrical, i.e. flat in one plane and curved in the one at right angles to it. Astigmatism may occur in long- or short-sighted people, and mixed astigmatism may exist in which the eye is long-sighted in one meridian and short-sighted in the other. In *presbyopia* changes due to age cause the lens to lose its ability to accommodate for near vision and glasses become necessary for reading; this is the case with most people after 45 and nearly all after 50. Dark glasses, although fashionable from time to time, are very rarely a medical necessity. *See also* Contact Lens.

Speculum: an instrument used to open a natural bodily passage so that the interior of a cavity can be directly inspected; a speculum differs from an endoscope, which is an instrument with a light at the end which is passed through natural passages so that the interior of a hollow organ can be seen through a system of lenses. An endoscope is the instrument used for looking into the bladder or into the stomach; a speculum is used for inspecting the interior of the vagina or rectum, the nasal cavity, or the outer ear.

Speech Disorders: *see* Stammering.

Spermatocoele: a cyst of the epididymis. Spermatocoeles are quite common, being usually found in men of middle age although they may form at other times of life. They are not dangerous, but they may attain quite a large size and become a nuisance; they may also become tense and painful, in which case they are best removed.

Sphenoid: although the word sphenoid means 'shaped like a wedge', the sphenoid bone in the base of the skull looks far more like a bat with its wings spread. The bone forms part of the floor of the middle fossa of the skull, and has in its body a depression (from its appearance called the sella turcica) which houses the pituitary gland. The body also contains the two sphenoidal sinuses, air spaces which communicate with the nose.

Sphincter: a ring of muscle fibres that closes a natural passage or the junction between two hollow organs, for example (*a*) the anal sphincter, (*b*) the pyloric sphincter between the stomach and the duodenum.

Sphygmomanometer: an instrument for measuring the pressure of the blood in the arteries.

Spica: a bandage put on like a figure-of-eight so that the turns overlap each other.

Spinal Column: the backbone. It is made up in the child of 33 bones, but in the adult the lowest four unite to form the coccyx and the five above them unite to form the sacrum, so that there are only 26 separate bones in the adult vertebral column. These are arranged as follows: 7 cervical vertebrae in the neck, 12 thoracic vertebrae with attached ribs in the thoracic or chest region, and 5 lumbar vertebrae in the small of the back. Below them are the sacrum, uniting the two hip-bones to form the pelvis, and the coccyx. The average length of the male vertebral column is about 70 cm; the cervical spine is 12 cm long, the thoracic spine 28, the lumbar 18 and the sacrum and coccyx 12 cm. The female spine is about 10 cm shorter. The spinal column when looked at from the side shows four curves. The cervical, or neck, curve is convex forwards, the thoracic curve concave forwards, the lumbar curve convex forwards and the pelvic curve concave forwards. The vertebral canal lies behind the bodies of the vertebrae, which are separated from each other by the inter-vertebral discs, and curves with the column. The spinal cord in the adult does not extend below the upper part of the second lumbar vertebra.

Fractures of the vertebrae are usually caused by forced flexion or extension (for example in motor accidents), direct violence, dropping on the feet from a height or diving on to the head. The most dangerous complication of a fractured spine is injury to the spinal cord, which can result in paralysis, and if there is any question that the victim of an accident has broken his spine he must not be moved by unskilled hands unless he is carried *exactly* in the position in which he was found. If this is not possible he may in grave emergency be carried face downwards so that the spine cannot flex, with the neck supported so that it cannot move. It is very important to remember that people who have sustained injuries to the head may very well have injuries to the neck as well, and if they are unconscious they cannot complain of pain or show the signs of paralysis. The two regions of the spinal column which are most often fractured are the cervical and lumbar, and the commonest type of fracture is the crush fracture of the body of a vertebra that results from violent

693

flexion. It is possible for people to recover from injury to the
cervical cord providing that the substance of the cord has not
been torn or cut.

Spinal Cord: this extends downwards from the brain to run
in the vertebral column as far as the second lumbar vertebra,
where it stops and is continued by the filum terminale, a
fibrous cord fastened to the second sacral vertebra. The spinal
cord is surrounded by membranes named meninges – pia,
arachnoid and dura – just the same as the brain, and the
membranes of the brain are continuous with those covering
the cord. Cerebro-spinal fluid is contained in the space
between the pia and arachnoid membranes (*see* Lumbar
Puncture). If the cord is cut across it is seen to be made up of
white matter surrounding a mass of grey matter which is
shaped like an H with ventral 'horns' pointing forwards towards the belly and dorsal horns pointing to the back. The
ventral horns are concerned with the motor part of the
nervous system (that part supplying the muscles), and the
dorsal horns are to do with the sensory system, which relays
sensory impulses to the brain. The intermediate part of the
grey matter between the first thoracic segment of the cord
and the third lumbar is part of the sympathetic system (*see*
Nervous System). The white matter is made of bundles of
nerve fibres running up and down the cord; they are all
arranged in a definite order according to their function. From
the spinal cord run 31 pairs of spinal nerves which between
them supply the muscles of the body except those of the head
and some of the neck, and bring sensory impulses back to the
brain. Each spinal nerve has an anterior root, through which
go the motor fibres, and a posterior root for the sensory fibres.
The posterior root has on it a ganglion. The two roots join,
emerge from the vertebral foramen, the space between the
vertebrae, and separate into two branches, one to supply the
back and the other, the ventral branch, to supply the front of
the body. The nerve also gives off sympathetic fibres to the
chain of ganglia that run down each side of the vertebral
column, and receives fibres back. The spinal nerves that are
to supply the arms and legs form large plexuses, the brachial
and lumbar plexuses, from which the limb nerves originate,
but the nerves of the abdomen and thorax run separately
round the body. Although the spinal nerves emerge from

between each vertebral bone and are named accordingly – the first thoracic nerve, for example, being related to the first thoracic vertebra – the spinal cord itself is shorter than the vertebral column, so that the lower spinal nerves run ever more obliquely inside the vertebral canal to their exit foramina (*see* Cauda Equina). The results of injury to the spinal column depend on the level; in the neck the effects – paralysis or loss of sensation or both – may include everything below the neck, while it is possible to crush bones in the lumbar spine without injuring the nervous system at all. Although it is not possible for nervous tissue to heal, it cannot at first be determined after a spinal injury how much irrecoverable damage has been done, and improvement, which usually begins to show in the first few days, can continue for many months.

Tumours, both benign and malignant, grow in and about the spinal cord, many of which can be removed by surgery; the commonest disease affecting the cord is multiple sclerosis (q.v.). *See* Nervous System.

Spirochaetes: micro-organisms which are shaped like spirals. Three genera include organisms that produce disease in human beings: Treponema, Borrelia and Leptospira. Treponema pallidum causes syphilis, an organism indistinguishable from it causes pinta, and T. pertenue causes yaws; Borrelia recurrentis and Borr. duttonii cause relapsing fever, and Borr. vincentii can cause Vincent's angina and severe inflammation of the gums; Leptospira ictero-haemorrhagiae causes Weil's disease (infective jaundice) and L. canicola causes canicola fever.

Spirolactone: spirolactones oppose the action of aldosterone on the kidney (*see* Corticosteroids) and so increase the loss of sodium from the body and tend to conserve potassium. They are used to a certain extent in the treatment of oedema in combination with other compounds.

Splanchnic: to do with any of the viscera (the large internal organs) but most often used of the abdominal organs. Splanchnology is the study of the internal organs.

Spleen: the spleen is an oblong flattened abdominal organ that lies behind the stomach on the left side of the abdominal cavity covered by the ninth, tenth and eleventh ribs and in contact with the under surface of the diaphragm. It is red, and measures about 12 cm by 6 cm by 4 cm. Normally it is protected by the ribs from injury except by considerable direct violence, but in some countries where malaria is common and the spleen is consequently enlarged a man can be killed by a shrewd blow in the left upper part of the belly. If injured the spleen bleeds freely, for its artery is a branch of the aorta through a short thick trunk called the coeliac artery, and the venous drainage is into the portal system which has no non-return valves. Moreover, the pulp of the spleen is full of blood, for its functions are concerned with the blood. It is part of the reticulo-endothelial system (q.v.), and its cells scavenge old red blood cells and fragments of matter from the bloodstream; if needed, new red cells can be made in the spleen, and it manufactures lymphocytes, other white cells, and antibodies. In some animals, but not in man, the spleen is able to contract and force the blood contained in it out into the general circulation in times of emergency.

Sometimes the spleen has to be removed, usually after an injury which has given rise to haemorrhage, but no lasting ill effects follow except in young children, who may become unduly susceptible to infections.

Splenectomy: the surgical removal of the spleen. *See* above.

Splenic Anaemia: (Banti's disease). A disease in which enlargement of the spleen, cirrhosis of the liver and anaemia are associated. The disease is caused by obstruction to the portal venous system, and one of the symptoms is therefore the vomiting of blood leaking from blown-out oesophageal veins or varices. The treatment is that of portal hypertension and cirrhosis of the liver; the condition is sometimes improved if the spleen is removed, particularly if the obstruction to the portal circulation is in the splenic vein, but in other cases it is necessary not only to remove the spleen but also to connect the splenic vein to the vein of the left kidney in order to make a short-circuit between the portal circulation and the circulation of the rest of the body.

Splenomegaly: enlargement of the spleen, which may be

696

found in a number of diseases but is very often due to malaria. Enlargement of the spleen may be associated with anaemia, and in such cases surgical removal of the spleen brings relief.

Splints: simple measures to keep fractures still are needed in the first-aid treatment of broken bones so that the patient can be removed to hospital without suffering unnecessary pain or further damage. A splint can be made from anything stiff which can be bound to a limb, but is only really essential when the forearm or wrist is broken, for the upper arm is best bound to the side and the lower limbs tied together if one is broken. If the forearm is bound to a splint it should be supported in a sling. *See* Thomas' Splint.

Spondylitis: inflammation of the vertebrae. Ankylosing spondylitis, or rheumatoid spondylitis, is a disease which affects young men and results in complete stiffening of the spine, which is bent forwards; the radiological appearance is called 'bamboo spine'.

Spondylolisthesis: in this condition the fifth lumbar vertebra slips forward on the sacrum, and the patient complains of low back pain and in some cases pain down the legs, for the intervertebral disc may protrude. The treatment is in the first place rest and physiotherapy, and a spinal support may help the discomfort; in advanced cases surgical operation is indicated. *See* Slipped Disc.

Spondylosis: a degenerative condition of the spine similar to the osteoarthritis which occurs in other parts of the body. CAUSE: it is associated with degeneration of the intervertebral discs, and is found locally in those parts of the spine which are most exposed to repeated minor damage or wear – the lower cervical and lower lumbar regions. It also follows accidental damage, perhaps some years after the original injury which may, for example, have been sustained in a car accident after which the patient noticed a stiff neck, as is by no means uncommon. (It may be that the provision of head rests in cars will lessen this type of injury.) SYMPTOMS: if the spondylosis is in the lumbar spine the symptoms resemble those of a prolapsed intervertebral disc, i.e. pain in the back and down the leg (sciatica). The pain is

697

relieved by rest and aggravated by movement. Spondylosis of the cervical spine, which is a very great deal more common than protrusion of an intervertebral disc in the neck, produces symptoms ranging from headache and pains in the arms to weakness of the legs and difficulty in passing water. Symptoms progress slowly over a period of years or months. TREATMENT: in cases of cervical spondylosis with symptoms the neck is kept still in a plastic collar, and the limitation of movement usually relieves the pain. Operation on the cervical spine is only undertaken if the disease is very severe; a laminectomy can be carried out and the dura mater over the cord split to allow backward displacement away from the compressing bony bar, or the cervical vertebrae can be fused to prevent further movement. In the lumbar spine physiotherapy and the provision of a spinal corset may help, not because a 'spinal support' can in any way support the spine, but because it prevents movement. If a spinal corset is worn the patient should carry out exercises designed to keep up the tone of the spinal muscles, otherwise the corset will do more harm than good. Surgical operation has little to offer, although the lumbar spine can be fused to stop movement. *See* Rheumatism.

Spores: in bacteriology, spores are variations of form which certain organisms assume in order to resist adverse environmental conditions that would kill the ordinary form. The organisms of medical importance that form spores include those that cause gas gangrene, anthrax and tetanus. Spores can resist temperatures up to about 100 °C., and this means that eradication of these organisms is much more difficult than the destruction of non-sporing organisms. They can survive in the absence of animal or human hosts in dust and in the soil.

Spotted Fever: a fever that is accompanied by spots on the skin; the term is applied to epidemic cerebro-spinal meningitis, Rocky Mountain spotted fever (*see* Rickettsiae), and typhus.

Sprains: injuries to a joint in which the ligaments are damaged, but without their being completely ruptured.

Sprue: a tropical disease in which there is deficient absorption of food, particularly of fat. It is not seen in Africa.

CAUSE: the causes are complicated and not fully understood; circumstances have variously suggested that the disease may be caused by a virus infection or by factors in the diet.

SYMPTOMS: diarrhoea with pale large motions, a sore tongue, loss of appetite and loss of weight. If the disease progresses unchecked the patient may develop osteomalacia (softness of the bones), peripheral neuritis, oedematous swelling of the extremities, and megaloblastic anaemia.

TREATMENT: the administration of folic acid and cyanocobalamin; if the diarrhoea continues, then a course of tetracycline can with advantage be given. Anaemia is corrected if necessary by intravenous transfusions, and iron can be used if there is any sign of iron-deficiency anaemia in addition to the megaloblastic anaemia.

Tropical sprue must be distinguished from gluten sensitivity. *See* Coeliac Disease.

Sputum: the substance that is coughed up from the lungs and air passages.

Squill: obtained from the bulbs of Urginea maritima, squill is used in expectorant mixtures.

Squint: a condition in which the two eyes do not point in the same direction; it results from the over- or under-action of one or more of the muscles which move the eyeball, and may have a number of different causes. Long-sightedness in childhood may cause an inward squint, especially on looking at objects close at hand, and if the refractive error in one eye is greater than that in the other the good eye alone is used, resulting in a greater or lesser degree of blindness in the other. Similarly short-sightedness may produce an outward squint when it has not been compensated for by proper glasses. Defective vision in one eye is a less frequent cause. Squint appearing in later life is usually the result of paralysis of the nerves supplying the eye muscles (four straight and two oblique) or disease in the brain affecting these nerves. Treatment must begin as early as possible in life with the wearing of suitable glasses, which may have one dark lens to stop the child using the good eye. This prevents the bad one from becoming worse. Orthoptic exercises to train the child to use its eye muscles correctly must be given at a later stage, and in more severe cases operation may be necessary to strengthen a poorly acting eye muscle or weaken an over-acting one.

Stammering: stammering and stuttering are common forms of speech disorder caused by inco-ordination of the muscles around the larynx. In stammering there is hesitation in the pronunciation of a syllable, in stuttering a repetition of the initial letters. Stammering may arise in childhood or make its first appearance in adolescence or later life; it is generally believed that the former type is predominantly physiological in origin, resulting from something wrong with the organization of the neuromuscular apparatus concerned with speech, and the latter type psychological. This is not to say that emotional factors may not exacerbate the first con-dition, but it is common to find a family history of stammering together with a history of left-handedness – which has given rise to the theory that the basic cause is an incomplete dominance of the leading hemisphere of the brain.

TREATMENT: in the physiological type of stammer this comprises speech therapy and training in breath control, coupled with psychological treatment to remove any emotional problems which may exacerbate the stammer or are present because of it. Some types of childhood stammer are mainly psychogenic and in Freudian terminology centre around conflicts of a deep-seated nature associated with the oral (mouth) region. The later-developing stammers are all psychogenic and essentially of a hysterical nature; they readily respond to treatment of the underlying anxiety state but are in any case usually of short duration.

Stapes: one of the small bones of the middle ear. It is shaped like a stirrup. *See* Ear.

Staphylococcus: a round micro-organism (coccus) which grows in clumps that look like bunches of grapes. It is Gram-positive, and the strain chiefly responsible for producing disease in man is the Staphylococcus aureus; the charac-teristic lesion is a circumscribed infection, for example a boil, and the organism is the chief contaminant of skin wounds and abrasions, in which it usually provokes the formation of pus. It also contaminates food, and in some cases grows in colonies which elaborate a poisonous toxin so that anyone who eats the food on which they are growing develops acute vomiting and diarrhoea (*see* Food Poisoning). Staphylococci have in many cases grown resistant to penicillin, and can present a difficult problem. Particularly difficult to deal with are those which flourish in hospitals and become resistant to tetracycline as well as elaborating penicillinase which destroys penicillins.

Starvation: if men are completely starved but have enough water they can survive for over 60 days; if they have even 500 calories worth of food a day it makes a very great difference to survival. Emergency food should be in the form of carbohydrate rather than protein because in conditions where there is not enough food and water the kidneys are able to conserve more water if they do not have to excrete the end products of protein metabolism. As men become starved they become apathetic and giddy, and behave more and more like 'zombies'; they can be reduced to the state of concentration camp prisoners by 6 months on a diet insufficient in calories, without any brutal treatment or threats. In infancy, undernutrition causes irreversible damage to the developing brain and will result in intellectual dullness. *See also* Fasting.

Status: in medicine, a state or condition; for example status asthmaticus, in which there is a continuous state of asthma with breathlessness and exhaustion, or status epilepticus in which the patient goes into a series of repeated epileptic attacks without regaining consciousness.

Steatopygia: the condition of having fat buttocks.

Steatorrhoea: the passage of excessive fat in the motions. There are many causes for this, ranging from gluten sensitivity to cirrhosis of the liver. The stools become large, pale, frothy and offensive, and the patient shows signs of deficient absorption of vitamins and other essential constituents of the food including iron. The treatment is the treatment of the cause. *See* Coeliac Disease, Sprue.

Stellate Ganglion: there are three sympathetic nervous ganglia in the neck; the uppermost is opposite the second and third cervical vertebrae, the middle is opposite the sixth cervical vertebra, and the lowest lies above the neck of the first rib. The lowest ganglion is often joined to the first thoracic ganglion, which lies below the neck of the first rib, and this large irregular formation is called the stellate ganglion. Its function is to supply sympathetic nervous fibres to the lowest two cervical nerves which run into the arm, to supply the heart through its cardiac branch, to send a small inconstant branch to the vagus nerve and to supply neighbouring blood vessels (branches of the subclavian artery). The upper thoracic sympathetic ganglia are sometimes removed surgically to produce dilatation of the blood vessels of the arm and hand in Raynaud's disease and other conditions, and to control excessive sweating, but if possible the stellate ganglion is left intact to prevent the onset of Horner's syndrome (q.v.).

Stenosis: narrowing of a natural orifice or passage, for example mitral stenosis, narrowing of the mitral orifice in the heart.

Stereoencephalotomy: the use of instruments to guide probes and electrodes accurately into deep structures in the brain and the consequent production of surgical lesions in predetermined places.

Stereoscopic Vision: the nervous pathways running from the retina of the eye, upon which light falls from the outside world, are so arranged that the right-hand field of vision is dealt with by the left cerebral hemisphere and vice versa. One effect of this is that perception in depth (stereoscopic vision) is possible, for although the eyes normally point in the same direction and look at the same thing, they do not look at it from the same point of view; the relative distance of objects from each other and from the eyes are judged from minute differences in the visual impressions derived from the left and right eyes, the stimuli from one half of each retina going to the same cerebral hemisphere for analysis. Stereoscopic vision is not possible with one eye alone, a fact which quickly becomes apparent to a normal person who covers up one eye.. All the same there are some very good one-eyed golfers.

Sterility: some people wish to be sterile, and undergo operations and take drugs to attain this end, while others complain that they cannot have children and ask the doctor for his advice. There are many reasons for a couple being sterile; on the male side, it is essential that the man shall be capable of intercourse, that the semen should be normal, and that the spermatozoa should move freely. In about 15% of cases the man is wholly at fault, and he contributes to the sterility of a further large number of marriages. On the female side, it is essential that ovulation should take place, that the ova should be able to find their way into the uterus through the uterine tubes, and that the lining of the uterus should be in a proper condition for the embedding of the fertilized ovum. In the investigation of cases of sterility the husband's semen is first examined, after the doctor has satisfied himself that copulation is being performed in a way that can result in pregnancy (it sounds odd, but there are enough cases of sterility resulting from inefficient intercourse to make it necessary to go into the matter); while the tests are being carried out, the woman's general health and her state of nutrition are considered, and a full examination is performed to see if there is any disease of the pelvic organs. If these investigations are negative, then more specialized gynaecological procedures become necessary for which specialist services are required. In the case of a young woman it is reasonable to wait two years after marriage before starting investigations for sterility, but in an older woman there may be more urgency.

Sterilization: (1) The destruction of bacteria contaminating instruments, dressings etc., by heat, the use of antiseptics or by irradiation. (2) The operation of rendering individuals incapable of reproduction, which can be carried out in men by tying and dividing the vas deferens on each side as it ascends from the scrotum, a simple operation; and in women by tying and removing part of the uterine tubes, an operation permissible if further pregnancies would endanger the patient's life. The use of contraceptive pills is a way of producing temporary sterility by the action of hormones.

703

Sternum: the breastbone. It has three parts, called from above downwards the manubrium, the body and the xiphoid process.

Steroid: one of a group of chemical substances that are like cholesterol and include sex hormones, bile acids and Vitamin D as well as the hormones of the adrenal glands. *See* Corticosteroids, Cholesterol.

Stethoscope: an instrument through which the physician listens to noises arising in the interior of the body, usually from the heart and lungs. It was invented by Laënnec, a French physician (1781–1826).

Stilboestrol: a synthetic oestrogenic hormone (*see* Ovary), which is used in preference to naturally occurring oestrogens, for example in treatment of cancer of the prostate gland.

Stillbirth: if a child is born after the 28th week of pregnancy and does not breathe or show any other sign of life it is said to be stillborn.

Stokes-Adams Attacks: a condition in which a patient with an abnormally low pulse rate suddenly loses consciousness. The cause is heartblock. *See* Heart.

Stomach: the stomach is a large pouch into which the oesophagus (gullet) conducts the food. It has a capacity of between half and one litre in health, and it secretes gastric juices which digest the food. It lies below the diaphragm in the left upper part of the abdomen, crossing over to the right below the liver, and the oesophageal end is called the cardia; the other end which is continuous with the duodenum is called the pylorus. The cardia lies to the right of an upward bulge called the fundus, which normally contains a bubble of air, and the part between the cardia and fundus and the pylorus is called the body of the stomach. The left border of the stomach, which is the longer, is called the greater curvature and the right, the shorter border, is called the lesser curvature. The part of the stomach just before the pylorus is sometimes known as the antrum. From the greater curvature of the stomach hangs the great omentum, and the stomach is connected to the under surface of the liver above by a fold of membrane called the lesser omentum. The stomach hangs comparatively free in the abdominal cavity, and moves with the breathing; it is tethered at the cardiac end by the oesophagus and at the pyloric end by the duodenum. It is lined by mucous membrane thrown up in folds (rugae) and the wall is well furnished with smooth muscle, the tone of which is affected by various factors, including the emotions.

The glands of the mucous membrane secrete hydrochloric acid, pepsin and various other enzymes, and when the food has been mixed with these secretions it is called chyme. The glands become active both because of the presence of food in the stomach and because of a reflex in the brain set in motion by the sight or the expectation of food. The emotions have a great deal to do with gastric secretions, and anger increases them while anxiety diminishes the volume. The stomach moves food towards the small intestine by peristaltic waves travelling along its muscular wall; acute emotion can bring on paralysis of the muscle and dilatation of the stomach, which gives rise to the sensation of the 'heart dropping into the boots' – substitute stomach for heart and pelvis for boots, and the phrase is probably accurate.

Stomach Disease: the commonest diseases of the stomach are gastritis, or inflammation of the lining, ulceration and cancer.

Acute gastritis. Caused by irritant chemicals, including aspirin, unsuitable food, and alcohol. It may be associated with excessive smoking.

SYMPTOMS: discomfort and loss of appetite, vomiting and occasionally bleeding.

TREATMENT: if the cause can be identified it must be avoided. Alkaline effervescent salts or milk of magnesia are suitable remedies.

Chronic gastritis. The causes in some cases are similar to those of acute gastritis, except that the patient perseveres in drinking alcohol or stewed tea or strong black coffee, or eating irritating substances, until the changes of acute gastritis become permanent. In other cases no cause can be identified.

SYMPTOMS: there may be no symptoms, or there may be loss of appetite and dyspepsia. The most important general

705

condition associated with chronic gastritis is pernicious anaemia, for the changes in the mucous membrane lining the stomach result in a decrease of the secretions, including hydrochloric acid and the intrinsic factor, a substance elaborated in the stomach without which Vitamin B_{12} cannot be absorbed.

TREATMENT: the treatment is to stop taking irritant food or drink. If pernicious anaemia is present Vitamin B_{12} is given by intramuscular injection. Iron-deficiency or simple anaemia may be present, and must be treated by giving iron.

Gastric and duodenal (peptic) ulcer. The exact cause is not known. Duodenal ulcers are about ten times more frequent than gastric ulcers, but both are conveniently considered here. Duodenal ulcers are more common in sedentary workers, particularly businessmen and doctors, and gastric ulcers are more common among manual workers. Duodenal ulcers are more common in men, among whom there are four peptic ulcers to every one found in women; women tend to develop their ulcers in the stomach. Obvious factors which seem to be related to the production of peptic ulcers are worry and irregular meals, but even here authorities disagree.

SYMPTOMS: *Gastric ulcer.* The classical symptoms are pain, vomiting and bleeding, of which the last is luckily the least common. On the whole the pain of gastric ulceration is felt to the left of the mid-line, and it comes on sooner after food than the pain of the duodenal ulcer.

Duodenal ulcer. The chief symptom is pain, which is felt towards the right side or in the middle of the upper abdomen under the ribs. It comes on an hour or two after meals, and characteristically wakes the patient up at about two in the morning. It is relieved by food of some sort – a biscuit will often be enough – by a drink of milk or by alkalies. Vomiting also relieves the pain, and there are spontaneous remissions.

TREATMENT: the treatment of an uncomplicated peptic ulcer is in the first instance medical. The patient should go to bed, and take small meals regularly at short intervals – the idea is that the stomach should never be entirely empty. Many people find that fried and spiced food brings on the pain, and there is little doubt that alcohol should not be taken on an empty stomach (if it should be taken at all). Ulcers heal more quickly in those who give up smoking. Alkalies can be taken with advantage, and satisfactory preparations include aluminium hydroxide and magnesium trisilicate, which may be combined with atropine in small doses. Carbenoxolone (Biogastrone), a substance obtained from liquorice, tends to hasten the resolution of gastric ulcers. It is not sensible to try to treat a peptic ulcer yourself.

COMPLICATIONS: the complications of gastric ulceration are perforation, scarring of the stomach (*see* Hourglass Stomach) and acute bleeding; and the complications of a duodenal ulcer perforation, bleeding, and scarring of the pylorus and duodenum resulting in obstruction to the passage of food.

TREATMENT OF COMPLICATIONS: haemorrhage, obstruction of the pylorus, and perforation are all indications for operation. If possible the surgeon performs a partial gastrectomy – removal of part of the stomach – for a gastric ulcer. For a duodenal ulcer he may perform the same operation or may combine division of the vagus nerves that supply the stomach with a plastic operation to widen the pylorus so that the stomach can empty quickly. The operations of partial gastrectomy and division of the vagus nerves both decrease the secretion of acid in the stomach by well over a half, and in the hands of a good surgeon are less dangerous than having an active ulcer.

Cancer of the stomach. A fairly common type.

CAUSE: in rare cases the growth follows chronic gastritis, but cancer usually develops in an otherwise healthy stomach. There is no agreement about the possibility of a simple gastric ulcer turning malignant; it is argued that when it appears to have done so the ulcer has been malignant from the beginning.

SYMPTOMS: insidious dyspepsia, slow loss of weight, loss of appetite and weakness, followed in time by nausea and vomiting. There may be pain resembling that of peptic ulcer, or pain may be constant.

TREATMENT: if possible, surgical removal of the growth.

INVESTIGATION OF THE STOMACH: the investigation of diseases of the stomach is similar in all cases. It includes X-rays taken after the stomach and duodenum have been outlined by a barium meal, and in many cases gastroscopy, the inspection of the interior of the stomach through a gastroscope (q.v.). In other cases a complete diagnosis cannot be made without an exploratory operation.

Stomatitis: inflammation of the mucous membrane lining the mouth. It may be caused by infection with Candida albicans (thrush), by infection with Vincent's spirochaete (Vincent's angina), or may be found in blood diseases such as leukaemia or poisoning with gold or mercury. In secondary syphilis the mucous membrane of the mouth is sometimes affected, and superficial ulceration is seen on the palate where it is said to look like snail tracks. Simple ulcers in the mouth are quite common, particularly in middle-aged women, but their cause is not known; they come and go spontaneously, and their disappearance can be hurried by the local use of hydrocortisone pellets which are sucked or allowed to dissolve in close proximity to the ulcers. Gly-oxide, 10% carbamide peroxide, is an effective healing agent in uncomplicated mouth conditions. It is applied locally four times a day.

Stone: (Calculus). Stones are found in the kidneys, bladder, gall-bladder, prostate and salivary glands and in other places. They are formed in the main as a result of inflammation, but in some cases follow desiccation. The symptoms and treatment of stones in the more important organs are described separately under the headings of those organs.

Stools: the faeces, the waste matter discharged from the bowels.

Strabismus: squint (q.v.).

Strangulation: 1. Compression of the windpipe in order to stop a person breathing.
2. Compression of a part which results in the cutting off of its blood supply, for example a strangulated hernia.

Strangury: a state in which the urine can only be passed in painful drops although there is a strong desire to urinate.

Streptococcus: a round Gram-positive micro-organism which forms straight chains. Some of the species produce disease in man, of which the most important are Streptococcus pyogenes (the β-haemolytic streptococcus), S. viridans (the α-haemolytic streptococcus), and S. pneumoniae. Streptococcus pyogenes is responsible for tonsillitis, scarlet fever, impetigo, erysipelas, rheumatic fever, acute nephritis, puerperal fever, and may infect wounds. It characteristically does not produce pus like the staphylococcus but tends to spread in the tissues and set up a cellulitis. Streptococcus viridans is normally present in the mouth, but infects damaged heart valves and produces subacute bacterial endocarditis; it may also be found in abscesses round the roots of the teeth. Streptococcus pneumoniae (formerly called Diplococcus pneumoniae) causes bacterial pneumonia. The drug of choice in treating streptococcal infections is penicillin.

Streptomycin: an antibiotic obtained from the soil mould Actinomyces griseus and discovered in 1944 by Waksman in the United States. It is active against certain Gram-negative organisms that are unaffected by penicillin in ordinary concentrations and, most important of all, it is effective against the germ of tuberculosis, the treatment of which was revolutionized by the discovery. Similarly valuable is its close relative dihydrostreptomycin. The main drawback of these drugs is their liability to create resistant strains of organisms, a disadvantage which can partly be overcome by combining streptomycin with P.A.S. (para-amino-salicylic acid) and isoniazid (q.v.). Both streptomycin and dihydro-streptomycin may cause giddiness and deafness as well as sensitivity reactions such as skin rashes and fever.

Stria: a line or groove. Striae atrophicae are the white lines seen on the abdominal wall after pregnancy, or after a great deal of weight has been lost. They are caused by rupture of the elastic fibres of the skin by stretching.

Stricture: the narrowing of a natural passage such as the urethra, bowel, or oesophagus by scarring after injury or infection, or by a new growth.

Stridor: the noise made by the breath passing an acute obstruction in the larynx, which may be caused by laryngo-tracheitis (usually a virus infection), diphtheria, or an inhaled foreign body.

Stroke: *see* Apoplexy.

Stroma: the tissue forming the framework of an organ, as distinct from the parenchyma, the functioning tissue.

Strongyloides: Strongyloides stercoralis is a roundworm found in subtropical and tropical countries. *See* Worms.

Strophanthin: the active principle of an African plant which is identical to ouabain and has an action very similar to digitalis (q.v.).

Struma: goitre.

Strychnine: an alkaloid derived from the seeds of Strychnos nux-vomica, an East Indian tree. It is a nervous stimulant which increases muscle tone, and was formerly used widely in tonics and as a bitter although it is much less used for these purposes now. Poisoning leads to convulsions very similar to those of tetanus; it is liable to be fatal. Barbiturates are injected as antidotes.

Stupor: a state of incomplete unconsciousness.

Stuttering: *see* Stammering.

Stye: infection of a sebaceous gland in the edge of the eyelid. The infecting organism is usually a staphylococcus, and the resolution of the small abscess may be helped by the removal of the eyelash which is commonly found protruding from its centre, hot bathing, and, if the infection shows signs of spreading, antibiotics.

Subacute Bacterial Endocarditis: infection of previously damaged heart valves.
CAUSE: the infecting organism is usually Streptococcus viridans; the valves have usually been damaged by rheumatic fever, but sometimes are the seat of congenital abnormality. Normal valves are only affected when the patient is weak as the result of chronic disease or drug addiction. Streptococcus viridans is often set loose in the bloodstream by the extraction of a tooth or the formation of a dental abscess, for the organism is normally present in the mouth in large quantities.
SYMPTOMS: the diagnosis is suspected when a patient known

to have valvar disease of the heart starts running a low-grade fever, looks pale and feels generally ill. Petechial haemorrhages (q.v.) occur in the skin and nodules may form as the result of tiny clots blocking the small arteries of the hands and feet. Various other symptoms may follow small embolisms in the kidneys, spleen or brain.

TREATMENT: the organisms are isolated from the blood and tested for drug sensitivity; they usually prove to be sensitive to penicillin, which is given in massive doses.

Subarachnoid Hemorrhage: bleeding into the subarachnoid space, which is normally filled with cerebro-spinal fluid (*see* Meninges).

CAUSE: aneurysms (q.v.) on the arterial circle of Willis at the base of the brain are the usual source of the bleeding; they are present at birth as small weaknesses in the wall of an artery which, with the passage of time, blow up into berry-shaped swellings with thin walls which may rupture. Angiomatous malformations of the arteries may also bleed into the subarachnoid space. (Subarachnoid haemorrhage may follow a head injury, but the presence of blood in the subarachnoid space is then only incidental.)

SYMPTOMS: a sudden severe headache stuns the patient, who may think he has been hit on the head. He may quickly lose consciousness; he will show rigidity of the neck, dislike of light and other signs of irritation of the meninges when he comes round. There may be a number of indications that the haemorrhage has damaged the brain and the cranial nerves, commonly those which run to the eyes, so that paralyses, squint, fixed pupil and altered reflexes may be found.

TREATMENT: once the diagnosis has been made patients should be admitted to a neurosurgical unit, where it may be thought best to perform an operation to stop the aneurysm bleeding. Subarachnoid haemorrhage usually attacks fit young people and recovery from one attack does not mean that there will not be others; surgery in cases where the aneurysm is suitable can be very successful. In some cases angiomatous tumours can also be treated with success.

Subclavian: under the collar-bone, for example subclavian artery.

Subclinical: it is possible for people to catch infections and overcome them without ever developing symptoms. Such hidden infections are referred to as subclinical, and this is the way in which most of us acquire resistance to common diseases.

Subcutaneous: under the skin, usually applied to injections.

Subdural Hematoma: bleeding under the dura mater, the outer membrane of the three enclosing the brain. In the same way that haemorrhage can occur between the arachnoid and pia mater (*see* Subarachnoid Hemorrhage), and outside the dura (*see* Extradural Hemorrhage), it can also occur between the dura mater and the arachnoid.

CAUSE: in this case the source of the blood is venous rather than arterial; the veins leak as the result of a blow on the head (often comparatively minor) or an injury sustained during birth. The bleeding is slow, for the pressure inside the head is high enough to stop blood escaping quickly from the veins, and it does not at first reveal its presence. As the collection of blood enlarges, however, it begins to produce symptoms; the blood breaks down, and because it forms an area of high osmotic pressure fluid from outside is attracted into the haematoma, which gradually swells at the expense of surrounding brain tissue.

SYMPTOMS: any time from a week to six months or more after a relatively trivial bump on the head the patient begins to suffer from headaches, and then becomes forgetful and dull. He may be confused and stuporous, or may fall into unconsciousness. The condition can be bewildering because it varies so much, and one of the characteristics of a subdural haematoma is fluctuation of the symptoms.

TREATMENT: the treatment is surgical. Once the diagnosis has been made by neurological examination, aided by arteriography, echo-encephalography, and if necessary ventriculography, the fluid is let out of the haematoma and steps are taken to ensure that the brain expands again. The treatment of a subdural haematoma is in most cases completely successful.

Subluxation: a dislocation which is not complete.

Submandibular Gland: this gland, which secretes saliva into the mouth, lies under cover of the lower jaw-bone just in front of the angle; it is about the size of a walnut. Its duct is 5 cm long, opening on top of a little papilla under the tongue. The submandibular duct is also known as Wharton's duct, and under that name figures in an unquotable mnemonic rhyme.

Subphrenic: under the diaphragm, for example subphrenic abscess, which is a collection of pus under the diaphragm arising from a ruptured appendix, perforated peptic ulcer, or some other cause of purulent peritonitis.

Subtemporal: beneath the temple. Usually used to mean beneath the temporal muscle in the phrase subtemporal decompression, which is the name of an operation designed to lower the pressure inside the skull in cases of inoperable intracranial tumour by removing that part of the wall of the skull which lies underneath the temporal muscle so that the brain can bulge under cover of the muscle.

Succussion: a sound of splashing that is heard when a patient who has fluid and air in a body cavity is shaken.

Suicide: paradoxically, suicide is a phenomenon of prosperity. Wherever one looks it becomes apparent that it is in the technically advanced and wealthy parts of the world (or even of countries and cities) where the suicide rate is highest. In underdeveloped lands it is so rare that few people know what the word means, or can even picture the idea of a person killing himself. Why this should be so nobody knows for certain although, in view of the facts that are available, it is fair to put forward some hypotheses. The first thing to point out is that the Industrial Revolution brought about a change in the structure of the family; whereas in an agricultural society every member of a large family plays a useful part – the grandparents looking after the young while the parents work in the fields and the children being social and economic assets from a very early age – this pattern was rudely reversed by the advent of heavy industry. Today children no longer represent useful help on the land, but have become economic liabilities until they leave school at

the age of 16 or possibly much later, and the old have become
a nuisance in our small houses. Once the man has retired and
his family gone elsewhere, an ageing couple are liable to feel
(and with justice) cast-off, useless, and doomed to live out a
lonely life in an otherwise deserted house, or worse still in an
old people's home.

Loneliness at all ages is an important factor in suicide, and
this is related to the high geographical and social mobility
rate of modern society. The single man who has to move
from one place to another to get a job and the student (perhaps from a foreign country) alone in his bed-sitter are high
among the number of those who kill themselves. There is a
close correlation between the number of single bed-sitting
rooms in an area and its suicide rate. Again, to take another
aspect of industrial society, it is obvious that the more importance we attach to success and the greater the stigma we
attach to failure, the worse we make things for even the
relative failure. The sayings 'the farther you rise the harder
you fall' and 'those who are down need fear no fall' are
substantially true; the former case is liable to suicide while
the other is not. Finally, among other false ideas which have
gained wide acceptance in the Western world is the over-
dramatized concept of Romance, which plays a considerable
part in cases of attempted suicide among adolescents and
married women whose sentimental attitudes towards love-
affairs or marriage have been shattered by hard realities.

Suicide and attempted suicide are not at all the same thing.
Suicide successfully accomplished is largely a male preserve.
Out of every four men who make the gesture, three succeed;
but out of every four women, only one. Attempted suicide
is typical of younger age groups and married women, for
much the same reason – disappointed 'love'. Thus, unlike
accomplished suicide in which social isolation is a common
feature, attempted suicide almost always occurs in a social
setting because basically it is an appeal to others, a threat, or
even a thinly disguised form of emotional blackmail. In
effect, the individual is saying: 'Look what you've made me
do – and I'll do it again if you don't give me more attention!'
But it would be a mistake to suppose that those who threaten
to commit suicide, whatever their motive, are unlikely to
carry out their threat. In one group of cases of death from
suicide, investigation showed that more than two-thirds had

told someone of their intention beforehand. Nor is it true, as is so often believed, that anyone who fails the first time is unlikely to succeed later; moreover, there are cases in which unwanted success is achieved by accident.

Sulphonamides: a group of compounds introduced in 1935 following the discovery of Prontosil by Domagk, the German physician who was a Nobel prizewinner for 1939. For some years sulphonamides saved countless lives, for they were active against bacteria that previously could not be controlled. They had, however, like all powerful and valuable drugs, drawbacks: in nearly one in ten patients treated with sulphonamides side effects were seen which included blockage of the kidneys by the formation of crystals, damage to the blood cellular system with consequent deficiencies in red and white blood corpuscles, and severe reactions in the form of skin rashes, fever, jaundice, nausea and vomiting. When antibiotics (q.v.) came into use sulphonamides were gradually dropped, until now they are only used in special cases.

Sulphones: chemical compounds which are active against leprosy when given by mouth. The most effective is dapsone (diaminodiphenylsulphone). Sulphones have the peculiar property of being slowly absorbed, then excreted in the bile and being absorbed again from the intestines; relatively cheap compounds, they can safely be given continuously for several years.

Sulphur: a non-metallic element used in medicine both in its uncombined form and as its salts. Sulphur lotions and ointments are used on the skin; sodium sulphate is Glauber's salts and magnesium sulphate Epsom salts.

Sunburn: the effect produced by ultraviolet rays on the skin, especially in fair-skinned people. Severe degrees of sunburn involving large blisters call for the attention of a doctor.

Sunstroke: *see* Heatstroke.

Superfluous Hair: if at all abundant superfluous hair is best removed by shaving, which does not, as is so often stated, cause it to grow more rapidly or to become coarser. Isolated hairs can be dealt with by electrolysis and various depilatory creams can be used in place of shaving. Care must be taken with these, since they are irritant to many skins and dangerous if they get in the eyes.

Supination: to lie supine is to lie with the face upwards; supination is a term usually applied to the movement of turning the forearm so that the palm of the hand is upwards or forwards. The opposite motion is pronation; to lie prone is to lie with the face downwards.

Suppository: cone made of glycerine jelly or some other easily melted substance combined with a drug for insertion into the rectum or vagina.

Suppuration: the process of forming pus. A suppurating wound is one discharging pus.

Suprapubic: above the pubic bone, i.e. at the bottom of the abdomen. Usually applied to operations performed through the lower abdominal wall, for example suprapubic prostatectomy, suprapubic cystotomy.

Suprarenal: *see* Adrenal.

Suprasellar: above the sella turcica, the bony depression in the sphenoid bone at the base of the skull that holds the pituitary body. Tumours of this region, which may be congenital (suprasellar cyst) or acquired (suprasellar meningioma), very often interfere with the function of the optic nerves, which join and cross in the optic chiasm just above the pituitary gland. They also interfere with various functions of the hypothalamic area of the brain and of the pituitary gland (q.v.).

Supraspinatus Tendinitis: the supraspinous muscle takes origin from the upper part of the shoulderblade, and its tendon is closely applied to the capsule of the shoulder joint and fastened to the upper part of the humerus, the bone of the upper arm. The tendon may become inflamed, and then the arm cannot be raised from the side for more than 30° without being rotated outwards, for the tendon comes into painful contact with the underside of the acromion, the bony point of the shoulder. Treatment for the condition of supraspinatus tendinitis includes injection of the area of tenderness with hydrocortisone and local anaesthetic, and physiotherapy. It is important that the shoulder joint should not be allowed to stiffen.

Suramin: (Germanin, Bayer 205). A drug active against trypanosomes when given by injection, preferably intravenous. It is used in the treatment of African sleeping sickness; because it is also active against Onchocerca volvulus it can be given in severe cases of onchocerciasis (African river blindness), but it is best reserved for cases which do not respond to other remedies, for Suramin can cause damage to the kidneys and produce peripheral neuritis and urticarial eruptions.

Suture: (*a*) surgical stitch. (*b*) A type of fibrous immovable joint between bones, seen for example between the bones of the skull.

Swab: a twist of cotton wool on a stick used for taking specimens from the surface of mucous membranes or discharging wounds for examination by the bacteriologist. Also used to mean pieces of gauze or other material with which the surgeon mops up blood during an operation.

Sycosis Barbae: barber's itch, an infectious staphylococcal invasion of the hair follicles, which used to affect the area of the beard, being spread by infected instruments in the barber's shop. It was almost completely confined to male adults, and has grown much rarer in the last thirty years. It is treated by antibiotics.

Symbiosis: a condition in which two organisms live together. If the arrangement is beneficial to one and detrimental to the other, it is called parasitism. If it is detrimental to both it is called synnecrosis, and if beneficial to both mutualism.

717

Sympathetic: in medicine this describes part of the autonomic nervous system. Sympathectomy is the operation for removal of part of the sympathetic nervous system. *See* Nervous System.

Symphysis: an immovable joint in which the bone ends in apposition are united by cartilage, for example symphysis pubis.

Symptom: evidence of functional change which indicates the presence of disease or disorder. It is usually applied to evidence that the patient himself has noticed, as opposed to *sign*, which is evidence of disease noted by an observer (the physician).

Synapse: the place where processes of different nerve cells meet, or where processes meet the bodies of other nerve cells; at the synapse transmission of nerve impulses occurs. *See* Nervous System, Spinal Cord.

Syncope: a faint, or sudden loss of consciousness due to a fall of blood pressure in the brain.

Syndrome: a set of signs and symptoms which occur together in a definite pattern always associated with a particular disease process.

Synousiology: the study of the science of sexual intercourse.

Synovitis: inflammation of the slippery synovial membrane which lines joint capsules and tendon sheaths.

Syphilis: a serious and important venereal disease.
CAUSE: sexual contact with an infected person, except when a foetus is infected by the mother. It is due to the microorganism Treponema pallidum, one of the spirochaetes, which is very easily killed by a change in temperature or in humidity.
SYMPTOMS: syphilis has three stages. In the first stage, which develops three or four weeks after infection, a hard sore (chancre) forms on the infected part – the genital organ, lip or finger; the local lymph glands are enlarged, but the sore is

not painful nor do the lymph glands hurt (*see* Hunterian Chancre).

Diagnosis is made on microscopical examination of discharge from·the sore, for blood tests cannot be relied on to become positive until the second stage, three or four weeks after the appearance of the chancre. In the second stage there is a generalized coppery rash which develops over a week or two on the trunk, the palms and the soles, and the forehead, where it is called the corona Veneris. Ulcers develop in the mouth and throat which are said to look like snail tracks, and there is a sore throat. The symptoms and signs may disappear and then recur; the blood tests – Kahn, V.D.R.L. and Wassermann – are by now positive. In the third stage the disease is no longer infectious, and the characteristic change is the development of a granuloma (q.v.) called a gumma. The most common site for this lesion is the aorta, where the granulomatous reaction can cause inflammation of the aorta, disorder of the aortic valve, narrowing of the mouths of the coronary arteries, and aneurysm. Gumma formation may also occur in the central nervous system in the meninges, the membranes that cover the brain, but the commonest syphilitic disorders of the central nervous system are G.P.I., or general paralysis of the insane (q.v.), and tabes dorsalis (locomotor ataxia) (q.v.).

Syphilis can mimic any number of diseases, for it spreads widely throughout the body, and it has been called the Great Imitator. Routine tests on the blood for syphilis must be done on all patients, whoever they are, or sooner or later the physician will be caught out. In particular all expectant mothers must have a blood test carried out, for in this way many cases of congenital syphilis – due to infection of the foetus in the womb – will be avoided. If this precaution is not taken, and the child is not seen to be infected at birth (such children have 'snuffles', infection round the lips, and rashes, but these may be so mild that they pass unnoticed), congenital syphilis may show itself many years later, very often as interstitial keratitis which interferes with vision.

TREATMENT: the drug of choice is penicillin, given by intramuscular injection. The usual dose is 6 mega units over ten days in primary syphilis, up to 20 mega units when the blood reaction is positive in primary and secondary syphilis, and 20 mega units in 20 days if necessary in repeated courses in tertiary syphilis. The patient's blood reactions are followed up and so is the reaction of the cerebro-spinal fluid. If the patient is sensitive to penicillin tetracyclines, erythromycin, or the organic arsenical drugs or bismuth may be used. It is very important that patients with other venereal infections should be regarded as having syphilis as well until it is proved that they have not, for otherwise cases will be missed which may progress to the crippling third stage without showing themselves.

Syringe: an instrument for injecting fluid directly into any orifice or cavity, or through a needle into skin, muscles or veins.

Syringomyelia: an uncommon disease of the spinal cord beginning between the ages of 15 and 30, in which cavities very slowly form in the substance of the cord in the region of the lower neck and interfere with the sensations of heat and pain in the arms and hands so that the patient tends to burn himself without realizing it. Examination by the physician shows that there is also interference with position and vibration sense. The disease progresses slowly; it may stretch up into the lower part of the brain stem and affect the sensation of the face. Very rarely the cavity in the cord, which is filled with fluid, undergoes sudden enlargement and the symptoms change rapidly to those of compression of the cord, with weakness or paralysis of the legs and difficulty in passing urine. In such cases operative exploration of the cervical spinal cord and evacuation of the fluid from the cavity may relieve symptoms, but otherwise no effective treatment is known. Nevertheless, most patients live a reasonable life and die from an unrelated disease.

Systole: contraction of the muscle of the heart, especially of the ventricles.

T

Tabes: in the general sense, not now much used, the word means a wasting disease; today the term is applied almost exclusively to tabes dorsalis. *See* Locomotor Ataxia.

T.A.B. Vaccine: vaccine containing micro-organisms of typhoid fever and paratyphoid A and B treated with phenol or acetone. Cholera may be included in the vaccine, which is then known as T.A.B.C.; 0.5 ml is given by subcutaneous injection, followed by a further 1 ml in a week's time. Immunization takes 2 weeks to develop, and it lasts for a number of months. Booster doses of 0.5 ml can be given.

Tachycardia: a rapid heartbeat, which may result from fever, emotion, exercise, chronic infection, anaemia, haemorrhage and certain drugs; in paroxysmal tachycardia (q.v.) the heart-rate doubles for no good reason.

Taenia: (1) A genus of tapeworms. *See* Worms. (2) Bands of fibrous tissue that run longitudinally along the colon, puckering it up. (3) In anatomy, strips of soft tissue.

Talipes: club-foot (q.v.).

Talus: the ankle-bone or the ankle itself.

Tannin: a pale brown powder with an astringent taste which is used to coagulate proteins. Small wounds can be treated with tannin to stop them bleeding, but the use of tannin on burns to provide an impermeable cover and stop the loss of tissue fluid is now not fashionable.

Tapeworm: a parasitic worm which is long and flat, like a piece of tape, and divided into segments. *See* Worms.

Tar: a black sticky substance which is obtained by heating coal or certain sorts of wood. It is used in medicine as an application to the skin, for it contains a number of valuable substances including cresol, phenol and toluene; it is particularly effective in the treatment of psoriasis and chronic eczema. Crude coal tar may be mixed with zinc paste in concentrations varying from 1 to 10%, or may be painted directly on to the skin either in its natural state or diluted with acetone and benzene. It is not carcinogenic to man except where contact is prolonged over a number of years, although cancers can be provoked on the skin of mice by painting them with crude tar. It does, however, make human skin sensitive to light.

Tarsorrhaphy: an operation in which the eyelids are sewn together to protect the eye, used in cases where the cornea has lost its sensitivity, for example after operations on the fifth cranial nerve for trigeminal neuralgia, or sometimes after herpes zoster.

Tarsus: (1) The ankle. (2) The flat, hard plate which supports the eyelid.

Tartar Emetic: a mixture of antimony and potassium tartrate, which was originally, as the name indicates, used as an emetic, a use not now recommended because it has a slow action and depresses the respiration and heartbeat. It is now sometimes used in the treatment of Schistosoma japonicum (*see* Bilharzia) and kala-azar.

Teeth: in man there are 32 permanent teeth, 16 in each jaw. These are divided up as follows on each side of the jaw: 2 incisors, 1 canine, 2 pre-molars, and 3 molars. The incisors are used for cutting, the canine (well-developed in carnivorous animals) for tearing and piercing, and the premolars and molars for grinding. The outer layer of a tooth is made of enamel which is a hard substance composed of calcium phosphate, magnesium phosphate, calcium carbonate and calcium fluoride, while the rest of the tooth is composed of dentine made up of the same materials but not so hard as the enamel. In the dentine are many small channels which communicate between the enamel and the pulp in the centre of the tooth, which consists mainly of blood vessels and nervous tissue. The root of the tooth is single in the incisors and canine and usually in the first premolar tooth, but the second premolar has two roots and the molars of the upper jaw three; the molars of the lower jaw have two roots each. The 'milk teeth' which precede the permanent ones are fewer, smaller, whiter and somewhat different in shape, the permanent teeth developing from the fifth to the twentieth year. The last and smallest molar is the 'wisdom tooth'.

Development of milk and permanent teeth

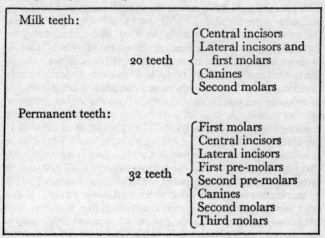

Milk teeth:

20 teeth
- Central incisors
- Lateral incisors and first molars
- Canines
- Second molars

Permanent teeth:

32 teeth
- First molars
- Central incisors
- Lateral incisors
- First pre-molars
- Second pre-molars
- Canines
- Second molars
- Third molars

Dental caries is essentially a disease of civilization caused in large measure by eating 'civilized' foods which are too soft and too sweet. These cause bacteria to multiply which disintegrate the enamel and attack the dentine, breaking down the tooth and destroying the pulp. One of the symptoms of this is toothache, and the infection may lead to a dental abscess or gumboil. The first aid treatment of toothache (which will afterwards require the dentist's attention) is to wash the mouth out with an alkali such as baking soda, give aspirin, and if a cavity exists plug it with a piece of cotton wool soaked in oil of cloves. Lack of dental care or infections of the mouth are the cause of gingivitis (inflammation of the gums) in which during the acute stage the gums are swollen, red and bleed easily on being brushed. A soft toothbrush should be used gently in cleaning, and the gums should be massaged daily; an antiseptic mouth-wash may help. Pyorrhoea alveolaris or paradontal disease differs from gingivitis in that pockets of pus are formed around the junction of the teeth and gums, but in both conditions the teeth tend to become loose in their sockets and the gums shrink, exposing the necks of the teeth. The ultimate treatment of gingivitis and pyorrhoea should be left to the dentist.

The teeth should be brushed in the morning and at night, and after each meal if possible, and those who wish to keep their mouths healthy would be well advised to discourage in themselves the use of excessive amounts of sweets, carbo-hydrate foods and sweet drinks. The effect of dental health upon the health of the body is a matter of controversy. Obviously in very severe cases of pyorrhoea it is undesirable to swallow the pus produced around the gums, but very few doctors nowadays believe that dental decay has the results it was once supposed to have. Thirty years or more ago it used to be thought that 'focal sepsis' could cause a multitude of diseases from rheumatoid arthritis to insanity – indeed, every disease which had no known cause was attributed to focal sepsis, and unfortunate schizophrenics and sufferers from rheumatism had their teeth ruthlessly drawn in the hope of improvement of their condition. This, of course, was rubbish; nor is there any reason to suppose that gastric diseases have any close relationship to dental disorders; for the obvious fact is that certain types of people are likely to get ulcers no matter what they do, or do not, eat, whereas others who may have no teeth at all eat (or at any rate swallow) any kind of food, chewed or unchewed, with im-punity. A more moderate attitude is that dental disease is largely confined to the mouth but is nevertheless unpleasant, unaesthetic and painful, and few normal people would wish to wear dentures if a little attention to their teeth from the early years could prevent it. The prevention of decay in the teeth by adding fluorine to drinking water is mentioned under the heading of Fluorine.

Teething: this is often given as the cause for numerous minor complaints of infancy, probably in the majority of cases quite wrongly. However, the irritation of pain caused by erupting teeth can cause loss of sleep and appetite with consequent loss of weight and fretfulness; that teething can also cause skin eruptions, cough and diarrhoea is rather more doubtful. If the child rubs its gums and salivates profusely, the best treatment is to give it rusks to chew, which will aid in the process of cutting the teeth.

Telangiectasis: spots on the skin formed by dilated capillary blood vessels.

Telemetry: the measurement of phenomena at a distance; in medicine, telemetry is sometimes advocated as a way of overcoming the chronic shortage of skilled nurses. *See* Monitor.

Temperature: *see* Fever.

Temperomandibular Joint: the joint between the temporal bone and the lower jaw-bone, the mandible. It is just in front of the ear, and the head of the mandible can be felt moving if a finger-tip is placed in the external auditory meatus (the ear-hole). The joint allows movement of the mandible from side to side, for it is not a simple hinge but rather a sliding hinge. There is a plate of cartilage in the joint which normally separates the bones, but it may become displaced or torn so that the joint clicks. Relatively minor incidents such as an excessively wide yawn can result in dislocation. If this happens the lower jaw-bone can be replaced by putting the thumbs on the back teeth inside the mouth and the fingers under the chin. The thumbs are pressed down, the fingers bring the chin up, and the jawbone snaps into place.

Tendinitis: inflammation of a tendon; tenosynovitis is inflammation of the tendon and its sheath. *See* below.

Tendon: the cord of dense fibrous tissue which joins muscle to bone. Injuries which affect tendons include rupture, dislocation and division in wounds and lacerations.

Tenesmus: straining painfully but ineffectively in trying to pass motions or pass urine.

Tennis Elbow: a condition in which severe pain is felt at the elbow, radiating down the forearm; examination of the elbow shows tenderness over the outer bony point (lateral epicondyle), and injection of local anaesthetic with hydrocortisone often relieves discomfort.

Tenosynovitis: inflammation of tendon and sheath. This may follow infection, but such a case is rare; more commonly it is the result of repeated minor injury, and housewives, for example, are not uncommonly affected in the forearms and wrist. The condition is painful and there is tenderness over the inflamed tendon sheath, but rest and immobilization will lead to a cure.

Tentorium: the tentorium cerebelli is the fold of dura mater that intervenes at the back of the skull between the undersurface of the cerebral hemispheres and the upper surface of the cerebellum.

Teratoma: a tumour composed of embryonic tissues including all three layers of developing cells – endoderm, mesoderm and ectoderm. A solid teratoma may contain pieces of bone, nerve or intestine, and is usually malignant; it arises in the testicle or the ovary, and must be removed. In the case of a cystic teratoma the outlook is not so bad, for such cysts, which contain various rudimentary tissues such as skin, hair and teeth, are not malignant and may be removed completely. Teratomatous cysts commonly contain ectoderm to the exclusion of other tissues, and are therefore called dermoid cysts.

Term: a definite period of time, in medicine usually applied to the duration of a pregnancy; full term is 282 days from the first day of the last menstrual period. The date on which birth can be expected is calculated by adding 7 to the date of the last menstrual period and taking away 3 calendar months.

Terramycin: *see* Tetracycline.

Testicle: the testis is smooth and oval, and measures about

726

4 cm × 3 cm × 2.5 cm. Each testis is covered by a membrane called the tunica vaginalis, which has two layers separated in health by a thin film of fluid; both testes lie in the scrotum, the left usually a little lower than the right. Along the back of the testis lies the epididymis, a long thin tube coiled and turned upon itself which has about fifteen ducts opening into it from the testis through which travel the spermatozoa. From the epididymis the spermatozoa pass into the vas deferens, which runs in the spermatic cord into the abdominal cavity through the inguinal canal and passes into the prostate gland at the base of the bladder. Here the vas joins the seminal vesicle, and from it the spermatozoa pass into the urethra through the ejaculatory duct. Each testis contains a large number of seminiferous tubules in which spermatozoa are formed, and interstitial cells in which testosterone, the male hormone, is elaborated. The testes also secrete small amounts of oestrogens, just as normal ovaries secrete a small amount of male sex hormone. The pituitary hormones involved in the control of the testis are the same as those in control of the ovary, i.e. F.S.H., which has to do with the formation of spermatozoa, and L.H., which is concerned with the secretion of the male hormone. There are, however, no cyclical changes in the male gonads (*see* Ovary).

Diseases of the testicle. (1) Inflammation causes epididymo-orchitis, the micro-organisms involved commonly being gonococcus, Escherichia coli or sometimes the tubercle bacillus. Symptoms are swelling and pain in the testicle, and treatment varies according to the cause. It is important to remember that epididymo-orchitis is usually secondary to disease elsewhere in the genito-urinary system, and investigations which may not at first seem relevant are often carried out by the doctor. Inflammation of the testis alone is not common and is usually caused by mumps. (2) There may be imperfect descent of the testis. *See* Orchidopexy. (3) Tumours of the testis may be malignant or simple. *See* Seminoma, Teratoma. (4) Hydrocoele, or fluid in the tunica vaginalis covering the testicle, may develop as a consequence of inflammation or the growth of a tumour or without any obvious cause. *See* Hydrocoele. (5) Injuries are not uncommon, but in civilian life are rarely severe enough to need surgical treatment, although a collection of blood (haematoma) may have to be let out if it is causing a marked increase of pressure inside the capsule of the testis. Even relatively slight blows dealt the gland are liable to cause great pain and shock.

Test Meal: a meal which is given to test the function of the stomach. The meal, composed of substances of known composition and amount, is left in the stomach for a given length of time, and then removed by aspiration through a stomach tube. At the present time the commonly used 'test meal' is not a meal at all; an injection of histamine is given to stimulate gastric secretion and the resulting gastric juice is aspirated, measured and analysed. It is, however, possible to determine if hydrochloric acid is being secreted by the stomach without using a stomach tube, for an ion-exchange resin containing quinine can be given by mouth which will free its quinine in exchange for hydrogen from free hydrochloric acid. If an injection of histamine is given, and more than a certain amount of quinine excreted in the urine over a measured period of time, then it is clear that free hydrochloric acid is being secreted by the stomach and the patient has been saved the unpleasantness of swallowing and retaining a stomach tube. A development of this test uses tablets of caffeine sodium benzoate to stimulate gastric secretion, and blue-coloured test granules. (Diagnex Blue azuresin diagnostic test.)

Testosterone: the male sex hormone. *See* Androgen.

Test Type: printed letters used to test acuity of vision. The letters are carefully designed to subtend a particular angle at the eye when the subject stands at a specified distance from the test type, or when he holds a test card at a given distance from his eye.

Tetanus: an acute disease of the nervous system.
CAUSE: the toxin of the micro-organism Clostridium tetani, which is found in soil, dust and the bowels of various herbivorous animals such as cows and horses.
SYMPTOMS: the organisms enter the body through a scratch or wound contaminated with animal droppings or with soil in which spores (q.v.) of the organism are dormant. About three weeks after the wound has been sustained the patient

becomes irritable and apprehensive, develops stiffness of the muscles and difficulty in opening his mouth (lockjaw). The neck is stiff, the face goes into spasm, and in a severe case the back is arched and the patient may raise himself into the position of opisthotonus (q.v.). Soon the smallest stimuli – a draught of cold air, the click of a light switch – may send the patient into convulsions, which are dreadfully painful and may lead to exhaustion and death.

TREATMENT: as soon as a wound has been sustained in circumstances which may make one suspect the possibility of tetanus (for example because of contamination with soil or cattle droppings) the advice of a doctor must be sought. If there is a history of active immunization against the disease the doctor will give a booster dose of vaccine; if not, each case will be considered on its merits, for passive immunization with horse serum is not without its own dangers; the use of human immune gamma globulin may be advisable. The only real way to be sure of avoiding tetanus is to undergo active immunization, and if a patient has not had the vaccine he should be given a dose at once. He must come back for a further dose 6 weeks later even if he feels well and is perfectly recovered from his wound. If the wound needs it, surgical exploration and cleaning will be carried out, and it may be necessary to give antibiotics; as the Clostridium tetani is sensitive to penicillin this may give protection.

If the full-blown disease develops then hospital treatment is absolutely essential. The patient is put under heavy sedation, given a dose of human immune gamma globulin with massive doses of penicillin, and nursed with care and quietness. It may be necessary for an anaesthetist to give a general anaesthetic and muscle relaxants.

Tetany: not to be confused with tetanus, tetany is a condition in which there is abnormal excitability of the nerves and muscles, shown by flexion of the wrist and ankle (carpopedal spasm), cramp and twitching of the limbs, and tingling, twitching and spasm of the face. It is caused by lack of calcium in the blood, which may be due to deficiency of the parathyroid glands or deficient absorption of calcium; it may occur through alkalosis of the blood because of the ingestion of too much alkali, as in overenthusiastic treatment of peptic ulcer, or after a bout of hysterical overbreathing.

Tetracyclines: these are a number of antibiotic drugs which were discovered by research into the properties of organisms found in soil (hence the proprietary name Terramycin for oxytetracycline). The drugs are derived from the same chemical substance; tetracycline, oxytetracycline and chlortetracycline are all very similar in formula, properties and activity. Other compounds are dichlortetracycline, methacycline and tetracycline-phosphate complex. The tetracyclines are usually given by mouth, although they can be given by intramuscular injection; rolitetracycline (Tetrex P.M.T., Syntetrin) is the best compound for parenteral use. The compounds are active against a number of bacteria (Gram-negative and Gram-positive), amoebae, Rickettsiae, and Bedsoniae, but do not affect viruses. It is important to realize that a great many pathogenic bacteria found in hospitals have become resistant to tetracyclines, but organisms outside institutions that are still sensitive to tetracyclines include Haemophilus pertussis (whooping cough), H. influenzae (meningitis, bronchitis etc.), pneumococci, meningococci, gonococci, Clostridia and others. Undesirable side effects are gastro-intestinal irritation, skin rashes, oedema and fever, and sometimes a drop in the number of white cells in the blood; tetracyclines can discolour the teeth of children and interfere with the growth of bones. This sounds a formidable list, but all powerful and valuable drugs have a number of undesirable side effects which must be balanced against the lives they save and misery they prevent. Such a list only means that drugs must be used with knowledge, skill and judgment.

Tetra-ethyl Lead: this substance is an organic compound of lead which may produce lead poisoning in man by absorption through the intact skin or through the lungs. It collects in the central nervous system where it produces delirium, delusions, depression, convulsions and in severe cases coma. The patient may become suicidal, and has to be nursed with care and judicious sedation. *See* Lead.

Tetraplegia: paralysis of all four limbs.

Thalamus: a large group of nuclei in the mid-brain, where the ascending sensory nerve fibres from the spinal cord and the brain stem relay to the cerebral cortex. It is here that stereotaxic surgical methods are used to influence various diseases, although the functions of the thalamus are not yet precisely understood. *See* Stereoencephalotomy.

Thalassaemia: an inherited blood disease.
CAUSE: there is a genetic defect in the formation of haemoglobin. The disease is found throughout the world, but occurs most often in people who come from the shores of the Mediterranean sea. It is found in two degrees of severity, called major and minor.
SYMPTOMS: *Major*. A profound and in the end fatal anaemia which does not allow its victims to survive into adult life. *Minor*. There is serious but not fatal anaemia. Both conditions are helped by removal of the spleen and transfusion.

Thalidomide: a sedative and hypnotic drug which appeared when first introduced to be safe, for the effects of a large overdose were not fatal. It was brought on to the market in West Germany in 1956, and two years later came to Great Britain, where it was used freely as a 'tranquillizer'. In 1960 it was suspected that thalidomide might be responsible for the development of myxoedema (thyroid deficiency) and neuritis, and it was therefore not allowed to be sold in the U.S.A. By 1961 it was clear that the drug had in fact been responsible for the birth of a number of deformed children, and it was withdrawn in December 1961; it had by then been the cause of something like ten thousand birth deformities in Europe. The only possible comment is that drugs must not be given to pregnant women except when strictly necessary; we do not understand the effects of well-known drugs on the foetus, let alone new compounds. How one is to tell when a woman is in the early weeks of pregnancy is another matter.

Theca: a sheath, usually used of the dura mater covering the spinal cord.

Theobromine: theobromine, theophylline and caffeine are alkaloids in tea, coffee and cocoa. They are all similar compounds. *See* Caffeine.

731

Theriac: a mixture once believed to heal the bites of wild animals and protect men from the effects of their poisons. The word is from Greek *theriake*, an antidote.

Thermography: variations of temperature over the surface of the body can be recorded by using photographic film sensitive to infra-red radiations (q.v.). The technique is named thermography, and the record a thermogram. Because the surface temperature of the body is determined by the local state of the circulation and other known factors, thermography may help in the diagnosis of certain disease processes.

Thermometer: on the whole an instrument better not applied to measuring the heat of the human body outside hospital and the doctor's consulting-room, for solitary observations made at home, if not actively misleading, are far less valuable than the subjective sensations of the patient. *See* Fever, Rigor.

Thiabendazole: a compound used in the treatment of infestation with the worms strongyloides and ankylostoma. *See* Worms.

Thiamine: Vitamin B_1; deficiency of this vitamin produces the disease beri-beri (q.v.).

Thiopentone: (Pentothal). A short-acting derivative of barbituric acid used as an intravenous anaesthetic.

Thiotepa: (Triethylene thiophosphoramide). A cytotoxic drug used in the treatment of cancer of the breast and cancer of the ovary.

Thiourea: a substance from which a number of drugs have been derived which interfere with the secretion of the thyroid hormone. These drugs are used in the treatment of toxic goitre, being given to prepare a patient for operation or used as the main form of treatment in patients who are not suitable for operation. *See* Goitre.

Thomas' Splint: a splint used to keep the knee straight and to transfer the weight of the body from the foot of the splint, which is in contact with the ground when the patient stands up, directly to the pelvis and spine via the ischial tuberosity – the bony part of the pelvis on which we normally sit. The foot can be tied to the lower end of the splint, and as the upper end is applied to the pelvis traction on the foot stretches the whole leg, including the thigh; in this way traction can be put on the femur. The splint is named after a nineteenth-century Liverpool surgeon.

Thoracic Duct: the large lymph vessel which collects lymph from the legs, abdomen, and left side of the chest, neck and head. It begins just under the diaphragm, runs up to the root of the neck through the thorax, and discharges the lymph into the left subclavian vein at its junction with the left internal jugular vein. It is about 40 cm long and 0.5 cm in diameter. The vessels from the right side of the head, neck and thorax drain into the right subclavian vein through the very short right lymphatic duct which, like the thoracic duct, has non-return valves to prevent the reflux of blood.

Thoracic Inlet Syndrome: a condition caused by pressure on the nerves and blood vessels of the arm as they cross the first rib on their way from the spinal cord and the great vessels of the thorax to pass through the armpit into the upper part of the arm. There are a number of local circumstances which may be involved: (1) the anatomical relationship of the scalenus anterior muscle, which runs between the spinal column to the first rib like a guy-rope, to the nerves and the artery, which can be nipped in the angle between the muscle and the rib; (2) the presence of an extra, abnormal, cervical rib; (3) an anatomical abnormality of the plexus of nerves in which it arises one segment lower than usual in the spinal cord, so that the lowest part of the plexus is liable to be stretched.

SYMPTOMS: pain and changes of sensation in the arm and hand, with gradual wasting of the muscles of the hand and weakness. The hand may show signs of a 'poor circulation' – it may go white and be abnormally sensitive to cold (*see* Raynaud's Disease). The symptoms are worse at night, when the patient is tired, and they are often brought on by carrying heavy weights in the hand so that the shoulder is depressed. The condition often affects middle-aged women, and the weight that is carried is frequently a bucket of water.

TREATMENT: rest. The arm and shoulder should be exercised and efforts made to build up the strength of the muscles of the shoulder girdle. Obviously it is silly to try to lift or carry heavy things on the affected side. If the condition persists, then it is possible for an operation to be carried out to try to relieve pressure by removing an extra rib, if it is present, or by dividing the anterior scalene muscle.

Thoracoplasty: plastic operation on the thorax, or chest wall; for example, the removal of a number of ribs in order to collapse the chest wall and the lung beneath.

Thoracotomy: the operation of opening the wall of the chest.

Thorax: the chest, which contains the heart and lungs and through which runs the oesophagus (gullet) carrying food from the mouth to the stomach. The walls of the thorax are supported by the ribs, 12 on each side, which are joined to the vertebral column at the back and in the case of the upper 7 ribs join the breastbone in front. Between the ribs are intercostal muscles, nerves, arteries and veins, the chest wall being covered by skin outwardly and by the parietal pleural membrane on its inner surface. The thorax is separated from the abdominal cavity by the diaphragm, and into right and left sides by a central membranous partition named the mediastinum, which contains the great vessels, oesophagus and heart, as well as the windpipe (trachea), the first parts of the right and left bronchi into which it splits, and a number of lymph glands. The heart is contained within a special membrane named the pericardium (q.v.) and the lungs are covered by the visceral pleural membrane, which moves upon the inner lining of the chest wall, the two layers of pleural membrane being separated by a very thin layer of fluid. The lungs are inflated by movements of the wall of the thorax and of the diaphragm; when the ribs are raised the volume of the thorax increases, and it is increased further by the downward movement of the dome of the diaphragm (q.v.) which accompanies contraction of the diaphragmatic muscle. The pressure within the thorax falls, and atmospheric pressure drives air into the lungs through the mouth and the windpipe. The breath is driven out of the lungs by the lowering of the ribs and relaxation of the muscle of the diaphragm. Contraction of the muscles of the abdominal wall will cause the dome of the diaphragm to rise still higher into the thorax as the abdominal organs are thrust back and upwards. *See* Pneumothorax.

Threadworm: (Pinworm). *See* Worms.

Thrill: in medicine, what is felt when a hand is placed on the surface of the body over an internal structure in which vibration is being produced; thus a hand placed on the chest wall over a heart with bad valvular disease, in which the blood passing through the damaged valve is setting up a vibration, will feel a thrill.

Throat and its Diseases: the main diseases considered here are acute pharyngitis and carcinoma of the oesophagus. *Acute pharyngitis* often follows the common cold or accompanies one of the infectious fevers such as measles, scarlet fever and diphtheria.

SYMPTOMS: slight fever and malaise, a burning sensation in the throat, cough at first dry and later moist, and a voice which may be hoarse.

TREATMENT: rest in bed, gargles and aspirin. In severer cases antibiotics may have to be used.

Although strictly speaking the throat does not include the oesophagus, disorder in swallowing is usually thought of as being connected with the throat. The oesophagus or gullet is the site of several disorders usually characterized by pain or difficulty in swallowing. *Oesophagitis* or inflammation may result from drinking irritant or too hot liquids. *Dysphagia* or difficulty in swallowing may be due to disorders of nervous control. But the most important disease affecting this area is *cancer of the oesophagus*. This is responsible for about 1% of all cancer deaths and usually occurs in men over the age of 50, the main symptoms being difficulty in swallowing and loss of weight. Until recently the outlook in this condition was absolutely hopeless and relatives had to stand by helplessly while the patient literally starved before their eyes as swallowing became more and more difficult. But now advances in chest surgery make it possible for an operation to be carried out in which the diseased area is removed and the stomach brought up into the chest and stitched to the remainder of the gullet.

In many cases difficulty in swallowing or a feeling of choking has a purely emotional cause. This condition is called globus hystericus and it must be treated psychologically. Often it is symptomatic of an intolerable situation facing the patient and is the body's way of saying, 'I can't swallow that', i.e. 'I can't stand this situation'.

Thrombin: *see* Blood Coagulation.

Thromboangiitis Obliterans: a rare condition in which the arteries in the legs of men of early middle age who are heavy smokers become blocked as the result of inflammatory changes in the walls. It is very likely that this disease does not exist as a separate entity, but is part of the picture of atheromatous arterial change; a few cases may have been due to polyarteritis nodosa.

Thrombocytopenic Purpura: bleeding from capillary vessels into the skin (purpura) may be the result of lack of platelets in the blood (thrombocytopenia), for the platelets are essential for the integrity of the vascular system and for efficient clotting of blood. There are a number of diseases which are associated with a drop in the normal number of platelets in the circulating blood; they include leukaemia, aplastic anaemia, kidney disease, heart failure, secondary carcinomatous growths in the bone marrow, very severe bacterial infections, collagen disease, malaria, bilharziasis, kala-azar and poisoning by various substances including certain drugs. It is also possible for patients to develop the condition without any obvious cause; in these cases the reason for the drop in blood platelets is thought to be the abnormal production of an antibody against them, so that they are destroyed in great numbers in the spleen and liver.

SYMPTOMS: there may be severe bleeding from the nose, kidneys or bowels, as well as the characteristic bruising of the skin, and the condition fluctuates a great deal.

TREATMENT: the treatment of the idiopathic disease, that is the disease for which no obvious cause can be found, is the administration of corticosteroids; if there is no satisfactory response the spleen may be removed, an operation which may result in a dramatic recovery.

Thrombophlebitis: inflammation of a vein with consequent thrombosis (formation of a clot). It is quite common in the superficial veins of the leg, particularly if they are varicose.
SYMPTOMS: the veins become red and tender, and often the surrounding tissues are inflamed. It can be painful enough to make walking difficult.
TREATMENT: the condition normally resolves by itself in two or three weeks, and treatment is confined to the use of analgesics for the pain and the use of a supporting bandage.

Thrombosis: the formation of a clot (thrombus) in the blood vessels. It may affect arteries, particularly those in which the walls have been damaged and roughened by atheroma (*see* Coronary Thrombosis), or may affect the veins. In deep veins, particularly those of the leg, the formation of a thrombus is attended by the danger that some of it will break off and be carried away in the circulation until it meets a vessel through which it cannot pass. This may be part of the circulation of the lungs, or rarely when there is a communication between the two sides of the heart (patent foramen ovale) may be on the arterial side of the vascular tree. Patients are liable to develop thrombosis of the deep veins of the leg after surgical operations, and any pain in the calf of the leg must be reported to the surgeon.
Pulmonary embolism, the lodging of a broken-off piece of clot in the pulmonary artery, is often suddenly fatal; it is a well-known post-operative complication, but if the surgeon knows that a clot has formed in the leg there is a good chance that he can take various steps to diminish the risk.

Thrush: (Candidosis, Moniliasis). An inflammation of the mouth.
CAUSE: infection with the micro-organism Candida albicans which is a fungus resembling yeast. The infection occurs in infants, being acquired during birth from an infected mother or being spread by dirty teats or bottles, and in patients suffering from severe chronic illness or being treated by antibiotics.
SYMPTOMS: the inside of the mouth becomes covered with a

white membrane which can be wiped off to leave a bleeding, ulcerated surface. Candidosis can affect the vulva in women or the oesophagus.

TREATMENT: nystatin or amphotericin B suspensions are applied locally, tablets may be sucked, and in the case of infection of the female genital tract suppositories are used.

Thymol: an antiseptic derived from oil of thyme, a common ingredient of mouth-washes and gargles.

Thymus: a gland which lies in the lower part of the neck and the upper thorax. It was until quite recently little understood, but it has now become clear that it is the most important organ in the lymphoid system, and that it secretes a hormone in the developing animal upon which the production of lymphocytes depends. After puberty the gland normally shrivels up and almost disappears, having reached the height of its development in the human being at the age of nine. In the adult the gland still functions and keeps the supply of lymphocytes constant; it is particularly valuable because the lymphocytes formed in the thymus are not affected by antigens until they are released into the circulation, when they are able to respond to new antigens. The gland plays a part in some auto-immune diseases; removal of the thymus in some cases of myasthenia gravis, a disease in which it may be enlarged in the adult, improves the condition considerably.

Thyroid: the thyroid gland is a ductless gland lying in the neck in front of the windpipe just below the Adam's apple. It has two lobes, one on each side of the windpipe, joined across the middle line by an isthmus. Two parathyroid glands (q.v.) are embedded in each lobe. The function of the gland is to regulate the metabolism of the body – the physical and chemical processes essential to life and activity. It secretes thyroid hormones into the blood, elaborating Thyroxine (T_4) and Tri-iodothyronine (T_3) from iodine and tyrosine. Without the thyroid hormones animals cannot grow, amphibia cannot undergo metamorphosis, the brain does not develop properly, and bone does not mature. *See* Goitre.

Thyrotoxicosis: *see* Goitre.

Thyroxine: *see* Thyroid, Goitre.

Tibia: the shin-bone, so called because it makes a good flute. (Tibia is Latin for pipe.)

Tic: a quick spasmodic movement, for example twitching of the face. The repetition of particular movements is also called a tic, and may be linked with mental disease as in saltatory mania or dancing mania. Tic douloureux is named after the spasm of the muscles of the face produced by the enormous pain of trigeminal neuralgia. *See* Neuralgia.

Tick: a blood-sucking parasite larger than a mite; soft ticks are Argasidae, hard ticks Ixodidae. Of the soft ticks Ornithodorus is a vector of relapsing fever, and the hard ticks carry typhus, spotted fever, Q fever (*see* Rickettsiae), Colorado tick fever and tularaemia, various viruses causing such diseases as louping-ill and Omsk haemorrhagic fever.

Tincture: alcoholic solution of a drug.

Tinea: term applied to various fungus infections of the skin, for example tinea pedis (athlete's foot), tinea capitis (ringworm), tinea corporis (ringworm of the body), tinea cruris (ringworm of the crutch). *See* Ringworm.

Tinnitus: name applied to the noises in the ears that are heard as a result of disease.

Tissue: the tissues are the substance of the body; particular tissues like connective tissue and fatty tissue are collections of cells all specialized in the same way to carry out a definite function. A tissue culture is a collection of cells removed from an organism set out to grow and multiply in artificial circumstances (in vitro).

Tobacco: *see* Smoking.

Tocopherol: Vitamin E, an alcohol or mixture of alcohols isolated from wheat-germ oil. Without Vitamin E rats cannot reproduce, but the same has never been shown to be true of human beings.

Tolbutamide: a sulphonylurea which is used in the treatment of diabetes mellitus in selected cases. It is given by mouth.

Tomogram: a special X-ray taken to show structures lying in a selected plane in the body and to exclude structures lying at a different depth. When the plane has been chosen the X-ray tube and the plate rotate about it, and so make an optical section of the body.

Tomomania: a madness for cutting; unkindly applied to some surgeons.

Tongue: the tongue is made up of the fibres of a number of muscles contained within its substance (intrinsic muscles) and a number arising outside and blending with the intrinsic muscles. The muscles that arise outside (mainly from the hyoid bone and the lower jaw-bone) are called the extrinsic muscles, and they move the tongue in relation to neighbouring structures; the intrinsic muscles are mainly concerned with altering the shape of the tongue. There is a fibrous partition running down the centre of the tongue, and very few blood vessels cross the mid-line. The nerve that supplies the muscles of the tongue is the hypoglossal nerve (the twelfth cranial nerve), and the sensory nerves are the lingual nerve for the front two-thirds and the glossopharyngeal nerve for the back. The artery is the lingual artery, and the tongue is covered by stratified squamous epithelium (q.v.). It is not possible to estimate the degree of constipation or otherwise of a patient by inspecting his tongue, for furring does not have the significance it was once thought to have, but the state of the tongue is a good indication of the level of hydration of the body.

The tongue is liable to certain diseases: *glossitis*, or inflammation, can result from excessive smoking, habitually eating hot or irritating food or drink, or neglecting septic teeth and gums. Sometimes small *ulcers* form at the edge and tip of the tongue which are very painful; they may be due to herpes. Other types of ulceration of the tongue may be serious and all ulcers should be shown to the doctor, for one of the manifestations of cancer of the tongue is ulceration. Ulcers of the tongue are also found in syphilis in all three stages, and in tuberculosis, diphtheria and leukaemia. Chronic irritation may produce an appearance of the surface of the tongue called *leukoplakia* because it is a white thickening often with splits or fissures. It is a pre-cancerous condition. *Cancer* of the tongue is not at all uncommon, and is often associated with bad teeth. It usually forms a hard ulcer on the edge of the tongue towards the front, and it is treated by radiotherapy, the implantation of radioactive material, or by removal. It may be necessary to remove neighbouring lymph glands as well.

Tonics: there is no such thing as a tonic; broadly speaking, anybody who feels unwell is either suffering from a specific disease for which he requires the appropriate treatment or is psychologically upset, i.e. suffering from depression, being 'fed-up', bored, etc. In the sense of a preparation which really makes one feel better the only tonics that work are drugs designed to combat depression (*see* Mental Illness, Tranquillizers). It is possible that mixtures containing bitters improve the appetite, but the indiscriminate use of iron only serves to turn the patient's motions black, and 'neurophosphates' and similar substances have no effect at all. Some have great faith in vitamins in spite of the fact that, unless used for some specific disease, they are only necessary to those who lack them. (It is unfortunately the case that the more overfed a nation is the more vitamin pills it consumes.) *See* Placebo.

Tonsillitis: inflammation of the tonsils, the two collections of lymphoid tissue that lie one on each side of the throat. They can be seen just behind the back of the tongue between two folds of membrane running up to the soft palate – the two pillars of the fauces.
CAUSE: inflammation of the tonsils is usually due to infection by Streptococcus pyogenes.
SYMPTOMS: a sore throat, raised temperature, pain on swallowing, and a greater or lesser degree of general malaise. The tonsils are seen to be inflamed if the mouth is opened wide, and in many cases spots of pus exude from them. Externally, the tonsillar lymph glands which lie just below and behind the angle of the jaw are tender and enlarged.
TREATMENT: the infecting organisms are tested for sensitivity and the appropriate antibiotic is used. The condition must

be treated energetically for it can result in scarlet fever, nephritis or rheumatic heart disease (q.v.).

Chronic tonsillitis is a term applied to cases in which there is enlargement of the tonsils accompanied by repeated attacks of infection, and it is often in such cases that the adenoids – masses of lymphatic tissue on the back wall of the pharynx behind the nasal cavity – become enlarged and obstruct the opening of the Eustachian tube, which connects the middle ear with the pharynx and equalizes the pressures on each side of the eardrum. Consequent deafness is taken to be an indication for removing a child's tonsils and adenoids, an operation which is now carried out far less frequently than it used to be. *See* Quinsy.

Tophi: deposits of sodium biurate which in gouty people may grow in the pinna of the ear or on the knuckles.

Torticollis: twisted neck, or wry neck, commonly caused by birth injury to the sternomastoid muscle which runs from the mastoid process of the skull behind the ear to the inner end of the collar-bone and the top of the breastbone (sternum). It may be recognized in the infant by preferential positioning of the head and a hard lump in the side of the neck. Remedial treatment may be started at once. If the injury is not recognized the muscle scars, with the formation of fibrous tissue. When this contracts over the course of time the head is turned to the opposite side and the neck twisted. The treatment is division of the fibrous tissue in the affected muscle and physiotherapy.

Tourniquet: a device for compressing a limb and thereby obliterating the arteries and veins. The purpose may be to stop bleeding from a wound, to provide a bloodless field for the surgeon, or to prevent the flow of poisons, for example snake venom, into the general circulation. If the artery to a limb is obliterated by a tourniquet it must not be left on for more than a certain time, for the tissues cannot survive if permanently deprived of their blood supply. It is usually said that a tourniquet must be loosened every half-hour and not kept on for more than two hours. It is very important to let everyone know that a patient has a tourniquet on, and never to let him go out of your sight into other hands without making absolutely sure that the new attendants know about the tourniquet and the length of time it has been on. It is good practice to mark a capital T on the patient's forehead with the time the tourniquet was applied. A tourniquet should not be put on a bleeding limb unless it is impossible to stop the haemorrhage by direct compression.

Toxaemia: a term meaning the presence of toxins in the blood. Toxaemia of pregnancy includes the states of pre-eclampsia and eclampsia (q.v.).

Toxicology: the study of poisons.

Toxin: a poison; the word is usually applied to a poison elaborated by bacteria.

Toxoid: a toxin so altered that has lost its poisonous properties, but can still act as an antigen to provoke the formation of antibodies, for example tetanus toxoid, which will provide active immunity against tetanus if injected but does not produce the symptoms.

Toxoplasmosis: infection with the protozoal parasite Toxoplasma gondii.
CAUSE: the Toxoplasma is carried by a large number of domestic dogs and cats – perhaps half the pet population – and passed in the eggs of the common worm Toxacara mystex. It is frequently possible for worm eggs containing Toxoplasma to contaminate food, and for man in this way to acquire the infection. The parasite is present in many mammals and in birds and the consumption of under-cooked infected meat may spread infection. In the circumstances it is not surprising that Toxoplasma gondii has been found to be a common parasite of man.
SYMPTOMS: a large number of infections give rise to no symptoms, or at the most mild enlargement of the lymph glands. If the infection affects a pregnant mother the foetus is invaded by the parasites, and the situation is much more serious. There may be a stillbirth or miscarriage; if it survives the child may have inflammation of the choroid layer of the eye (*see* Eye) which damages the retina and affects the vision, inflammation of the brain producing convulsions or hydrocephalus, and lesions in the liver, spleen and lungs.

TREATMENT: in the great majority of cases the infection is not recognized, and in most diagnosed cases in which the parasite produces symptoms they are not bad enough to require any treatment. In the case of congenital toxoplasmosis, fortunately rare, the treatment used is a combination of sulphonamide and pyrimethamine.

Tracheitis: inflammation of the trachea, usually part of a general infection of the respiratory tract and commonly associated with bronchitis.

Tracheotomy: an operation in which an opening is made in the windpipe through the lower part of the neck in the middle line; it is commonly carried out to make an artificial passage for the breath in cases where there is, for example, an obstruction to the larynx, and in such cases the opening itself is called a *tracheostomy*. After the windpipe has been exposed, usually under local anaesthetic, and an oval piece cut out of the third and fourth cartilaginous rings, a tube is passed through the tracheostomy and tied to the neck with tape. It is changed and cleaned at regular intervals. Although the obvious reason for making a tracheostomy is laryngeal obstruction, there are a number of less obvious reasons which include brain damage leading to coma, nervous diseases which cause paralysis of the muscles used in breathing, and injuries of the chest when the ribs are no longer supported and the chest wall cannot move to draw out the lungs. The advantages of tracheostomy in such cases are: it decreases the 'dead space', i.e. the space in the mouth and upper windpipe through which the air merely goes in and out without reaching the lungs; it gives the attendants an approach through which excess secretions can be sucked out of the lungs; it provides a wide, unobstructed airway; and it makes it possible to connect the patient to a positive-pressure breathing machine. The hole in the trachea heals up quickly when the patient recovers, and the technique has saved many lives.

Trachoma: an eye disease, caused by Bedsoniae (*see* Ornithosis), affecting the cornea and the conjunctiva. It results in deformity of the eyelids, ulceration and blindness, and is prevalent in tropical countries, for it is a disease of dirt and poverty, spread by flies. It is common among American Indians and Mexican immigrants of the south-west of the United States.

Tranquillizers: a group of drugs which have the property of quelling undue anxiety and calming excited patients. They suppress symptoms of disease rather than cure the underlying condition, and should be used with care and discrimination. In fact, tens of millions of prescriptions for tranquillizers are issued every year – in 1967 in the National Health Service in Great Britain alone 14·7 million such prescriptions were filled. Tranquillizers may be divided into two groups, major and minor. The major tranquillizers are those which are used to treat delusions, agitation and hallucinations in the psychoses, and the minor tranquillizers are used to quieten neurotic anxieties. It is not surprising that the majority of prescriptions are for the minor tranquillizers, which are thought by most patients to be more respectable than alcohol. *See* Mental Illness.

Transfusion: the introduction of fluids into the circulation, usually applied to the infusion of blood into the veins. *See* Blood Groups, Cross Match.

Transplant Surgery: kidneys, livers and hearts have all been transplanted from those who had no further use for them into patients who but for irrecoverable disease of the one organ would be healthy, and some cases have survived long enough to make it clear that spare-part surgery can be a practical proposition. The great difficulty is to make sure that the body into which the new organ is grafted does not treat it as an antigen and elaborate antibodies to destroy it. The problem has largely been overcome in 'transplanting' blood from one individual to another by cross matching (*see* Blood Groups), and there is every hope that it will be over-come in a similar way in the more complicated case of grafting whole organs. Another approach is to use artificial means to damp down the reaction of immunity, but this has grave drawbacks; it would appear that a combination of testing to ensure the most complete matching possible and restraining the immune reaction is best employed. There is no foreseeable future possibility that the central nervous system

745

will lend itself to grafting or transplantation. *See* Death.

Transvestism: a sexual perversion in which the individual chooses to wear the clothes of the opposite sex.

Trauma: an injury or wound.

Traveller's Diarrhoea: a term applied to the short attacks of diarrhoea which many people suffer when they first arrive in a foreign country. Although some cases are due to bacillary infection, it is thought that a great number are due simply to a change in the normal bacteria present in the bowel; treatment, if the severity of the condition warrants treatment, should always be simple, for example kaolin mixture. It is not sensible to treat oneself with antibodies or sulphonamides in the absence of a diagnosis which includes the isolation and identification of a pathogenic micro-organism.

Travel Sickness: *see* Motion Sickness.

Trematodes: flukes. The flukes important in medicine include Schistosoma (bilharzia), Paragonimus and Clonorchis, the Chinese liver fluke. *See* Flukes, Worms.

Tremor: shaking, which may be fine, as in hyperthyroidism, or coarse as in Parkinson's disease. It may only appear when the patient is reaching out for something (intention tremor), or it may disappear on purposeful movement and be present only at rest. It may be caused by disease, hysteria or alcohol (tremor potatorum).

Trephining: an old term for making a hole in the head. The trephine, an instrument for removing a small disc of bone from the skull, is not now much used, but a very small trephine may be used to remove a disc of tissue from the sclera or the cornea in eye surgery.

Treponema: a genus of spirochaetes, micro-organisms that are formed of a fine coiled thread which can bend and spin on its axis. The medically important treponemata are Treponema pallidum, the organism of syphilis, T. pertenue, which causes yaws, and T. carateum, which is found in pinta (q.v.)

Trichinella: Trichinella spiralis is a parasite found in un-cooked pork that can infest man. The disease is called trichinosis, and the worms invade the muscles. *See* Worms.

Trichlorethylene: (Trilene). A volatile liquid used as a general anaesthetic; the vapour is inhaled and produces a light anaesthesia with marked analgesia. The drug often makes the heart rate slow down and the rate of breathing increase, and it is commonly used in combination with nitrous oxide in suitable cases. It is widely used in obstetrics, being self-administered through a face mask by the woman in labour, who is instructed to take a few deep breaths during the pains of delivery.

Trichomonas: a protozoal parasite of a number of animals including man. Trichomonas vaginalis is a species which can cause inflammation of the vagina in the female and of the urethra in the male. It is commonly passed on by sexual intercourse, but is about the only organism affecting the genito-urinary system which can genuinely be picked up from a lavatory seat. The treatment is metronidazole (Flagyl).

Trichuris: whipworm, a roundworm. *See* Worms.

Trigeminal Nerve: the fifth cranial nerve, the sensory nerve of the face. It has three branches, described as ophthalmic, maxillary and mandibular or first, second and third divisions. It also has a motor branch which supplies the muscles used in chewing. *See* Cranial Nerves, Neuralgia.

Trilene: *see* Trichlorethylene.

Triorthocresyl Phosphate: an organophosphorus compound used in industry as an anticorrosion agent which can if taken internally produce irreversible damage to the central nervous system.

Trismus: spasm of the muscles which move the jaw; lockjaw.

Trocar: a sharp instrument for piercing the wall of a cavity, usually used with a cannula, which is a shorter hollow tube

747

fitting over the trocar so that the sharp end protrudes. When the trocar and cannula have been passed, for example, into a hydrocoele (q.v.) through the skin of the scrotum, the trocar is withdrawn and the fluid allowed to escape through the cannula.

Trombicula: a genus of mite, Trombicula akamushi carries the diseases Japanese river fever and scrub typhus, and T. deliensis carries Tsutsugamushi disease.

Tropical Sore: a skin infection with Leishmania tropica. *See* Leishmaniasis, Kala-azar.

Truss: a device used to keep hernias under control and to prevent them from protruding. *See* Hernia.

Trypanosomes: a genus of protozoa which cause the diseases sleeping sickness and Chagas' disease. African sleeping sickness is transmitted by the tsetse fly and the South American disease by bloodsucking bugs. *See* Sleeping Sickness.

Trypanosomiasis: *see* Sleeping Sickness.

Tryparsamide: a drug used for many years in the treatment of trypanosomiasis, but now superseded by melarsoprol (Mel B) because it was liable to damage the optic nerve and the liver.

Tsetse Fly: *see* Glossina, Sleeping Sickness.

Tubal Pregnancy: a pregnancy taking place not in the uterus but in one of the uterine tubes. *See* Ectopic Pregnancy.

Tuberculosis: a disease characterized by the production of tubercles, which are lesions originally about a millimetre across containing special cells called epithelioid cells and giant cells. Often many tubercles join to form a larger mass, and grow from their original small size to become abscesses, called cold abscesses because they are full not of pus but of cheesy (caseous) matter. In time the caseous matter in the middle of a tuberculous mass may become liquid, so that a cavity is formed, or it may become calcified and fibrotic as it heals.

CAUSE: infection with the tubercle bacillus, Mycobacterium tuberculosis. There are various kinds of tubercle bacillus, but those which infect man are the human and the bovine types. The human type usually infects the lungs; the bovine type, which is now quickly disappearing because of improved public hygiene, the pasteurization of milk and the prevention of tuberculosis in cattle, usually infects children and causes inflammation of the lymph glands and the bones. Infection is spread in the case of the human type by infected sputum and by coughing, and in the case of the bovine organisms by infected milk. The most important single factor in the spread of pulmonary tuberculosis is overcrowding; as standards of living improve the incidence of tuberculosis falls.

SYMPTOMS: these vary according to the site of the disease.

Tuberculosis of the lungs. When infection first takes place it is often unrecognized, frequently being taken for an attack of influenza or some other minor illness. There may be fever and cough, and perhaps a little pain in the chest; the area affected, called the primary focus, heals up, often becoming calcified, and the local lymph glands become scarred. The primary lesion (Ghon focus) and the infected lymph glands are called the primary complex, and signs of inactive primary complexes are found in a large proportion of healthy people. If secondary tuberculous infection occurs, or tubercle bacilli spread from the primary focus, the symptoms are the spitting of blood (haemoptysis), a chronic cough, pain in the chest on breathing, tiredness, loss of appetite, sweating, especially at night, and in women cessation of the periods. As the disease progresses the patient loses weight.

Tuberculosis of the lymph glands. The glands of the neck are commonly affected in children. They are enlarged without much tenderness or pain, but are liable to break down and discharge through the skin. The sinuses that form in this way are difficult to heal (*see* King's Evil). If the abdominal glands become infected there may be discomfort, but often these glands heal up satisfactorily without giving rise to symptoms. Fortunately abdominal tuberculosis rarely spreads, but it can cause tuberculous peritonitis.

Tuberculosis of bones. Secondary infection from the primary focus in lung, intestines or tonsils is carried to the bones by the blood. The disease, like tuberculosis of the lymph glands, is usually found in children, who develop pain, loss of appetite and general ill health. A characteristic symptom is the 'night-start'; at night the muscles which by contracting have prevented movement in diseased joints during the day, relax, and the pain of slight movement in sleep wakes the child up. If the vertebrae are infected they may collapse and cause spinal deformity; infection of joints, often the knee or the hips, results in stiffening or disorganization and deformity.

Other sites of infection. Tuberculosis may be found in the kidneys, bladder, testicles and prostate gland, and the symptoms it causes are characteristic of infection of the urogenital system. *See* Cystitis, Pyelonephritis.

Miliary tuberculosis. It may happen that there is widespread dissemination of infective matter, especially in children and young adults. In such a case a large number of small tubercles develop which are called miliary because they look like millet seeds. They may fill the lungs, or invade the meninges, the membranes covering the brain, where they cause tuberculous meningitis.

TREATMENT: the treatment of tuberculosis has been revolutionized by the discovery of streptomycin, para-aminosalicylic acid (P.A.S.) and isoniazid (I.N.H.). While the old principles of rest, good air and good food still prevail, the use of effective drugs has cut the death rate down enormously, and surgical treatment, which was at one time employed freely, is now not often required. It is possible to produce active immunization by the injection of attenuated tubercle bacilli (B.C.G.).

Tularaemia: an infection of rodents caused by Pasteurella tularensis, named after Tulare in California where the disease was first identified. It resembles plague, and can be transmitted to human beings, particularly those engaged in handling the skins or the bodies of infected creatures. An ulcer forms at the site of infection, lymph glands are enlarged, and the patient feels generally ill and runs a temperature. Antibiotics are used in treatment.

Tulle Gras: a net of pliant material impregnated with soft paraffin, balsam of Peru, and other substances, used for dressing raw surfaces.

Tumour: any swelling; it may be benign, malignant or inflammatory.

Twilight Sleep: the induction of a state of partial anaesthesia and analgesia in childbirth by giving the mother scopolamine and morphine. It diminishes pain, but also diminishes the force of contraction of the uterus and sometimes causes difficulty with the breathing of the child after birth.

Tympanum: the cavity of the middle ear. *See* Ear.

Typhlitis: inflammation of the caecum. It may be due to actinomycosis, a diverticulum, an ulcer inside the caecum, a malignant growth or appendicitis. It is usually diagnosed as appendicitis (once named perityphlitis) and discovered at operation.

Typhoid Fever: an enteric fever.
CAUSE: infection with the micro-organism Salmonella typhi, a Gram-negative bacterium. Infection is spread by contamination of water and food by sewage. After a patient has had the disease (perhaps in a very mild form) the bacteria may survive in the gall-bladder for years, so that the patient becomes a carrier, and if such a carrier is employed in preparing or serving food the infection can spread unless standards of hygiene are very high.
SYMPTOMS: the incubation period is one or two weeks, and the onset of the disease is insidious. The patient has headaches, feels ill and dizzy, has pains in the limbs, and sometimes a sore throat and a cough. Classical signs are bleeding from the nose and a slow pulse, which may go with a raised temperature, higher in the evenings. The patient takes to his bed; about the end of the first week his tongue becomes sore and his cheeks flushed. He is increasingly fatigued, and may develop a rash on the skin composed of 'rose-spots', each about 3 or 4 mm across; there are usually only about a dozen of them on the abdomen and thorax, and they fade in two days to be succeeded by another crop. By now the patient is beginning to be very ill, and soon he may go into the 'typhoid state', classically with a low muttering delirium; he passes a great number of typhoid bacilli in his motions and urine and

is highly infectious. The motions become loose, perhaps showing a little blood from ulcers of the bowel, which may perforate. If the condition is allowed to continue the patient may die.

TREATMENT: antibiotics are effective, and the use of steroids aids their action. Active immunization is provided by injections of a combined vaccine containing heat-killed Salmonella typhi and S. paratyphi A and B (T.A.B. vaccine). *See* Food Poisoning.

Typhus: a disease transmitted by the louse and therefore most prevalent in wartime and in conditions of gross overcrowding.

CAUSE: infection with the micro-organism Rickettsia prowazeki. The disease is common in the East, on the shores of the Mediterranean, in North Africa, and in other parts of the world.

SYMPTOMS: the incubation period is five to twenty-one days and the onset sudden with headache, pains in the back and limbs, and shivering. The rash, which is called 'mulberry rash', appears on the fourth day and consists of pink spots with larger papules and a mottled appearance under the skin, spreading from the trunk to the limbs and disappearing in the second week. The temperature rises to over 40 °C., falling suddenly by 'lysis' about the end of the second week. Typhus is a disease which causes great prostration, and delirium is a common feature, the mind nearly always remaining clouded while the fever lasts.

TREATMENT: tetracyclines are remarkably effective, and the disease is controlled by the destruction of lice by D.D.T. Brill's disease is the name given to recurrent typhus, and scrub typhus is a rickettsial infection transmitted by mites which live in jungle grass and scrub in the Far East and the South-west Pacfic. *See* Rickettsia.

Tyrosine: an amino acid which is essential for life.

U

Ulcer: a chronic defect in an epithelial surface exposing the tissues below the skin or mucous membrane. It is formed by the interaction of a number of factors which include poor blood supply or inefficient drainage, infection by micro-organisms, damage by physical agents such as heat, cold, chemicals, pressure or irradiation, malignant growths, and diseases of the nervous system which by abolishing the sensation of pain make the skin the site of continued minor trauma. Examples of ulceration: *varicose ulcers*, caused by poor blood supply, poor drainage, and injury; *syphilitic ulcer*, caused by infection with the micro-organism Treponema pallidum; *rodent ulcer*, caused by the malignant growth, basal-cell carcinoma; *perforating ulcer* of the sole of the foot, caused by lack of sensation resulting from syphilitic damage to the central nervous system; *bedsore*, caused by pressure, a poor blood supply and poor drainage. The treatment of an ulcer is the removal of the cause. Where the cause cannot be removed the ulcer in most cases will not heal; in the case of malignant ulcers the growth must be removed together with the ulcerated portion, and in some other cases where destruction of the underlying tissues and damage to the surrounding skin edges have made it impossible for the ulcer to heal, excision and skin graft may be best. Antibiotics do not help except where the ulcer is the result of infection with a sensitive organism, as in syphilis.

Ulcerative Colitis: chronic inflammation and ulceration of the colon and rectum.

CAUSE: unknown.

SYMPTOMS: the patient, usually a young adult, develops diarrhoea and bleeding which may give way to constipation. In time diarrhoea becomes the principal symptom, there is abdominal pain and tenderness, and when the condition is severe, dehydration may be marked enough to call for intravenous fluids. The illness is incapacitating and weakening, and the patient becomes introspective, anxious and depressed. There may be remissions, but the disease pursues

753

a chronic course and the patient is always liable to relapse. TREATMENT: complete rest in bed, with a high-protein diet. If there is severe anaemia blood transfusion is carried out, and doses of iron added to the diet. Corticosteroids may be given in the form of retention enemas. If there is no lasting response surgical removal of the affected bowel is advised even if it means the construction of an artificial anus or ileostomy; for life with an ileostomy is entirely practical, but one with ulcerative colitis may be almost unbearable.

Ulna: the inner of the two bones of the forearm. It is thinner in its lower part than at the upper end, which takes part in the formation of the elbow joint with the lower end of the humerus – the point of the elbow is the olecranon process of the ulna. The bone may be fractured with the radius at its lower end by falls on the outstretched hand (*see* Colles' Fracture), and the olecranon may be fractured by direct violence to the point of the elbow.

Ultrasonics: the outlines of various interfaces in the body between surfaces having different acoustic properties can be demonstrated by ultrasound; an ultrasonic beam is bounced back from the interface and a record made to show the distance the beam travelled from its source of origin to the deflecting surface. This technique is particularly useful in examining the brain through the intact skull, for the walls of the ventricles in the brain, which contain cerebro-spinal fluid, can be detected and displacement from their normal positions demonstrated without disturbing the patient.

Ultraviolet: rays which lie beyond the violet end of the spectrum up to the wavelength of X-rays are said to be ultraviolet (wavelengths between 1,800 and 3,900 ångströms). The sun is a natural source of ultraviolet rays, which produce suntan; but they can also burn, and are used to sterilize the air in operating theatres and sterile laboratories. *See* Infra Red.

Umbilicus: the navel.

Unconsciousness: in all cases of unconsciousness the first and the most important thing to do is MAKE SURE THE AIRWAY

IS CLEAR. If the unconscious man has swallowed his tongue, put your fingers in his mouth and pull it forwards. If he seems to be choking, put your fingers down his throat and see if there is anything there. These simple measures can save life. If the airway is clear, then turn the patient on to his front and turn his head to one side so that his tongue falls forward and any vomit or secretions drain out of his mouth instead of down into his lungs. If he is injured in such a way that you cannot or dare not turn him over, then put your fingers behind the angle of the patient's lower jaw below his ear and pull the jaw forwards, a measure which, you will find, carries the tongue forwards and prevents it falling back. You must keep the jaw forwards, and if possible turn the head sideways. If you have to carry or move an unconscious man who has been injured carry him 'all of a piece' without moving his position until you know what his injuries are; but it is always best to leave an injured man where he lies until skilled help comes. Do not try to force any drink down an unconscious man's throat, for you have a good chance of pouring it into his lungs where it will do him no good at all. If the unconsciousness is not the result of injury, look through the man's pockets in case he suffers from diabetes. If he is a known case he will probably carry a card and some sugar with him. Epilepsy is usually obvious and more frightening and dramatic than dangerous, and the only thing you have to do is make sure the patient neither chokes nor hurts himself. In all cases direct your efforts to making sure the airway is clear and keeping it clear, and keep the man reasonably warm.

Undecylenic Acid: a substance used in the treatment of ringworm.

Undine: a small, specially shaped glass flask which is used for irrigating the eye.

Undulant Fever: (Brucellosis).
CAUSE: infection with the micro-organism Brucella abortus, melitensis or suis. Infection with Br. abortus is acquired from cow's milk, Br. melitensis (Malta fever) from sheep and goats, and Br. suis from pigs.
SYMPTOMS: the symptoms of undulant fever are various, but

in general the patient feels unwell, sweats, has pains in the joints and feels continually tired. The temperature may be undulant or may be intermittent, low in the morning and rising to 38 to 40 °C. (101 or 104 °F.) in the evening. The disease can last for a matter of months on and off, for there are often remissions and exacerbations. The diagnosis of this vague fever, which has no really characteristic clinical signs, is difficult, and the patient has a good chance of being labelled neurotic unless the pattern of the fever is made clear, for quite often he looks to be in good health.

TREATMENT: tetracycline and if necessary streptomycin. Preventive treatment includes the testing and the slaughtering of animals carrying the infection, as well as the use of vaccines to immunize cattle and goats.

Upper Respiratory Tract: includes the nose, mouth and throat as far down as the trachea, and 'infection of the upper respiratory tract' is confined to these structures, for example the common cold.

Urates: the salts of uric acid. They are found normally in the blood and urine, but in gout are deposited in the skin of the ear and in the joints and kidneys. *See* Gout, Tophi.

Urea: *see* Uremia.

Uremia: (also spelt uraemia) the condition of having too much urea in the blood.

CAUSE: it is in most cases an indication of failure of the kidneys, for urea is the chief waste product that they normally remove from the blood.

SYMPTOMS: urea is an inert chemical substance deriving mainly from the breakdown of proteins, and although it does no harm itself its presence in various body secretions has disagreeable consequences; it is secreted in the saliva, where it gives rise to a bad taste in the mouth and a characteristic smell on the breath because it is broken down into ammonia by micro-organisms, and it is secreted in the gastric juice where on being broken down it provokes ulceration and bleeding of the lining of the stomach, which makes the patient vomit and feel nauseated. Other symptoms are headache, dizziness, intractable hiccuping, and in the more severe degrees of uraemia convulsions and coma, which occur because of other results of renal failure.

TREATMENT: uraemia may be caused by any type of kidney failure, and the treatment is the treatment if possible of the underlying condition with the use in selected cases of the artificial kidney. In chronic cases dialysis may have to continue for a lifetime.

In a few cases high levels of urea in the blood are due to factors which lead to poor kidney function without there being any kidney disease. In such cases the condition is called pre-renal uraemia, and the treatment is of the pre-cipitating cause, which is often disorder of fluid and electro-lyte balance particularly in the post-operative period or after severe injury.

Ureter: the muscular tube that connects the kidney to the bladder.

Urethra: the tube passing from the bladder to the exterior through which urine is discharged from the body. It is subject to a number of troubles. Inflammation of the urethra is called urethritis, and the most common cause is gonorr-hoea; the next most common cause is the passage of instru-ments or the presence of a catheter left in place to drain the bladder over a period of time. Inflammation can lead to stricture, the formation of a scar in the urethra which con-stricts the tube and blocks the passage of urine. Strictures are uncommon in women; in men they follow injury as well as inflammation. Congenital strictures are sometimes found in children, but they occur at the external orifice and are easily dealt with, unlike the narrow and tortuous strictures arising from old inflammation through which it may be difficult to pass an instrument. Abscesses may form round a stricture, burst through the skin, and so form a fistula between the urethra and the skin of the perineum. In favourable cases of stricture treatment involves only instrumental dilatation with bougies and sounds; in other cases operations have to be carried out. In all cases sounds have to be passed at intervals to ensure that the stricture does not narrow again. Injuries of the urethra occur in men, and are treated by passing a catheter through the ruptured or lacerated section, either blind or by open operation, and draining the bladder through the abdominal wall until healing has taken place. The urethra must afterwards be dilated regularly to guard against the formation of a stricture.

Urethritis: *see above*; *see also* Reiter's Disease.

Uric Acid: *see* Urates.

Urine: the fluid secreted by the kidneys, passed thence through the ureters into the bladder where it is stored, and from the bladder discharged to the exterior through the urethra. In health it is of constant composition – that is, constant within well-defined limits – and examination and analysis of the urine is an invaluable aid to the diagnosis of illness. Urine specimens are tested for protein sugar reaction and specific gravity; the sediment is collected on the centrifuge, and examined under the microscope for red and white blood cells, micro-organisms and cellular débris. It is then cultured; from the culture in infected cases are isolated the micro-organisms of disease, which can be tested for drug sensitivity. In addition to this a number of chemical tests can be carried out on the urine. In health the colour of urine is amber; it has a characteristic smell, a slightly acid reaction, and a specific gravity of about 1·024, with normal limits of 1·005 and 1·030. There should be no protein, blood or sugar. If normal urine is allowed to stand it may cloud over with a precipitation of phosphates which are of no significance; they disappear on boiling. The normal man secretes during an average day about 1,500 ml of urine, which contains about 50 g of solids, but the amount of urine secreted depends upon the amount of drink taken, among other things, and the weather.

Urology: the branch of medicine that deals with diseases of the urinary system in both the male and female, and those of the genital organs in the male.

Urticaria: a condition in which there are wheals on the skin.
CAUSE: a generalized antibody-antigen reaction set off by sensitivity to various substances from penicillin to shellfish, physical agents such as ultraviolet light, heat or violent exercise, and angio-neurotic oedéma (q.v.). The specific

mechanism is thought to be the liberation of histamine into the skin, for the reaction of the skin if histamine is injected intradermally resembles the development of urticaria – redness followed by itching and the appearance of a white raised area in the centre of the red patch.

TREATMENT: antihistamine drugs, one of the best of which is chlorpheniramine (Piriton or Chlortrimeton). If the urticaria is severe it may be necessary to give adrenaline injections subcutaneously.

Uterus: the womb. It is a hollow pear-shaped organ 7 cm long, 5 cm in breadth and about 2·5 cm thick. It is divided into a body, a cervix or neck, and a fundus. At the upper end of the body, at each corner, the two uterine tubes extend outwards towards the ovaries; the part of the uterus lying above the opening of the tubes is the fundus. At its lower end the cervix projects into the upper part of the front wall of the vagina; the opening in the cervix is called the os uteri. The outside of the body of the uterus is covered with peritoneum, and at each side the broad ligaments extend towards the wall of the pelvis. The uterus lies in most cases with the fundus directed forwards, while the body bends forwards slightly from the cervix. It may be displaced, but a backward position (retroversion) or an exaggerated forward position (anteflexion) in a woman who has not borne children are not of consequence by themselves. More important displacements are those which follow weakening of the supports of the uterus and the pelvic floor in childbirth – descent of the uterus into the vagina (vault prolapse), or descent of the front wall of the vagina with the uterus (cystocele). These conditions are treated by the insertion of a supporting pessary or in bad cases by operation. Other conditions affecting the uterus are fibroids (q.v.), or cancer, which may affect either the body of the uterus or the cervix, the latter type being 30 times more common than the former and occurring usually in women who have borne children. Cancer of the body is more common in those who have never been pregnant. Early symptoms include blood-stained discharge, and it is therefore important that any woman who has excessive loss at the periods or irregular bleeding should see her doctor at once, since cure either by radium or surgery depends for its success upon early diagnosis.

Such symptoms of course do not necessarily indicate that cancer is present, but it is as well to make sure. The cervix may be lacerated in childbirth, and the body of the uterus may be torn in attempts to procure abortion.

Uveitis: inflammation of the uvea, a name given to the choroid coat of the eyeball, the ciliary body and the iris. *See* Eye.

Uvula: the prolongation of the soft palate which hangs down in the middle of the throat over the root of the tongue.

V

Vaccination: vaccinia is a disease of the cow (cowpox) which, when inoculated into man, produces local pocks at the site of inoculation and slight general symptoms, thus conferring protection, as Jenner discovered in 1796, against smallpox. The exact nature of the condition produced by vaccination is not known for certain, but the two possibilities are (1) that it is smallpox modified by passing through the calf, and (2) that it is a similar but separate disease. Most authorities believe that vaccinia (cowpox) and variola (smallpox) are really the same disease and that the difference between them results from the susceptibilities of the animal in which they occur.

Vaccination is normally performed in Great Britain on infants at the age of 6 weeks and every 7 years thereafter. In the United States infants are not vaccinated until their second year. The material used is lyophilized or glycerinated sterilized calf lymph. The site of the vaccination should not be allowed to become wet, and if a pustule develops a dry dressing should be applied. There are three possible reactions:

Primary reaction in people who have not been vaccinated before – a red papule developing in 4 days, blistering in 6 days and becoming pustular in 8 days. A scab forms in 11 days and separates by the end of the third week.

Accelerated reaction, in people who have been vaccinated before – the same as above, the blistering occurring on the third day and the scab separating in just over a week.

Immediate reaction, in people who have been vaccinated before – a red spot forming on the first day and fading without forming a blister after 3 days.

The duration of the immunity conferred is about 12 years; it diminishes the liability to contract smallpox and, even if the disease occurs, it is much milder and less likely to be fatal. Although orthodox advice is to repeat vaccination every 7 years, the International Certificate of Vaccination has to be renewed every 3 years. Those in a particular position of risk should be vaccinated every 3 years or even yearly.

Complications of vaccination are now very rare, those described being (*a*) generalized vaccinia; (*b*) cellulitis from secondary infection by other germs entering the arm at or after the time of vaccination; (*c*) encephalitis, which is the rarest complication of all. Whatever its critics may say there is no doubt that vaccination has caused a great decrease in the mortality of the disease; thus in Sweden, which made vaccination compulsory in 1816 and practised it widely from 1801, there were 2,049 deaths per million population in 1800, 623 per million yearly between 1802 and 1811, and in the years 1890–9 only 1 death per million. The term vaccination has been extended to cover the production of active immunity against other diseases.

Vaccine: a preparation of attenuated (weakened) or killed micro-organisms or infective material injected into the body for the purpose of provoking an active immunity to disease without producing the symptoms of disease. *See* Immunization.

Vaccinia: cowpox. *See* Vaccination.

Vagina: the female genital passage. Some discharge from the vagina is normal in health, and is more plentiful during pregnancy, but any discoloured or offensive discharge should be reported to the doctor. *See* Vaginitis.

Vaginismus: spasm of the vagina on attempted intercourse. In a few cases this is due to pain from a local condition but the vast majority of cases are psychological.

Vaginitis: inflammation of the vagina. A common cause is infection with the micro-organism Trichomonas vaginalis, which produces a yellow discharge and is transmitted by intercourse (in men the organism infects the urethra). It is treated by metronidazole. Candida albicans is another infecting organism, which is found most frequently during pregnancy and produces white patches; it is treated by local application of nystatin. In children vaginitis is usually due to a mixed infection with bacteria and cocci and occurs because of lack of cleanliness, and in old age a variety of organisms may be found. Treatment in both cases includes appropriate antibiotics and the administration of stilboestrol. Other causes of vaginitis include irritation from contraceptive devices and chemicals and the presence of a malignant growth.

Vagotomy: surgical division of the vagus nerve, a treatment used in cases of peptic ulcer in which it is desired to cut down gastric movements and secretions.

Vagus: the tenth cranial nerve, called 'vagus' or 'wanderer' because its branches spread from the skull to the abdomen. It is the principal outflow of the cranial parasympathetic part of the autonomic nervous system (q.v.). It travels out of the skull into the neck, where it gives off branches to the larynx, through the thorax and into the upper part of the abdomen and gives off branches to the bronchi, heart, oesophagus, stomach and small intestine.

Valerian: the root of valerian – a common plant in Europe – was once much used in the treatment of hysteria. There is no evidence that it had any pharmacological effect, but the smell of it is appalling.

Valgus: genu valgum is knock-knee. *See* Club-foot.

Valvar Disease: disease of the heart valves. The main causes of valvar disease are rheumatic fever, syphilis, atherosclerosis and congenital heart disease, and the valves affected are either rendered incompetent because they cannot shut properly or are narrowed (stenosed) by scar tissue. In the first case the blood regurgitates, in the second it cannot pass freely through the orifice of the valve. Valves can obviously be both stenosed and incompetent. Structural alteration of a heart valve disturbs the blood flow and sets up vibrations in the chest which can be heard through the stethoscope. These noises are known as murmurs, but they have far less significance than one would think, for the important thing is the function of the heart, not the noise it makes; it is possible for a patient to own a massive heart murmur and not to know that it is there. Consequences of valvar disease can include heart failure (*see* Heart), and infection of the damaged valves (*see* Subacute Bacterial Endocarditis). The outlook for patients suffering from valvar disease of the heart has greatly changed in the last twenty-five years with the rapid development of open heart surgery.

Valvotomy: the operation of cutting a valve, usually applied to the operation of cutting the mitral valve of the heart when it is narrowed (stenosed) to such an extent that the efficiency of circulation is impaired.

Varicella: chickenpox (q.v.).

Varicocele: varicosity of the veins of the pampiniform plexus, a plexus of veins which lies round the spermatic cord. The cause is not known; occasionally the patient complains of pain, but the majority of cases are found on routine medical examination and have no significance. If there is discomfort a suspensory bandage can be worn.

Varicose Veins: these occur in about one out of every two women and one out of every four men over the age of 40 years, although they may also make their appearance in much younger people.

CAUSE: in large measure varicose veins are the penalty man has to endure for standing upright, since only then does the problem arise of returning the blood to the heart against the pull of gravity. Normally this is done by contraction of the leg muscles, which pump the blood upwards, a process dependent on the integrity of the valves in the veins of the leg which by their one-way action keep the blood flowing in the right direction. When the valves fail, the veins swell and the blood stagnates within them; this is the condition described as varicose veins. The damage may be caused by pregnancy in women, by constipation or other causes which partially block the veins in the pelvis, and by jobs which involve a great deal of standing without much movement, for example dentistry, haircutting, etc.

SYMPTOMS: the veins affected are not the deep ones embedded in the muscles but those of the superficial saphenous system (*see* Saphenous Veins) which can be seen running directly beneath the skin. The result of failure of their valves is a heavy, tired feeling in the legs, swelling of the ankles, and frequently skin rashes, ulcers and phlebitis. *See* Thrombo-phlebitis.

TREATMENT: elastic stockings or pressure bandages are recommended for the old, those who cannot or do not wish to undergo an operation, and pregnant women. The best treatment is, however, surgical, and there are three possible operations: injection, cutting and ligation, ligation and stripping. In injection a sclerosing solution is injected into the veins to produce a clot which causes the blood to change its course and travel through unaffected veins; this gives relief in mild cases, but in a large number of cases the veins recur. Stripping means threading a long wire through the vein from the groin to the ankle, the vein then being tied securely to the wire and pulled out. This is an effective operation. Cutting and ligation is a rather less effective operation in which the main saphenous vein and its branches are tied and divided at the groin, and incisions made along the course of the veins in order to tie off the communications connecting superficial and deep veins. *See* Veins.

Variola: smallpox.

Varus: genu varus means bow-legs. *See* Club-foot.

Vas: a hollow tube carrying fluid in the body, usually used to mean the vas deferens, the tube that carries spermatozoa from the epididymis into the abdominal cavity and so through the prostate gland at the base of the bladder into the urethra. The vas has thick muscular walls that make it feel like whipcord; it has an outside diameter of 2·5 mm, of which the muscular coat accounts for 2 mm, and is about 45 cm long. In the operation of male sterilization the vas deferens is tied off and cut between ligatures as it leaves the scrotum and passes through the inguinal canal, a relatively simple and safe operation if carried out properly. The vas deferens is also named the ductus deferens.

Vasodilator: a substance which makes blood vessels dilate. Vasodilators are used in conditions in which the blood flow is diminished by arterial disease, not because they can make diseased arteries relax, but because they sometimes help to open up an alternative circulation by keeping anastomotic or connecting blood vessels open. Drugs which have this action include inositol nicotinate (Hexopal) and phenoxy-benzamine (Dibenzyline). Chlorpromazine (Largactil or Thorazine) is a vasodilator, and is particularly useful in cases of severe circulatory trouble where the anxieties of the patient may need calming.

Vasomotor Rhinitis: (Allergic rhinitis). A condition like hay fever, but distinguished from it by the fact that it occurs in winter as well as summer. Another distinguishing mark is that there is no conjunctival injection, or reddening of the eyes. The symptoms are persistent congestion of the nasal mucous membrane with sneezing, watery discharge from the nose and obstruction, and the patient may suffer from nasal polyps and sinusitis. No one sensitizing agent is found, and it is thought that the condition is a response to many stimuli. Treatment includes the use of antihistamines, ephedrine and nasal sprays, and it is sometimes necessary to treat infection of the sinuses. Cauterization of the inferior turbinate bones inside the nose has been tried, but it is better to use local applications of cortisone; surgical removal of polypi helps relieve nasal obstruction.

Vasovagal Attack: (Fainting attack). In this common type of loss of consciousness the patient feels hot and cold, yawns and has a 'sinking' sensation in the stomach. The blood pressure falls, the heart beats slowly and the patient collapses. The symptoms are those of unopposed action of the parasympathetic system, hence the name (*see* Vagus). The fall of blood pressure stimulates sympathetic activity which turns the face white, makes the heart beat more quickly and with more force, and starts the patient sweating.
Recovery is usually fairly quick, and is aided by lying down or putting the head between the knees. *See* Fainting.

V.D.R.L.: Venereal Disease Research Laboratories. The initials are used to signify a particular blood test for syphilis.

Vector: an animal carrying infective organisms, e.g. the mosquito in malaria (q.v.).

Veins: the blood vessels in which blood drains from the tissues back to the heart. Venous blood is used blood, and it is therefore dark – the only exception is the blood in the pulmonary veins, for they bring bright red oxygenated blood from the lungs to the heart. The walls of the veins have three coats, like the walls of the arteries, but there is very much less elastic and muscular tissue and the coats are thin so that the vessel collapses easily. Veins, unlike arteries, have valves which are designed to let blood pass only one way, so that when the veins in the limbs are compressed by the surrounding muscles the blood is actively pumped towards the heart. Pressure in the veins is about 5 mm positive at the level of the heart, and in the rest of the body is determined by the distance above or below the heart – when a man is standing up it is positive in the leg, and negative in the skull. There are two venous systems in the body, the systemic in which the veins accompany the arteries and take the blood directly into the superior and inferior venae cavae and so to the heart, and the portal, in which the veins that drain blood from the internal abdominal organs join in to form the portal vein which takes the blood to the liver, where it is passed through sinusoids – dilated venous spaces – before it drains back to the inferior vena cava. Disorders of the veins include varicosities (*see* Varicose Veins) and thrombosis (*see* Thrombophlebitis); thrombosis of the deep veins, especially those of the leg, may be a serious condition both because the drainage of blood is obstructed and because pieces of clot may break off and become obstructions in the pulmonary arteries. *See* Thrombosis.

Vena Cava: the two largest veins in the body are the superior vena cava, into which blood drains from the head, neck, arms and chest, and the inferior vena cava which receives blood from the legs and abdomen. Blood from the intestines and abdominal organs passes into the portal system of veins and so through the liver before draining in the hepatic veins into the inferior vena cava. Both the superior and the inferior vena cava empty into the right atrium of the heart.

Venepuncture: puncture of a vein for the purpose of withdrawing blood.

Venereal Disease: it is continually being pointed out by journalists of all sorts that the incidence of venereal disease is on the increase; unlike many of the depressing tales which are alone thought newsworthy this one is true. The main venereal diseases are gonorrhoea, syphilis and chancroid (soft sore), which have already been described under their own headings (more than one venereal disease can be picked up at the same time). The fact that makes a disease venereal – that is, a disease contracted by sexual intercourse – is that the organisms are too delicate to survive away from the heat and moisture of the genital organs, where they find conditions ideal. Syphilis is, of course, a killer, which can spread to any part of the body; gonorrhoea, on the other hand, tends (although by no means always) to be localized. Both are easy to diagnose in a man, who can hardly fail to notice the hard sore of the former on his penis, or the thick pus exuding from his urethra in the latter. Unfortunately, although easily diagnosed by a doctor, the symptoms of both diseases are much less obvious to a woman, who may therefore go on infecting others unknowingly; the fact that about one female attends a V.D. clinic for every four males suggests that many women are unaware of their condition, and that the incidence of V.D. in women is higher than the figures would suggest. As pointed out in connection with the individual diseases, the end results of syphilis (both for the individual and the next generation) are very serious indeed, and gonorrhoea, if less serious in most cases, can also have very unpleasant consequences. Neither disease is ever contracted from cups, towels or lavatory seats; sexual intercourse and, rarely, kissing someone with an active sore on the lip are almost the only sources of infection. Cure is relatively simple; in the earlier stages of syphilis penicillin is almost invariably successful, and a single penicillin injection often suffices for gonorrhoea.

Nevertheless, the figures are disquieting and obviously it is necessary to explain them before deciding what practical measures to take. Most authorities are agreed that there are two minor and one major cause for the explosive increase in V.D. The first minor cause is that nowadays, when less social stigma is attached to these diseases and cure is known to be relatively simple, fewer cases are concealed and that therefore part of the increase is more apparent than real; the second is the greater social mobility of people in the modern world which makes it possible for an infected person to infect others in widely separated areas – the car has supplanted the bicycle. The major cause, however, as is evidenced by the increases in the lower age-groups, is the increasing sexual activity of the young. The only feasible solution is more and better sex education both by parents and teachers. This should be objective and based on discussion rather than preaching. Many of the adolescents who become infected with V.D. are doubtless children with delinquent tendencies, but the great bulk are ordinary youngsters who would not run the risks of pregnancy and disease had they been better informed and treated with greater understanding. It is not only sexual desire that causes juvenile promiscuity – many adolescents fornicate for the same reason that they smoke: to prove that they are adults and because grown-ups threaten them and tell them that these are things they must not do. Their behaviour is in the nature of a 'dare' or challenge. Thus the headmaster of a school where smoking was rife called his pupils together and gave them a factual, truthful and unemotional talk about the risk attached to the habit, following his talk with a statement that all those who wished to do so could smoke in a small room in the school during the last half-hour of the lunch break, but at no other time. So far from increasing, smoking practically ceased altogether, because (a) those who went to the room to smoke were caused to feel rather silly and cut off from the rest of their school-mates, and (b) the daring aspect of the habit had been removed. We are not suggesting that exactly the same procedure should be carried out in relation to sex, but it is suggested that those who lead public opinion should take into account psychological research; that there should be a far wider spread of factual information; and that thundering from the pulpit or parliamentary bench is likely to spread the very evil it is intended to curb.

Venesection: letting blood by cutting a superficial vein.

Ventricle: a 'small belly' (ventriculus); applied to a small cavity, e.g. the ventricles of the heart.

Ventriculography: a technique used in neurosurgery whereby the ventricles of the brain are outlined by the injection of air or oxygen introduced through a needle passed *via* a burr hole in the skull. Any deformity of the outline, or displacement of the ventricles from their normal position, reveals the presence of a tumour or collection of blood. In some circumstances Myodil, a radio-opaque heavy oil, is used to show the ventricular outlines, especially when the third and fourth ventricles are to be examined.

Verruca: a wart (q.v.).

Version: in obstetrics, a manipulation carried out in order to change the position of a foetus in relation to the mother. It may be external or internal. External version is usually carried out at or about the 36th week in cases of breech presentation, or during labour in the case of a second twin lying awkwardly after the first twin has been born. Internal version is nowadays rarely tried.

Vertebra: one of the bones of the spinal column, of which there are 33, some fused together. *See* Spinal Column.

Vertigo: the feeling that the world is revolving round the patient, who cannot keep his balance. It is produced in many ways ranging from disease of the inner ear (Menière's disease) to epilepsy and hysteria. The word is wrongly used as a synonym for dizziness; the treatment depends upon the cause.

Vesical: to do with the bladder, for example vesical stone.

Vesicle: a little blister.

Viable: something that is capable of living. It is applied to the foetus from the 28th week of pregnancy, for it is then capable of living outside the womb.

Vibrio: two species of the family Spirillaceae important to medicine are the Vibrio cholerae and the V. eltor. Both produce cholera; the V. eltor was first isolated at the Egyptian quarantine station at El Tor. *See* Cholera.

Villus: a small protrusion from the surface of a membrane. (From the Latin word meaning tuft.)

Vincent's Angina: term applied to an infection of the mouth and gums in which there is ulceration of the mucous membrane. The cause is Vincent's organism, a spirochaete named Borrelia vincentii, which is normally present in the mouth in health. When the health is poor, the mouth dirty and the teeth neglected, Vincent's organisms multiply and together with spindle-shaped bacteria are found in the ulcerated parts of the mouth and gums. The symptoms are sore mouth and throat, and a foul breath; the local lymph glands are enlarged, and there is a fever. The infection responds to penicillin.

Virilism: the appearance of masculine characteristics in the female which may be caused by tumours of the adrenal glands or by the use of anabolic drugs (q.v.).

Virus: particles too small to be seen with a light microscope, viruses consists of either D.N.A. or R.N.A. surrounded by a protein coat. They can only reproduce themselves in living cells, and cannot exist without the ribosomes of the host cell, for they have none themselves (*see* Cell). Viruses are responsible for smallpox, poliomyelitis and yellow fever as well as a number of lesser diseases, and are not affected by antibiotics. It is, however, possible to induce active immunity to virus diseases by the injection of attenuated or killed viruses, and in this way poliomyelitis, smallpox and yellow fever have been controlled and are not now the great plagues that once they were. There are three groups of viruses; they have as their hosts animals, plants and bacteria (*see* Phage), and those which produce disease in man and animals are classified by using four characteristics: (1) the type of nucleic acid; (2) the structure of the protein coat; (3) whether there is an envelope or not; (4) whether the virus is stable in the presence of ether. The names given to viruses are in general descriptive, for example herpesviruses, poxviruses, arboviruses (ARthropod-BOrne viruses).
Virus diseases besides those mentioned above include the common cold, foot and mouth disease, dengue fever, influenza, encephalitis, mumps, rabies, chickenpox, measles and rubella. *See* Interferon.

Viscera: the large internal organs, for example lungs, liver, intestines.

Visual Purple: *see* Rhodopsin.

Vitamins: organic substances that occur in very small quantities in the food and are necessary for life and health. They must be supplied in the diet, for the body by itself cannot make them.

A: a fat-soluble vitamin found in cod liver oil, other fish livers, cheese, butter, egg-yolk, milk and green vegetables. Deficiency: night blindness, lessened resistance to infection and opacity of the cornea of the eye (keratomalacia). Thousands of children in poor countries still go blind with keratomalacia every year.

B complex: a group of water-soluble vitamins including thiamin, riboflavine, nicotinic acid, Vitamin B_6 group, pantothenic acid, biotin, inositol, folic acid, choline, para-aminobenzoic acid, Vitamin B_{12} (cyanocobalamin). Deficiencies: thiamin – beri-beri; nicotinic acid – pellagra; Vitamin B_{12}, folic acid – pernicious anaemia.

C: ascorbic acid; found in fresh fruit and vegetables and raw meat. Deficiency: scurvy.

D: calciferol, a fat-soluble sterol found in liver oils, herrings and dairy produce, and formed by the action of sunlight on the skin. Deficiency: rickets in children, osteomalacia in adults.

E: tocopherol; found in wheat-germ oil, egg-yolk, liver and cereals. A vitamin without which rats cannot reproduce.

K: found in spinach, cabbage, egg-yolk. Deficiency: prothrombin, necessary for the clotting of the blood, is not formed in the liver. The vitamin is normally synthesized by bacteria that inhabit the bowels, and is generally given in cases where haemorrhages are associated with disease of the liver or intestines.

There are also Vitamins F, G, H, J, L, M, P (which is found in lemon juice and paprika), R, S, V and X (the same as P). *See* Diet.

Vitiligo: *See* Leucoderma.

Vitreous Humour: a transparent thin jelly that fills the vitreous chamber of the eye. It lies behind the lens. *See* Eye.

Vocal Cords: *see* Larynx.

Volvulus: a condition in which a loop of bowel twists round itself. *See* Obstruction.

Vomiting: this has many causes, both physical and psychological. Many acute fevers, especially in children, begin with vomiting, and any form of gastric irritation, whether from disease or irritant substances taken into the body, has the same effect. Other abdominal conditions not connected with the stomach such as intestinal obstruction, peritonitis, pregnancy, renal and biliary colic, and brain disorders such as tumour, abscess, injury and meningitis are associated with vomiting and retching. Certain drugs such as apomorphine have the same effect. A common cause of vomiting is travel sickness. The danger of vomiting, especially in children, is loss of water and salts and consequent dehydration and imbalance of electrolytes in the body. If the vomit is inhaled the consequences are very serious.

Vulva: the female external genital organs.

Warfarin: a compound that stops the clotting of blood. It is named after the Wisconsin Alumni Research Foundation, and is used more as a rat poison than an anticoagulant in human beings.

Warts: (Verrucae). Extremely common both in childhood and later life, warts are considered to be a virus infection and are capable of spread. Freezing with carbon dioxide snow is the best treatment, since it leaves no scar, but in mild cases glacial acetic acid applied on a stick wrapped in cotton wool or the use of silver nitrate will cure the condition. Plantar warts are painful, appearing on the soles of the feet and usually contracted in swimming-baths, etc.; they may occur in epidemics in schools and are treated by incision, scraping out, and cauterization. Care should be taken against infecting others. Warts often disappear spontaneously and are therefore sometimes treated successfully by charms.

Wassermann Reaction: a serological test used in the diagnosis of syphilis. It was introduced by the Berlin bacteriologist Wassermann (1866–1925), and remains an accurate and valuable test. *See* Kahn Test.

Waterbrash: sudden appearance in the mouth of clear fluid, associated particularly with peptic ulcer. The fluid is from the salivary glands. *See* Heartburn.

Wax: quite frequently waxy secretions collect in the external auditory meatus (the earhole) and deaden the hearing. It is not safe to try to pick the wax out; it must be syringed by someone who knows what he is doing. If the wax is particularly hard it can be softened by drops of olive oil put into the ear twice a day for a week.

Weber's Test: the foot of a vibrating tuning fork is put on the centre of the forehead. If the fork seems to be making a noise in the middle of the head, the result is normal, but if it seems to be coming from one or the other ear the result is abnormal, and the test is called positive, the side of the ear in which the noise is heard being noted as 'Weber right' or 'Weber left'. The sound is referred to the side of the ear in which bone conduction is better than air conduction because of disease of the middle ear or otosclerosis; in fact the damaged ear. *See* Ear, Rinne's Test.

Weights and Measures: these are the principal units in medical and pharmaceutical use in the United Kingdom and the United States.

Length (Metric)
1,000 millimetres (mm) = 1 metre (m)
100 centimetres (cm) = 1 metre
10 decimetres (dm) = 1 metre

Weight (Metric)
1,000 micrograms (m) = 1 milligram (mg)
1,000 milligrams = 1 gram (g)
1,000 grams = 1 kilogram (kg)

Liquid (Metric)
1,000 millilitres (ml) = 1 litre (l)
1,000 (approx.) cubic
   centimetres (cc) = 1 litre

Weight (Avoirdupois: avdp)
16 drams (dr) = 1 ounce (oz)
16 ounces = 1 pound (lb)
14 pounds = 1 stone (U.K. only)

Liquid (British and U.S.)
16 fluid ounces (fl oz) = 1 U.S. pint (pt)
20 fluid ounces = 1 imperial (British) pint
2 pints = 1 quart (qt)

Weight (Troy: t)
480 grains (gr) = 1 ounce (oz)
12 ounces = 1 pound (lb) (U.S. only)
240 pennyweight (dwt) = 1 pound
(*See* also Apothecaries' Weights)

Approximate Equivalents
25 millimetres (mm),
   2·5 centimetres (cm) = 1 inch (in)
1 metre (m) = $39\frac{1}{3}$ inches

1 milligram (mg)	$=\frac{1}{60}$ grain (gr)
60 milligrams	= 1 grain
1 gram (g)	= 15 grains ($\frac{1}{30}$ ounces)
30 grams	= 1 ounce (oz)
1 kilogram (kg)	= $2\frac{1}{4}$ pounds (lb)
6·5 kilograms	= 1 stone (14 lb)
1 millilitre (ml)	= 15 minims (min)
30 millilitres	= 1 fluid ounce (fl oz)
600 millilitres	= 1 imperial pint (pt)
1 litre (l)	= 35 fluid ounces
175 troy ounces (oz t)	= 192 avoirdupois ounces (oz avdp)

1 grain (60 milligrams) is the only unit identical in the troy (t), apothecaries' (ap) and avoirdupois (avdp) systems.

Weil's Disease: a form of leptospirosis.

CAUSE: Leptospira icterohaemorrhagica, a spirochaete which is a danger wherever men work in places where they can come into contact with rat's urine or water which has been contaminated by infected rats. Leptospira canicola, which gives rise to canicola fever, is almost identical and is found in the urine of pigs, dogs and cattle; the disease it produces is less severe.

SYMPTOMS: there is sudden high fever with shivering, vomiting, and cramp in the muscles. Before the end of the week, the patient becomes jaundiced and begins to pass blood and albumin in the urine. There is abdominal pain and the skin shows small haemorrhages. In L. canicola infection there is no jaundice, but the patient complains of severe headache and shows signs of meningism. The infection resolves in about two weeks.

TREATMENT: the organisms of Weil's disease are sensitive to penicillin, but the liver and kidneys and rarely the brain are liable to have sustained damage in the early stages of the disease which penicillin cannot cure.

Weir-Mitchell Treatment: a régime consisting of absolute rest and a nourishing and easily digested diet, formerly used in the treatment of neurosis; the patients got well out of boredom.

Wen: *see* Sebaceous Cyst.

Wharton's Jelly: a gelatinous material that fills the umbilical cord.

Whiplash Injury: in an automobile accident that involves sudden acceleration, for example when the car is struck from behind, the head is jerked backwards and then flicks forwards like a whiplash, and the cervical spine is injured. A headrest or high seat back helps to minimize this type of injury.

Whipworm: *see* Worms.

Whites: popular name for a white vaginal discharge.

Whitlow: (Felon). A purulent infection of the finger tip, which should always receive skilled attention. *See* Pulp Infection, Paronychia.

Whooping Cough: pertussis.
CAUSE: the micro-organisms Bordetella pertussis and Bord. parapertussis, of which the first gives rise to the more severe infections. The disease is very infectious and is spread by droplet spray; various adenoviruses, para-influenza and respiratory viruses are associated with whooping cough.
SYMPTOMS: the incubation period is between one and two weeks, and the quarantine period three weeks. The disease commonly affects infants during the first year of life, although many cases occur in children up to 5 years old. The infant develops a cold with a marked cough which, failing to get better in a few days, becomes more severe and spasmodic until at the end of a spasm the child gives out the characteristic whoop. As the paroxysms of coughing increase the disease becomes less infective, but the patient may vomit and burst small blood vessels in the nose or the conjunctiva of the eye under the strain, or may even rupture himself. Broncho-pneumonia is always a danger, as is infection of the middle ear, and convulsions occur in severe cases. The disease may last a matter of weeks.
TREATMENT: ampicillin is given in full doses for 2 weeks; precautions are taken to see that the child does not inhale its

vomit in a coughing attack, and the mother must know how to hold the child upside down and pat it on the back to help it cough the stringy mucus out of its lungs and throat.

PREVENTION: an effective vaccine is available consisting of the organism Bord. pertussis killed by formalin. It is usually combined with vaccines against diphtheria and tetanus in a triple injection given when the child is between 3 and 6 months.

Windpipe: the trachea, a cartilaginous pipe which runs from the Adam's apple in the throat to the point of bifurcation where it branches into the right and left main bronchi which run to the lungs. It is about 25 cm long, and has between 16 and 20 rings of cartilage which are incomplete behind, where the wall contains smooth muscle. Behind the trachea runs the gullet (oesophagus), and in the neck the thyroid gland lies to each side with its isthmus crossing the mid-line. In the chest the trachea comes into relationship with the aorta and the thymus gland, and at its division into right and left bronchi there are important groups of lymph glands. *See* Tracheotomy, Tracheitis.

Wireworm: *see* Worms.

Witches' Milk: the milk secreted from the breasts of a new-born baby in response to the hormones of its mother.

Witch-hazel: made up into a lotion or ointment, witch-hazel is mildly astringent. It is sometimes recommended as ung. hamamelidis for external application to piles.

Womb: the uterus (q.v.).

Worms: (Helminths). The worms that infest human beings are divided into two large groups, roundworms and flatworms. Flatworms can be divided into flukes and tapeworms. The following list gives the common worms of man, their length, the disease they cause, the method of transmission and the treatment. *See* also Flukes, Tapeworms.

Roundworms

Ascaris lumbricoides	15–25 cm	Inflammation of the intestine and lungs
		Eating contaminated food
		Piperazine

Enterobius vermicularis 10–15 mm (Pinworm, threadworm)		Itching anus Dirty fingers and food Piperazine, Viprynium (Vanquin) Povan
Trichuris trichiura 30–50 mm (Whipworm)		No symptoms, or mild enteritis Dirty fingers or food Thiabendazole (Mintezol)
Trichinella spiralis 1 mm		Trichinosis, muscular pain and weakness Undercooked pork No specific treatment
Ancylostoma duodenale 10 mm Necator americanus (Hookworms)		(Tropical and subtropical) Anaemia, nutritional disorders Through skin from infected water Bephenium compounds (Alcopar)
Wuchereria bancrofti Up to 50 mm Brugia malayi		(Tropical) Filariasis, q.v. (elephantiasis) Mosquitoes Diethylcarbamazine (Banocide, Hetrazan)
Loa loa 2–50 mm		(Tropical) Filariasis (Calabar swellings) Chrysops, a blood-sucking fly Diethylcarbamazine
Onchocerca volvulus 2–50 mm		(Tropical) Filariasis (African river blindness, lumps in the skin) Simulium, the Buffalo gnat Diethylcarbamazine
Strongyloides stercoralis 2 mm		(Tropical) Creeping skin eruptions and enteritis Larvae penetrate skin Thiabendazole
Dracunculus medinensis 50–75 cm (Guinea Worm)		(Tropical) Infestation of the skin Intermediate host (a freshwater crustacean) is swallowed in water Removal, thiabendazole, niridazole
Flatworms; flukes Schistosoma japonicum 10–20 mm mansoni haematobium		(Tropical and subtropical) Schistosomiasis (Bilharziasis, q.v.) Larvae penetrate skin in water Niridazole (Ambilhar) etc.
Paragonimus westermani 7–10 mm		(Far East) Cysts of the lung Undercooked crab Bithionol (Biotrase)

Clonorchis sinensis	10–12 mm	(Far East) Liver inflammation Raw fish Bithionol
Fasciola hepatica	3–4 cm	Inflammation of the liver Watercress, vegetables Bithionol etc.
Tapeworms Taenia solium	1 or 2 metres	Inflammation of intestine, cysticercosis Underdone pork Dichlorophen (Anthiphen) Niclosamide (Yomesan), male fern extract
Taenia saginata	Several metres	Inflammation of the intestine Underdone beef Treatment as above
Diphyllobothrium latum	Up to 18 metres	Inflammation of the intestine Raw fish Treatment as above
Echinococcus granulosus	2 mm	Hydatid disease Food contaminated by dogs No specific treatment

Wounds: wounds may be classified as incised, punctured, contused, lacerated and perforating.

Incised. Wounds made by cutting, as with a knife; the wound tends to bleed a good deal and the edges gape. After such a wound has been cleaned, the edges are stitched and allowed to heal by 'first intention'. The gap between the incised surfaces fills with serum and blood clot, and as long as the wound does not become infected it heals in a week or two.

Punctured. Punctures are dangerous because it is usually impossible to tell how far the puncturing instrument has penetrated. If there is any question of deep penetration, as there must be in all punctured wounds of the abdomen, the patient must be watched carefully for signs of internal bleeding or peritonitis. The size of the hole in the skin bears no relation to the possible depth of the puncture.

Contused. Severe contusions (bruises) sustained, for example, by being run over, may indicate serious underlying injury, for the extent to which crushed tissues have been killed becomes clear only slowly, and if dead tissue is contaminated and infected it is liable to gas gangrene. Moreover, a great deal of blood and fluid can be lost in a crushing injury without obvious external signs, and the patient can, without fluid replacement, go into severe shock.

Lacerated. Torn wounds are the most likely to be infected, and the most likely to be sustained in road accidents. All lacerated wounds must be seen by a surgeon, who will clean them thoroughly, if necessary removing dead and damaged tissue under general anaesthetic until he is quite certain that what is left is clean, living and has a good blood supply. In some cases it will be necessary to carry out plastic surgery in order to close the wound satisfactorily, for an important amount of skin may have to be removed.

Perforating. Through-and-through wounds caused by foreign bodies such as bullets and fragments of metal are called perforating. They tend to show a small entry wound and a large exit wound, and the tissues in between are extensively damaged. *Penetrating* wounds are caused by foreign bodies that are retained. In both cases surgical attention is needed, and the surgeon opens up the track made by the missile, removes all dirty and damaged tissue, and takes away all the foreign material (clothes, etc.) introduced into the wound as well as removing the bullet or metallic fragments.

Complications of wound healing are bleeding, infection and necrosis (death of tissues). Collections of blood must be let out, and infected wounds have to be opened and pus and dead tissue removed. They may have to be left to heal by 'second intention' – granulation, which is the slow formation of fibrous tissue – or may sometimes be closed by secondary suture. In all cases of wounding the possibility of tetanus (q.v.) must be remembered, and appropriate action taken.

Wrist: the complicated joint between the forearm and the hand. The skeleton of the wrist has eight small bones which articulate with the radius and ulna proximally and the metacarpal bones of the hand distally. Sprains and inflammation of the tendons passing over the wrist are not uncommon; for fractures of this region *see* Colles' Fracture.

Wryneck: *see* Torticollis.

Wuchereria: *see* Filariasis, Worms.

X

Xanthoma: a small deposit or lump of yellow material sometimes found in the skin in diseases involving a disorder of metabolism of fat or carbohydrates.

Xenopus Test: a test for pregnancy that used to be carried out by injecting a specimen of urine into a toad (Xenopus laevis) from South Africa. Simpler tests have rendered the toads redundant.

Xeroderma: a disorder of the skin characterized by the formation of scales on a dry rough surface.

Xerophthalmia: a type of dry conjunctivitis due to lack of Vitamin A.

Xeroradiography: a method of producing X-ray pictures by a dry photoelectric process, using metal plates coated with a semiconductor.

Xiphisternum: the tip of the breastbone which lies between the seventh ribs over the upper abdominal cavity.

X-rays: electromagnetic waves of the same type as radio, heat or light waves but much shorter, able to penetrate bodies opaque to ordinary light. The absorption of X-rays depends upon the nature of the atoms they meet, so that the heavier the atoms the greater the absorption. Thus a thin sheet of lead will absorb much of a beam of hard X-rays that would easily penetrate several feet of wood. A beam of X-rays passing through the body is less easily absorbed by the flesh than by the bone, and if a fluorescent screen is placed behind the body the bones will be revealed by the shadows they cast. Other parts of the body can be made opaque to X-rays by injecting or otherwise introducing appropriate substances, for example barium to outline the intestines or iodine compounds to outline the gall-bladder and kidneys. Permanent X-ray records are obtained by using a photographic plate which is sensitive to X-rays.

X-rays are used in the treatment of many types of cancer as well as certain other diseases. *See* Ionizing Radiation.

Xylocaine: (Lignocaine). A powerful synthetic local anaesthetic which is absorbed by mucous membranes and active when given by injection. It is usually used with adrenaline because it tends to dilate the blood vessels.

Y

Yaws: (Framboesia). A chronic disease of the tropics.
CAUSE: Treponema pertenue, a micro-organism very like the organism that causes syphilis. Yaws is not a venereal disease, although it is passed on by close physical contact. Blood tests for syphilis are positive in yaws.
SYMPTOMS: a pimple develops where the infectious contact has resulted in inoculation, and this enlarges to the size of a raspberry. There follow in the secondary stage multiple excrescences on the skin, and in the third stage there is ulceration which may affect the face. The disease may be widespread and disfiguring, and is seen at its worst in primitive rural people.
TREATMENT: the disease is cured by one injection of a long acting penicillin such as P.A.M. (procaine benzyl penicillin with 2% aluminium monostearate), but it leaves scars. Tetracycline is also active against T. pertenue.

Yeast: yeasts are one-celled fungi that reproduce by budding. Yeasts and yeast-like fungi that produce disease in man include Candida albicans, the organism of thrush, and Cryptococcus neoformans, which causes cryptococcosis, a chronic granulomatous disease once named torulosis.

Yellow Fever: an acute, often fatal, disease found in Central Africa and parts of South America.
CAUSE: infection with a virus carried by the mosquito Aedes aegypti.
SYMPTOMS: the incubation period is less than a week; the patient develops fever, has a slow pulse, begins to vomit and passes albumin in the urine. He then develops haemorrhages

and jaundice; the mortality of the disease is 25%.

TREATMENT: there is no specific treatment for yellow fever.
PREVENTION: one attack of yellow fever gives immunity for life, and inoculation with a vaccine made from attenuated virus provides active immunity for a number of years, variously estimated by different authorities as between three and ten. Revaccination is called for every six years. Although the A. aegypti is mainly a 'domestic' mosquito, it can pick up and transmit the disease from monkeys, which form a reservoir of infection in the tropical African forests and spread the virus when they come near villages. In South America, the monkeys are infected by the mosquito Haemagogus spegazzini in the wet season, and the infection is preserved in the dry season by another mosquito, Sabethes chloropterus. It is obviously important that the control of mosquitoes in aircraft and the inoculation of travellers 10 days before they go through an endemic zone should be rigidly enforced, for there is otherwise a real risk that the yellow fever virus could spread to countries where there are uninfected Aedes aegypti mosquitoes and the disease is at present unknown.

Z

Zinc: many zinc salts are used in medicine, although they can be toxic if they are absorbed, producing symptoms which resemble lead poisoning. Zinc preparations used as external applications include zinc oxide made up as an ointment or cream which is used in many skin conditions, zinc oxide used as a dusting powder, zinc undecenoate used as an ointment for fungus infections of the skin, zinc acetate used as an astringent solution, zinc salicylate, zinc sulphate and zinc iodide. Very small quantities of zinc are necessary in the diet because it is needed in several enzyme systems.

Zygomatic Bone: the cheek-bone, which forms part of the outer wall and floor of the eye-socket (orbit).

Zygote: the fertilized ovum.